# Intensive Care Nursing

## A framework for practice

## Second edition

Philip Woodrow

*Clinical Scenarios by Jane Roe*

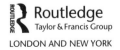
Routledge
Taylor & Francis Group

LONDON AND NEW YORK

To the States or any one of them, or any city of the States,
Resist much, obey little,
Once unquestioning obedience, once fully enslaved,
Once fully enslaved, no nation, state, city, of this earth, ever afterwards
    resumes its liberty.

Walt Whitman

Fashion, even in medicine.

Voltaire

First published 2000
by Routledge
Second edition published in 2006
by Routledge
2 Park Square, Milton Park, Abingdon, Oxon OX14 4RN

Simultaneously published in the USA and Canada
by Routledge
270 Madison Ave, New York, NY 10016

Reprinted 2000, 2001, 2003 (twice) and 2004

*Routledge is an imprint of the Taylor & Francis Group*

Main text © 2006 Philip Woodrow
Clinical scenarios © 2006 Jane Roe

Typeset in Sabon and Futura by
Newgen Imaging Systems (P) Ltd, Chennai, India
Printed and bound in Great Britain by
The Cromwell Press, Trowbridge, Wiltshire

*British Library Cataloguing in Publication Data*
A catalogue record for this book is available from the British Library

*Library of Congress Cataloging in Publication Data*
A catalog record for this book has been requested

ISBN10: 0–415–37322–0 (hbk)
ISBN10: 0–415–37323–9 (pbk)

ISBN13: 9–78–0–415–37322–7 (hbk)
ISBN13: 9–78–0–415–37323–4 (pbk)

# Contents

*List of illustrations*                                                    ix
*Preface*                                                                 xiii
*Acknowledgements*                                                         xiv
*List of abbreviations*                                                   xvii

Part I

## ■ Contexts of care                                                      1

1   Nursing perspectives                                                   3
2   Humanism                                                              11
3   Psychological care                                                    17

Part II

## ■ Fundamental aspects                                                  29

4   Artificial ventilation                                                31
5   Airway management                                                     47
6   Sedation                                                              59
7   Pain management                                                       70
8   Pyrexia and temperature control                                       81
9   Nutrition and bowel care                                              87
10  Mouthcare                                                             98
11  Eyecare                                                              108
12  Skincare                                                             114
13  Children in adult ICUs                                               122
14  Older patients in ICU                                                131
15  Infection control                                                    138
16  Ethics                                                               148

Part III

## ■ Monitoring                                                          157

17  Respiratory monitoring                                               159
18  Gas carriage                                                         170

19   Acid–base balance and arterial blood gas analysis          182
20   Haemodynamic monitoring                                     195
21   Blood results                                               209
22   ECGs and dysrhythmias                                       223
23   Neurological monitoring                                     247

Part IV

## ▌ Micropathologies                                           **259**

24   Cellular pathology                                          261
25   Immunity and immunodeficiency                               269
26   Disseminated intravascular coagulation (DIC)                277

Part V

## ▌ Respiratory                                                **285**

27   Acute respiratory distress syndrome (ARDS)                  287
28   Severe acute respiratory syndrome (SARS) and Legionella     297
29   Alternative ventilatory modes                               304

Part VI

## ▌ Cardiovascular                                            **313**

30   Acute coronary syndromes                                    315
31   Cardiac surgery                                             327
32   Shock                                                       343
33   Sepsis, SIRS and MODS                                       354
34   Fluid management                                            362
35   Inotropes and vasopressors                                  372
36   Vascular surgery                                            382

Part VII

## ▌ Neurological                                              **389**

37   Central nervous system injury                               391
38   Peripheral neurological pathologies                         406

Part VIII

## ▌ Abdominal                                                 **411**

39   Acute renal failure                                         413
40   Haemofiltration                                             422
41   Gastrointestinal bleeds                                     432
42   Hepatic failure                                             441
43   Obstetric emergencies in ICU                                450
44   Transplants                                                 458

Part IX
## ■ Metabolic                                              471

| 45 | Pancreatitis | 473 |
| 46 | Diabetic crises | 480 |
| 47 | Overdoses | 488 |

Part X
## ■ Professional                                           499

| 48 | Professionalism | 501 |
| 49 | Managing the ICU | 508 |
| 50 | Cost of intensive care | 517 |

| *Glossary* | 523 |
| *References* | 531 |
| *Index* | 571 |

# Illustrations

## Figures

| | | |
|---|---|---|
| 5.1 | ETT just above carina | 49 |
| 5.2 | High and low pressure ETT cuffs | 51 |
| 5.3 | Nasal cavity | 52 |
| 7.1 | Referred pain | 73 |
| 7.2 | Dermatomes | 77 |
| 9.1 | Krebs (citric acid) cycle | 89 |
| 9.2 | Bristol stool form chart (after Heaton, 2000) | 93 |
| 10.1 | Oral (buccal cavity) | 100 |
| 11.1 | External structure of the eye | 112 |
| 12.1 | Pressure sore grading | 117 |
| 17.1 | Auscultation sites for breath sounds (anterior chest wall) | 162 |
| 17.2 | Normal (self-ventilating) breath waveform | 163 |
| 17.3 | Pressure:volume (hysteresis) graph | 164 |
| 18.1 | Oxygen dissociation curve | 174 |
| 18.2 | Carbon dioxide dissociation curve | 176 |
| 19.1 | Origin of acid–base imbalance | 185 |
| 20.1 | Arterial trace | 198 |
| 20.2 | Main central venous cannulation sites | 199 |
| 20.3 | CVP waveform | 200 |
| 22.1 | Normal sinus rhythm | 226 |
| 22.2 | Chest lead placement | 227 |
| 22.3 | Action potential | 229 |
| 22.4 | Sinus arrhythmia | 232 |
| 22.5 | Atrial (supraventricular) tachycardia | 233 |
| 22.6 | Premature atrial ectopic | 235 |
| 22.7 | Atrial fibrillation | 235 |
| 22.8 | Atrial flutter | 236 |
| 22.9 | Wolff–Parkinson–White syndrome | 237 |
| 22.10 | Nodal/junctional rhythm | 237 |

| | | |
|---|---|---:|
| 22.11 | First degree block | 238 |
| 22.12 | Second degree block (Type 1) | 239 |
| 22.13 | Second degree block (Type 2) | 239 |
| 22.14 | Third degree block | 240 |
| 22.15 | Bundle branch block | 240 |
| 22.16 | Multifocal ventricular ectopics | 241 |
| 22.17 | Bigeminy and trigeminy | 242 |
| 22.18 | Ventricular tachycardia | 243 |
| 22.19 | Torsades de pointes | 243 |
| 22.20 | Ventricular fibrillation | 244 |
| 23.1 | Pressure/volume curve | 249 |
| 23.2 | Intracranial hypertension and tissue injury: a vicious circle | 250 |
| 23.3 | Cross-section of the cranium showing Foramen of Monro | 255 |
| 23.4 | Normal ICP waveform | 255 |
| 24.1 | Cell structure | 262 |
| 30.1 | Coronary arteries, with inferior myocardial infarction | 317 |
| 31.1 | Intra-aortic balloon pump – inflated (a) and deflated (b) | 331 |
| 31.2 | Arterial pressure trace showing augmented pressure from use of an intra-aortic balloon pump | 332 |
| 31.3 | Ventricular assist devices (left and right) | 333 |
| 34.1 | Perfusion gradients | 366 |
| 41.1 | Sengstaken tube | 434 |

## Tables

| | | |
|---|---|---:|
| 1.1 | Levels of care | 4 |
| 4.1 | Commonly used abbreviations and terms | 33 |
| 4.2 | Recommended PEEP to $FiO_2$ settings | 39 |
| 6.1 | Ramsay | 63 |
| 6.2 | Addenbrookes | 63 |
| 6.3 | Newcastle scale | 64 |
| 6.4 | New Sheffield | 64 |
| 9.1 | Normal anthropometric chart | 92 |
| 10.1 | Normal contents of saliva | 100 |
| 10.2 | The Jenkins oral assessment tool | 102 |
| 10.3 | Jiggins & Talbot's (1999) oral assessment | 103 |
| 17.1 | Sputum colour – possible causes | 161 |
| 18.1 | Partial pressures of gases at sea level | 171 |
| 18.2 | Some factors affecting oxygen dissociation | 173 |
| 19.1 | Some symbols commonly found on blood gas samples | 189 |
| 19.2 | Main electrolyte + metabolite results measured by most blood gas analysers | 189 |
| 20.1 | Normal flow monitoring parameters | 203 |
| 21.1 | Erythrocyte results | 211 |
| 21.2 | Some types of anaemia | 212 |
| 21.3 | Normal white cell counts | 213 |

22.1   Framework for ECG interpretation                                    228
22.2   Antidysrhythmic drug classification                                 231
27.1   Complications of prone positioning                                  291
30.1   TIMI risk score (Antman *et al.*, 2000)                             318
34.1   Summary of fluids                                                   364
35.1   Main target receptors for drugs                                     375
36.1   Common complications of open surgery to the aorta
       (after Prinssen *et al.*, 2004)                                     386
37.1   Possible main aspects of medical management of moderate/
       severe head injury                                                  396
37.2   Priorities of care during fitting                                   399
39.1   Functions of the kidney                                             414
40.1   Renal replacement therapies – commonly used terms                   424
42.1   Main liver function tests                                           444
44.1   Code of practice: preconditions (DOH, 1998)                         460
44.2   Brainstem death tests                                               460
45.1   Priorities of nursing care                                          475

# Part I

# Contexts of care

Chapter 1

# Nursing perspectives

## Contents

Introduction                         4
Technology                           4
The patient...                       5
...their relatives...                5
...and the nurse                     6
Stress                               7
Breaking bad news                    8
Duty of care                         8
Implications for practice            9
Summary                              9
Further reading                      10
Clinical questions                   10

## Introduction

What is the purpose of nurses in an ICU? What does critical illness and admission to intensive care cost patients and their families? In the busyness of everyday practice, these fundamental questions can be too easily forgotten. Yet an ICU is expensive: staffing accounts for half of the ICU budgets, and nursing accounts for most staffing costs (Edbrooke *et al.*, 1999). So ICU nurses need to clarify their value and 'articulate the importance of their role in caring for patients and their relatives' (Wilkinson, 1992: 196). This book explores issues for ICU nursing practice; this section establishes core fundamental aspects of ICU nursing. To help readers articulate the importance of their role, this chapter explores what nursing means in the context of intensive care, while Chapter 2 outlines two schools of psychology (Behaviourism and Humanism) that have influenced healthcare and society.

Acknowledging and continuously re-evaluating our beliefs is part of human growth. Examining nursing's values and beliefs, within the context of our own area of practice, is part of our professional growth (Sarvimaki & Sanderlin Benko, 2001).

In the UK, Comprehensive Critical Care (DOH, 2000a) identified four levels of care (see Table 1.1), used throughout the National Health Service (NHS). This text is about level three (critically ill) patients; a companion book (Moore & Woodrow, 2004) focuses on level 2 patients.

## Technology

Intensive care is a young speciality. The first purpose-built intensive care unit (ICU) in the UK opened in 1964 (Ashworth, personal communication). ICUs offer potentially life-saving intervention during acute physiological crises, with emphasis on medical need and availability of technology.

Technology provides valuable means of monitoring and treatment. Continuous observation of critically ill patients is important (RCN, 2003a), but should not become a substitute for care. To achieve a patient-centred focus,

### *Table 1.1* Levels of care

| | |
|---|---|
| *Level 0* | Patients whose needs can be met through normal ward care in an acute hospital |
| *Level 1* | Patients at risk of their condition deteriorating, or those recently relocated from higher levels of care, whose needs can be met on an acute ward with additional advice and support from the critical care team |
| *Level 2* | Patients requiring more detailed observation or intervention including support for a single failing organ system or post-operative care and those 'stepping down' from higher levels of care |
| *Level 3* | Patients requiring advanced respiratory support alone or basic respiratory support together with support of at least two organ systems. This level includes all complex patients requiring support for multi-organ failure |

*Source:* **DOH, 2000a**

patients, not machines, must remain central to each nurse's role (Internal Council of Nurses (ICN), 2000). Yet the 'tyranny of busyness' keeps nurses isolated from each other, preventing them from expressing their feelings to each other (Manias & Street, 2000: 381), and presumably also from patients and their families. While acknowledging the need for technical roles, ICU nurses should develop therapeutic and humanistic environments which help the patient as a whole person towards their recovery (Jastremski, 2000; Jewitt, 2002).

## The patient...

Patients are admitted to intensive care because a physiological crisis threatens one or more body systems, and their life. Care therefore needs to focus primarily on supporting failed systems. Whatever merits nursing models may have for other specialities, they have usually proved problematic for the ICU. The Mead model (McClune & Franklin, 1987), adopted or adapted by most ICUs, derives from Roper's model, yet arguably owes more to the much-maligned 'medical model'. Although this book discusses various aspects of technological and physiological care, many chapters focussing on specific systems and treatments, these aspects should be placed in the context of the whole person.

Intrinsic needs derive from patients' own physiological deficits, including many 'activities of living' (e.g. communication, comfort, freedom from pain). Meeting these needs is fundamental to nursing.

People are influenced by, and interact with, their environment. Extrinsic needs for

- dignity
- privacy
- psychological support and
- spiritual support

define each person as a unique individual, rather than just a biologically functioning organism.

Unlike all other medical and paramedical professions, nurses do not treat a problem or set of problems. Uniquely amongst healthcare workers, nurses are with the patient throughout their hospital stay. A fundamental role of nurses is therefore to be with and be for the patient, as a whole person.

## ...their relatives...

Relatives, including friends and significant others, are an important part of each person's life (Burr, 1998), giving patients courage to struggle for survival (Bergbom & Askwall, 2000). In contrast of the often high-tech focus of staff, families of intensive care patients often focus on fundamental aspects of physiological needs, such as shaving (Ryan, 2004), pain relief and communication (Danis, 1998). Rather than ruminate by bedsides, afraid to touch their loved ones incase they interfere with some machine, relatives should be offered opportunities to be actively involved in care (Azoulay *et al.*, 2003), without being made to feel guilty or becoming physically exhausted. Letting relatives participate in care can help them psychologically (Dyer, 1991; Hammond, 1995).

Physiological crises of patients often create psychological crises for their relatives. Holistic patient care should include caring for their families and other significant people in their life (Greenwood, 1998; Whyte & Robb, 1999). Too often, focus on tasks, however futile, can lead ICU nurses to neglect the support needed by families (Brenner, 2002).

Relatives may be angry. They are usually angry at the disease, but it is difficult to take anger out on a disease. Instead, anger, complaints or passive withdrawal may be directed at those nearby, who are usually nurses (Maunder, 1997). Most relatives display symptoms of anxiety or depression (Pochard *et al.*, 2001; Jones *et al.*, 2004), yet these symptoms too often remain unnoticed. Relatives often experience unnecessary suffering (Jastremski & Harvey, 1998). They may blame themselves, however illogically, for their loved one's illness. Feeling guilty and distressed, they may stay in a penance-type vigil (Dyer, 1991), neglecting their own physical needs, such as rest (Van Horn & Tesh, 2000) and food. Facilities for relatives should include a waiting room near the unit, somewhere to stay overnight and facilities to make refreshments (DOH, 2000a).

Relatives need information, both to cope with their own psychological crisis and to make decisions. They often have a psychological need for hope, but with one quarter of patients dying on the unit, and additional post-discharge mortality and morbidity, there may be little hope to offer. If death seems likely, relatives need to know so they can start grieving (Eastland, 2001). Families may experience information overload, at a time they are least able to cope with it (Curry, 1995). Communication by staff is often ineffective (Azoulay *et al.*, 2000). Printed information can provide useful reminders (Plowright, 1995), but should not be a substitute for discussion – relatives need human support and contact. Information given should be consistent and should be recorded in multidisciplinary notes. As most communication is not verbal, nurses should be sensitive to both their own and relatives' non-verbal cues, such as posture, eye-contact and tone of voice (Maunder, 1997). Of all staff, nurses are best placed to meet relatives' needs, yet the needs are not always met (Holden *et al.*, 2002).

## ...and the nurse

Nurses monitor and assess patients, but they also provide care. Assessment is fundamental to providing care, but sometimes a plethora of paperwork prevents care. Nursing assessments should therefore remain patient-focussed, enabling nurses and others to deliver effective care.

Nurses should collaborate with doctors (and other members of the healthcare team) (Nursing and Midwifery Council (NMC), 2004). Traditional nurse to patient ratios of 1:1 for UK ICUs are higher than in most other countries, but UK ICU patients are also sicker (Ryan, 1997; Depasse *et al.*, 1998). The Department of Health (2000a) recommends the flexible use of beds for level 2 and level 3 patients. Widely accepted nurse–patient ratios for high dependency are 1:2, which the BACCN (2005) position statement identifies should be the maximum number of patients per nurse. While this may reflect acuity of disease, it often fails to reflect nursing workload: level 2 patients are usually conscious but may be acutely disorientated/ confused, whereas level 3 patients are often unconscious, so more nursing time may be consumed maintaining safety for level 2 patients. Decreasing staffing levels increases complication rates (Dang *et al.*, 2002; Whitman *et al.*, 2002) and mortality (Tarnow-Mordi *et al.*, 2000; West *et al.*, 2004).

Psychological stress caused or accentuated by intensive care has been widely discussed in nursing literature since Ashworth's seminal study of 1980. Patients' own reports of experiences in the ICU, such as Sawyer (1997), make salutary reading. Dyer (1995) compares ICU practices to torture, while Johns (2005) illustrates how dehumanising nursing can become when machines, rather than people, become the focus of attention. Unable to speak, make decisions, or alter their environment, ICU patients are confronted with a barrage of unusual, and deficit of usual, sensory inputs (discussed further in Chapter 3). The ICU dehumanises patients (Calne, 1994). Nurses control ICU environments, so they can rehumanise it for their patients (Todres *et al.*, 2000).

Nurses, and nursing, have valuable roles within intensive care. But staff are an expensive commodity. Even if economic pressures are ignored, the global shortage of nurses and ageing workforce (Buchan, 2002) limit supply. A pragmatic solution to both economic and recruitment limitations has been to develop support worker roles. Most units employing support workers have found they provide valuable contributions to teamwork, provided skillmix of nurses is not reduced inappropriately (RCN, 2003a). BACCN guidelines should protect patients, nurses and support workers from inappropriate delegation (Pilcher & Odell, 2000).

Intensive care can support failing physiological systems, but too often opportunities to prevent physiological deterioration before life-threatening crises are missed. ICU Outreach (Medical Emergency Teams in Australia) aims to enable earlier detection and support of problems to prevent ICU admission becoming necessary, and to follow-up patients discharged from ICU to help their recovery. ICU Outreach is discussed in Higgs (2004). Similarly, pre-surgical high dependency units enable optimisation (noninvasive ventilation, aggressive fluid management, inotropes), and so reduced complications (Wilson *et al.*, 1999). Pre-surgical high dependency has not so far been widely adopted in the UK.

## Stress

Patients, their relatives and nurses all suffer stress. Stress is both a psychological and physiological phenomenon. Psychology and physiology interact. Critically ill patients suffer physiological stress from their illness, and psychological stress from negative emotions such as fear. The stress response is a primitive defence mechanism, activating the hypothalamic–pituitary–adrenal (HPA) axis (Marik & Zaloga, 2002). The pituitary gland releases adrenocorticotrophic hormone (ACTH), which stimulates adrenal gland production of adrenaline (epinephrine) and noradrenaline (norepinephrine), with increased production of other hormones, including cortisol. This 'fight or flight' response, discussed further in Chapter 32, increases

- heart rate
- stroke volume
- systemic vascular resistance
- respiration rate
- blood sugar and
- fluid retention.

While protective in an acutely life-threatening confrontation, all factors are frequently detrimental with critical illness.

Patients are admitted to the ICU with acute physiological crises, so intervention necessarily focuses care on physical needs. Critically ill patients share their relatives' suffering, and feel guilty because of it (Bergbom & Askwall, 2000). Caring for both physical and psychological needs, nurses can add a humane, holistic perspective into patient care, preparing for recovery and discharge. Supporting relatives provides valuable psychological support for patients.

## Breaking bad news

One-fifth of ICU patients die (Young & Ridley, 2002). ICU staff often have to break the bad news to relatives and friends. Changes may be rapid and unpredictable, but if patients are dying their family need to be aware of the impending bereavement to begin grieving (Eastland, 2001).

Where possible, both the nurse caring for the patient and a senior doctor should inform the family of anticipated outcomes, away from the patient's bedside, preferably in a room where discussion will not be interrupted by others, including telephones. The door should be closed for privacy, but access to doors should not be obstructed incase distressed relatives need to escape. Everyone should sit down, as family members may faint, and staff should not stand above relatives. Posture, manner and voice should be as open as possible. Tissues should be available. Having witnesses is useful incase relatives later complain. Detailed records of discussions should be recorded.

Relatives should be given time to think about information, express their emotions, ask anything they wish, and offered the opportunity to return if they wish. An information book, including details of who to contact, support groups (such as CRUSE), is useful. Further information on bereavement can be found in Woodrow (2004a).

## Duty of care

Nurses' primary duty of care should be to their patients. Relatives' values and priorities often differ from that of nurses' (Gelling & Provest, 1999; Priestly, 1999).

Where relatives' needs conflict with patients', nurses should put patients first. The most frequent conflict experienced is lack of time and resources to care for both (Farrell, 1999). Conflict can also include issues of confidentiality. Nurses have a duty to maintain confidentiality (NMC, 2004), so should not disclose sensitive information to anyone not directly involved in their patient's care, or if it is unnecessary to do so. Especial care should be taken with telephone conversations, both because the other person may not be who they claim to be, and because reactions are unpredictable.

## Implications for practice

- Nurses need technical knowledge and skills, but nursing is more than being a technician.
- ICU nurses have a unique role in providing holistic, patient-centred care that can humanise a hostile environment for their patients.
- Nurses have a professional duty of confidentiality to their patients, which remains even after their patients die.
- Physiology and psychology interact, so although the physiological crisis necessitating ICU admission is the focus of treatment, holistic care includes meeting physical and psychological needs. Reducing psychological distress reduces the stress reponse, and so promotes physiological recovery.
- Relatives experience psychological distress. Holistic patient care should include care of relatives and significant others.
- Nursing values underpin each nurse's actions; clarifying values and beliefs helps each nurse and each team increase self-awareness.
- Patient experiences are central to ICU nursing, so consider what patients are experiencing.

## Summary

Much of this book necessarily focuses on technological/pathological aspects of knowledge needed for ICU nursing, but the busyness of clinical practice brings dangers of paying lip service to psychological needs in care plans and course assignments, while not meeting them in practice. Psychological care is not an abstract nicety; it affects physiology, and so remains fundamental to nursing care. This chapter is placed first to establish fundamental nursing values before considering individual pathologies and treatments; nursing values can (and should) then be applied to all aspects of holistic patient care.

Intensive care is labour intensive; nursing costs consume considerable portions of budgets. ICU nursing therefore needs to assert its value by

- recognising nursing knowledge
- valuing nursing skills and
- offering holistic patient/person-centred care.

Person-centred care involves nurses being there for each patient, rather than the institution.

Having recognised the primacy of the patient, nurses can then develop their valuable technological skills, together with other resources, to fulfil their unique role in the multidisciplinary team for the benefit of patients. ICU nurses should value ICU nursing on its own terms: to humanise the environment for their patients. Relatives are an importance part of the person's life, and have valuable roles to play in holistic care. But relatives also have needs which are often exacerbated by their loved one's critical illness, and which may remain unmet. The beliefs, attitudes and philosophical values of nurses will ultimately determine nursing's economic value.

## Further reading

Much has been written on what nursing is or should be. *Comprehensive Critical Care* (DOH, 2000a) has profoundly influenced recent developments. Pilcher and Odell (2000) and the RCN (2003c) offer guidelines for staffing levels.

Sawyer (1997) describes experiences of being a patient in the ICU, while Johns (2005) provides a useful reminder of humane perspectives. www.routledge.com/textbooks/0415373239

For clinical scenarios, clinical questions and the answers to them go to the support website at www.routledge.com/textbooks/0415373239

## Clinical questions

Q.1 Identify environmental, cultural, behavioural and physiological factors from your own clinical area that may contribute to the suffering and dehumanisation of patients in the ICU.

Q.2 Outline specific resources and nursing strategies, which can minimise the suffering and dehumanisation of patients.

Q.3 Consider the role of a Consultant Nurse within the ICU. What are the responsibilities of a Consultant Nurse and how may their contribution to patient care be evaluated?

Q.4 Reflect upon the assessment of patient dependency in your own clinical area. Does this consider

- patients' need for nursing interventions
- medical interventions and
- Level of technology?

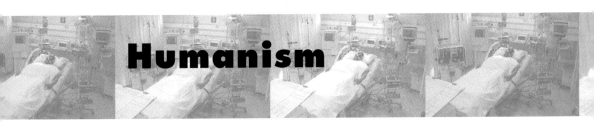

# Chapter 2

# Humanism

## Contents

| | |
|---|---|
| Introduction | 12 |
| Behaviourism | 12 |
| Behaviourism in practice | 13 |
| Time out 1 | 13 |
| Humanism | 14 |
| Lifelong learning | 14 |
| Problems | 15 |
| Implications for practice | 15 |
| Summary | 15 |
| Further reading | 16 |
| Clinical scenarios | 16 |

## Introduction

Philosophical beliefs affect our values. Our values may be either explicit or implicit, and influence both individual attitudes and the culture we work in (Sarvimaki & Sanderlin Benko, 2001). Values therefore influence care. Chapter 1 identified the need to explore values and beliefs about ICU nursing. This chapter describes and contrasts two influential philosophies to supply a context for developing individual beliefs and values. This is not a book about philosophy, so descriptions of these movements are brief and simplified; readers are encouraged to pursue their ideas through further reading.

The label 'Humanism' has been variously used through human history, probably because its connotations of human welfare and dignity sound attractive. The Renaissance 'Humanistic' movement included such influential philosophers as Erasmus and More. In this text, 'Humanism' is a specifically twentieth-century movement in philosophy, led primarily by Abraham Maslow (1908–1970) and Carl Rogers (1902–1987).

The Humanist movement, sometimes called the 'third force' (the first being psychoanalysis, the second Behaviourism), was a reaction to Behaviourism. This chapter therefore begins by describing Behaviourism. Two World Wars, and other traumatic events of the twentieth century, have however replaced some of Humanism's classical optimism by an emphasis on recovering humane values from the impersonality of bureaucratic and technological systems (Walter, 1997).

## Behaviourism

Behaviourist theory was developed largely by Watson (1924/1998), drawing on Pavlov's famous animal experiments: if each stimulus eliciting a specific response could be replaced by another (associated) stimulus, the desired response (behaviour) could still be achieved ('conditioning').

Behaviourism therefore focuses on outward, observable behaviours. Behaviourist theory enabled social control and so became influential when society valued a single, socially desirable, behaviour. For Behaviourists, learning *is* a change in behaviour (Reilly, 1980).

Holloway and Penson (1987) suggest nurse education contains a 'hidden curriculum' controlling behaviour of students and their socialisation into nursing culture. Through Gagné's (1975, 1985) influence, many nurses have accepted and adopted a Behaviouristic competency-orientated culture, without always being made aware of its philosophical framework. Hendricks-Thomas and Patterson (1995) suggest this Behaviouristic philosophy is often covert, masked under the guise of Humanism. So Roper *et al.*'s (1996) use of Maslow's hierarchy of needs does not necessarily reflect adoption of Humanistic philosophy.

Behaviourist theory relies largely on animal experiments, but humans do not always function like animals, especially where cognitive skills are concerned. Focus on outward behaviour does not necessarily change inner values.

People can adopt various behaviours in response to external motivators (e.g. senior nursing/medical staff), but once stimuli are removed, behaviour may revert; when no external motivator exists, people are usually guided by internal motivators, such as their own values. So if internal values remain unaltered, desired behaviour exists only as long as external motivators remain.

Behavourism relies on a series rewards and punishments to motivate individuals to conform to the desired behaviour. The rewards and punishments used by Behaviourism are public, external to the individual, such as essay grades, job promotion, salary or loss of privileges. Humanism also uses on rewards and punishments, but the Humanist relies on internal ends, such as self-actualisation and individual conscience. Humanism is therefore dependant on the individual valuing a moral code.

## Behaviourism in practice

### Time out 1

A patient in the ICU attempts to remove his endotracheal tube. There have been no plans to extubate as yet.

*Options:*

> explanation (cognitive)
> accepting extubation
> analgesia and sedation (control)
> restraint (e.g. chemical sedation)

*Comment:*

Here, 'pure' Behaviourism has already been tempered with humanitarianism: to try and comfort. Nevertheless, description remains deliberately Behaviouristic, seeing the problem as behaviour (extubation). While extubation causes justifiable concern, behaviour is a symptom of more complex psychology. The patient attempts extubation because the tube causes distress. Until underlying problems are resolved, they remain problems; restraint only delays resolution.

No philosophy is ideal for all circumstances, and few are without some merit. In this scenario, Behaviourism may justifiably 'buy time' until underlying pathophysiology is resolved or reduced, when extubation will be desirable rather than a problem. Behavioural approaches can be useful, but they can also be harmful, dehumanising others to lists of task-orientated responses. Pre-registration courses emphasise learning outcomes, creating passive learners (Romyn, 2001). Analysing values and beliefs, understanding the implications they have for practice and selecting appropriate approaches to each context enables nurses to provide humanistic, individualised care.

## Humanism

The Humanist movement was concerned that Behaviourism overemphasised animal instincts and attempted to control outward behaviour. Humanism emphasises inner values that distinguish people from animals, a 'person-centred' philosophy. Rather than emphasising society's needs, Humanism emphasised the needs of the individual self. Maslow's *Motivation and Personality* (1954/1987) popularised the concept of 'holism' (the whole person). Humanists believe people have a psychological need to (attempt to) achieve and realise their maximum potential. Maslow (1954/1987) described a hierarchy of needs, self-actualisation being the highest. Roper *et al.* (1996) adopted Maslow's hierarchy into their nursing model, although arguably to Behaviouristic ends. Simplistically, Behaviourism can be viewed as attempting to control, whereas Humanism attempts to empower. People who are controlled too often learn to become helpless (Seligman, 1975). Patients believe empowerment helps their recovery (Williams & Irurita, 2004).

Emphasis on inner values led Humanist educationalists to concentrate on developing and/or attempting to change inner values. Values that are internalised will continue to influence actions after external motivators are removed. Changes in nursing practice made to conform with desires of one person may not continue after that person has left, or even when they are not present (e.g. days off), but changes made because the staff wish for change to occur will continue as long as consensus remains.

Concern for inner values and holistic approaches to care makes Humanism compatible with many aspects of healthcare and nursing, although familiarity with terms can reduce them to levels of cliché. Humanism has much to offer nurses analysing their philosophies of care and practice, but no ideas should be accepted uncritically.

## Lifelong learning

Where Behaviourist education aimed to achieve conformity, Humanist education sought to promote individuality; this reflects the training versus education debate. Training seeks to equip learners with a repertoire of behaviours responses to specific stimuli, usually with a 'hidden curriculum' of indoctrinating conformity. Such training is often time-limited. In animals, stimulus-response reactions are often simple (as with Pavlov's dogs). Training equips the learner to be reactive to problems (stimuli) rather than proactive (to prevent potential problems occurring). Conditioned responses can be life-saving during a cardiac arrest, but 'training' fails to develop higher skills to work constructively through actual and potential human problems.

Facts and ideas are quickly outdated (Rogers, 1983), so are less valued by Humanists than the development of skills to enable personal growth (Maslow, 1971) and learning (Rogers, 1983). Humanism seeks to develop higher cognitive and affective skills to analyse issues according to individual needs, most valuable human interactions occurring above stimulus-response levels. For healthcare, Humanism promotes a person-centred philosophy that enables learning to continue beyond designated courses; each clinical area becomes a place for learning, and nurses should be extending and developing their skills through practice.

Many nursing actions have (literally) vital effects. Professional safety is necessary (Rogers, 1951), and most countries have professional regulatory bodies (e.g. NMC), but emphasis on individualised learning (e.g. learning contracts), reflection and life-long learning (DfEE, 1998) recognise that learning processes must be meaningful for each individual rather than determined by Behaviourist objectives and outcomes. NMC requirements for re-registration emphasise that attendance during study days does not ensure learning has taken place.

## Problems

Humanism has a weak research base, so acceptance or rejection of its philosophy remains largely subjective. Arguably, research-based approaches conflict with Humanism's fundamental beliefs in individualism; Rogers' early work did attempt to adapt traditional scientific research processes to Humanism, but his later work adopts more discursive, subjective approaches.

Much learning occurs through making mistakes; individualistic learning necessarily means making mistakes. Accepting the possibility of mistakes involves taking risks. Human fallibility should be recognised – expecting that mistakes will not occur, and so treating them as unacceptable, is unrealistic (DOH, 2000b). However, errors with critically ill patients can cause significant, potentially fatal, harm. ICU staff, especially managers, need to achieve the difficult balance between facilitating positive learning environments and maintaining safety for patients and others.

## Implications for practice

- Philosophy (beliefs and values) influences practice. So to understand our practice, we need to understand our underlying beliefs and values.
- Changing inner values, rather than just outward behaviour, ensures continuity when external stimuli are removed.
- Healthcare, nursing and the ICU retain Behaviouristic legacies that can undermine individualistic, patient-centred care.
- Humanism emphasises inner values and individualism, so Humanistic nursing helps humanise the ICU for patients.
- Humans are fallible, so mistakes will occur. Accepting this fallability encourages errors to be acknowledged, learnt from and so limits future risks.

## Summary

Philosophy is not an abstract theoretical discipline, but something underlying and influencing all aspects of practice, so it is relevant to every chapter in this book. Our beliefs, even if we are unaware of their source, influence our practice. Nurses can humanise care by

- being there
- sharing
- supporting
- involving
- interpreting and
- advocating.

(Andrew, 1998)

This chapter has outlined two influential and opposing philosophies; applying these beliefs to nursing values (see Chapter 1) helps clarify our own and others' motivation.

## Further reading

Skinner (1971) gives interesting late perspectives on Behaviourism, while Gagné (1975, 1985) significantly influenced nurse education.

Maslow (1954/1987) is a classic text of Humanistic philosophy. Rogers is equally valuable, and more approachable; his 1967 text synthesises his ideas, while his 1983 book valuably discusses educational theory.

Many texts identified in Chapter 1 reflect (often unacknowledged) Humanistic philosophy. Andrew (1998) offers valuable applications of Humanistic principles to intensive care nursing.

## Clinical scenarios

Mr Oliver is a 35-year-old who was admitted to ICU with a GCS of 6 following an unsuccessful attempt at suicide. He is invasively ventilated, but without sedation in order to facilitate the weaning process. He continually reached towards his orally endotracheal tube (ETT). This behaviour causes the nurse to respond.

Q.1 Describe a 'Behaviourist' response by the nurse to Mr Oliver reaching for his ETT.

Q.2 Explain how a 'Humanistic' response would differ from a 'Behaviourist' response in this situation. Consider the values that underpin each response, for example, safety, duty of care, autonomy, motivation of Mr Oliver, needs of Mr Oliver.

Q.3 Review your own practice and evaluate typical responses to this patient's gesture. What are your own and others' motivating values? How might the presence of a nurse with Mr Oliver influence his and the nurse's responses?

Chapter 3

# Psychological care

## Contents

| | |
|---|---|
| Introduction | 18 |
| Confusion | 18 |
| Time out 1 and 2 | 19 |
| Sensory input | 19 |
| Reticular activating system | 21 |
| Rubbish in – rubbish out | 22 |
| Circadian rhythm | 23 |
| Sleep | 23 |
| Noise | 24 |
| Music | 25 |
| Post-traumatic stress disorder (PTSD) | 25 |
| Recovery | 26 |
| Implications for practice | 26 |
| Summary | 27 |
| Further reading | 27 |
| Clinical scenarios | 27 |

## Fundamental knowledge

Sensory receptors and nervous system
Motor nervous system
Autonomic nervous system
Stress response (see Chapter 1)
Psychological coping mechanisms – e.g. denial

## Introduction

In the busyness of attempting to resolve acute physiological crises, psychological care may be relegated to afterthoughts. But physiology and psychology interact; psychological stressors cause physiological stress responses (see Chapters 1 and 32):

- tachypnoea
- tachycardia
- hypertension
- hyperglycaemia
- immunocompromise and
- oedema formation

all usually complicating critical illness.

Factors causing acute confusion and psychological distress to critically ill patients include

- acute cerebral hypoxia/ischaemia/damage
- sensory imbalance
- sleep deprivation and
- fear/anxiety.

Hazzard (2002) found that ICU patients respond with

- intense, unremitting anxiety
- emotional volatility (hope, despair) and
- violent cognitive readjustment towards catastrophic possibilities.

Extreme psychological distress may cause post-traumatic stress disorder (PTSD). Incidence of PTSD among ICU survivors is increasingly recognised as a major problem. Complete solutions remain elusive, but good psychological care may reduce incidence of subsequent psychological ill-health.

## Confusion

Many ICU patients suffer delirium (acute confusion) (Ely *et al.*, 2001; Roberts, 2001; Lin *et al.*, 2004), especially if they smoke or are normally hypertensive (Dubois *et al.*, 2001). Modifiable factors in ICU include

- sensory imbalance (overload or deprivation), also called ICU syndrome, ICU psychosis
- sleep disturbance/deprivation
- drugs, including acyclovir and digoxin and
- incomplete memories.

Delirium increases mortality (Ely *et al.*, 2001; McCusker *et al.*, 2002).

Sedation may provide anxiolysis (see Chapter 6), but is also a (chemical) restraint, so it should not become a substitute for nursing care.

ICU environments are abnormal, exposing patients both to excessive and deficient sensory stimulation, and causing psychological and physiological problems. Environments are interpreted through our five senses – sight, hearing, touch, taste and smell. Misinterpreted or imbalanced sensory inputs can cause confusion/delirium ('rubbish in – rubbish out').

## Time out 1

Take 2–3 minutes to list your own impressions of your environment at this moment; complete this before reading any further.

Review your list, noting down beside each item whether impressions were perceived through sight, hearing, touch, taste or smell. Some items may be perceived by more than one sense. How often was each sense used?

Most items are probably listed under sight, followed by a significant number under hearing. Touch is probably a poor third, with few (if any) under taste or smell. This reflects usual human use of senses: most input is usually through sight and hearing, with very limited inputs perceived from other senses.

## Time out 2

Imagine yourself as a patient in your own ICU. Jot down under each of the five senses any inputs you are likely to receive.

When finished, review your lists, analysing how many of these inputs are 'normal' for you. Remember that people usually rely most on visual and auditory inputs.

## Sensory input

Even if eyes are/can open, ICU patients often have distorted vision from

- drugs, e.g. opioids may cause blurred vision
- absence of glasses (if normally worn) or
- restricted visual field from positioning of head or equipment such as ventilator circuits.

Absence of vision may be caused by

- periorbital oedema (preventing eye opening) or
- exposure to keratinopathy (see Chapter 11).

Walls and ceilings are usually visually unstimulating; overhead equipment may be frightening. Attempts to rationalise such sensory inputs, especially if unprepared for this environment before admission, are likely to cause bizarre interpretation. Watching overhead monitors detracts from eye contact (non-verbal communication), and becomes dehumanising. Nurses should actively develop nonverbal skills (e.g. open body language, quality touch). Windows with views help maintain orientation to normality, so views should not be obscured by blinds, or beds placed so patients are unable to see out of windows.

Patient recall of ICU suggests that *hearing* remains unaltered by critical illness, so staff and visitors should assume patients can hear normally. Communication is fundamental to nursing care, yet aural communication may be impaired if

- patients are unable to respond to cues
- hearing aids are missing, faulty or not switched on
- the cochleal nerve is damaged by ototoxic drugs (e.g. gentamicin, furosemide) or
- English is not understood, or is not the person's first language.

Conversation is too often confined to either instructions or others' conversation (e.g. medical/nursing/team discussions, sometimes spoken across patients). Instructions, although valid in themselves, should be supplemented by quality conversation. Patients learning about their own condition and progress (or misinterpreting conversation as being about them) may become understandably anxious. Half-heard discussions and misunderstood terms are likely to increase anxiety. Unfamiliar sounds, such as alarms, also cause anxiety (Casbolt, 2002). Quality communication from nurses, explaining environments and strange noises, what is happening and providing information can reduce anxiety (Moser *et al.*, 2003).

*Touch* is a major means of non-verbal communication, especially with impaired vision. Touch is central to caring (Edvardsson *et al.*, 2003), yet is frequently underused in the ICU. Overload of abnormal tactile sensations may be caused by

- unfamiliar bedding (e.g. people used to duvets)
- pulling from tubes/drains/leads
- oral endotracheal tubes
- endotracheal suction or
- pressure area care, passive movements and body positioning.

Most touch in ICU remains task-orientated. Task-orientated touch is necessary, but reduces individuals to commodities, reinforcing their dehumanisation. Comfort (reassuring) touch significantly improves well-being (Butts, 2001), so patients may appreciate their pillow being turned or their hand being held. Human touch is valuable, especially if provided by loved ones.

Various receptors sense information about the body's internal and external environment. Proprioceptors, in the musculoskeletal system, provide information about body movement. Prolonged intervals between movement, common in most unconscious patients, result in lack of signals. Any movement sensed, such as movement in hoists or for procedures, may cause abnormal prioceptive stimulation.

Isolation can be physical (e.g. siderooms) or social; social isolation may be overt (e.g. gowns and masks, emphasising subhuman 'untouchable' status, restricting visiting) or covert (e.g. avoidance of patients who have nit infestation, or depriving patients of quality touch and meaningful conversation).

Caring touch is individual, and used inappropriately may suggest intimacy (Davidhizer & Giger, 1997) or power (Davidhizer *et al.*, 1995). Touch should be used sensitively, respecting individual wishes (Edvardsson *et al.*, 2003). Touching hands, forearms and shoulders is usually acceptable (Schoenhofer, 1989). Sensitive use of touch can offer positive proprioceptive stimulation, rehumanising care in a potentially dehumanising environment (Wilkin, 2003).

Warm environments (above 24°C) contribute to poor sleep, as probably experienced by readers during warm summer nights. Ambient temperature in most ICUs usually exceeds 24°C.

Few ICU patients receive oral diets, so *taste* is limited to drugs (e.g. metronidazole causes a metallic taste) and anything remaining in the mouth such as

- blood
- vomit
- mucus
- mouthwash (reminiscent of dentists)
- toothpaste or
- fungal infections (*Candida albicans* – 'thrush'), stomatitis.

Taste relies largely on smell, so reduced olfactory input (from intubation) reduces perception of taste.

Air turbulence over four nasal conchae (or tubinates) exposes *smells* to olfactory chemoreceptors. Intubation bypasses this mechanism, so sense of smell is usually reduced, although not absent. ICU smells are often abnormal:

- 'hospital' smells (disinfectant, diarrhoea, body fluids)
- human smells (perfume, body odours)
- putrefying wounds or
- nasogastric feeds.

## Reticular activating system

Sensory information is filtered by the reticular activating system, near the medulla. This normally discards nearly all inputs, only passing on meaningful (for the individual) information to the cerebral cortex. This prevents sensory overload thereby maintaining sanity. Reticular activating system dysfunction may be caused by drugs (e.g. ketamine, lysergic acid – LSD, ecstasy – see Chapter 47)

- reduced sensory input
- relevance deprivation
- repetitive stimulation
- unconsciousness

(O'Shea, 1997)

resulting in sensory overload ('psychedelic' effects) and hallucinations.

## Rubbish in – rubbish out

The senses provide the cerebral cortex with information to make sense of the individual's environment. Abnormal sensory input is likely to cause abnormal cerebral interpretation, resulting in abnormal responses, such as hallucinations and psychosis. Responses depend on both *reception* (sensory stimuli) and *perception* (sensory transmission to, and interpretation by, higher centres). Hallucinations vary, often being vivid and usually terrifying. Sensory deprivation can cause acute psychoses, delusions and severe depression, which may persist for many days. Delirium is undesirable from humanitarian perspectives, but it also has physiological costs – ICU mortality increases with delirium (Lin *et al.*, 2004).

Reasons behind nursing actions may appear mysterious to many patients (relevance deprivation). Explanations may reduce anxiety and psychological (and so physical) pain (Hayward, 1975). Reality orientation can be useful, but can also provoke aggression; people who are disempowered by being expected to passively accept contradiction are likely to respond with aggression.

Understanding patients' perceptions and interpretations is not always possible, but can make sense of hallucinations and bizarre actions: lying on moving beds may resemble cross channel ferries. Reported experiences often suggest profound fear; nurses (and other healthcare professionals) may become devils/tormentors, so nurses attempting to explore fears or reassure patients may meet resistance.

Intubation prevents ICU patients from speaking, and conscious ICU patients often have psychomotor weakness, which makes writing difficult. Unable to communicate fully and normally, patients often experience frustration. Gestures, facial expression and physiological signs (e.g. tachycardia) may be attempts to communicate, or indicate comfort, pain or anxiety. Etchels *et al.* (2003) describe a machine to enable intubated patients to 'talk', but so far this research technology appears to be languishing unused.

Delirium is problematic to manage. Haloperidol is widely used. Ely *et al.* (2004) suggest haloperidol has few side effects, although as it affects many different receptors it can cause various problems, and only changes the behavioural response (delirium).

Bergeron *et al.* (2001) describe a screening tool for delirium which, if used constructively, may help identify problems. However, if screening becomes one additional time-consuming task taking nurses away from giving human interaction, it may become counter-productive.

## Circadian rhythm

Circadian rhythm (change in body function over a day) is individual to each person, with normal slight variations between each day. Critical illness and abnormal environments (ICU) can severely disrupt one's circadian rhythm. Circadian usually peaks at about 6 pm hours and ebbs between 3 and 6 am. Most nurses working night duty experience the ebb stage (Muecke, 2005), so should avoid high-risk actions (e.g. extubation) at this time. During this ebb, reduced peripheral circulation may cause ischaemia ('night cramps'). Nursing assessment should identify whether patients normally suffer from night cramps, and what they do to relieve it.

Circulating catecholamine and cortisol levels peak around 6 am (Chassard & Bruguerolle, 2004). Sympathetic stimulation from catecholamines (increased heart rate, vasoconstriction) prepares for increased physical activity, but results in highest risk from myocardial infarctions and strokes between 6 and 10 am (Soo *et al.*, 2000). Early morning stimulation (e.g. washes) are best avoided with vulnerable patients.

## Sleep

Sleep is restorative and essential to health. Disrupted sleep can cause ill-health – most major accidents, such as Chernobyl, Three Mile Island and Bhopal, have been linked to night work, and most sleep-related vehicle accidents occur between 2 and 6 am (Rajaratnam & Arendt, 2001). Most ICU patients suffer sleep disruption (Bourne & Mills, 2004).

Sleep patterns can vary widely, cycles being controlled by the suprachias-matic nucleus ('biological clock') in the hypothalamus. Release of many hormones (e.g. melatonin, serotonin, growth hormone, glucagon, cortisol, catecholamines, ADH) increases during sleep. Inadequate sleep causes,

- catabolism
- immunocompromise
- respiratory dysfunction and

(Bourne & Mills, 2004)

can delay weaning (Higgins, 1998) and increase morbidity and mortality (Parthasarathy & Tobin, 2004).

Most people normally enjoy 4–5 sleep cycles each night, each lasting about 90 minutes. Cycles consist of two main phases:

- non-rapid eye movement (non-REM), sometimes called orthodox and
- rapid eye movement (REM), sometimes called paradoxical, due to increased levels of cerebral activity.

Non-REM sleep has four stages, Stages 3 and 4 being the most essential, restorative part of sleep (Dodds, 2002). Dreams normally occur in late stages, but arousal is easier (Bourne & Mills, 2004), and if sudden may cause

23

disorientation (Dodds, 2002). Sleep is often disrupted by ICU drugs, which reduce REM sleep, which include benzodiapines (e.g. midazolam), opioids, clonidine and noradrenaline (Bourne & Mills, 2004).

One of the most important nursing interventions at night is usually to allow patients to sleep, so nursing care should facilitate sleep. Pain is the main cause of disturbed night sleep in ICU patients (Frisk & Nordström, 2003), but nursing tasks also often disturb sleep. Nursing activities should be clustering to facilitate undisturbed stretches of two hours (one sleep cycle) whenever possible. Lights are usually dimmed overnight to maintain circadian rhythm, but commencing nursing activities early each morning (e.g. 6 am) may deprive patients of their final sleep cycle.

Dimming lights mimics day/night cycles, but 'dimmed' lighting often exceeds levels most nurses would choose for their own bedrooms at night. At night environments should generally be as dark as is safely possible, while during day sunlight, rather than artificial light, promotes psychological wellbeing. Florescent lighting makes a poor substitute for windows.

Sleeping during abnormal times in the circadian rhythm reduces both quantity and quality of sleep, as experienced with jet lag (Rajaratnam & Arendt, 2001). Morning rest is mainly REM sleep, which increases cerebral blood flow, recovery of brain tissue and emotional healing. Morning sleep is therefore especially useful for patients with traumatic brain injury. During afternoon rest non-REM sleep predominates. As non-REM sleep increases release of growth hormone, afternoon rest is especially beneficial following trauma, surgery or myocardial infarction.

## Noise

Noise in the ICU has been much studied, perhaps because it is relatively easy to measure, although environmental noise does not appear to be a major cause of sleep disturbance in ventilated patients (Bourne & Mills, 2004). Noise (undesired sound) is subjective: what is useful or enjoyable for one person can annoy others. But sustained noise

- impairs quality and quantity of sleep
- increases adrenocorticotrophic hormone release, triggering the stress response (see Chapter 1) (Christensen, 2002)
- reduces motivation and cognition (Stansfeld & Matheson, 2003).

ICUs are noisy. Much of the noise is unavoidable, inevitably continuing overnight. However, 'unnecessary noise is the most cruel absence of care which can be inflicted on either sick or well' (Nightingale, 1859/1980: 5). Nurses should therefore actively reduce unnecessary noise.

Sound is measured in decibels (dB), every 10 dB representing a tenfold increase in intensity. Sounds of 0 dB are barely perceptible by the human ear, but 10 dB has 10 times this intensity and 20 dB has 100 times. Healthy human ears can detect changes as small as 0.1–0.5 dB whereas 130 dB causes physical pain. While equipment and interventions in ICU rarely reach this level, they constantly breach the International Noise Council's recommended upper limit of 45 dB for ICU during daytime and 20 dB overnight (Granberg et al., 1996), and often the upper UK legal limit of 85 dB for noise at work. Prolonged exposure to 85–90 dB causes hearing loss (Stansfeld & Matheson, 2003). Overall ICU noise levels are often 61.3–100.9 dB (McLaughlin et al., 1996). Conversations can measure 90 dB (Ros et al., 2000), while even whispers usually cause 30 dB, enough to disturb sleep (Wood, 1993). Not all conversations are necessary.

## Music

Not all sound is undesirable. Music therapy can reduce anxiety (Chlan, 1998; Wong et al., 2001; Wang et al., 2002), but should

- reflect patients' choices (rather than staffs')
- use comfortable volume levels (this varies between individuals, choosing the right level for someone unable to speak can be problematic)
- be varied rather than repeated
- allow rest periods (especially if using headphones, which can quickly become uncomfortable).

## Post-traumatic stress disorder (PTSD)

Follow-up studies of ICU experiences consistently identify traumatic memories (Simini, 1999; Roberts & Chaboyer, 2004). Up to half of ICU patients may develop post-traumatic stress disorder (PTSD), compared with only 1 per cent of the general population (Jones & Griffiths, 2002; Jones et al., 2004). Following discharge, some patients need mental health services (Daffurn et al., 1994), but are often reluctant to seek help (Maddox et al., 2001). Relatives may also experience PTSD.

Memories of the ICU are often incomplete and compressed. Unlike normal sleep, sedation and critical illness can cause partial or total amnesia (Backmän & Walther, 2001), leaving patients with incomplete, abnormal and often traumatic memories, and the psychological trauma of missing or lost time (Perrins et al., 1998). Patients consider that their recovery is improved if they have personal control (Williams & Irurita, 2004), so 'missing time' can be psychologically traumatic. 'Patient diaries' recording significant events during their illness which patients may want to find out about can be a valuable way to come to terms with 'missing time' (Bergbom et al., 1999; Combe, 2005). Professional duties of confidentiality, other ethical issues and time factors may limit whether staff can or should keep patient diaries, but they could be kept by families, who are more likely to record what would interest patients.

Sensitive, humane nursing care can reduce some of the trauma. This may be through attending to fundamental physiological needs, such as oral hygiene, or through considering how actions and conversations may be interpreted by patients. Feedback from Outreach and ward nurses should be used to change problem practices (Hazzard, 2002).

## Recovery

Despite complications, most ICU patients survive critical illness. Transfer to wards can cause relocation stress (Strahan & Brown, 2005). Weaning care by reducing

- time spent with patients or
- monitoring (equipment, frequency)
- helps adjustment to non-intensive care environments.

## Implications for practice

- Sensory imbalance is a symptom of psychological pain, provoking a stress response; alleviating pain provides both humanitarian and physiological benefits, so should be fundamental to nursing assessment and care.
- Sensory imbalance can be reduced by

  - creating environments that minimise sensory monotony or overload
  - provide patients with explanations, and help them to understand what they are experiencing
  - where patients are able to participate in care, encouraging them to take active roles.

- Monitors should be sited unobtrusively.
- Facilitating sleep is usually the nurse's most important role overnight, and can be optimised by:

  - individual assessment of sleeping pattern/needs
  - minimising interventions
  - allowing three to four undisturbed two-hour periods
  - dimming lights as much as is safely possible overnight.

- Afternoon rest periods of 90–120 minutes should also be provided.
- Relatives should be encouraged to participate in care, and encouraged to share news and use touch. They should not be made to feel guilty or exhausted. Open visiting, facilities and information can give relative much-needed support.
- Patient diaries can be a useful means for patients to come to terms with 'missing time' and PTSD.
- Patients should be offered psychological support following ICU discharge
- Problems identified from Outreach visits and post-discharge surveys/audits should be used to change practice.
- With recovery, care should be weaned to prepare patients for ward environments.

## Summary

Many critically ill patients experience acute psychoses, some developing persistent post-traumatic stress disorder. Critical illness and ICU are stressful, but nurses can actively reduce stressors, positively contributing to the psychological, and so physiological, health of their patients.

The significance of psychology is often acknowledged in academic assignments, but not so often translated into practice. Critical care nurses necessarily prioritise resolving physiological crises, so inadequate staffing may cause neglect of psychological care (Williams & Irurita, 2004). But, despite limitations from macroeconomics, aspects of psychological care can be improved.

Sensory imbalance includes both sensory overload and sensory deprivation. Maintaining sensory balance helps maintain psychological health, reducing complications from stress responses. Quality sensory inputs to humanise care may include the reassurance, caring touch and presence of relatives.

Sleep facilitates health and healing, yet many critically ill patients suffer sleep deprivation. Nurses should individually assess each patient's needs, attempting to provide a humanised and healthy environment for recovery.

## Further reading

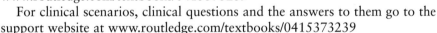

McInroy and Edwards (2002) identify problems and practical strategies, while Roberts (2001) and Roberts and Chaboyer (2004) identify patients' psychological needs. Christensen (2002) reviews the continuing problem of noise and Bourne and Mills (2004) review sleep disruption. Casbolt (2002) discusses communication, while Bergbom *et al.* (1999) show the value of patient diaries. Dodds (2002) summarises normal sleep patterns and problems in the ICU. www.routledge.com/textbooks/0415373239

For clinical scenarios, clinical questions and the answers to them go to the support website at www.routledge.com/textbooks/0415373239

## Clinical scenarios

Mr Robert Duke is 67 years old and was admitted to the ICU 26 days ago following an emergency abdominal surgery. His past medical history includes COPD, smoking and heavy alcohol use. Mr Duke has a tracheotomy and his respiratory support has been weaned to bilevel NIV. He continues to have copious secretions requiring clearance and twice daily 5 mg nicotine patch applications. Mr Duke refuses to co-operate with nursing care and avoids eye contact with everyone except his wife.

27

He appears sleep deprived and, as observations indicate, he takes 15 minute naps at night, with a total of 2 hours sleep recorded in 24 hours.

Q.1 Note the best methods to determine Mr Duke's psychological state, for example, mood, anxiety, understanding, consent to treatments, pain, discomfort, etc. How will you assess Mr Duke's communication abilities and understanding of his situation?

Q.2 Identify risk factors associated with development of sensory imbalance and delirium in the ICU for Mr Duke. How can these risks be minimised?

Q.3 Consider strategies to improve his experience of critical care and include specific interventions for psychological and physical comfort.

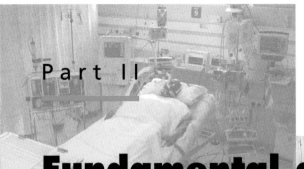

Part II

# Fundamental aspects

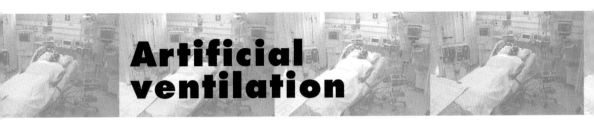

# Chapter 4

# Artificial ventilation

## Contents

| | |
|---|---|
| Introduction | 32 |
| Respiratory failure | 32 |
| Artificial ventilation | 34 |
| Care of ventilated patient | 35 |
| Safety | 35 |
| Physiological complications | 36 |
| Ventilator associated lung injury (VALI) | 37 |
| Tidal volume | 38 |
| Positive end expiratory pressure (PEEP) | 38 |
| Trigger | 39 |
| Sigh | 40 |
| Assisted mandatory ventilation (AMV) | 40 |
| SIMV | 40 |
| Airway pressure release ventilation (APRV) | 40 |
| Dual control modes | 41 |
| Proportional assist ventilation (PAV) | 41 |
| Inspiratory:expiratory ratio | 41 |
| Inverse ratio ventilation | 42 |
| Independent lung ventilation | 42 |
| Weaning | 42 |
| Noninvasive ventilation (NIV) | 44 |
| Implications for practice | 45 |
| Summary | 45 |
| Further reading | 45 |
| Clinical scenarios | 46 |

## Fundamental knowledge

Respiratory anatomy & physiology
Normal (negative pressure) breathing & mechanics of
    normal breathing
Deadspace and normal lung volumes
Experience of nursing ventilated patients
Local weaning protocols/guidelines

## Introduction

Ventilation is the process by which gases move in and out of the lungs. When self-ventilation is, or is likely to be, inadequate due to disease or drugs, artificial ventilation may be required. Artificial ventilation may fully replace patient's own ventilation, or support self-ventilation.

Intensive care units developed from respiratory units. Providing mechanical ventilation, and so caring for ventilated patients, is fundamental to intensive care nursing. Nurses should have a safe working knowledge of whichever machines and modes they use – manufacturers' literature and company representatives are usually good sources for information. This chapter discusses the main components of ventilation, more commonly used modes, and identifies complication of positive pressure ventilation on other body systems. Table 4.1 lists commonly used abbreviations and terms, but terminology of modes varies between manufacturers and authors (Branson & Campbell, 2001). Additional ventilatory options are discussed in Chapter 29. Negative pressure ventilation is rarely used in ICUs, so is not discussed in this book. Oxygen toxicity is discussed in Chapter 18. NIV is briefly discussed.

Invasive ventilation can be life-saving, but dying sedated and intubated on a busy ICU is not a dignified death. Invasive ventilation should therefore only be used for potentially recoverable conditions. When patients cannot make competent decisions for themselves, nurses (as patients' advocates) should contribute actively to multidisciplinary decisions. A useful ethical maxim is whether proposed interventions are likely to prolong life or prolong death.

## Respiratory failure

Respiratory failure causes inadequate oxygenation, and may cause inadequate carbon dioxide removal. There are two types of respiratory failure:

- Type1: Oxygenation failure – hypoxia ($PaO_2 < 8$ kPa) with normocapnia ($PaCO_2 < 6$ kPa).
- Type 2: Ventilatory failure – hypoxia ($PaO_2 < 8$ kPa) with hypercapnia ($PaCO_2 > 6$ kPa).

(British Thoracic Society, 2002)

## *Table 4.1* **Commonly used abbreviations and terms**

| | |
|---|---|
| AMV | assisted mandatory ventilation |
| APRV | airway pressure release ventilation |
| APV | adaptive pressure ventilation |
| ASV | assisted support ventilation |
| barotrauma | damage to alveoli from excessively high (peak) airway pressure |
| CMV | controlled mechanical ventilation |
| $FiO_2$ | fraction of inspired oxygen (expressed as a decimal fraction, so $FiO_2$ 1.0 = 100% or pure oxygen) |
| I:E | inspiratory to expiratory ratio (on ventilator) |
| MMV | mandatory minute ventilation |
| open lung strategies | strategies to keep alveoli constantly open, and so prevent atelectasis |
| PAV | proportional assist ventilation |
| permissive hypercapnia | tolerating abnormally high arterial carbon dioxide tensions ($pCO_2$) to enable smaller tidal volumes |
| pressure support | self-ventilating (triggered) breaths have volume augmented by the ventilator until preset airway pressure is reached |
| PRVC | pressure regulated volume control |
| PS | pressure support |
| respiratory failure | Type 1: oxygenation failure – hypoxia ($PaO_2 < 8$ kPa) with normocapnia ($PaCO_2 < 6$ kPa); Type 2: ventilatory failure – hypoxia ($PaO_2 < 8$ kPa) with hypercapnia ($PaCO_2 > 6$ kPa) |
| SIMV | synchronised intermittent mechanical ventilation |
| trigger | when patient-initiated breaths generate sufficient negative pressure, trigger initiates inspiratory phases through ventilators |
| V/Q | (alveolar) ventilation to (pulmonary capillary) perfusion ratio; normal V/Q = 0.8 |
| VALI | ventilator-associated lung injury (see VILI) |
| VILI | ventilator-induced lung injury (see VALI) |
| volutrauma | damage from alveolar distension (excessive volume); also called 'volotrauma' |

Gas exchange in lungs is determined by three factors

- ventilation (V) – breath size
- perfusion (Q) – pulmonary blood flow
- diffusion – movement of gases across tissue between pulmonary blood and alveolar air.

Normal adult alveolar respiration is about four litres each minute; normal cardiac output is about five litres each minute, creating a ventilation:perfusion (*V/Q*) ratio of 4:5, or 0.8. Perfusion without ventilation is called a *shunt*. Shunting can also occur at tissue level (reduced oxygen extraction ratio – see Chapter 20).

Carbon dioxide is 20 times more soluble than oxygen. In health distance between alveolar air and pulmonary blood is miniscule – 0.2–0.4 micrometers (erythrocyte diameter is about 7 micrometers). So in health, poorer solubility of oxygen is insignificant. However, diseases increasing distance between alveolar air and pulmonary blood (such as pulmonary oedema) inhibit oxygen transfer, causing Type 1 respiratory failure.

Air contains virtually no carbon dioxide (0.04 per cent). Carbon dioxide in blood is a waste product of metabolism. If metabolism and carbon dioxide production remain constant, blood levels depend on its removal, which is mainly affected by breath size, flow ('washout') and frequency (rate). Type 2 respiratory failure may be caused by any disease which limits breath size, such as neuromuscular weakness (e.g. Guillain Barré Syndrome), bronchoconstriction (chronic obstructive pulmonary disease) or extensive alveolar damage (emphysema, ARDS). Carbon dioxide production can be altered by nutrition – Pulmocare® causes less carbon dioxide production than standard feeds.

## Artificial ventilation

Artificial ventilation attempts to temporarily replace or support patients' own ventilation. This may be planned as part of post-operative care, or necessitated by existing or potentially imminent severe respiratory failure.

Ventilators are traditionally classified as

- time (controlled by rate or I:E ratio)
- volume (delivers gas until preset tidal volume is reached)
- pressure (delivers gas until present airway pressure reached)
- flow (rarely used)

cycled. Fully regulating ventilation through one of these means created *controlled mandatory ventilation (CMV)*, but this is now rarely used in ICUs. Modern ventilators usually provide various mandatory and self-ventilating modes, many being 'dual control' – able to switch automatically to other modes. Ventilators also have various safety features, including apnoea backup, which changes self-ventilating modes to mandatory ones if apnoea persist beyond preset limits (often 20 seconds). Modes and options used depend largely on patients' needs, but also on available technology, which varies slightly between manufacturers. All settings should be considered in the context of individual patient needs and problems, and other ventilator settings.

Oxygenation relies on functional alveolar surface area, so is determined by

- mean airway pressure
- inspiration time
- PEEP
- $FiO_2$
- pulmonary blood flow.

Carbon dioxide removal requires active tidal ventilation, so is affected by

- inspiratory pressure
- tidal volumes

- expiratory time
- frequency and flow of breath.

Manipulating these factors can optimise ventilation while minimising complications.

## Care of ventilated patient

Caring for ventilated patients should be holistic, the sum of many chapters in this book. Artificial ventilation causes potential problems with

- safety
- replacing normal functions (see Chapter 5)
- system complications.

## Safety

Individual patient handover is usually at the bedside. During handover, and frequently during their shift, nurses should observe their patients'

- general appearance (e.g. colour, position, facial expression)
- level of sedation
- comfort (signs of pain, body position/alignment, coughing/gagging from tube).

Following handover, respiratory observations include

- chest wall movement (bilateral)
- lung auscultation to identify air entry (see Chapter 17) and lung sounds. If secretions (rattles) are heard, suction is usually needed
- size and position of tube
- cuff pressure (see Chapter 5)
- effectiveness of sedation and analgesia (usually through scoring systems).

Additional observations should be individualised to the patient, but may include

- Glasgow Coma Scale
- arterial blood gas analysis.

Following handover, the ventilator should be checked for

- all settings, and whether they are appropriate for the patient
- alarm limits
- what effort/breaths (if any) the patient is making, and size of self-ventilating tidal volumes.

Layout of bedareas should minimise nurses having to turn their backs on their patients. Alarms do not replace the need for nursing observation, but are useful adjuncts, so should be narrow enough to provide early warning of significant changes, but with sufficient leeway to avoid causing patients or family unnecessary distress.

Safety equipment and backup facilities incase of ventilator, power or gas failure should include

■ manual rebreathing bag, with suitable connections
■ oxygen cylinders
■ reintubation and suction equipment.

Additional safety equipment may also be needed (e.g. tracheal dilators). Nurses should check all safety equipment at the start of each shift.

Physical restraint, used in some countries to prevent self-extubation and ensure safety, is generally unacceptable in the UK. Physical restrains should only be used as a last resort (RCN, 1999), limited to manual restraint, using minimum force necessary, and released as soon as possible. Chemical restraint (sedation) is discussed in Chapter 6.

## Physiological complications

All body systems are affected by artificial ventilation. Managing artificial ventilation focuses on avoiding or limiting ventilator-induced damage rather than achieving 'normal' gases. Although this description is reductionist, and further complications are identified in Chapter 5 and elsewhere, cumulative effects on the whole person should be remembered.

*Respiratory* The main complication, ventilatory-associated lung injury (VALI), is discussed later. Other respiratory complications include increased resistance from narrow, rigid tubes causing increased work of breathing (with self-ventilating breaths). Artificial support should therefore be increased if patients show signs of exhaustion or becomes tachypnoeic with low tidal volumes. If severe respiratory muscle causes prolonged weaning, patients may benefit by 'resting' overnight on ventilator-initated modes, to resume weaning the following day.

*Cardiovascular* Normal respiration aids cardiac return through negative intrathoracic pressure. Conversely, positive pressure ventilation

■ impedes venous return
■ increases right ventricular workload
■ causes cardiac tamponade.

So positive pressure ventilation increases venous while reducing arterial pressures, potentially causing

■ oedema (including pulmonary)
■ hypoperfusion/failure of all organs.

*Oedema* may be caused by

■ venous congestion
■ renin–angiotensin–aldosterone response
■ antidiuretic hormone secretion
■ atrial natriuretic peptide.

*Liver* dysfunction from

■ diaphragmatic compression (raised intrathoracic pressure)
■ portal congestion and hypertension (impaired venous return)
■ ischaemia (arterial hypotension)

reduces

■ albumin production
■ drug/toxin metabolism
■ clotting factor production
■ complement production (infection control)

so causing

■ reduced colloid osmotic pressure (hypovolaemia, hypotension, oedema)
■ toxicity (e.g. ammonia can cause coma)
■ coagulopathy
■ opportunistic infection.

*Neurological* Reduced cerebral bloodflow predisposes to confusion/delirium.

## Ventilator associated lung injury (VALI)

Positive pressure can cause chronic lung damage (Cooper *et al.*, 1999). Identified or speculated causes of VALI include:

■ barotrauma, from high airway pressure
■ volutrauma, from overdistension, usually caused by large tidal volumes
■ atelectrauma, possible damage from continual opening and closure of alveoli
■ biotrauma, proinflammatory cytokine release from alveolar distortion
■ oxygen toxicity (see Chapter 18).

(Pinhu *et al.*, 2003; Cooper, 2004)

Most recent changes in ventilatory practice aim to prevent VALI.

Barotrauma can be reduced by pressure-limiting ventilation, and adjusting ventilatory patterns. Lung function is affected by the way positive pressure is applied, so maximising tidal volume while minimising peak pressures optimise gas exchange while limiting barotrauma (Bigatello *et al.*, 2005), which can be adjusted using pressure:volume waveforms. However, it remains unproven whether mean, peak or end expiratory pressures cause most damage (Cooper, 2004). Barotrauma occurs more frequently in lateral positions (Cooper, 2004).

Cooper (2004) recommends that VALI can be minimised through

- Open lung strategies: PEEP + prone position (or continuous lateral rotation therapy if prone contraindicated)
- semi-recumbent position
- low tidal volumes
- pressure-limited ventilation.

Peak airway pressure (PAP) should, if possible, be limited to 30 cmH$_2$O (Acute Respiratory Distress Syndrome Network, 2000; Hess, 2002).

## Tidal volume

Tidal volume affects gas exchange, but can also cause shearing damage to lungs; settings therefore balance oxygenation and carbon dioxide removal against limiting lung injury. Patients at greatest risk from alveolar trauma usually have poor compliance, low functional lung volumes and hypoxia. The Acute Respiratory Distress Syndrome Network (2000) recommend tidal volumes between 4 and 8 ml/kg, with a 'target' of 6 ml/kg (420 ml for 70 kg patients), which may necessitate accepting permissive hypercapnia. Gas exchange may be improved through adjusting other aspects (e.g. inspiratory flow, mean airway pressure, PEEP).

## Positive end expiratory pressure (PEEP)

Normally, respiratory muscles relax passively with expiration, leaving residual gas within airways, usually exerting 2–2.5 cmH$_2$O pressure. This is variously called 'auto-PEEP', 'intrinsic PEEP', 'natural PEEP', 'air trapping' and 'breath stacking'. Intubation prevents upper (but not lower) airway closure, so measured airway pressure returns to *zero-PEEP* at the end of expiration.

PEEP resists expiratory flow, which

- prevents atelectasis
- recruits collapsed alveoli
- facilitates oxygen exchange during expiratory pause thereby improving oxygenation.

However PEEP can

- cause barotrauma
- cause gas trapping and hypercapnia

**Table 4.2 Recommended PEEP to FiO$_2$ settings**

| FiO$_2$ | PEEP |
|---------|------|
| 0.3 | 5 |
| 0.4 | 5 |
| 0.4 | 8 |
| 0.5 | 8 |
| 0.5 | 10 |
| 0.6 | 10 |
| 0.7 | 10 |
| 0.7 | 12 |
| 0.7 | 14 |
| 0.8 | 14 |
| 0.9 | 14 |
| 0.9 | 16 |
| 0.9 | 18 |
| 1.0 | 20 |
| 1.0 | 22 |
| 1.0 | 24 |

**Source: Acute Respiratory Distress Syndrome Network (2000)**

- reduce venous return (increasing cardiac workload)
- increase work of breathing on self-ventilating modes by increasing resistance to expiration.

Optimal PEEP with artificial ventilation is debated. The Acute Respiratory Distress Syndrome Network (2000) recommends increasing PEEP according to FiO$_2$ (see Table 4.2).

Disconnection from ventilators causes loss of PEEP and so atelectasis. Some ventilators include very short-term lung recruitment manoeuvres, often lasting less than one minute, to re-recruit alveoli after disconnection (Pinhu *et al.*, 2003).

# Trigger

This senses patient-initiated breaths. Making trigger levels less negative makes it easier to initiate breaths through the ventilator, so can be useful for weaning. With most modes, triggered breaths are additional to preset volumes.

Intermittent positive pressure breathing (IPPB – e.g. the 'Bird') is effectively a ventilator cycled solely by triggering. IPPB encourages deep breathing and alveolar expansion, and is sometimes used for physiotherapy.

At rest, self-ventilation negative pressure is approximately $-3$ mmHg, trigger levels below this can cause discomfort (fighting). Settings close to zero are usually used (e.g. 0.5–2). Settings of zero can cause autocycling, the ventilator triggering itself at the end of each expiratory phase. Trigger/sensitivity settings normally allow for PEEP (but check manufacturers' information), so trigger of $-0.5$ cmH$_2$O with PEEP of 5 allows triggering at $+4.5$ cmH$_2$O.

Self-ventilating modes rely on patient-initiated breaths. If patients are gas-trapping (e.g. asthma), they may generate insufficient negative pressure to trigger ventilators.

## Sigh

Normal breathing includes a physiological *sigh* every few minutes, preventing atelectasis during shallow breathing, increasing compliance, and so preventing infection. Ventilator sighs usually double tidal volumes. The use of the ventilator sigh was rapidly abandoned in the UK (although not in all countries), as it seemed to have no proven benefit and could cause barotrauma. However, use of smaller tidal volumes has revived interest in the sigh to recruit alveoli in ARDS (Pelosi *et al.*, 2003).

## Assisted mandatory ventilation (AMV)

This provides controlled mandatory ventilation, while allowing patients to trigger breaths. Modern ventilators include trigger with almost all modes, making AMV almost obsolete.

## SIMV

Synchronised intermittent mechanical ventilation (SIMV) is a primitive weaning mode, creating 'gaps' between mandatory breaths, allowing blood carbon dioxide to accumulate, so stimulating the respiratory centres. Reducing SIMV rate increases duration of 'gaps'. Total minute volume therefore depends on size and number of self-ventilating breaths.

The 'synchronised' component recognises patient-initiated breaths, delaying any imminent mandatory breath to prevent 'stacking' – hyperinflation of mandatory breath volume on top of triggered breath volume, which might cause barotrauma. Adding pressure support to SIMV increases size of triggered breaths, reducing work of breathing and assisting weaning. However, most ventilators now include better weaning modes.

## Airway pressure release ventilation (APRV)

This self-ventilating mode provides continuous positive airway pressure (CPAP), with periodic release of pressure to a lower level (Habashi, 2005). This makes it an 'open lung' approach, with ventilation occurring during release rather than inspiratory phases, release allowing clearance of carbon dioxide. Reducing the pressure difference encourages spontaneous ventilation, and so can be useful for weaning.

### Pressure limit

To prevent barotrauma, peak pressure limit prematurely terminates inspiration once preset limits are reached. Peak pressure limit should usually be 30 cmH$_2$O (Acute Respiratory Distress Syndrome Network, 2000).

### Pressure support

This is a self-ventilating, flow-cycled, 'mode. Once a breath is triggered, pressure support delivers gas until preset pressure is reached, adding volume to weak breaths, so compensating for respiratory muscle weakness. Pressure support is often commenced at 20 cmH$_2$O, then decreased usually in increments of 2 cmH$_2$O, until extubation usually at 10 cmH$_2$O.

Pressure support (PS) can by used as a self-ventilating mode, or a support to patient-initiated breaths in mandatory modes. Whenever patients are making some respiratory effort, pressure support is usually useful. Spontaneous negative pressure breathing also increases venous return to the heart, and so reduces cardiac compromise.

### Dual control modes

Duel modes combine advantages of volume control ventilation (constant minute volume) and pressure-controlled ventilation (rapid, variable flow). However, depending on settings, some ventilators may fail to control minute volume.

A widely used dual control mode is *Pressure Regulated Volume Control* (PRVC), also called *Adaptive Pressure Ventilation* (APV). This controls volume, but ceases if maximum preset pressure is reached.

More recent dual control modes include *Adaptive Support Ventilation* (ASV), which adjusts various aspects (mandatory rate, tidal volume, inspiratory pressure, inspiratory time, I:E ratio) to maintain preset minute volume. This makes weaning easier to manage (Petter *et al.*, 2003), while ensuring apnoeic patients are fully ventilated.

### Proportional assist ventilation (PAV)

PAV allows ventilators to adjust (proportion) airway pressure according to patients' effort (Hess, 2002), thus compensating for changes in lung compliance and resistance. It is currently not available on many ventilators.

### Inspiratory:expiratory ratio

A breath has three active phases:

■ inspiration
■ pause/plateau/inspiratory pause
■ expiration

and a fourth passive phase

■ expiratory pause.

Some ventilators determine breath pattern by adjusting two of the parts as percentages of the whole breath; other ventilators set an I:E (inspiratory to expiratory) ratio, with separate control for pause/plateau time. Whichever used, these are different ways to express the same equation. This text uses I:E ratios. I:E ratio cannot be regulated in self-ventilating modes.

Adjusting mandatory breath pattern affects ventilation. Oxygen transfer occurs primarily during inspiration and plateau; incomplete expiration (e.g. short expiratory phase; gas trapping) increases alveolar carbon dioxide concentrations, reducing diffusion from blood. Changing I:E ratio therefore manipulates alveolar gas exchange.

Normal I:E ratios are about 1:2. Awake patient's are unlikely to tolerate significantly different ratios. However, reduced airflow (poor lung compliance, e.g. ARDS), necessitates relatively longer inspiratory time. Prolonging pause/plateau time has similar effects to PEEP – increasing gas exchange, but also increasing intrathoracic pressure. Bronchospasm (e.g. asthma) reduces expiratory flow, needing longer expiratory time.

## Inverse ratio ventilation

Inverse ratio ventilation (IRV) uses ratios of 1:1 or below, making expiratory time abnormally short. Advantages of IRV are:

- alveolar recruitment from prolonged inspiration time
- alveolar stabilisation from shorter expiratory time (like PEEP)
- increased mean airway pressure (increased ventilation) without raising peak pressure (barotrauma).

However, IRV is physiologically abnormal, so can only be used with mandatory ventilation and usually necessitates additional sedation and often paralysis. IRV further increases intrathoracic pressure, compromising cardiac output.

## Independent lung ventilation

With single-lung pathology, patients may benefit from different modes of ventilation being used to each lung. Independent lung ventilation requires double lumen endotracheal tubes, one lumen entering each bronchus. Independent ventilators, each using any available mode, may then be used for each lung.

Independent lung ventilation may be impractical due to:

- insufficient available ventilators
- increased costs and workload (e.g. ventilator observations are doubled)
- danger to safety (access to patient, consuming more nursing time).

## Weaning

With severe respiratory failure, artificial ventilation may be life-saving. But prolonging ventilation unnecessarily is costly, both to patients (morbidity, risks) and to ICUs (workload, financial). While early extubation is desirable, premature extubation increases morbidity and mortality, often necessitating reintubation. Daily 'sedation holds' (see Chapter 6) helps assess likely success of extubation.

Recently, various weaning protocols have been introduced, claiming to reduce both number of ventilator-dependent days and length of ICU stay (Brock et al., 1998; Brochard, 1999). Ely et al.'s (2001) protocol specifies how to regulate a spontaneous breathing trial. However, over-rigid use of protocols may delay more proactive, and equally (or more) successful, weaning using skilled clinical judgement (Blackwood et al., 2004; Krishnan et al., 2004). Locally preferred weaning methods are more likely to succeed (Blackwood et al., 2004).

Debate persists over what are the most reliable weaning criteria, but frequently used ones include:

- underlying pathologies resolving
- appropriate ventilator settings (e.g. PEEP 5, $FiO_2 < 0.5$)
- measured respiratory function (e.g. blood gases, pH 7.3–7.45, $PaO_2$:$FiO_2$ ratio $> 26$; rapid shallow breathing index $< 100$)
- other respiratory assessments (e.g. CXR, auscultation)
- stability and function of other systems (especially cardiovascular)
- sedation score/status
- therapeutic drugs – usually sedatives and inotropes are discontinued before weaning; paralysing agents should always be discontinued before weaning
- any other risk factors (e.g. bleeding).

There is no generally accepted ideal weaning mode. Widely used modes are

- Assisted spontaneous breathing (ASB)
- Pressure support (PS) (Brochard, 1999; Koksal et al., 2004)
- T-piece (Brochard, 1999)
- CPAP (Koksal et al., 2004)
- Noninvasive ventilation (Dasgupta et al., 1999; Ferrer et al., 2003).

However well-planned, weaning may take longer than anticipated, especially if patients have underlying chronic lung conditions. If initial short-term weaning plans fail, slower weaning plans should be instigated. Occasionally patients may need referral to centres specialising in long-term ventilation.

Where further aggressive intervention would be inappropriate, teams may plan a 'one way wean'. This may be part of terminal care or with hope of survival but recognising futility of reintubation, but raises ethical issues about certainty of prognosis and value of life. Ideally, patients would participate in decision-making, but this is not always possible. Where expected outcome of a one-way wean is rapid death, withdrawal of life-prolonging treatment should not mean withdrawal of all treatment. Terminal care, however brief, should aim to provide patients with the best possible death that can reasonably, and legally, be offered. However, what makes a 'good death' is value-laden, so may vary greatly between patients – some patients might choose to die fully sedated and analgesied, while others might choose consciousness even at the cost of possible pain.

## Noninvasive ventilation (NIV)

Negative pressure ventilation is noninvasive, but is seldom used in acute care. There are two main types of noninvasive positive pressure ventilation:

- continuous positive airway pressure (CPAP)
- bilevel (or 'biphasic') positive airway pressure.

Both options can be useful, but can also cause complications. Generally higher pressures create more complications, so a rule of thumb is 'start low and work up' according to individual patients' needs.

CPAP is a self-ventilating form of PEEP. Stand-alone CPAP technology is available and is used in many clinical areas; although stand-alone equipment may be available in ICUs, CPAP is more often a self-ventilating option available on ventilators. CPAP stabilises and recruits alveoli, enables gas exchange to continue between breaths and can resolve pulmonary oedema. On ventilators it may be used for weaning usually shortly before extubation. CPAP is often commenced at 5 cmH$_2$O.

Bilevel positive airway pressure, often known after brand-name products such as BiPAP®, is like two alternating CPAP circuits, the higher pressure occurring during inspiration (Inspired Positive Airway Pressure – IPAP), and the lower during expiration (Expired Positive Airway Pressure – EPAP). EPAP provides all the benefits of PEEP/CPAP, while higher inspiratory pressures increase tidal volume. Increased pressure during inspiration and decreased resistance during expiration enables more carbon dioxide clearance making bilevel ventilation a useful self-ventilating option with Type 2 respiratory failure. Increasing differences between IPAP and EPAP (sometimes this difference is called 'pressure support') increases carbon dioxide clearance. Initial settings are often 8 cmH$_2$O (IPAP) and 4 cmH$_2$O (EPAP).

Noninvasive ventilation may prevent the need for invasive ventilation, avoiding need for sedation, reducing risks from ventilator associated pneumonia and so reducing morbidity and mortality (Plant *et al.*, 2001; Conti *et al.*, 2002). NIV may also provide a useful support when poor prognosis contraindicates invasive ventilation.

NIV technology used in community and ward settings is relatively simple, but more complex technology may be seen in some ICUs, allowing more of the options and monitoring familiar from invasive ventilators.

For further discussion of NIV see Woodrow (2004b).

## Implications for practice

- Most patients admitted to ICU suffer from respiratory failure, many needing mechanical ventilation.
- Nurses have a central role in managing ventilation, so they need technical knowledge of equipment to care safely and effectively for their patients.
- Any machine can be inaccurate or fail; nurses should check all alarms and safety equipment at the start of each shift. Ventilator function should be checked through recorded observations (at least hourly) and continuously by visual observation and setting appropriate alarm parameters (often within 10 per cent); remember alarms may also fail.
- Check the patient – air entry, appearance.
- Ventilators include default settings – know your machine and check these.
- Positive pressure ventilation affects all body systems; function of other systems should be continuously and holistically assessed.
- Ventilated patients depend on nurses to provide fundamental aspects of care (e.g. mouthcare).
- All intubation/mask equipment can cause damage – ties/tapes can occlude venous flow or cause direct trauma (e.g. tapes across open corneas); CPAP or other close fitting masks and endotracheal cuffs can cause pressure sores.
- In addition to maintaining safe technological environments, nurses should provide psychological care through explanations and reassurance.
- Early weaning reduces morbidity, but premature weaning creates complications. Ability to wean should be assessed. Weaning necessitates close monitoring and observation, revising plans if patients appear unable to cope.

## Summary

Breathing is vital to life. Patients rely on nurses and others to maintain safety. When breathing is wholly or partly replaced by mechanical ventilation, maintaining safety includes ensuring adequate ventilation.

Most ICU patients need ventilatory support. Many modes and options are available, although not all modes discussed are available on all machines. Choice should be adapted to individualised patient needs, which relies on nurses to continually monitor and assess their patients. Nurses therefore need a working knowledge of equipment on their unit and should be familiar with local protocols.

Positive pressure ventilation compromises function of other body systems. Nurses should assess complications from artificial ventilation, preventing risks where possible, minimising risks that cannot be avoided and replacing lost functions through fundamental care.

## Further reading

Manuals/information on machines used on the unit should be read. Most specialist texts include sections on ventilators and ventilation. Branson and Campbell's chapter (2001) provide an accessible overview. Pinhu (2004) reviews ventilator-associated lung injury. Cooper (2004) provides a useful nursing review about optimising ventilation. www.routledge.com/textbooks/ 0415373239

For clinical scenarios, clinical questions and the answers to them go to the support website at www.routledge.com/textbooks/0415373239

## Clinical scenarios

Mr Robert Hook is 32 years old with acute pancreatitis, bilateral pleural effusions, hypoxia, metabolic acidosis, tachypnoea and renal impairment. He was admitted to ICU for mechanical ventilation following four days of noninvasive ventilation and worsening respiratory function. He is orally intubated, weighs 106 kg, has copious white secretions via ETT and is draining thick sinus fluid into his oropharynx.

**Ventilator settings**

Mode SIMV – pressure cycled
Respiratory rate 18 bpm
Airway pressure 22 cmH$_2$O
PEEP 9 cmH$_2$O
I:E ratio 1:2
FiO$_2$ 0.6

**Patient initiated variables**

Respiratory rate 26 bpm

Airway pressure 24 cmH$_2$O
TV 710 to 750 ml
MV 18 to 19.5 l/min
SpO$_2$ 100%

| **Arterial blood gas result** | **Other blood results** | **Vital observations** |
|---|---|---|
| pH 7.41 | Hb 9.8 g/dl | Temperature 39.6°C |
| PaO$_2$ 14.5 kPa | WBC 15.5 × 10$^{-9}$/litre | Heart Rate 118 bpm |
| PaCO$_2$ 6.69 kPa | Platelets 132 × 10$^{-9}$/litre | BP 140/55 mmHg |
| HCO$_3^-$ 27.6 mmol/litre | CRP 83 mg/litre | CVP 15 cmH$_2$O |
| BE 4.5 mmol/litre | Albumin 13 g/litre | |
| SaO$_2$ 97% | Phosphate 1.23 mmol/litre | |
| | Magnesium 0.6 mmol/litre | |
| | Chloride 117 mmol/litre | |

Q.1 With this mode of ventilation, list other parameters which may be set and specify alarm limits. What other observations should be documented?

Q.2 Interpret Robert's results and suggest changes to the ventilator settings. Identify potential complications of mechanical ventilation and strategies to minimise these for Robert.

Q.3 Assess Robert's readiness to wean using evidence based criteria, estimate PaO$_2$/FiO$_2$ ratio and Rapid Shallow Breathing Index (RSBi = f / V$_T$). Devise a weaning plan for Robert including modes, parameters and indicators of success.

Chapter 5

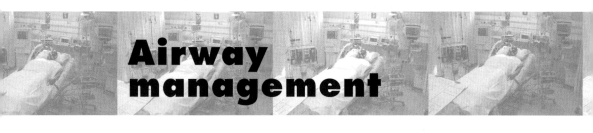

# Airway management

## Contents

| | |
|---|---|
| Introduction | 48 |
| Intubation | 48 |
| Tracheostomy | 49 |
| Problems | 50 |
| Humidification | 52 |
| Suction | 53 |
| Catheters | 55 |
| Saline | 55 |
| Hyperinflation | 56 |
| Extubation stridor | 56 |
| Implications for practice | 56 |
| Summary | 57 |
| Further reading | 57 |
| Clinical scenarios | 57 |

## Fundamental knowledge

Glossopharyngeal nerves
Oropharynx, and proximity of oesophagus to trachea
Tracheal anatomy, mucociliary mechanism ('ladder')
Cricoid anatomy
Carina + positions of right and left main bronchi
Differences between paediatric and adult trachea
Alveolar physiology
Deadspace

## Introduction

Ventilatory support usually necessitates endotracheal tubes (ETTs) or tracheostomy. ICU nurses therefore are responsible for ensuring patency of, and minimising complications from, artificial airways. This chapter describes types of tubes usually used in the ICU, main complications of intubation and controversies surrounding endotracheal suction.

Physiological airways

- warm
- moisten
- filter

inspired air. Bypassing part of physiological airways necessitates replacing lost functions, as well as minimising complications. Airway management has been much-studied, resulting in many changes to technology and practice. Older literature therefore often has limited value for current care. But evidence is often limited or questionable for many aspects making recommendations necessarily tentative.

## Intubation

Traditionally intubation could be

- oral
- nasal
- tracheostomy.

Oral tubes cause gagging, but are easier to insert. ETTs are rigid, limiting lumen size and increasing airway resistance (especially nasal tubes).

Nasal tubes are narrow, increasing airway resistance, so are rarely used unless oral intubation is contraindicated (e.g. dental or head/neck surgery).

Nurses assisting with intubation may be asked to apply cricoid pressure. Cricoid cartilage (just below the 'Adam's Apple') is the only complete ring of cartilage in the trachea, so cricoid pressure (pressing cricoid cartilage down with three fingers towards the patient's head) compresses the pharynx against cervical vertebra, preventing gastric reflux and aspiration. Pressure is maintained until the endotracheal tube cuff is inflated.

To ventilate both lung, ETTs should end above the carina (see Figure 5.1); this should be checked by

- X-rays
- auscultating for air entry
- ensuring chest movement is bilateral.

If available, capnography is reliable and immediately and continuously available. Accidental single bronchus intubation usually occurs in the right main bronchus, which is more vertical to the trachea than the left main bronchus. Misplaced tubes should be repositioned by anaesthetists and reassessed.

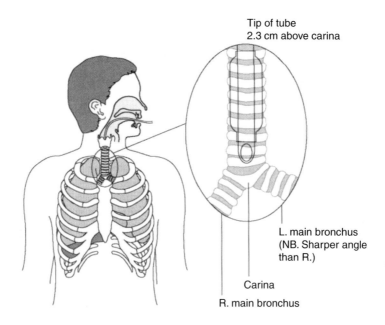

Tip of tube
2.3 cm above carina

L. main bronchus
(NB. Sharper angle
than R.)

Carina

R. main bronchus

**Figure 5.1 ETT just above carina**

Endotracheal tubes are manufactured in a single (long) length, so almost invariably require cutting to minimise ventilatory deadspace, usually to 21 cm (female) and 23 cm (male).

Childrens' airways differ from adults (see Chapter 13) so to prevent excessive pressure on tracheal tissue, uncuffed endotracheal tubes should be used with children under 8 years old (Bennett, 1999).

## Tracheostomy

Tracheostomy avoids many complications of oral and nasal intubation and reduces deadspace by up to half, so where artificial ventilation is likely to be prolonged, causing respiratory muscle weakness and delayed weaning, endotracheal tubes are usually replaced by tracheostomies within 7–14 days (Bodenham & Barry, 2001), or earlier if indicated.

Tracheostomies are usually formed percutaneously rather than surgically (Walz et al., 1998; Freeman et al., 2000). Percutaenous insertion is quicker, simpler, reduces risks of infection and haemorrhage and leaves a smaller scar (Walz et al., 1998). However, surgical tracheostomies may be created if percutaenous approaches are contraindicated; Astle (2003) lists many contraindications, including ARDS, coagulopathy, cervical injury preventing extension of the neck, enlarged thyroid gland, neck tumour, neck oedema, significant burns to the head or neck and active infection at the tracheostomy site.

Percutaneous stomas take 7–10 days to mature (Bodenham & Barry, 2001; Broomhead, 2002), so if replaced before this time the stoma may occlude more rapidly than surgical stomas. With early displacement of either surgical or percutaenous tubes it is safer to reintubate (Broomhead, 2002).

Emergency bedside equipment should include:

- tracheal dilators
- spare tubes – one the same size and one the size smaller
- suction
- syringe.

Tracheostomies are seldom stitched into skin, but if they are, a stitch cutter is also needed. Nurses caring for patients with a tracheostomy should check this emergency equipment that is easily accessible at the start of their shift.

Frequency of tracheostomy dressing depends on both the wound and the type of dressing used. If the stoma looks infected, it should be redressed. Otherwise, some tracheostomy dressings are designed to be replaced daily, others are designed to remain in place considerably longer (some up to one week).

Because tracheostomies reduce deadspace, decannulation significantly increases work of breathing, by 30 per cent (Chadda *et al.*, 2002). Weaning from a tracheostomy should therefore be a carefully planned and staged process to minimise need for recannulation:

- remove or minimise CPAP and pressure support (CPAP no more than $5\,cmH_2O$)
- initially use a T-piece rather than tracheal mask; T-pieces provides some PEEP and a reservoir of oxygen-rich gas.

Minitracheostomies (crichothyroidotomy), initially developed to facilitate removal of secretions, can also be used for high frequency, but not conventional, ventilators. Noninvasive positive pressure ventilation may avoid necessity for intubation.

## Problems

Intubation is often a necessary medical solution that creates various nursing problems.

*Coughing* is a protective mechanism, removing foreign bodies, including respiratory pathogens, from the airway. This reflex can also be triggered by oral endotracheal tubes and suction catheters, causing distress, possibly necessitating sedation.

Artificial airways can *damage tissue*, especially lips, gums, damage cilia and mucus-producing goblet cells (nonspecific immunity). Condition of lips and gums should be assessed and tissues protected as necessary – various commercial products can cushion pressure from tapes on lips. Tube position on the lips/gums should be changed at least daily.

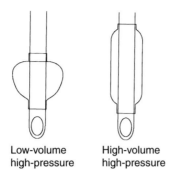

Low-volume          High-volume
high-pressure       high-pressure

■ *Figure 5.2* **High and low pressure ETT cuffs**

If cuff pressure exceeds capillary occlusion pressure, tracheal tissue will not be perfused, causing *tracheal ulcers*. 'High volume low pressure' 'profile' cuffs (see Figure 5.2) reduce cuff pressure by exerting lower pressure over an extended area. Unlike pressure sores on skin, tracheal epithelium is not directly visible. Average capillary occlusion pressure is about 30 mmHg, but can be lower (see Chapter 12), especially in hypotensive ICU patients. Cuff pressures should be checked at least once each shift and whenever cuff volume is changed. Most cuff pressure manometers display 'safe' ranges of 20–25 mmHg.

Impaired cough and swallowing reflexes may cause *aspiration* of saliva and gastric secretions. Profile cuffs rarely completely seal lower airways, making some aspiration almost inevitable. Risks of aspiration pneumonia can be reduced by nursing patients at 45° (Drakulovic *et al.*, 1999).

Oral ETTs cause *hypersalivation* and impair swallowing reflexes (see Chapter 10), with drying of mucosa near the lips and saliva accumulation (and potential aspiration) in the throat. 'Bubbling' sounds during inspiratory phases of ventilation indicates need to remove secretions and check cuff pressure. Nasal intubation and tracheostomy prevent hypersalivation, but tracheal secretions may still accumulate.

Tubes bypass and damage nonspecific immune defences (e.g. cilia). *Immunocompromise*, together with impaired cough reflex, predisposes patients to infection. Endotracheal intubation displaces the isothermic saturation boundary further down the trachea, further impairing mucociliary clearance (Ward & Park, 2000).

Sympathetic nervous stimulation from intubation and suction initiates *stress responses* (see Chapter 1). Direct *vagal* nerve stimulation (anatomically close to the trachea) can cause bradycardic dysrhythmias and blocks, especially during intubation.

Oral ETTs cause discomfort and *anxiety*; nasal tubes and tracheostomies are usually tolerated better. Patients' inability to speak due to intubation through their vocal cords should be explained.

## Humidification

The upper airway

- warms
- moistens
- filters

inspired air (see Figure 5.3). Endotracheal intubation bypasses these normal physiological mechanisms, necessitating artificial replacement. Oxygen is a dry gas, so inadequate humidification dehydrates exposed membranes (below the endotracheal tube), damaging cilia and drying mucus. Stickier, thicker mucus and impaired cilial clearance reduces airflow and increases infection risks.

During inspiration, airways warmed air to body temperature. This is normally reached by the carina, sometimes called the 'isothermic saturation boundary'. Warm air transports more water vapour than cold air, so fully saturated room air/gas (100 per cent relative humidity) will not be fully saturated once warmed to body temperature. Ideally, tracheal gas temperature should be 32–36°C.

Humidification may be achieved by

- heat moisture exchange (HME) filters
- cold water humidifiers
- hot water humidifiers
- nebulisers (e.g. saline).

*Heat moisture exchangers* (HMEs) use hydrophobic membranes to repel airway moisture, and are very efficient bacterial filters (95–100 per cent efficacy (Lawes, 2003)), and reflect heat. Nakagawa *et al.* (2000) suggest that

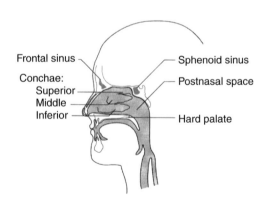

Frontal sinus

Conchae:
Superior
Middle
Inferior

Sphenoid sinus

Postnasal space

Hard palate

**Figure 5.3 Nasal cavity**

HMEs and water bath humidifiers have similar effects on mucus transport, although temperature of the water they used was only 32.6°C, and they did not address concerns about infection.

Heat moisture exchangers increase deadspace and resistance (Hilbert, 2003), although efficacy varies, increases often being insignificant for adults (Lawes, 2003). HMEs are usually best avoided in children (Ward & Park, 2000) and patients with COPD (Girault *et al.*, 2003). HMEs have improved since many early (1980s) studies (Lawes, 2003), so early literature now has limited value.

HMEs present the lowest infection risk. They should be changed daily (or more frequently if soiled).

*Hot water humidifiers* warm inspired air to preset temperatures, usually 37°C. Most systems are auto-filling, avoiding the need to break circuits. Like HMEs, significant technological improvements invalidate many early studies. Nurses should monitor and record humidifier temperature, keep fluid bags easily visible and replace them when empty. Circuits should be changed according to manufacturers' instructions.

*Cold water humidifiers* provide less efficient humidification, but fewer risks from infection and tracheal burns. Water bottles should be replaced when empty and circuits changed according to manufacturers' instructions.

*Nebulisation* delivers particles initially into airways, so where drugs effects are desired primarily within airways, such as bronchodilation (e.g. salbutamol) or pulmonary vasodilators (prostacyclin), nebulisation is often the best route, although it may create the paradox that drugs mainly reach open parts of lungs, whereas effect may be needed most in collapsed airways. This makes nebulisation a poor choice for antibiotics. Nebulising saline (2–5 ml) delivers droplets directly to airway epithelium.

Different types of nebulisers create different sized droplets. Droplets of 5 microns will be deposited in the trachea, whereas droplets of 2–5 microns will reach the bronchi. Droplets <2 microns reach alveoli. Most nebulisers deliver 2–5 micron droplets, but some (e.g. ultrasonic) deliver smaller droplets.

Nebulisers should ideally be placed near the patient, just before the Y connection, with no HME between the nebuliser and the ETT. Some ventilators include nebuliser circuits, but if using oxygen/air flow meters, 6–8 litre flow is needed to generate effective droplets. HMEs should be placed on return circuits to protect ventilators. Nebulisers should be cleaned or replaced after use, as static fluid is a medium for bacterial growth. Nebulisers should be cleaned in sterile (not tap) water and left to air-dry.

## Suction

Endotracheal suction is usually necessary to remove accumulated secretions, but can cause

- distress
- infection

- trauma
- hypoxia
- atelectasis

so should be performed when needed, not routinely (Ashurst, 1997). Indications include:

- rattling/bubbling on auscultation
- sudden increases in airway pressure
- audible 'bubbling'
- sudden hypoxia (e.g. in $SpO_2$).

Suction is uncomfortable – Sawyer (1997) describes experiencing a 'sink plunger technique'. Nurses should warn patients before suction, passing tubes steadily, but not aggressively.

Closed circuit suction (see later) reduces infection risk, but can still transport bacteria down the upper airway.

Negative (suction) pressure damages delicate tracheal epithelium (Maggiore et al., 2003), causing possible

- haemorrhage
- oedema
- stenosis
- metaplasia.

Negative pressure should be sufficient to clear secretions, but low enough to minimise trauma. Suction pressures, usually measured in kilopascals (kPa) but sometime in millimetres of mercury (mmHg), should be displayed on equipment. Many ICU nurses limit negative pressure to 20 kPA, although Ashurst (1997) recommends 16 kPa (120 mmHg).

Suction removes oxygen from airways and can cause atelectasis. Suction should therefore be as brief as possible (maximum 10 seconds). Nurses are recommended to hold their own breath during each pass: when they need oxygen, so will their patient.

Hypoxia from bronchoconstriction (sympathetic stress response) usually follows endotracheal suction. Although closed-circuit suction enables ventilation to continue during insertion, suctioning itself prevents alveolar ventilation, causing possible desaturation, especially when patients are dependant on high levels of oxygen. Although Wood's review (1998) found no proven benefit to routine preoxygenation, evidence is sparse, and failure to preoxygenate is probably more dangerous than routine preoxygenation, so preoxygenating all patients (100 per cent oxygen for 3–5 minutes) is recommended. Most ventilators include time-limited control for delivery of 100 per cent oxygen, preventing inadvertent delivery of toxic levels continuing after stabilisation. If $FiO_2$ is increased manually, it should be returned to baseline levels once $PaO_2$ is restored.

Care, and problems, should be fully recorded, to help later staff decide how and when to suction.

## Catheters

Oral secretions are often best removed with Yankauer catheters (Dean, 1997). Closed-circuit suction is almost always used with intubated ICU patients, 'open' suction largely being limited to self-ventilating patients who have a tracheostomy but whose cough reflex is too weak to effectively clear secretions. Open suction is discussed further in Moore (2004). Closed circuit systems maintain ventilation and PEEP when passing catheters, enabling slower (less traumatic) catheter introduction. In-line circuits should be changed according to manufacturers' instructions.

Closed circuit systems are manufactured in various sizes. Smaller catheters cause less trauma, but remove fewer secretions. For adults, standard catheter sizes are French Gague (FG) 10, 12 and sometimes FG 14. Removing very tenacious secretions with small catheters (below FG 12) can be difficult, but watery secretions can usually be removed effectively with FG 10. FG 14 catheters are very traumatic, and no larger sizes should be stoked. Smaller sizes will be needed for children. Many texts (usually anecdotally) recommend catheters should not exceed half to two-thirds ETT diameter; Odell *et al.* (1993) recommend:

$$\text{catheter size} = (\text{endotracheal tube size} - 2) \times 2$$

for ETTs above 6 Ch size.

## Saline

Instilling bolus saline into ETTs causes many problems, including

- dislodging bacteria (Hagler and Travers, 1994)
- hypoxia (Ackerman, 1993)
- not reaching distal bronchi (Hanley *et al.*, 1978)
- most of the saline remaining not being recovered (Hanley *et al.*, 1978).

Saline bolus may stimulate a cough reflex, but so should passing a catheter. Yet Schreuder and Jones' (2004) eight patient study advocates instilling saline to increase sputum clearance. Secretions may be mobilised through

- physiotherapy
- humidification
- nebulised saline.

Substantial research evidence is needed before saline instillation can be recommended (Blackwood, 1999).

## Hyperinflation

Muscle recoil following hyperinflation mimics the cough reflex (Sivasothy *et al.*, 2001). However, it also

- raises intrathoracic pressure
- reduces cardiac return
- causes (mechanical) vagal stimulation (resulting in bradycardia)
- causes barotraumas.

Hyperinflation can be achieved with manual ('rebreathe') bags, but is usually best controlled through ventilators (e.g. manual sigh), where tidal volume and pressure can be accurately monitored. Hyperinflation has largely been abandoned, as barotraumas can provoke ARDS.

## Extubation stridor

Laryngeal oedema often causes hoarseness following extubation, making patients temporarily hoarse or speechless on extubation. Children, having smaller airways, are especially liable to oedematous obstruction. Jaber *et al.* (2003) found than extubation stridor, an asthma-like wheeze, occured in more than one tenth of their ICU patients, although this incidence seems exceptionally high. Stridor may be treated with

- nebulised adrenaline (1 mg in 5 ml saline)
- dexamethasone
- Heliox (see Chapter 18).

If stridor cannot be rapidly reversed, reintubation is usually necessary.

## Implications for practice

- Nurses assisting with intubation may have to perform crichoid pressure, so should be familiar with how to perform it.
- ETT cuff pressures should be checked each shift, and whenever any change in pressure is suspected. Pressures should not exceed 25 mmHg (3.3 kPa).
- Unless other positions are specifically indicated, patients should be nursed semi-recumbent.
- Airway humidification is essential to maintain effective mucociliary clearance.
- Suction should never be 'routine', but performed when indicated.
- Negative pressure should not exceed 20 kPa.
- Bolus saline should not be instilled into airways. Secretions may be mobilised through physiotherapy, water humidification systems (preferably heated) and nebulised saline.
- Hyperinflation and preoxygenation are more safely performed through ventilators.

## Summary

Intubation remains a medical intervention, but nurses monitor and manage artificial airways, so they should also

- maintain safe environments, including ensuring safety equipment
- replace lost/impaired physiological functions, including humidification and clearing secretions
- individually assess each patient for risk factors caused by intubation and plan individualised care accordingly. No aspect of airway management is routine.

## Further reading

Tracheostomy care is discussed in greater detail in Woodrow (2004c). Bodenham and Barry (2001) review tracheostomies, while Lawes *et al.* (2003) identifies problems with HMEs. Drakulovic *et al.* (1999) provide convincing evidence for semi-recumbent positioning. Blackwood (1999) highlights problems from instilling saline. www.routledge.com/textbooks/0415373239

For clinical scenarios, clinical questions and the answers to them go to the support website at www.routledge.com/textbooks/0415373239

## Clinical scenarios

Tony Richards is 45 years old, very hirsute with a thick bushy beard and weighs 160 kg. He was admitted to the ICU following elective surgery for closer airway management. He was a difficult intubation (Grade 3) and mechanically ventilated via a size 9 ETT, with length 21 cm marking at his lips and cuff pressures of 35 cmH₂O. Tony is ready for extubation and biting on his ETT.

Q.1 List the equipment and process used to prepare Tony for extubation. Identify the most suitable type of respiratory support for Tony. Provide a rationale for your suggestion.

15 minutes after extubation Tony develops an audible stridor with intermittent gurgling noises from his throat. His respiratory rate changes from 18 to 28 bpm.

Q.2 Analyse possible causes of Tony's added airway sounds and changed respiratory rate. Interpret the significance of these results and implications on his airway management.

On expectoration, Tony's sputum is thick with brown discolouration. He has a weak cough with high risk of sputum retention.

Q.3 Review the range of methods used to mobilise and clear sputum from both lower and upper airways. Select the most suitable approach for Tony.

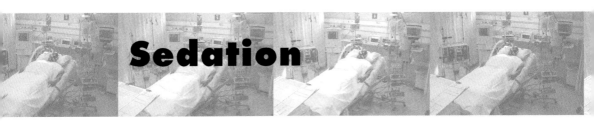

# Chapter 6

# Sedation

## Contents

| | |
|---|---|
| Introduction | 60 |
| Drugs | 60 |
| Bolus sedation | 62 |
| Assessing sedation | 62 |
| Ramsay | 62 |
| Addenbrookes/Cambridge | 63 |
| Newcastle | 63 |
| New Sheffield | 64 |
| Bispectral index | 65 |
| Sedation hold | 65 |
| Neuromuscular blockade | 65 |
| Implications for practice | 67 |
| Summary | 67 |
| Further reading | 68 |
| Clinical scenarios | 68 |

## Fundamental knowledge

Psychological distress in the ICU (see Chapter 3)

## Introduction

Critical illness, many interventions used in intensive care and the intensive care environment itself can all cause distress and psychoses (see Chapter 3). There are sound humanitarian reasons for sedating many patients in ICU, especially as many sedative drugs induce amnesia.

But sedation also deprives the individual of their autonomy, and to some extent their current awareness of being alive. Sedative drugs therefore create ethical dilemmas. Increasingly, sedative drugs have been viewed as 'chemical restraint' (Bray *et al.*, 2004), an intervention only justified when there is a specific indication, and within the limits of that indication.

Adverse effects vary between sedatives, but problems include:

- hypotension
- reduced gut motility (malabsorption, constipation), especially opioids
- prevention of REM sleep
- amnesia
- delirium (Pandharipande *et al.*, 2004).

Although drugs are mentioned, this chapter focuses on nursing assessment and care, including for neuromuscular blockade (paralysing agents).

## Drugs

Shehabi and Innes (2002) identify five groups of sedative agents:

- benzodiazepines
- opioids
- anaesthetics
- alpha 2 agonists
- antipsychotics.

### Benzodiazepines (e.g. diazepam, lorazepam, midazolam)

Gamma-aminobutyric acid (GABA) is the main cerebral cortex inhibitory neurotransmitter, hence GABA stimulation (by benzodiazepines) induces sedation, *anxiolysis* and hypnosis (Eddleston *et al.*, 1997). Prolonged benzodiazepine use causes receptor growth and down-regulation (tolerance), necessitating higher doses (Eddleston *et al.*, 1997).

Midazolam has largely superseded other benzodiazepines in the ICU because it acts relatively rapidly and has the shortest half-life. Midazolam is largely hepatically metabolised and renally excreted, so failure of these organs may unpredictably increase half-life, especially with older people who usually have reduced renal clearance. Some ICU patients take one week to wake after prolonged use of midazolam (Shehabi & Innes, 2002). Concurrent use of opioids and midazolam substantially reduces dose requirements of both drugs (Shehabi & Innes, 2002).

The antagonist for benzodiazepines is flumazenil. Flumazenil's effect is far shorter than benzodiazepines (half-life under one hour) so although useful to assess underlying consciousness, resumption of sedation necessitates caution if changing any treatments (e.g. extubation).

### Opioids (e.g. morphine, fentanyl, remifentanil, alfentanil, sufentanil)

Opioids have sedative effects. Normally considered a 'side effect', for ICU management this combination of strong analgesia and sedation makes opioids useful. Preferred opioids vary between units. Morphine remains widely used, but the more expensive fentanils cause less accumulation and fewer side-effects. Opioids are discussed in Chapter 7.

### Anaesthetic agents (e.g. propofol, ketamine)

Propofol is the most widely used ICU sedative (Murdoch & Cohen, 2000). Its lipid emulsion easily crosses the blood–brain barrier, giving rapid sedation. This, together with its metabolites being inactive, makes its half-life short. Propofol reduces cerebral metabolism, so may be useful for treating epilepsy. It is relatively expensive, so some units restrict use to when sedation is planned to one day. Currently, licensed use of propofol is limited to 72 hours. Using any drug or equipment beyond manufacturers' licence places onus of legal liability on users (see Chapter 48). Propofol is available in both 1 and 2 per cent concentrations, so labels should be checked especially carefully.

Propofol can cause

- profound hypotension
- prolonged clotting (Fourcade *et al.*, 2004)
- hypertriglyceridaemia, delaying return of cerebral function if used >72 hours (Eddleston *et al.*, 1997)
- 'creaming', accumulation of emulsifying fat in lungs and serum (Spencer & Willats, 1997), is visible with blood samples, can affect analyses (e.g. blood gases) and damage analysers
- immunocompromise from inhibition of phagocytosis (Krumholz *et al.*, 1995)
- greenish urine which, although probably clinically insignificant, may make relatives anxious.

It contains no preservative, but its lipid base may facilitate bacterial growth. Propofol has no analgesic effect, so concurrent analgesia should be given.

### Alpha 2 agonists (e.g. clonidine)

Although not widely used, some centrally acting alpha 2 antagonists are sometimes used for sedation.

### *Antipsychotics (e.g. haloperidol)*

Many ICU patients experience delirium and acute psychoses (see Chapter 3). Antipsychotics are sometimes used to relieve these problems.

## Bolus sedation

Shorter-acting sedatives are often infused continuously. However, many units use morphine and midazolam for prolonged sedation. Continuous infusions of these drugs can accumulate, delaying weaning and recovery, so bolus sedation may be more effective, given when accumulated effects start to fade. Bolus morphine can also control sudden pain, or anticipated pain from procedures, in self-ventilating patients. Bolus doses of morphine and midazolam are often 1–2 mg, with effect being assessed, and further increments usually given, if necessary, at 5–10 minute intervals. Most infusion pumps can deliver fixed boluses (often called 'piggyback').

## Assessing sedation

Over- and under-sedation are relative concepts. Over-sedation delays weaning and recovery, compromises perfusion to, and so function of, all organs and increases financial costs. Under-sedation exposes patients to pain and stress. Achieving optimum sedation is a humanitarian necessity; professional autonomy and accountability makes each nurse responsible for ensuring that their patients are appropriately (i.e. not over- or under-) sedated. Assessing sedation enables nurses to effectively titrate drugs to ensure optimal sedation.

Gently brushing tips of eyelashes can usefully identify if someone is sedated deeply enough to tolerate traumatic interventions (e.g. intubation). Many sedation scales and other means of assessment have been developed, but many are unsatisfactory for clinical use (De Jonghe *et al.*, 2000). A recent thorough, but complex, addition is the Minnesota Sedation Assessment Tool (Weinert & McFarland, 2004). Many scales are lists – relatively simple, but potentially subjective, and usually variants of the Ramsay scale. Reliable assessment necessitates familiarity and confidence with whatever is used, so limiting number of tools used on one unit promotes reliable assessment. Some scales necessitate inflicting pain, so for regular assessment, observation-orientated tools may be more appropriate. Some scales are known both by their developer's names and the place where they were developed.

Paralysis, whether from paralysing agents or pathology, prevents patients expressing awareness, invalidating almost all means of assessing sedation. Hence infusions of any paralysing agents should be stopped long enough before sedation assessment to ensure they will not influence results.

## Ramsay (Table 6.1)

Originally designed for drug research, this is the oldest of the scale discussed here. It is also the most widely used (Murdoch & Cohen, 2000). It offers a

### *Table 6.1* Ramsay

Ramsay *et al.* (1974)

Awake levels:
1    patient anxious and agitated or restless or both
2    patient cooperative, orientated and tranquil
3    patient responds to command only

Asleep levels:
4    brisk response
5    sluggish response
6    no response

**Source: Ramsay et al., 1974**

simple choice between six descriptions. Variants of Ramsay include Cohen and Kelly (1987), the Bloomsbury (Armstrong *et al.*, 1992), University College Hospital (Singer & Webb, 1997), Brussels (Detriche *et al.*, 1999) and Riker (Riker *et al.*, 2001) scales.

## Addenbrookes/Cambridge (O'Sullivan & Park, 1990; Table 6.2)

Although derived from Ramsay, unlike most scales above, this was developed for clinical practice and from substantial clinical experience. O'Sullivan and Park (1990) recommend scoring sedation every hour. Their scale generally facilities scoring from nursing care, although hourly suction cannot be supported just to assess sedation.

### *Table 6.2* Addenbrookes

agitated
awake
roused by voice
roused by tracheal suction
paralysed
asleep

**Source: O'Sullivan & Park, 1990**

## Newcastle (Cook & Palma, 1989; Table 6.3)

Adapted from the Glasgow Coma Scale, this was developed to evaluate propofol (Olleveant *et al.*, 1998), although descriptors are applicable for any sedated patient. Being based on a tried and trusted neurological assessment tool, it has proved reliable. The scoring system is more complex than Ramsay-like scales, which can make it time-consuming, but also more comprehensive.

### Table 6.3 Newcastle scale

| | | |
|---|---|---|
| eyes open | spontaneously | 4 |
| | to speech | 3 |
| | to pain | 2 |
| | none | 1 |
| responds to | obeys commands | 4 |
| nursing | purposeful movement | 3 |
| procedure | non-purposeful movement | 2 |
| | none | 1 |
| cough | spontaneously strong | 4 |
| | spontaneously weak | 3 |
| | on suction only | 2 |
| | none | 1 |
| respirations | extubated | 5 |
| | spontaneous intubated | 4 |
| | SIMV triggering respiration | 3 |
| | respiration against ventilator | 2 |
| | no respiratory effort | 1 |
| loading for spontaneous communication | | 1 2 |
| | awake | 17–19 |
| | asleep | 15–17 |
| | light sedation | 12–14 |
| | moderate sedation | 8–11 |
| | deep sedation | 5–7 |
| | anaesthetized | 4 |

*Source:* **Cook & Palma, 1989**

## New Sheffield (Laing, 1992; Table 6.4)

This Ramsay adaptation was developed for ICU nursing practice. However Ramsay's subjectivity is replaced by descriptions of each level, enabling greater objectivity (descriptions are omitted from Table 6.4). Olleveant *et al.*'s (1998) evaluation resulted in minor modifications, the Modified New Sheffield. They claim this modification is more reliable, although potential researcher bias necessitates further objective measurement to support their claim.

### Table 6.4 New Sheffield

New Sheffield (Laing, 1992)

1 awake
2 agitation
3 optimal level (i)
4 optimal level (ii)
5 sluggish level
6 flat level

*Source:* **Laing, 1992**
**The scale includes a description of each level (see Laing, 1992)**

## Bispectral index

Bispectral Index (BIS) uses a forehead sensor for adapted EEG monitoring, deriving a numerical level of sedation between 1–100:

| | |
|---|---|
| Awake patients | 90–100 |
| Conscious sedation (responds to noxious stimuli) | 60–80 |
| General anaesthesia | 50–60 |
| Deep hypnotic state | <40 |
| Very deep sedation | <20 |
| Absence of any brain activity | 0 |

Although many ICU patients will be managed in the 60–80 range, <60 is usually desirable if patients are paralysed. Reliability has been debated, but Deogaonkar *et al.*'s study (2004) suggests that current technology is reasonably reliable.

Other similar adaptations of ECG, less widely used than bispectral index, include evoked potentials, cerebral function monitors (CFM) and cerebral function analysing monitors (CFAM).

## Sedation hold

Stopping sedation daily, usually in the morning before ward rounds, enables thorough assessment of

- neurological state
- effectiveness of and need for sedation and analgesia
- readiness to wean.

Sedation holds reduce ventilator time, and so enables earlier discharge (Kress *et al.*, 2000; Schweickert *et al.*, 2004). Sedation holds should be carefully planned to ensure adequate comfort for procedures such as X-rays, physiotherapy and line insertion, and be long enough for effects of sedatives previously given to fade. Time of sedation holds and observed effects should be recorded.

Sedations holds are usually excluded with

- head injury
- paralysis (from drugs or disease)
- patients in prone positions or on kinetic beds
- patients awaiting procedures, such as CT scans or tracheostomy insertion.

## Neuromuscular blockade

Improvements in ventilator technology have largely removed the need to prevent patients making respiratory effort. Neuromuscular blockade (chemical paralysis) is usually only used if there is a specific indication to prevent muscle work, such as hyperpyrexia (see Chapter 8).

Paralysing agents cannot cross the blood–brain barrier, hence have no sedative or analgesic effects. Paralysed patients cannot alert staff if they are inadequately sedated, making it the most hazardous form of chemical restraint (Bray *et al.*, 2004). Some studies have found up to two-fifths of patients who remembered being paralysed (Arbour, 2000), although Sandin *et al.* (2000) found that only 0.18 per cent of patients chemically paralysed during surgery remained aware of what was happening. Paralysing agents should not be used until patients are adequately sedated (Arbour, 2000).

Blocking release of acetylcholine (a neurotransmitter) at the neuromuscular junction causes skeletal (but not smooth) muscle relaxation. Paralysing agents may be classified as

■ depolarising
■ non-depolarising

Depolarising drugs act on motor endplate, whereas non-depolarising drugs act on the post-synaptic endplate. Whichever site is affected, acetylcholine transmission is blocked, causing muscle paralysis. Suxemethonium is a depolarising muscle relaxant; most other paralysing agents used in ICU are non-depolarising.

Most paralysing agents are metabolised hepatically or excreted unchanged in urine, giving them a relatively long duration of effect. Atracurium and suxamethonium hydrolyse spontaneously in plasma, hence are relatively short-acting (Rang *et al.*, 1999). Atracurium is the most widely used paralysing agent in ICU (Murdoch & Cohen, 2000). Effect is prolonged with acidaemia (Rang *et al.*, 1999), hence the cited 15–35 minute duration of action may be considerably extended in many ICU patients. Pancuronium is less likely to cause hypotension, so may be chosen where cardiovascular instability is especially problematic.

Paralysing agents should be stopped to assess sedation, but removing paralysis may cause undesirable physiological effects, hence, like sedatives, paralysing agents should be stopped for no longer than is pharmacologically necessary.

Effectiveness of neuromuscular blockade should be assessed. The extrinsic eye muscle is the first muscle affected by paralysing agents, and the first to recover (Rang *et al.*, 1999), so brushing the eyelid indicates effectiveness. Extrinsic eye muscle paralysis may cause double vision and contribute to sensory imbalance. Paralysis is usually tested by absence of reflexes, such as peripheral electrical nerve stimulation. A relatively low (non-painful) voltage is usually sufficient to stimulate nerve reflexes. Users can benefit by trying out such tests on themselves so they know what they are inflicting on their patients. The ulnar nerve is the most frequently used site (Arbour, 2000) and should cause thumb adduction, although no evidence exists to justify any site as being best (Rowlee, 1999). Arbour (2000) describes the 'train of four':

- 4 twitches = neuromuscular blockade occupies <75 per cent of receptors
- 3 twitches = 75 per cent blockade
- 2 twitches = 75–80 per cent blockade
- 1 twitches = 90 per cent blockade
- 0 twitches = 100 per cent blockade.

BIS monitoring provides continuous monitoring of paralysis (Arbour, 2000), without inflicting potentially painful electric shocks.

### Implications for practice

- Undersedation and oversedation cause complications, hence sufficient sedation should be provided to achieve comfort.
- Nurses should assess efficacy of sedative and paralysing agents for their patients at least once every shift.
- Because there is no ideal sedation score, units should select one means, so that all staff are competent to use and understand it.
- Daily sedation holds enable thorough reassessment.
- Sedation needs of each patient should be individually reviewed daily by the multidisciplinary team to meet each patient's need, evaluating

  - humanitarian needs
  - therapeutic benefits
  - side effects (e.g. hypotension).

- For brief procedures (e.g. intubation), absence of blink reflexes confirms patients are adequately sedated.
- Paralysing agents should be stopped for sufficient time prior to assessing sedation.
- Nerve stimulators are potentially painful/uncomfortable, so if used, nurses should try tests on themselves (where safe to do so) so that they are aware of what they are subjecting their patients to.

### Summary

Critical illness often causes sedation. How far, if at all, this should be compounded by chemical sedation is a question of balancing benefits and burdens. These issues cutting across professional boundaries, plans for sedation should be agreed by nurses and doctors, using advice from pharmacists.

Sedation can relieve much psychological trauma caused by ICU admission, potentially providing physiological as well as humanitarian benefits. However, hypotension and other side effects can cause problems, while deep coma inhibits orientation and compliance with requests, removes patient autonomy and may contribute to post-traumatic stress disorder.

Although chemical sedatives are prescribed by doctors, they are (normally) given by nurses; so the professional accountability of each nurse ensures that patients receive adequate (but not excessive) sedation.

Use of paralysing agents has declined; where used, there are usually specific therapeutic indications. Therefore nurses should monitor and assess their effects.

## Further reading

The BACCN guidelines on restraint, including chemical restraint (Bray *et al.*, 2004) should be essential reading for all nurses working in intensive care. Much literature is medical rather than nursing, such as Murdoch and Cohen's (2000) telephone survey of national practice and Kess *et al.*'s (2000) influential work on sedation holds. Arbour (2000) offers nursing perspectives on paralysing agents. www.routledge.com/textbooks/0415373239

For clinical scenarios, clinical questions and the answers to them go to the support website at www.routledge.com/textbooks/0415373239

## Clinical scenarios

Peter Renton is a 30-year-old builder who was admitted to ICU 10 days ago with crush injuries from an industrial accident. He has multiple lung contusions, difficult to ventilate and his clinical observations and bio-chemical results suggest that he is developing acute renal failure and sepsis. In order to facilitate ventilation and other interventions, Peter has been sedated with intravenous infusions of

| | |
|---|---|
| Midazolam | 10 mg/hour for 10 days |
| Alfentanil | 5 mg/hour for 10 days |
| Propofol | 250 mg/hour for 7 days |

In addition Peter received intravenous vecuronium at 10 mg/hour for 8 days, which was changed to bolus administration of pancuronium on Day 8.

Q.1  Calculate the total amount of sedation given to Peter in relation to the recommended dosage, drug metabolism and elimination (pharmacokinetics). Evaluate possible long-term complications and outline some nursing strategies which can minimise these.

Q.2 Review the appropriateness of sedation hold with Peter. Plan how this is best managed, for example, time of day, reduction in infusion rates, order in which to stop infusions, which infusions should continue, assessment of sedation level, goals of sedation.

Q.3 Consider the actions (pharmodynamics) of vecuronium and pancuronium and provide the rationale for changing paralysing agents on Peter's eighth day.

# Chapter 7

# Pain management

**Contents**

| | |
|---|---|
| Introduction | 71 |
| Physiology | 72 |
| Psychology | 72 |
| Assessing pain | 74 |
| Managing pain | 75 |
| Opioids | 75 |
| Epidurals | 76 |
| Patient-controlled analgesia (PCA) | 77 |
| Non-opioids | 78 |
| Antiemetics | 78 |
| Implications for practice | 79 |
| Summary | 79 |
| Further reading | 79 |
| Clinical scenarios | 80 |

**Fundamental knowledge**

Anatomy and physiology of the nervous system, including
  sympathetic and parasympathetic, central and peripheral,
  motor, sensory
Spinal nerves – position of thoracic and lumbar nerves
Stress response (see Chapter 1)
Pain as a physical and psychological phenomenon
Local protocols/policies for epidural and PCA management

### Introduction

Pain is undesirable, a physical and psychological phenomenon that can cause physiological as well as psychological complications. Physiological problems caused by pain include

- stress responses (see Chapter 1)
- reluctance to breathe deeply (if self-ventilating), contributing to atelectasis and respiratory failure
- immunosuppression (Cheever, 1999).

Alleviating and relieving pain is fundamental to nursing care. Nurses therefore should understand

- physiological and psychological processes of pain
- how to assess pain
- how to control pain.

Nurses should be familiar with indications, contraindications, usual doses, preparation, benefits and adverse effects of drugs they use. Much literature on pain management focuses on pharmacology, and specific information can be found in manufacturer's Summary of Product Characteristics (SPC) and pharmacopoeias (e.g. British National Formulary), both of which should be available in all clinical areas. This chapter discusses some drugs, but focuses mainly on mechanisms and assessment of pain.

Causes of acute pain may be obvious (e.g. surgery), but patients may also suffer pre-existing chronic pain (e.g. arthritis). Chronic pain is usually less amenable to analgesia, and drugs that do work often create complications, such as immunosupression. Many interventions can cause pain, including

- suction (the most commonly reported cause of pain in intubated patients)
- line insertion
- drain removal
- repositioning
- physiotherapy.

Individual nursing assessment may identify ways to minimise discomfort, information which should be shared with colleagues (verbally, nursing records).

Many ICU patients are unable to perform even fundamental activities of living, so managing pain should include comfort measures, such as

- smoothing creases in sheets
- relieving prolonged pressure
- turning pillows over
- limb placement (e.g. with arthritis)
- reducing noise and light
- touch, explanations, reassurance, empowerment.

## Physiology

Pain is both a physiological and a psychological phenomenon. Pain signals, which may originate from physical or psychogenic stimuli, are transmitted to and received by the cerebral cortex, where they are perceived (interpreted) by higher centres in the brain. Pain is therefore necessarily individual to each sufferer, a complex interaction between physiology and psychology. Pain relief can therefore block either reception or perception of pain signals.

Pain is sensed by nociceptors, specialised nerve endings found throughout the body, especially skin and superficial tissues. Two main types of nerves (A and C fibres) transmit pain signals.

A fibres are large, with thick myelin sheaths that enable rapid conduction – up to 20 metres/second (Grubb, 1998). Four subgroups have been identified: alpha, beta, gamma and delta. A delta are found mainly in skin, skeletal muscle and joints, producing sharp and well-localised impulses and defensive motor reflex withdrawal (Melzack & Wall, 1988).

C fibres are small and unmyelinated, conducting impulses <2.5 metres/second (Grubb, 1998). C fibres transmit dull, poorly localised, deep and prolonged pain signals, causing guarding movements and immobility. Sharp impulses from the fast A delta fibres are superseded by slower, dull and prolonged impulses from C fibres.

Melzack and Wall (1988) describe a 'gate' (in the substantia gelatinosa capping grey matter of the spinal cord dorsal horn) which may be

- open
- closed
- blocked.

When open, impulses pass to higher centres (where they are perceived). A closed gate prevents impulses passing, leaving nothing to perceive. Endogenous chemicals control this gate (e.g. serotonin increases pain tolerance), so manipulating, supplementing or replacing these chemicals can control pain. The gate can also be blocked by other signals. A delta and C fibres share pathways, so A delta stimulation (e.g. skin pressure) can block the slower, dull, prolonged C fibre pain. Hence scratching itches, pressure bracelets and transcutaneous electrical nerve stimulations can relieve pain.

Pain may be referred (e.g. phantom limb pain, cardiac pain in left arm, appendix pain in loin – see Figure 7.1) where embryonic nerve pathways were shared or where residual nerve pathways remain intact.

## Psychology

Perception of signals received is influenced by various psychological factors, including

- culture
- anticipation – e.g. past experience, misinterpretation
- emotional vulnerability – e.g. fear
- distraction.

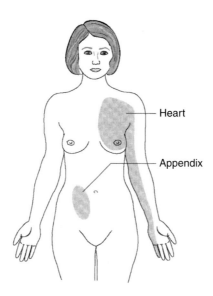

■ *Figure 7.1* **Referred pain**

The word 'pain' derives from the Latin 'poena' (punishment); perceiving pain as retribution may be partly a psychological coping mechanism, but also encourages physiologically harmful stoic attitudes of endurance. Culture also influences whether, when and how it is acceptable to admit to pain.

While recognising cultural influences, especially when pain is denied, stereotyping people is unhelpful and dehumanising. For example, older people may require less analgesia due to slower metabolism of analgesics and reduced pain sensation, but also grew up before the NHS existed, when stoicism was more widely expected. Postoperative pain is underassessed and undertreated in older people (Rakel & Herr, 2004). Even if pain impulses were comparable, pain experiences are unique to each individual, necessitating individual assessment.

Anticipation is influenced by previous exposure to similar stimuli (e.g. endotracheal suction) and expectations. Readers may experience this for themselves when visiting dentists.

Critically ill patients are vulnerable. They feel, and are, disempowered. Such negative emotions exacerbate pain (Hawthorne and Redmond, 1998). Fear can create self-fulfilling prophecies (something hurts because we expect it to hurt), but uncertainty increases fear, so clear, honest explanations before actions, warning them how long they will have to endure it, help patients prepare for pain. Hayward's (1975) classic study found information reduced pain, analgesia needs and recovery time.

Distraction may help people cope with pain by blocking the gate. Distraction and guided imagery can be useful nursing strategies, although impaired consciousness and verbal responses can limit their value in the ICU.

## Assessing pain

Pain relief and providing comfort are fundamental to nursing. Ideally, assessment of pain and effectiveness of pain management begins by asking patients, but communication may be limited by intubation, sedation, impaired psychomotor skills and sometimes denial. Family/friends and nursing/medical notes may provide useful information, especially about chronic pain and individual coping mechanisms.

Pain experiences and analgesia needs frequently change significantly, necessitating frequent reassessment. There is no ideal ICU pain assessment tool (Bird, 2003), but if patients are able to respond, they should be asked about their pain:

■  site (including any radiation)
■  type (intensity, frequency)
■  whether anything relieves it.

Nurses should observe whether pain is related to any activity, such as breathing (including artificial ventilation) or movement.

Most pain assessment tools provide structured (often numerical) questions for patients to answer. Pain rulers, widely used elsewhere, rely on consciousness, vision and psychomotor skills, which are often impaired in ICU patients. McKinley *et al.* (2003) describe a 'faces' scale for use in ICU, which is similarly problematic if vision is impaired (Bird, 2003). Adapted from paediatric pain management, some patients may find this patronising. Good pain management requires teamwork, so whatever means are used to assess and manage pain should be shared by all staff.

Non-verbal cues can be as reliable as verbal reports of pain (Feldt, 2000), so are especially useful if patients cannot talk. Sudden pain provokes a stress response (autonomic nervous system), with sudden

■  tachycardia (+ shallow breathing)
■  hypertension
■  tachypnoea
■  vasoconstriction (clammy, pale peripheries)
■  sweating.

Other non-verbal signs include

■  facial grimacing – clenched teeth, wrinkled forehead, biting lower lip, wide open or tightly shut eyes
■  position – doubled up, 'frozen', writhing

- facial grimacing
- pupil dilation.

(Blenkharn *et al.*, 2002; Murdoch & Larsen, 2004)

However, weakness/immobility and pathology may mask any or all of these signs. Prolonged pain may also cause parasympathetic-mediated hypotension and bradycardia.

## Managing pain

Opioids rightly remain the mainstay of acute pain management, but pain may be relieved through alternative or supplementary means. Pain is individual to each patient, so pain management should be individualised. Some generalisations can be made, provided practitioners remember to adapt generalisations to meet individual needs. Options will also be limited by what is available.

Where patients are conscious, or able to visit pre-operatively (or be visited on wards), discussing individual needs and preferences can provide nurses with valuable information, empower patients and reassure them. Where possible, open rather than closed questions should be used. Patient-controlled analgesia is discussed later.

## Opioids

Opioids bind to receptors in the central nervous system. Five types of receptors have been identified:

- mu 1(analgesia)
- mu 2 (respiratory depression, sedation, bradycardia, itch)
- kappa (spinal analgesia, sedation, meiosis, psychomimetic effects)
- delta (emotional effects)
- sigma (psychomimetic).

Common side effects include

- nausea
- respiratory depression
- sedation
- euphoria
- constipation
- urinary retention
- histamine release (pruritis)
- dysphoria
- hypotension.

(Macintyre & Ready, 2001)

75

Continuous intravenous infusions can cause accumulation of longer-acting opioids, or if metabolism is impaired (renal failure, hepatic failure). *Morphine* remains the 'gold standard' opioid against which others are judged. It suppresses impulse from C fibres, but not A delta, so relieves dull, prolonged pain. Its relatively long effect makes bolus administration feasible, which also reduces problems from accumulation.

*Diamorphine* (heroin) is metabolised to morphine, but being highly lipophilic it is more potent.

*Fentanyl* is twice as lipid-soluble as diamorphine (Hewitt & Jordan, 2004), so acts rapidly. Although more potent than morphine, it does not cause histamine release, so causes less hypotension. Fentanyl derivatives include alfentanil and remifentanil.

*Alfentanil's* shorter duration of action (1–2 hours) makes continuous infusion safer; its metabolites are inactive, making it useful for patients in renal failure, although liver failure prolongs its half life.

*Remifentanyl* is rapidly metabolised (by plasma), so has few, if any, complications from accumulation. It is, however, relatively expensive.

*Pethidine* is rarely used because it is very short-acting, produces the toxic metabolite norpethidine, is highly addictive and provides no greater pain relief than morphine (McQuay & Moore, 1998).

## Epidurals

Epidural analgesia can provide effective relief for severe pain. Infusions usually combine opioids (diamorphine or fentanyl) with local anaesthetic (bupivacaine). Dangers include

- dural puncture
- haematoma
- abscess
- catheter misplacement/migration
- hypotension.

Nurses should check the epidural site at each shift. Most Trusts have protocols and specific observation charts for managing epidurals. Most local protocols recommend hourly observation of

- vital sign monitoring (HR, BP, RR, oxygen saturations)
- pain
- nausea
- sedation level
- level of sensory block (see later).

Observation charts usually show 'dermatomes' – levels affected by each spinal nerve (see Figure 7.2). Where used, readers should be familiar with these.

Level of block is tested with cold spray or ice. A quarter of all epidurals fail to provide effective analgesia, often due to catheter misplacement

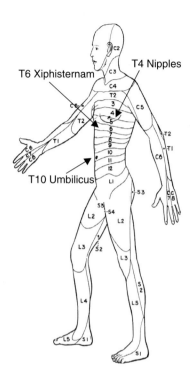

■ *Figure 7.2* **Dermatomes**

(Ballantyne *et al.*, 2003). Block should be sufficiently high to analgese, but not unnecessarily high or uneven. Blocks reaching T4 (nipple area) may paralyse respiratory muscles, so should be stopped immediately. Hypotension should *not* be managed by tilting head down, as this allows drugs to travel up the spine.

Removing epidural lines can cause infection and haematoma, so removal should be aseptic and only when clotting time is normal. The tip should be inspected to check it is intact; it is coloured (often blue) to make it distinctive. Heparin should usually be avoided before and after removal – times should be identified in local Trust policies.

## Patient-controlled analgesia (PCA)

Giving patients control of administering their own opioids, within maximum preset lock-out limits, usually achieves effective analgesia (McLeod *et al.*, 2001), and is preferred by patients (Snell *et al.*, 1997). PCA is unsuitable if patients cannot control devices due to

■  sedation/paralysis
■  impaired psychomotor function

- muscle weakness
- visual deficits
- confusion/forgetting how to control the machine.

Many Trusts produce specific observation charts for PCAs. These usually include:

- vital sign (HR, BP, RR, oxygen saturations)
- pain
- nausea
- sedation level.

As with epidurals, most Trusts recommend hourly observations.

PCA should be given through custom-made devices. These include a number of safety features, recording:

- set programs, including background rate and lockout time
- amount delivered
- unsuccessful attempts.

These should be recorded to enable continuing assessment. Unsuccessful attempts (demand within lockout time) indicates that analgesic needs are not being fully met, and so regimes should be reviewed.

## Non-opioids

Non-opioids, such as paracetamol, inhibit the neurotransmitter prostaglandin E$_2$ (PGE$_2$). Some non-opioids (but not paracetamol) are anti-inflammatory, making them effective against musculoskeletal pain. Most have synergistic effects when combined with opioids (McCaffery & Pasero, 1999), achieving similar analgesia with smaller opioid doses, and so reducing adverse effects, such as constipation and itching. NSAIDs (e.g. ibuprofen) are mainly used for chronic musculoskeletal pain, but are sometimes used for post-operative pain. They can cause renal failure.

## Antiemetics

Opioids, given by any route, may induce nausea, both through delayed gastric emptying and directly stimulating the vomiting centre in the brain. Nurses should observe for signs of nausea, assess likely causes, and give appropriate prescribed antiemetics. Most commonly used antiemetics, such as ondansetron, cyclizine and prochlorperazine (stemetil) primarily affect the vomiting centre. Maxalon (metoclopramide) primarily increases gastric motility, hence is useful where nausea is caused by gastric contents, but less useful when nausea is caused by vomiting centre stimulation (e.g. post-operative nausea and vomiting).

## Implications for practice

- Promoting comfort and removing/minimising pain are fundamental to nursing.
- Pain is a complex phenomenon involving both physiological transmission of pain signals and cognitive interpretation.
- Pain is individual to each person, so requires individual nursing assessment.
- Currently there is no ideal pain assessment tool for the ICU, but verbal questions and visual observations can indicate comfort.
- Good pain management involves teamwork, so means of assessing and managing pain should be shared by the team. Where possible, this team should include the patient – discussing options and effectiveness, and offering PCA.
- Nociceptor signals (reception) are interpreted as pain in the cerebral cortex (perception); pain can be managed by removing either component.
- Opioids remain the mainstay of ICU analgesia, but supplementary ways to relieve pain and provide comfort should also be used.
- Simple analgesics, such as paracetamol, have opioid-sparing properties, and so reduced adverse effects of opioids.
- Analgesia should be given before tasks which are likely to cause pain.
- Nurses should evaluate effectiveness of pain relief to optimise its effect and minimise its complications.
- Nurses should observe for signs of nausea, assess likely causes, and give appropriate prescribed antiemetics.

## Summary

Suffering is an almost inevitable part of critical illness, but this should not make pain acceptable. Pain is a complex phenomenon, involving both physiological transmission of pain signals and cognitive interpretation. Pain is culturally influenced and individual to each person, so should be assessed and managed individually. Promoting comfort and achieving effective pain management is fundamental to nursing, yet many patients continue to suffer unnecessary pain. Understanding physiological and psychosocial effects, together with pharmacology of drugs used, enables nurses to plan effective pain relief. Acute pain often needs opioids, although non-opioid drugs can provide useful synergy with opioids, and non-pharmacological approaches should be considered. Evaluating and documenting effectiveness of pain relief helps optimise its effect and minimise its complications.

## Further reading

Classic books on pain management include Melzack and Wall (1988), McCaffery and Pasero (1999) and Hayward's (1975) classic study on postoperative pain. Wall and Melzack (1999) is a comprehensive reference text. Bird

(2003) reviews pain assessment tools. Feldt (2000) and Blenkharn *et al.* (2002) describe assessing pain from nonverbal signs. Readers should be familiar with local policies and guidelines. www.routledge.com/textbooks/0415373239

For clinical scenarios, clinical questions and the answers to them go to the support website at www.routledge.com/textbooks/0415373239

## Clinical scenarios

Ms Persad is a 38-year-old legal secretary, who was admitted to ICU for respiratory management following her second bariatric weight loss surgical procedure. She has no immediate family in the area and has given her employer as next of kin. Ms Persad has a PCA of Morphine Sulphate 1 mcg/ml; her pain is poorly controlled. Ms Persad had previously had her pain controlled with pethidine and developed an urticaric rash. She dislikes the PCA and is requesting additional pethidine and medication to relieve itchiness.

Q.1 Identify type, location and source of pain Ms Persad has been experiencing along with other influencing factors. Select the most appropriate pain assessment tools to use.

Q.2 Review the range of approaches used to administer analgesia in the ICU. Analyse the use of pethidine versus morphine in managing Ms Persad's acute pain and discuss alternative approaches and drugs which could be effective in managing her pain.

Q.3 Consider other non-pharmacological interventions that can be implemented to effectively manage Ms Persad's pain.

# Chapter 8

# Pyrexia and temperature control

**Contents**

| | |
|---|---|
| Introduction | 82 |
| Pyrexia | 82 |
| Hyperpyrexia | 83 |
| Measurement | 83 |
| Treatment | 84 |
| Malignant hyperpyrexia | 85 |
| Implications for practice | 85 |
| Summary | 85 |
| Further reading | 85 |
| Clinical scenarios | 86 |

**Fundamental knowledge**

Thermoregulation – hypothalamic control, shivering, sweating and heat loss through vasodilatation

## Introduction

Human bodies can only function healthily within narrow temperature ranges. Body temperature, normally 35–37°C, is controlled by the thermoregulatory centre in the hypothalamus, responding to central and peripheral thermoreceptors. If cold, vasoconstriction and shivering responses conserve and produce heat; if hot, sweating and vasodilatation responses increase heat loss. Body temperature normally varies up to 0.5°C during each day (Weller, 2001).

Body heat is produced

■ by metabolism
■ in response to pyrogens.

Metabolism (chemical reactions) produces heat. Most post-operative pyrexias are caused by hypermetabolic tissue repair, not infection (O'Grady et al., 1998; Perlino, 2001). Blood transfusion similarly usually causes low-grade pyrexia. With metabolic pyrexia people usually feel hot, as experienced during heavy exercise.

Pyrogens, released by infection, typically cause higher temperatures than metabolism. Pyrogens (e.g. TNFα, interleukin-1) increase hypothalamic thermoregulatory setpoint, initiating heat production to achieve the higher level (= pyrexia). With infective pyrexias people usually feel cold/shivery, so attempt to conserve warmth (e.g. extra bedding/clothing).

Infants are especially prone to rapid pyrexial fluctuations, due to hypothalamic immaturity, higher metabolic rates and having more brown fat (which generates heat). Thermoregulatory impairment may cause febrile convulsions, so pyrexial children should be monitored frequently. The body surface area of children is proportionately larger than adults, making them also prone to more rapid heat loss.

Immunocompromise prevents heat-producing responses occurring, so older people (Watson, 2000a), people with immunocompromise diseases and people receiving immunosuppressive drugs do not always develop pyrexia with infection. Age-related reduction in metabolism produces less bodyheat, so older people may appreciate additional bedding.

Pyrexia is therefore a symptom, not a disease. It can be present without infection, and infection can be present without pyrexia.

## Pyrexia

The American Society of Critical Care Physicians (ACCP) defines clinically significant (i.e. probably from infection) temperatures as > 38.3°C (Isaac & Taylor, 2003), although hypermetabolism can cause severe hyperpyrexia.

Pyrexia can be protective,

■ *inhibiting bacterial and viral growth* – most micro-organisms cannot replicate in temperatures above 37°C (Henker et al., 2001) ('nature's antibiotic')

- *inhibiting proinflammatory cytokines* (Wong, 1998)
- promoting *tissue repair* through hypermetabolism but every degree centigrade also increases
- oxygen consumption
- metabolic waste – carbon dioxide, acids, water by about 10 per cent. Nurses should therefore assess both the likely cause of pyrexia and its cost to the patient.

## Hyperpyrexia

Hyperpyrexia (also called 'heatstroke' and 'severe hyperthermia') is a temperature above 40°C. At 41°C convulsions occur and autoregulation fails, death usually following at about 44°C, necessitating urgent ('first aid') neuroprotective cooling.

## Measurement

Hypothalamic temperature (where the thermoregulatory centre is) is the ideal core measurement. Being impractical, other choices are necessarily a compromise.

*Pulmonary artery* temperature, the closest measurable site to hypothalamic temperature, remains the 'gold standard' (O'Grady *et al.*, 1998). Catheters being highly invasive, temperature measurement alone does not justify their use. Debate persists about accuracy of alternative sites and equipment.

*Mercury-in-glass thermometers* are banned in many countries, and rarely used elsewhere. Mercury releases neurotoxic vapour and broken glass is hazardous. Latman (2003) considers that no other currently available thermometers compare favourably with mercury-in-glass.

*Rectal* measurement, undignified and unreliable, is rarely justified in the ICU.

*Axillary* measurement is theoretically unreliable for the ICU (Fulbrook, 1997; O'Grady *et al.*, 1998), but is often used for disposable *chemical thermometers* (e.g. Tempadots™). Board (1995) found chemical thermometers accurate, but their range is limited to 35.5–40.4°C (O'Toole, 1997), making them unsuitable for measuring hypothermia or hyperpyrexia. Chemical thermometers rely on visual interpretation, so can be subjective.

*Electronic thermometers* provide quick, less subjective (digital) measurement. Carotid arteries supply both the hypothalamus and *tympanic* membranes. Tympanic measurement may (Dowding *et al.*, 2002) or may not (O'Grady *et al.*, 1998; Craid *et al.*, 2002) be accurate. Poor techniques, such as not pulling back the pinna fully, taking temperature in an ear that has been resting on a pillow, or placing thermometers where earwax (cerumen) obstructs the canal, cause inaccuracy.

Probes on urinary catheters can measure *bladder* temperature. One quarter of cardiac output flows through renal arteries, so if urine flow is good

(60 ml/hour), bladder temperature indicates core temperature (O'Grady *et al.*, 1998). As ICU patients are usually catheterised, bladder measurement avoids additional invasive equipment. However, oliguria makes bladder temperature measurement unsuitable for many ICU patients.

*Nasopharyngeal* and *oesophageal* probes provide relatively noninvasive measurement, but nasopharyngeal measurement is affected by air leaks past endotracheal cuffs. Either probe may cause distress and discomfort, so cannot be recommended.

Infrared measurement of *forehead* temperature may (Harioka *et al.*, 2000) or may not (Sessler, 2002) be reliable.

Noninvasive skin probes, usually on patients' feet, measures *peripheral* temperature. Comparing differences between peripheral and central temperature indicates perfusion/warming – difference should be <2°C if well perfused. Limb reperfusion should be monitored following vascular surgery to the leg.

## Treatment

Appropriateness of treating pyrexia necessitates individual assessment and evidence-based practice. With pyrexias of infective origin, micro-organisms can often be destroyed more safely by antibiotics than by endogenous pyrexia.

Cooling may be

- central (altering hypothalamic set point)
- peripheral (increasing heat loss).

Peripheral cooling (reducing bedding, tepid sponging, fans) stimulate further hypothalamus-mediated heat production (shivering) and conservation (vasoconstriction). Shivering increases metabolism, increasing oxygen and energy consumption, while vasoconstriction traps heat produced in central vessels, creating hostile environments for major organs. Cooling also shifts the oxygen dissociation curve to the left, reducing oxygen delivery. Peripheral cooling is therefore fundamentally illogical (Marik, 2000). Paralysing and sedative drugs can reduce metabolism.

Antipyretic drugs (e.g. aspirin, paracetamol, nonsteroidal anti-inflammatory drugs – NSAIDs) inhibit prostaglandin synthesis, hence restoring normal hypothalamic regulation. Infective pyrexias usually respond to anti-pyretic drugs, while pyrexias from hypermetabolism or hypothalamic damage will not.

Sweat evaporation, vasodilatation and increased capillary permeability cause hypovolaemia and hypotension, necessitating additional fluid replacement. Electrolyte and acid–base imbalances should be monitored and treated.

If infection is suspected, appropriate cultures should be taken (e.g. blood) and empirical antibiotics prescribed. Suspected sources of infection (e.g. cannulae) should be removed if possible. Samples usually take days to culture, so recording samples sent on microbiology flow sheets help ensure results are promptly acted upon.

## Malignant hyperpyrexia

Malignant hyperpyrexia, a genetic skeletal muscle disorder (Redmond, 2001), may be triggered by drugs (e.g. anaesthetic agents such as suxamethonium, ecstasy) and stress (e.g. massive skeletal injury, strenuous exercise). Untreated malignant hyperpyrexia is fatal.

Precipitating causes should be removed. The only available drug to treat malignant hyperpyrexia is Dantrolene sodium (1 mg/kg) (Ellis & Halsall, 2002) which, being a calcium channel blocker, relaxes skeletal muscle. Neuromuscular blockade (paralysis) may be used to prevent shivering (heat production).

## Implications for practice

- Pyrexia is a symptom, not a disease. Pyrexia should be managed in the context of individual patients (cost/benefit analysis).
- Current evidence for thermometers is limited and inconsistent, but tympanic and chemical thermometers are probably preferable options.
- Pyrexia may be metabolic or infective in origin.
- Clinically significant pyrexia (infection) usually >38.3°C.
- Pyrexia inhibits micro-organisms, but increases oxygen and energy consumption, while increasing metabolic waste.
- Infection should be treated with appropriate antibiotics.
- Peripheral cooling of infective pyrexia is usually illogical and counterproductive.
- Central cooling (antipyretic drugs) can restore normal hypothalamic thermoregulation.
- Microbiology specimens should be recorded on a flow sheet to facilitate prompt review.

## Summary

Pyrexia is a symptom, not a disease. Patients, not observation charts, should be treated. Low-grade pyrexia may be beneficial, so managing pyrexia should be individually assessed for each patient – cause, cost, benefit. Clinically significant pyrexia (>38.3°C) usually indicates infection and excessive cost, so should usually be reversed with paracetamol while infection is treated with antibiotics. Unidentified infections should be traced through culture.

## Further reading

O'Grady *et al.*'s (1998) guidelines are authoritative. Useful reviews include Marik (2000), Dowding *et al.* (2002) and Isaac and Taylor (2003). www.routledge.com/textbooks/0415373239

For clinical scenarios, clinical questions and the answers to them go to the support website at www.routledge.com/textbooks/0415373239

## Clinical scenarios

Fiona Clarke, a 35-year-old known asthmatic was admitted to ICU with severe dyspnoea and rash on upper body and arms. Fiona's core (central) body temperature is 38.2°C with shell (skin) temperature is 33°C. She has started to shiver.

Q.1 (a) List potential causes of her increased core temperature.
    (b) Identify the blood cells and mediators responsible.
    (c) Explain the shivering response and its effects on metabolism.

Q.2 Compare various approaches to temperature assessment in your own clinical area; include common sites used in temperature assessment as well as the equipment available. Which would be the most appropriate method to monitor Fiona's core temperature (consider accuracy, time resources, safety, comfort, minimal adverse effects)?

Q.3 Review effective nursing strategies for managing Fiona's temperature, select most suitable pharmacological interventions, laboratory investigations, physical cooling methods (their value, limitations, necessity), comfort therapies.

Chapter 9

# Nutrition and bowel care

## Contents

Introduction                    88
Nitrogen (protein)              88
Energy                          88
Trace elements                  90
Enteral nutrition               90
Parenteral nutrition            91
Nutritional assessment          92
Bowel care                      92
Diarrhoea                       93
Constipation                    94
Colostomies                     95
Implications for practice       95
Summary                         96
Further reading                 96
Clinical scenarios              96

### Fundamental knowledge

Gut anatomy and physiology

## Introduction

Nutrition is fundamental to health, yet Nightingale's (1859/1980) claim that thousands starve in hospitals has been echoed in many recent reports, including *Essence of Care* (DOH, 2001a). Feeding within 24–48 hours of disease/surgery significantly improves outcome (McClave *et al.*, 2002a). Nutrition has improved, possibly to the extent of overfeeding some patients. However, prescribed feeds are often not fully completed (McClave *et al.*, 1999; De Beaux *et al.*, 2001) – incomplete administration of prescribed antibiotics would be considered unacceptable.

## Nitrogen (protein)

Metabolising (oxidation) 6.3 grams of protein produces one gram of nitrogen (Reid & Campbell, 2004). Serum nitrogen is transported mainly as ammonia ($NH_3$), which the liver converts to urea. So measuring urinary nitrogen indicates protein metabolism. Unless diet is especially protein-rich, excessive protein metabolism indicates malnourishment-induced muscle atrophy, which delays weaning. So

- neutral nitrogen balance = dietary nitrogen matches urinary loss
- negative nitrogen balance = excess urinary nitrogen catabolised for energy
- positive nitrogen balance = protein building (anabolism).

Nitrogen balance is normally measured by 24 hour urine collections, but abnormal nitrogen metabolism and loss makes urinary nitrogen unreliable during critical illness. Faecal loss of nitrogen, normally about 4 grams each day, increases with diarrhoea, so routine 24 urine collections in the ICU have little value.

## Energy

Cells need energy to function. They use adenosine triphosphate (ATP) produced in cell mitochondria. In health, ATP is mainly produced from aerobic glucose metabolism:

$$C_6H_{12}O_6 + 6O_2 \rightarrow 36\ ATP + waste\ (6CO_2 + 6H_2O)$$

Some energy is also derived from fats. Fat metabolism is more complex – Krebs' or the 'citric acid' cycle (Figure 9.1). Each stage of Krebs' cycle releases ATP and two carbon atoms. Carbon combines with coenzyme A, forming acetyl-CoA which enables further reactions. Fat metabolism produces much energy, but also much waste, each stage releasing acids (ketones, lactate), carbon dioxide and water. Carbon dioxide and water combine to form carbonic acid ($H_2CO_3$).

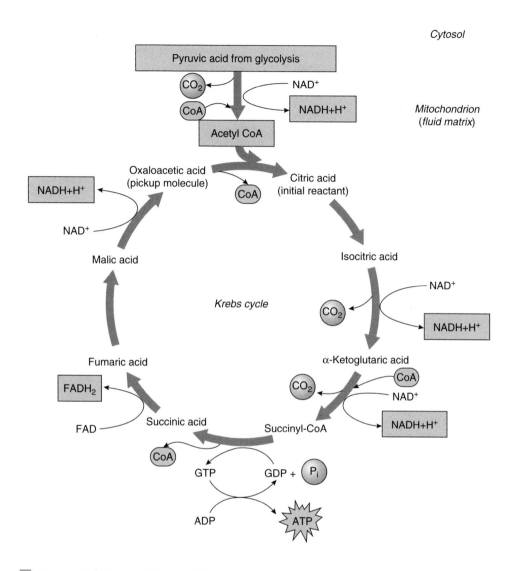

Cytosol

Mitochondrion
(*fluid matrix*)

**Figure 9.1 Krebs (citric acid) cycle**

Hypoperfusion (shock) deprives cells of normal energy sources (oxygen and glucose) and waste removal. Anaerobic metabolism of alternative energy sources (such as bodyfat) increases waste, causing hypercapnia and metabolic acidosis, and creating increasingly hostile, acidic environments for cells.

Energy is measured in *calories* (cal), kilocalories/*Calories* (kcal/kCal) or *joules*/kilojoules (J/kJ) (see glossary for definitions). One kilocalorie is approximately 4.2 joules (J). Carbon dioxide production from energy sources is expressed as the **respiratory quotient** (RQ). RQ of carbohydrate is 1.0, compared with 0.8 for protein and 0.7 for fat. RQ exceeding 1.0 indicates fat synthesis from excessive carbohydrates (Reid & Campbell, 2004) and thus overfeeding. Energy from non-feed sources, such as propofol, should be included in nutritional assessment (Bowling, 2004).

## Trace elements

Speculation persists over value of various trace elements. Glutamine has attracted particular interest – it may inhibit mediators of critical illness (Kudst, 2003), but does not improve survival from severe sepsis (Hall *et al.*, 2003).

## Enteral nutrition

The gut contains many bacteria. Immunoglobulins (IgA, IgM) prevent bacterial translocation into blood, but hypoperfusion (shock) rapidly causes atrophy of gut villi, releases proinflamatory cytokines (Zarzaur *et al.*, 2000; Guzman & Kruse, 2001; Harkin *et al.*, 2001; Kudst, 2003), and enables bacterial translocation. Enteral nutrition increases blood flow to the gut, preserving normal function (Revelley *et al.*, 2001) and may reduce pneumonia McClave *et al.*, 2002b).

Wide-bore gastric tubes (e.g. Ryles®) are easier to insert than fine-bore tubes, but cause more inflammation (Bowling, 2004). Nasogastric tube placement should be checked by X-ray (Metheny & Titler, 2001). Although testing aspirate pH (with pH paper – not litmus (NPSA, 2005)) is widely used, gastric aspirate may be unobtainable, or neutralised by antacids. Fine-bore tubes can usually be aspirated, sometimes by injecting air to dislodge the tube from stomach folds (Metheny *et al.*, 1993), although aspiration can cause collapse, blockage or rupture, so should not be routinely practised (Williams & Leslie, 2005) Tube placement is sometimes confirmed by capnography. Injecting air through tubes ('whoosh test') should not be used (NPSA, 2005), as transmitted sound can give falsely positive results. Marking nasogastric tubes enables any external tube migration to be detected (Metheny, 1993).

Nasojejunal tubes should have alkaline aspirate, which makes it impractical to distinguish between jejunal and pleural aspirates. Position should always be checked by radiography, before removing guidewires. 'Tiger' tubes have small projections, so peristalsis 'feeds' them into the jejunum.

Gut surgery, or absence of bowel sounds, do not contra-indicate enteral feeding (Hartsell *et al.*, 1997; Lewis *et al.*, 2001). Paralytic ileus seldom affects ileal motility, so if gastric feeding fails, jejunal tubes usually enable enteral nutrition. Jejunal tubes can regress into the stomach unless placed after the beyond duodenojejunal flexure (Bowling, 2004).

Absorption is often tested by measuring aspirate volumes, often 4–6 hourly although frequency and residual volumes vary greatly (Williams & Leslie, 2004; McClave *et al.*, 2005). Gastric aspirate contains nutrients, digestive juices and electrolytes, but is also needed to stimulate peristalsis and ileal secretions, so volumes of up to 200 ml are usually returned. Williams and

Leslie (2005) recommend reassessing but continuing feeding with aspirates of 200–500 ml. Drugs such as metoclopramide may increase gut motility (Booth *et al.*, 2002).

Some units rest feeds to restore gastric pH <3, so reducing bacterial colonisation. Rest times vary, four 4 being common, often overnight to follow physiologically normal circadian rhythm. Other units feed continuously to facilitate nutrient delivery (Williams & Leslie, 2004) and stabilise glycaemia, as illustrated in this chapter's clinical scenario. With current emphasis on tight glycaemic control, continuous nutrition also reduces risk of hypoglycaemia occuring.

Type and rate of feeds should be prescribed by dieticians, although most ICUs have protocols for commencing standard feeds at incremental rates. Feeds available include:

- standard – carbohydrate-rich
- fibre – may reduce diarrhoea
- 'respiratory' feeds – produce less carbon dioxide
- 'renal' feeds – produce less (nitrogen) waste
- pre-digested feeds – for malabsorption
- immune-modulating/enhancing feeds – contain substrates which alter immune/inflammatory responses – e.g. glutamine.

Risk of aspiration can be reduced by prokinetics (e.g. metoclopramide) and nursing patients at 45° (Drakulovic *et al.*, 1997).

## Parenteral nutrition

Enteral nutrition is preferable, but if unable to absorb sufficient enteral nutrition, supplementary or (total) parenteral nutrition (TPN) may prevent muscle atrophy. Supplemental TPN does not appear to reduce mortality (Heyland, 1998). TPN can cause:

- gut atrophy, enabling translocation of gut bacteria
- infection
- hyperglycaemia
- impaired neutrophil function
- lipid agglutination in capillaries (increased afterload)

and is costly.

TPN based on 50% glucose (14g and 9g Nitrogen formulations) should be given centrally (including peripherally inserted central catheters – PICCs). 'Peripheral' TPN (9g Nitrogen) often causes thrombophlebitis, so is best given centrally, especially if perfusion is poor. Gut function of patients receiving TPN should be closely monitored to enable weaning onto enteral nutrition as soon as possible.

**Table 9.1 Normal anthropometric chart**

| | | |
|---|---|---|
| Mid-upper arm circumferences | male | 26–29 cm |
| | female | 26–28.5 cm |
| (Below = overall weight loss) | | |
| Triceps skinfold thickness | male | 11–12.5 mm |
| | female | 16–16.5 mm |
| (Below = significant loss of fat stores) | | |
| Mid-arm muscle circumference | male | 23–25 cm |
| | female | 20–23 cm |
| (Below = protein depletion) | | |

## Nutritional assessment

Mortality increases with underfeeding (Kennedy, 1997) and overfeeding (Bowling, 2004). Simple nutritional assessments (*anthropometry*) include:

■ height
■ weight
■ mid upper arm circumferences (= overall weight loss)
■ triceps skinfold thickness (= energy reserves; fat loss)
■ mid-arm muscle circumference (= muscle bulk; protein loss).

See Table 9.1. However, gross oedema and deceptive increases in body weight may mask muscle atrophy (Say, 1997).

Metabolic analysers, included in some ventilators, calculate energy expenditure by comparing inspired and expired oxygen ('indirect calorimetry'). However, expense and doubts about their value have limited their use in the ICU.

Plasma albumin indicates protein synthesis (Say, 1997), but hypoalbuminaemia in critically ill patients is multifactorial.

Urinalysis may identify abnormalities such as ketonuria (from fat metabolism, e.g. starvation, diabetes mellitus (Say, 1997)). Periodic urinalysis is cheap, simple and quick, although abnormalities may have various causes.

## Bowel care

In contrast to eating and oral care, bowel function is often a social taboo. Despite its importance for nursing care, it can often be given relatively low priority. ICU patients are prone to bowel dysfunction from

■ immobility
■ abnormal diet
■ abnormal peristalsis
■ fluid imbalances
■ effects of many drugs on the bowels (e.g. antibiotics, opioids, diuretics).

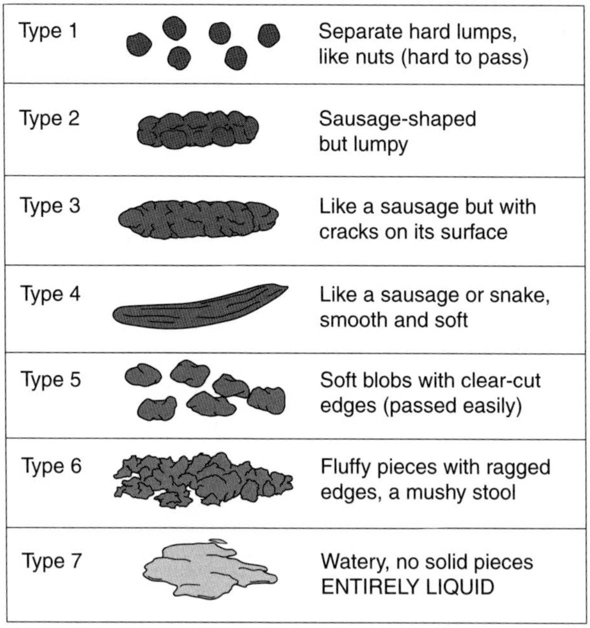

| Type 1 | | Separate hard lumps, like nuts (hard to pass) |
|--------|--|-----------------------------------------------|
| Type 2 | | Sausage-shaped but lumpy |
| Type 3 | | Like a sausage but with cracks on its surface |
| Type 4 | | Like a sausage or snake, smooth and soft |
| Type 5 | | Soft blobs with clear-cut edges (passed easily) |
| Type 6 | | Fluffy pieces with ragged edges, a mushy stool |
| Type 7 | | Watery, no solid pieces ENTIRELY LIQUID |

**■** *Figure 9.2 Bristol stool form chart (after Heaton, 2000)*

Commensal bacteria and yeasts in the colon assist digestion. Critical illness may facilitate their translocation across gut mucosa, causing endogenous infection. Translocation, and the controversial management of selective digestive decontamination, are discussed in Chapter 15.

Bowel care should include recording frequency, type and amount of faeces (Lewis and Heaton, 1997), and listening for bowel sounds (at least once each shift). The Bristol Stool Form chart (see Figure 9.2) provides objective descriptions.

## Diarrhoea

Many ICU patients develop diarrhoea – 50 per cent incidence is often cited, although Montejo (1999) found only 14.7 per cent. Diarrhoea is simply more fluid entering the colon than can be reabsorbed, and may be caused by

- ■ antibiotics (destroy gut flora): 41 per cent of patients on antibiotics develop diarrhoea with enteral feeds, compared to 3 per cent without antibiotics (Guenter *et al.*, 1991)
- ■ excessive fluid (colonic absorption is limited to about 4.5 litres each day)
- ■ reduced water reabsorption from hypoalbuminaemia or hypoperfusion (both common in ICU)

■ sorbitol (used in some elixirs, such as paracetamol suspension): exerts higher osmotic gradients than plasma, drawing fluid into the bowel (Yassin & Wyncoll, 2005).

Likely causes of diarrhoea should be identified and where reasonably possible treated. If treatment is not reasonably possible, nurses should attempt to alleviate problems and risks. Enteral feeds seldom cause diarrhoea, so should not usually be stopped if diarrhoea occurs.

Diarrhoea can be a homeostatic way to remove pathological bowel bacteria, so reducing motility may cause/prolong infection. The most common pathogenic cause of diarrhoea in the ICU is *Clostridium difficile* (O'Grady *et al.*, 1998). Pathogen removal should not be inhibited, but samples should be sent for culture, and appropriate antibiotics prescribed.

Diarrhoea not caused by pathogens may be managed by

■ reducing gut motility – e.g. codeine phosphate, loperamide
■ adding fibre to enteral feeds (Spapen *et al.*, 2001)
■ probiotics, such as *Saccharomyces boulardii*, if diarrhoea is caused by antibiotics (D'Souza *et al.*, 2002).

Bowel contents are normally rich in electrolytes, including potassium and bicarbonate (Yassin & Wyncoll, 2005), so diarrhoea may cause hypokalaemia and metabolic acidosis. Metabolic imbalances should be treated.

Diarrhoea is distressing and socially embarrassing for patients (and visitors), may excoriate skin, and spread bacteria into wounds, lines or urinary catheters. Patients should therefore be reassured, washed and given clean linen. Faecal collections systems may reduce psychological distress and physiological risks. Previously, various systems were improvised, some potentially causing rectal trauma from over-rigid tubes, and many exceeding manufacturers' recommendations (and so indemnity). The Zazzi Bowel Management System™ is a custom-made faecal tube, which is effective and reduces infection (Echols *et al.*, 2004; Yassin & Wyncoll, 2005), but is relatively expensive.

## Constipation

Contrary to popular belief, most people do not open their bowels once every day (Heaton *et al.*, 1992). Constipation is often defined as bowels not moving for 3 or more days (Locke *et al.*, 2000), but normal frequency ranges from three times a day to once weekly (Watson, 2001). Factors contributing to constipation in the ICU include lack of diet, dehydration, immobility and constipating drugs (e.g. opioids). Mostafa *et al.* (2003) found 83 per cent of ICU patients were constipated, nearly half of whom failed weaning from artificial ventilation.

Bowel management should include assessment of possible constipation through

■ identifying when bowels were last opened, and type of stool passed
■ observing and palpating for abdominal distension

- possibly, digital rectal examination ('PR')
- if shard stools are present in the rectum, giving stool softeners, enemas or (sometimes) manual evacuation of faeces.

RCN (2000) advise that nurses can undertake these procedures if they are competent to do so, but should ensure that they are allowed to be local policies and/or their contract of employment. The RCN guidelines also list contra-indications and cautions to digital rectal examination.

Laxatives may be

- bulk-forming, stimulating peristalsis
- direct peristaltic stimulants (e.g. senna)
- osmotic/softening (e.g. lactulose).

(Thorpe & Harrison, 2002)

Bulk-forming laxatives are usually impractical in the ICU and, increasing intra-abdominal pressure, reduce perfusion of abdominal organs. Osmotic laxatives should be avoided in hypovolaemic patients, or patients with poor gut perfusion. Stimulant laxatives, such as senna, are usually the best option. Normal gut transit time is often 12–24 hours, so senna is usually best given late at night.

## Colostomies

Major bowel surgery often necessitates colostomy formation. Colostomy care is the same in the ICU as elsewhere, except that ICU patients can seldom care for their own colostomies. Colour and perfusion of stomas should be checked at least once every shift, and any concerns reported. Most Trusts employ stoma nurses, who should be actively involved.

## Implications for practice

- Early and adequate nutrition hastens recovery and reduces endogenous infection.
- While multidisciplinary expertise is useful, nurses should both assess their patients' nutritional needs and co-ordinate care to ensure patients are adequately nourished.
- If the gut works, use it – enteral feeding is *usually* preferable.
- Nurses may need to initiate standard protocol feed regimes, but dieticians should individually assess patients as soon as reasonably possible.
- Success in establishing feeds should be assessed through

  - delivering prescribed regime
  - absence of high gastric aspirates or vomiting
  - absence of diarrhoea
  - absence of hyperglycaemia or other metabolic disturbances.

- If nasogastric feeding fails, other options include

  - prokinetic drugs (e.g. maxalon)
  - jejunal tubes
  - percutaneous endoscopic gastrostomy/jejunostomy (PEG/PEJ) tubes
  - pre-digested feeds.

- Diarrhoea is rarely caused by nasogastric feeding, so it is not an indication to stop feeds.
- Bowel function should be assessed on admission and reviewed each shift. Frequency, type and amount of stool should be recorded.
- The Bristol Stool form assessment provides a useful way to quantify bowel evacuations.
- Senna is usually the best laxative for ICU use.
- Stoma nurse specialist should be involved in the care of all patients with newly-formed stomas.

## Summary

Malnutrition causes much ill-health, delays recovery and increases mortality. Early and appropriate nutrition is fundamental to care. Protecting the gut may prevent sepsis. Nurses therefore should assess nutritional needs. Feeding should be enteral whenever possible.

Many ICU patients are unable to identify need to defecate, or report constipation, yet are prone to bowel dysfunction. Nurses should therefore monitor bowel function. Diarrhoea frequently occurs in ICU patients, usually being caused by disease or treatments.

## Further reading

Most ICU texts include substantial chapters on nutrition, and articles on nutrition frequently appear in medical and nursing journals. Bowling (2004) is a useful medical review, while Metheny and Titler (2001), Holmes (2004) and Williams and Leslie (2004, 2005) provide useful nursing reviews of enteral feeding. Websites such as that of the *British Association of Parenteral and Enteral Nutrition (BAPEN)* contain current and often useful material.

RCN guidelines (2000) on digital rectal examination provide valuable information for nurses and their managers. www.routledge.com/textbooks/0415373239

For clinical scenarios, clinical questions and the answers to them go to the support website at www.routledge.com/textbooks/0415373239

## Clinical scenarios

Richard Lewis is 71 years old, weighs approximately 70 kg, with arm span of 1.88 metres. He was admitted to the ICU 15 days ago following emergency surgery for a perforated appendix. He is a smoker and has a tracheotomy to facilitate weaning from mechanical ventilation. His glycaemic control maintains his blood sugar at 4.7 mmol/litre with intravenous insulin infusion of 0.5 iu/hour.

Richard is fed via a nasojejunal (NJ) tube in his right nostril. He receives 75ml/hour of enteral nutrition combining two pre-digested feed of 750 ml Peptamen® (1 kcal/ml) with 1 litre Nutrison Protein Plus® (1.25 kcal/ml). He has diarrhoea >800 ml/day, which is infected with *Clostridium difficile* and treated with IV vancomycin.

Q.1 Calculate Richard's Body Mass Index (BMI). Assess his nutritional status and requirements in the ICU. Identify other information needed to complete assessment.

Q.2 Analyse Richard's feeding regime including total daily calories, the potential benefits and risks of feeding approach and type of enteral feed.

Q.3 Consider strategies to manage Richard's diarrhoea and prevent cross infection. Review the range of faecal containment systems available in your clinical area and other resources used to manage patients' diarrhoea. Evaluate effectiveness of these strategies.

Chapter 10

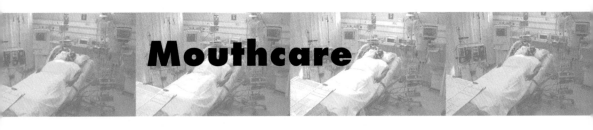

# Mouthcare

## Contents

| | |
|---|---|
| Introduction | 99 |
| Anatomy | 99 |
| Plaque | 100 |
| Infection | 101 |
| Assessment | 101 |
| Lotions and potions | 104 |
| Teeth | 104 |
| Lips | 105 |
| Pressure sores | 105 |
| Dentures | 105 |
| Implications for practice | 106 |
| Summary | 106 |
| Further reading | 106 |
| Clinical scenarios | 107 |

## Fundamental knowledge

Oral anatomy
Composition of dental plaque

## Introduction

Hygiene is a fundamental activity of living, yet oral health remains largely neglected (White, 2000), qualified nurses often lacking adequate knowledge to perform mouthcare (Adams, 1996). Limited ICU-specific literature on mouth-care has appeared since the first edition of this text. Poor oral care in the ICU predisposes to short-term complications such as ventilator-associated pneumonia (Dennesen *et al.*, 2003) and long-term effects such as dental decay (O'Reilly, 2003).

Oral hygiene provides psychological comfort (O'Reilly, 2003). The mouth is used for communication – lip-reading is possible despite intubation, while following extubation, oral discomfort may make speech difficult. The mouth is also associated with intimate emotions (smiling, kissing). Patients with, or thinking they have, dirty mouths or halitosis may feel (psychologically) isolated.

Providing oral hygiene merely replaces activities ICU patients would perform for themselves, if able. Mouthcare should therefore

- maintain hygiene
- keep the oral cavity moist
- promote comfort
- protect from infection
- prevent trauma
- prevent dental decay.

## Anatomy

Saliva is released from glands (see Figure 10.1). Secretion increases with

- oral pressoceptor stimulation (from anything in the mouth, including endotracheal tubes)
- oral chemoreceptor stimulation (especially acids)
- thoughts of food
- smelling food (in environment, on clothing)
- lower gut irritation.

However, ICU patients may develop dry mouths (xerostomia) from

- absence of oral intake
- reduced saliva from drugs (e.g. morphine, diuretics) and sympathetic nervous system stimulation
- drying (convection) from mouths wedged open by oral endotracheal tubes.

So saliva secretion may be excessive or diminished. Saliva contains many chemicals (see Table 10.1), including immune defences, so excess or deficits can cause colonisation/infection and ulceration. Normally slightly acidic (pH 6.75–7.0 (Marieb, 2004)), Treloar (1995) found mean salivary pH of 5.3 in ICU patients, which is more likely to cause tooth decay.

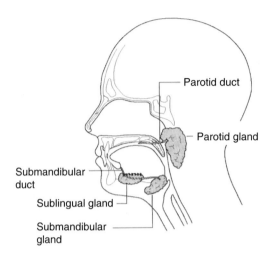

Parotid duct

Parotid gland

Submandibular duct

Sublingual gland

Submandibular gland

**■ *Figure 10.1* Oral (buccal cavity)**

**Table 10.1 Normal contents of saliva**

Water (97–99.5 per cent)
Linguinal lipase, ptyalin/salivary amylase (digestive enzymes)
Mucins (lubricate food, protect oral mucosa)
Immunoglobulin A (immunity)
Lysozyme (immunity; NB not lysosome)
Lactoferrin (immunity)
Growth factor (promoting healing)
Proline-rich proteins (protecting tooth enamel)
Metabolic waste (urea, uric acid)

Saliva may be serous (containing ptyalin, which digests starches) or mucous (containing mucin, a lubricant). Sympathetic vasoconstriction and dehydration reduce salivary gland perfusion, making saliva viscous and mucin-rich – dry mouths are familiar from 'fight and flight' responses. Endogenous sympathetic stimulation from stress may be compounded by exogenous catecholamines (adrenaline/noradrenaline). Saliva production also decreases with age – most ICU patients are old.

## Plaque

Plaque (sugar, bacteria and other debris) metabolises to acids, especially lactic acid. Plaque can contain $10^8$–$10^{11}$ bacteria per gram (Murray *et al.*, 1994). Accumulated plaque calcifies into calculus or tartar, disrupting seals between gingivae and teeth. Gingivitis (sore, red and bleeding gums) occurs within 10 days of plaque formation (Kite & Pearson, 1995).

Plaque is not water soluble, so mouthwash solutions are not a substitute for brushing. Oral neglect enables bacteria to multiply around teeth and dissolve bone (periotonitis/periodontal disease). Periodontitis is the main cause of adult tooth loss, so neglect in ICU can have rapid and enduring effects.

## Infection

Micro-organisms grow readily in ICU patients' mouths because

- mouths are warm, moist and static
- saliva accumulates at the back of throats, especially if gag/swallowing reflexes are impaired
- blood and plaque provides protein for bacterial growth (O'Reilly, 2003)
- normal flora is often destroyed by antibiotics
- immunosuppression facilitates growth.

Infection is usually bacterial, but candidiasis, the most common fungal infection, can be recognised by white spots (Clarke, 1993). Herpes simplex, the major oral virus (susceptible to aciclovir cream), creates sores and cysts around mouth and lips. Most oral fungi, including Candidasis, are susceptible to nystatin.

Excessive or purulent secretions should be removed with suction. Yankauer catheters are often best for the front of the cavity, but deep oral suction is often easier with a soft catheter. Removal of tenacious secretions may necessitate lubricating the mouth with clean water from a 5 ml syringe, usually best directed at the side of the mouth. Frequency of moistening or removing secretions should be assessed individually for each patient.

Micro-organisms may bypass low-pressure endotracheal cuffs. Scannapieco et al. (1992) found respiratory pathogens in 64 per cent of ICU patients, compared with 16 per cent of dental clinic patients. Endotracheal tube tapes are often heavily contaminated by bacteria (Hayes & Jones, 1995). Oral trauma, such as from suction, enables pathogens to enter the bloodstream. So ICU nurses should regularly reassess oral health and hygiene.

Oral decontamination (similar to selective digestive decontamination – see Chapter 15) may prevent spread from oral to respiratory infection. Pugin et al. (1991) found topical oropharyngeal antibiotics reduced oral infections from 78 to 16 per cent, but oral decontamination has not been widely adopted.

## Assessment

Oral assessment should include each aspect of the cavity:

- lips
- gums
- teeth
- tongue
- hard palette
- soft tissue

**Table 10.2 The Jenkins oral assessment tool**

| Patient's age | Score |
| --- | --- |
| 15–29 | 4 |
| 30–49 | 3 |
| 50–69 | 2 |
| 70+ | 1 |
| *Normal oral condition* | |
| Good | 4 |
| Fair | 3 |
| Poor | 2 |
| Very poor | 1 |
| *Mastication ability* | |
| Full | 4 |
| Slightly impaired | 3 |
| Very limited | 2 |
| Immobile | 1 |
| *Nutritional state* | |
| Good | 4 |
| Fair | 3 |
| Poor | 2 |
| Very poor | 1 |
| *Airway* | |
| Normal | 4 |
| Humidified oxygen | 3 |
| ET tube | 2 |
| Open-mouth breathing | 1 |

**Source: Jenkins (1989)**
Notes: Score 15 and above = 3 hourly care
　　　　12–14 = 2 hourly care
　　　　Below 12 = hourly care
　　　　If the patient has either/or:
　　　　　1 large-dose antibioticc steroid therapy
　　　　　2 diabetes mellitus
　　　　　3 low Hb
　　　　　4 immunosuppression
　　　　then the score of 1 should be substracted from the previous 'at risk' calculator score.

- salivary production
- evidence of any infection
- evidence of any cuts/purpura/blood.

These should be assessed against risk factors from

- overall condition
- underlying pathology
- treatments (including effects of drugs).

Viewing the oral cavity requires a good light (e.g. pentorch).

Although assessment should be individualised to each patient, assessment tools can provide a useful structure. Most tools are lists (e.g. Heals, 1993;

Treolar, 1995; Rattenbury *et al.*, 1999; Xavier, 2000) which may provide useful triggers, but are often subjective. Tools designed specifically for ICU include Jenkins (1989; see Table 10.2) and Jiggins and Talbot's (1999; see Table 10.3) paediatric assessment. However, Fitzpatrick (2000) considers that no oral assessment tools are valid or reliable.

### Table 10.3 Jiggins & Talbot's (1999) oral assessment

*Tongue* – feel and observe appearance of tissue
0 = pink, moist – papillae present
1 = coated/shiny appearance, increased decreased redness
2 = blistered or cracked

*Lips* – feel, observe appearance of tissue
0 = smooth, pink, moist
1 = dry or cracked
2 = ulceration or bleeding

*Mucous membranes* – observe appearance
0 = pink, moist
1 = reddened or coated – increased whiteness
2 = spontaneous bleeding or bleeds with pressure

*Gingiva* – gently press tissue with thermometer cover
0 = pink, firm, strippled
1 = observations – redness
2 = spontaneous bleeding or bleeds with pressure

*Saliva* – touch centre of tongue & floor of mouth with thermometer cover
0 = watery
1 = thick or ropy
2 = absent

*Teeth or gum line* – observe appearance
0 = clean – no debris
1 = plaque/debris in localised area
2 = plaque/debris along gum line

Risk assessment
*Ventilated*
0 = no/via tracheostomy
1 = nasally ventilated
2 = orally intubated
3 = ventilated >1 week
4 = ventilated >2 weeks

*Paralysed*
0 = no
1 = yes

*Sedated/comatose*
0 = no
1 = yes

*Immunocompromised*
0 = no
1 = yes, but receiving Nystatin
2 = yes, not receiving Nystatin

*(continued)*

***Table 10.3 (Continued)***

*Antibiotics*
0 = no
1 = yes
2 = yes >1 week

*Fluid restricted*
0 = no
1 = yes
2 = yes >2ml/kg

*Haemofiltered/PD*
0 = no
1 = yes
2 = yes >1 week

*Diuretics*
0 = no
1 = oral
2 = IV bolus
3 = IV infusion × 1
4 = IV infusion × 2

*Other factors* e.g. dental decay, fixed braces, Candida, chemotherapy
0 = no
1 = yes × 1
2 = yes × 2

## Lotions and potions

Many mouthcare solutions and other aids have been marketed, most with little support beyond custom and practice. Few remove or prevent plaque, or provide other significant benefits, and many leave unpleasant tastes (nurses can understand patients' experiences by tasting non-prescription products themselves).

Although tap *water* may be used, immunocompromise often encourages ICU nurses to use sterile water; whether this is treating patients or staff is unclear. Some mouthwashes are antibacterial: pharmacists can advise which solution is best for each patient.

*Foam sticks* are useful for moistening the mouth between cleaning (O'Reilly, 2003), but do not remove debris from surfaces or between teeth, so plaque accumulation progresses (Pearson, 1996). Frequency of moistening mouths should be individualised to patients.

*Chlorhexadine* (Corsodyl®) prevents bacterial and fungal growth (Fourrier *et al.*, 2000; O'Reilly, 2003). It is available as both a mouthwash and a gel.

## Teeth

Teeth should be brushed at least twice daily. Between brushing, additional comfort cleaning/refreshing will usually be needed. Toothbrushes (with or without toothpaste) remain the best way to clean patients' teeth, loosening debris trapped between teeth and removing plaque. Technique should reflect brushing one's own teeth: brush away from gums to remove, rather than impact, plaque from gingival crevices. Manipulating toothbrushes in others' mouths, especially when orally intubated, can be difficult, so smallheaded toothbrushes are often most effective for brushing others' teeth (Jones, 2004). Angling toothbrushes at 45° to gingival margins, using very small vibratory movements, collects and remove plaque (Dougherty & Lister, 2004). With limited mouth opening (trismus), interspace toothbrushes may be better for removing plaque. Toothbrushes can clean heavily coated tongues, and gums and tongue of endentitious patients (O'Reilly, 2003).

Fluoride toothpaste is preferable (Rattenbury *et al.*, 1999) although patients may find the taste of their usual brand comforting. Most toothpastes dry the mouth (Jones, 2004), so should be rinsed out thoroughly – sterile water from a 5 ml syringe, and continuous suction, are usually the best way to achieve this. Yankaur catheters can stimulate a cough/gag reflex, so should be used sparingly; soft catheters are usually more effective for mouthcare.

Vigorous brushing may cause bleeding, especially if patients have coagulopathies (e.g. DIC); oral care should therefore be planned holistically. If nystatin is prescribed, this should be administered following mouthcare.

## Lips

Lips are highly vascular, with sensitive nerve endings. Mucosa being exposed, it can dry quickly. Lips are even more closely associated with communication (e.g. lip-reading) and intimacy (e.g. kissing) than the mouth. Lipcare can therefore prevent drying/cracking, while providing psychological comfort. Lip balm or white petroleum jelly is often used to keep lips moist (Bowsher *et al.*, 1999). Contrary to circulating myths, petroleum jelly neither explodes nor burns (Winslow & Jacobson, 1998).

## Pressure sores

Any body surface area may develop pressure sores (see Chapter 12). Treloar's (1995) small study found multiple lip, tongue and mucosal lesions, as well as very dry mouths, in ICU patients. Endotracheal tubes and tracheostomies place pressure on various tissues, including the mouth. Gingival surfaces are more susceptible to sores than teeth (Liwu, 1990), and tube tapes can lacerate lip. Pressure from tapes can be reduced by placing them away from lip corners, supporting pressure points with gauze or sponge pads, and moving tapes and tubes (Clarke, 1993). Teeth can usually be cleaned most effectively when changing endotracheal tapes.

## Dentures

About half of older people do not have their own teeth (Watson, 2001). Intubation and impaired consciousness normally necessitates removal of any dentures, but property should be checked on admission so that dentures are not lost. Nursing records should include whether patients normally wear partial or complete dentures, and relevant care.

Dentures may easily be damaged or warp, especially if left dry or cleaned in hot water (Clarke, 1993). Dentures should usually be left soaking-overnight in cold water (Xavier, 2000; Clay, 2002; O'Reilly, 2003). Toothpaste should not be used on dentures, as it can damage their surfaces (Clarke, 1993). Patients, or their family, may be able to supply their normal cleaning agents which, if available, should be used (Xavier, 2000).

## Implications for practice

- Mouthcare should be individually assessed, rather than following routine/rituals.
- Toothbrushes (with or without toothpaste) are the best means for providing mouthcare.
- Teeth should (usually) be brushed with toothpaste twice daily, with additional comfort cleaning inbetween, according to individual assessment.
- Fluoride toothpaste helps prevent decay.
- Rinse toothpaste out thoroughly, using sterile water and continuous suction.
- Mouthwashes or moist swabs moisten the mouth but do not remove plaque.
- If antibacterial washes or gels are needed, consult pharmacists.
- If patients wear dentures, maintain their normal care if possible, and record where they are stored.
- White petroleum jelly protects lips from cracking.

## Summary

Mouthcare is too easily forgotten in the physiological crises of critical illness, but problems developing from their time in the ICU can cause long-term or permanent oral/dental disease. The current paucity of material on mouthcare in the ICU makes evidence-based practice difficult.

## Further reading

Jiggins and Talbot's (1999) paediatric ICU article is largely applicable to adults. White (2004) provides a useful collection of general nursing articles on mouthcare. Dougherty and Lister (2004) give practical and substantiated advice, although from onconology rather than intensive care perspectives. Recent articles on mouthcare in the ICU includes O'Reilly (2003), Fourrier et al. (2000) and Furr et al. (2004). www.routledge.com/textbooks/0415373239

For clinical scenarios, clinical questions and the answers to them go to the support website at www.routledge.com/textbooks/0415373239

## Clinical scenarios

Michael Dodd is a 22-year-old gentleman who has a past medical history of poorly controlled asthmatic. He presents with left lower lobe pneumonia. This is his third admission to the ICU for respiratory support. He weighs 90 kg, is receiving enteral nutrition at 75 ml/h and has been mechanically ventilated for 7 days. Michael's oral endotracheal tube length is 23 cm at lips, positioned on the right side of his mouth and balancing on his teeth. He has visible dental decay at gum margins with white spots on his tongue and hard palate.

Michael's intravenous drug therapy includes sedative infusions of propofol and midazolam, antibiotic infusions of vancomycin and rifampicin and hydrocortisone. He has a temperature of 38.5°C, Hb 10.4 g/dl, WBC 9.3 g/dl, CRP 207 mg/litre.

Q.1  List the equipment needed to inspect and assess Michael's oral status to include gums, tongue, salivary glands, teeth, palate, lips and jaw.

Q.2  Identify Michael's risk factors for developing oral complications. Use a published oral assessment tool to calculate and interpret Michael's oral assessment score.

Q.3  Develop a plan for Michael's mouthcare including frequency of interventions, method of brushing teeth and tongue, lip lubrication and use of any topical lotions or creams.

Chapter 11

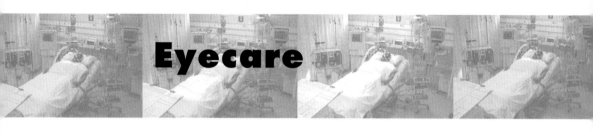

# Eyecare

## Contents

Introduction                          109
Ocular damage                         109
Assessment                            110
Interventions                         111
Implications for practice             112
Summary                               112
Further reading                       113
Clinical scenarios                    113

## Fundamental knowledge

Anatomy – cornea, lens, tear production, blink reflex

## Introduction

Patients are seldom admitted to ICU for ocular pathologies, but one-third to two-thirds of critically ill patients suffer eye surface disease (Dawson, 2005), especially drying of the cornea and eye surface. Exposed eye surfaces are at increased risk of infection (keratitis) and abrasion, while positive pressure ventilation increases intraocular pressure, so causing potential 'ventilator eye'. This chapter does not discuss specialist ocular pathophysiologies, but reasons for and types of eyecare needed by most ICU patients.

In health, the eyelid protects the eye surface. Tear production and frequent blinking maintains health and moistens eye surfaces. While many ICU patients can maintain their own ocular health, incomplete eyelid closure inevitably causes corneal damage (*keratopathy*) (Suresh *et al.*, 2000). Problems can occur from

- increased intraocular pressure or periorbital oedema (especially prone positioning)
- impaired blink reflex, such as from paralysis (disease or chemical)
- decreased tear production
- patient being unable to move their head
- eye infection.

If patients are unable to maintain their own ocular health, nurses should meet this need for them.

Nurses may feel squeamish about touching eyes, but eyecare maintains physiological and psychological health. Ocular abnormalities often make patients and relatives anxious. For most people, vision is the most used sense, eye contact helping communication. So visual deficits contribute significantly to sensory imbalance. ICU nurses should therefore evaluate:

- visual appearance
- eyecare performed
- how care is described.

Eyecare in ICU varies greatly, with limited supporting evidence (Dawson, 2005). Substantive research being needed, suggestions here necessarily remain tentative.

## Ocular damage

The cornea, the eye's outer surface, has no direct blood supply, otherwise sight would be impaired. It is therefore vulnerable to drying, trauma and lacerations (e.g. from pillows, endotracheal tapes, dust and particles). Blink reflexes and tear production, which normally protect and irrigate corneal surfaces, may be absent/weak. Drugs (e.g. atropine, antihistamines, paralysing agents) also inhibit tear production.

Bacteria can cause blepharitis, inflammation of eyelash follicles and sebaceous glands, resulting in redness, swelling and crusts of dried mucus collecting on the lids. Crusts may cause corneal trauma on eyelid closure with blinking. If ocular infection is suspected, it should be reported and recorded; swabs may need to be taken and topical antibiotics prescribed.

Incomplete eyelid closure or loss of blink reflexes causes corneal drying (exposure keratopathy), and can cause infection (keratitis) or corneal ulceration (Dawson, 2005). The cornea is richly supplied with sensory nerves (Patil & Dowd, 2000), making lacerations very painful. Corneal damage exposes deeper layers to infection, while avascularity delays healing, often leaving opaque scar tissue. Ocular trauma may remain unrecognised until patients regain consciousness, finding their vision permanently impaired.

Normal intraocular pressure is 12–20 mmHg (average 15 mmHg). Drainage of aqueous humour, and so intraocular hypertension, subconjunctival haemorrhage and other damage, may be caused by positive intrathoracic pressure (positive pressure ventilation), tight ETT tapes, oedema, poor head alignment or prone positioning. Hypercapnia increase intraoccular pressure (Patil & Dowd, 2000), a potential complication of permissive hypercapnia. ICU patients are therefore at high risk of intraocular hypertension. More than half the patients in Suresh *et al.*'s (2000) small study (n = 34) developed 'ventilator eye'. Head elevation (e.g. 30° if supine) assists venous drainage.

Contact lenses are removed pre-operatively, but with emergency admissions may still be in place. Contact lenses or glasses, if removed, should be stored safely, and recorded in nursing notes incase of loss.

## Assessment

Structured eye assessment tools are not generally used in ICUs, but nurses assess ocular needs through

- existing documentation
- visual observation of patients
- knowledge of normal ocular anatomy
- verbal questions (to patients or family).

Cues to consider include:

- contact lenses/glasses
- abnormalities (e.g. eyelids, lashes, exophthalmus); are abnormalities unilateral/bilateral?
- periorbital oedema
- patient positioning, venous drainage
- muscle weakness ('droopy eye')
- eye closure – do lids cover cornea completely?
- do eyes look infected/inflamed?
- do eyes look sore ('redeye')?

- tear production (excessive/impaired) – moist/dry eyes
- blink reflex (absent, impaired, slow)
- eye pain (flinching during eye care/interventions)
- visual impairment (double, cloudy, difficulty focusing)
- how does the patient feel (e.g. are eyelids heavy).

Closed questions are often easier for intubated patients to answer.
Unless patients have specific ocular disease, eyecare should

- maintain ocular health
- replace lost functions
- ensure comfort
- protect from trauma/infection.

To perform eyecare

- nurse patients supine, with head tilted down (Dougherty & Lister, 2004) –
this helps nurses see what they are doing and keeps solutions in the eye
- use a good light (Dougherty & Lister, 2004), but avoid shining light
directly into patients' eyes.

Frequency of eyecare should be individualised to needs.
While assessing and caring for patients' eyes, nurses can also make
neurological assessment of

- pupil size and reaction
- accommodation for near and long vision: place a finger near the patient's
nose; when moved away, pupils should diverge.

Ocular damage may invalidate any or all of these tests.

## Interventions

Dry eyes should be lubricated, although optimal solution or frequency remains
unclear (Dawson, 2005). *Artificial tears* seem a logical replacement if tear production is inadequate. They should be dropped into the outer side of the lower
fornix (see Figure 11.1), which is less sensitive than the cornea (Dougherty &
Lister, 2004). Over-vigorous use of eyedrops on corneas resembles water torture.
To minimise infection risk, solutions should be stored in a clean area. If reusable,
they should be labelled with date and time of opening. Local hospital policies
will identify how long solutions can be used for after opening.

If eyelid *closure* is incomplete, and patients cannot blink, corneal surfaces
should be kept moist and covered. Cleaning should be performed with sterile
water, eye surfaces being very susceptible to infection. Saline should not be
used, because it can irritate and sting. Excess moisture should be removed
delicately, but no method is ideal – cotton wool and gauze can both scratch

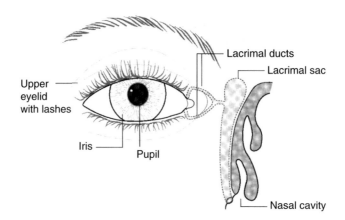

Upper eyelid with lashes

Lacrimal ducts

Lacrimal sac

Iris

Pupil

Nasal cavity

**■ *Figure 11.1 External structure of the eye***

delicate corneal surfaces, while sticks on cotton buds can cause trauma. Many people are especially squeamish about eyes, so relatives may become especially anxious when eyes are covered.

*Geliperm®*, an occlusive gel wound dressing, has been used to protect eyes (Dawson, 2005), although this is not included among its indications, and concerns about legal liability have almost made its use for eyecare obsolete. Geliperm® is waterbased, so should be replaced (not rehydrated, as this can introduce infection). Geliperm® is not available on NHS tariff.

## Implications for practice

- Many ICU patients suffer 'ventilator eye'.
- Care for each patient should be individually assessed.
- If patients are unable to maintain their own ocular health, eyecare should keep eyes clean, moist and covered.
- Nursing semirecumbent helps venous drainage.
- Prone positioning can damage eyes; elevating bedhead by as little as 10° and careful head alignment can reduce complications.
- Eyecare solutions are potential media for infection, so should be changed regularly (check unit/hospital policy; if not specified, change at least one each shift).
- Exposed corneas are vulnerable to trauma, so keep pillow edges, endotracheal tape and other equipment away from eyes.

## Summary

Although patients are seldom admitted for ocular conditions, diseases and treatments can expose the ICU patients to ocular damage. Yet eyecare in the

ICU is often given low priority, and there is little reliable and substantiated literature to guide interventions. Care inevitably relies heavily on custom, practice, rituals and anecdotal support. As part of their fundamental patient care, nurses should support/provide what their patients need. Nurses should therefore assess their patients' ocular health and risks, planning individualised care accordingly.

### Further reading

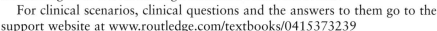

Eyecare in the ICU is much under-researched, and little other specialist literature exists. Ocular literature rarely discusses care of critically ill patients, although the Joanna Briggs Institute (2002) has synthesised what little knowledge is available. Patil and Dowd (2000) and Suresh *et al.* (2000) are among the few relatively recent medical articles. *The Royal Marsden NHS Trust Manual of Clinical Nursing Procedures* (Dougherty & Lister, 2004) offers sound advice for nursing care. www.routledge.com/textbooks/0415373239

For clinical scenarios, clinical questions and the answers to them go to the support website at www.routledge.com/textbooks/0415373239

### Clinical scenarios

Mr Jonathan Hopkins is 48 years old and works as a computer programmer. Jonathan wears non-gas permeable contact lenses and has a severe stigmatism in one eye. He recently required treatment for recurrent conjunctivitis. Jonathan was admitted with community acquired pneumonia. In the first 24 hours he received respiratory support via facial mask CPAP of 10 cmH$_2$O with FiO$_2$ of 0.5.

Q.1 Identify factors which can cause ocular damage or complications with Jonathan's vision.

Q.2 Jonathan developed bacterial keratitis and corneal ulceration associated with exposed cornea from an over-tightened head harness securing his CPAP face mask. Consider how this affected his recovery in relation to his perceptions, vision, communication interactions and pain. Reflect on the legal, ethical and professional responsibilities towards Jonathan. (Has substandard practice or negligence occurred? If yes, who might be responsible?)

Q.3 Review eye care in your own clinical area. Is the ocular assessment and associated interventions

■ systematic (in both approach and documentation)
■ based on a local or published guideline
■ knowledge and/or evidence-based
■ effective at identifying risk patients, and before complications occur?

Chapter 12

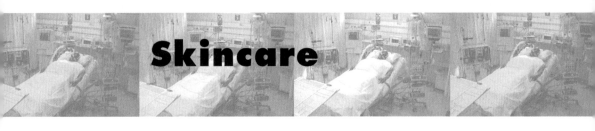

# Skincare

## Contents

| | |
|---|---|
| Introduction | 115 |
| Pressure sores | 115 |
| Assessment | 116 |
| Prevention | 118 |
| Necrotising fasciitis | 119 |
| Implications for practice | 119 |
| Summary | 120 |
| Further reading | 120 |
| Clinical scenarios | 120 |

## Fundamental knowledge

Structure and anatomy of skin
Functions of skin
Pressure sore (decubitus ulcer) formation
Stages of wound healing

## Introduction

Pender and Frazier (2005) found one-fifth of their ICU patients developed pressure sores, although mean arterial blood pressures averaging 47 mmHg in those developing sores and 52 in those that did not, generalisability of this finding is questionable. Up to a quarter of pressure sores in hospitals originate perioperatively, especially with vascular surgery (Scott *et al.*, 2001). Pressure sores increase

- morbidity (human costs)
- recovery time
- mortality
- financial costs (prolonged stay, additional treatments, litigation).

Epidermis cells take one months to migrate from basal layers to skin surfaces (Casey, 2002), so healing is slow, exposing deeper tissues to potential infection.
ICU patients at 'high risk' for developing pressure sore because of

- prolonged peripheral hypoperfusion
- oedema
- anaerobic metabolism
- immunocompromise
- malnutrition.

This chapter revises pressure sore development, identifies some assessment systems available and describes some ways of preventing pressure sores. Wound dressings are not discussed, as rapid changes in practice and availability makes inclusion in this book impractical. Necrotising fasciitis, a dermatological condition often proving fatal, is also discussed. Much literature originates, or is sponsored/promoted by, people and commercial companies with vested interests, so should be treated cautiously.

## Pressure sores

When external pressure exceeds capillary pressure, perfusion fails, leading to necrosis. *Capillary occlusion pressure*, the amount of pressure required to occlude capillaries, is often cited at 30–32 mmHg. This originates from Landis' 1930 study, which measured 21–48 mmHg in normotensive volunteers (mean 32 mmHg) (Lowthian, 1997). ICU patients are not volunteers, and seldom normotensive. So 20–25 mmHg is generally a safer upper limit for any unrelieved pressure on any tissue. Visible signs of pressure sores may appear on skin surfaces, but pressure in solid tissue near bony prominences can be 3–5 times that exerted on skin (Houwing *et al.*, 2000).
Pressure sores can be caused by intrinsic factors such as

- age
- malnutrition

- dehydration
- incontinence
- medical condition
- medication

and extrinsic ones:

- unrelieved pressure
- shearing
- friction.

(Waterlow, 1995)

Extrinsic factors are usually more easily modified.

Excessive moisture or dryness hastens skin breakdown. Urine is acidic, so leaks around urinary catheters excoriate skin. Perspiration makes skin excessively moist, and contains urea. Faeces also contains acids (Lowery, 1995). Diarrhoea, inability to alert nurses to the need for bedpans, and gathering sufficient staff to turn patients can result in anal areas being exposed to evacuated faeces, causing excoriation. Barrier creams can reduce risks of breakdown, so are useful adjuncts to, but not substitutes for, nursing care. Prompt hygiene and 'comfort' washes reduces risks, and lubricating dry skin (e.g. aqueous cream) can prevent breakdown.

Traditionally, pressure sores are associated with skin over bony prominences – elbow, heels, sacrum. These are risk areas for ICU patients, but other possible sites for sores include:

- head (especially the back)
- ears
- lips/mouth (around ETTs)
- beneath invasive equipment (e.g. hubs of arterial lines)
- skinfolds (e.g. breasts, groin, abdomen)
- chest and face if prone positioned.

Hair may hide sores on backs of heads, until blood is found on pillows. Nurses should therefore proactively assess all risk areas.

## Assessment

The UK has at least 14 grading systems for pressure ulcers (Harker, 2000). Many visually grade ulcers from one to four (see Figure 12.1).

The Braden tool (Bergstrom et al., 1987) is the most widely used assessment in the USA (Ayello & Braden, 2002), but is unreliable for the ICU (Pender & Frazier, 2005). Waterlow (1985, updated 2005) is most widely used in the UK. Most UK nurses are familiar with it, but not being designed for ICU it classifies most patients as 'high risk'. Scores between different staff can also be very discrepant (Cook et al., 1999). Despite a 1992 consensus conference, the 'Stirling' Scale (Reid & Morison, 1994) proved difficult to use (Harker, 2000).

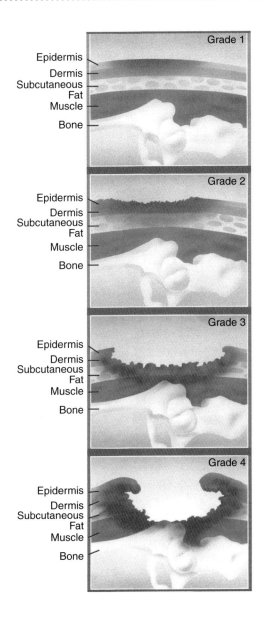

**Figure 12.1 Pressure sore grading**

A few tools have been developed specifically for ICU, but none have been widely adopted. Birty's tool (Birtwistle, 1994) uses colour rather than numerical codes. While visually clear and simple, colour printing is expensive, and absence of scores necessitated incorporating the whole tool into each nursing record. Cubbin and Jackson (1991; revised Jackson, 1999) spawned Lowery's

(1995) 'Sunderland' scale. Bateson *et al.*'s (1993) more sensitive scale was published after a substantial pilot study, but the promised follow-up does not seem to have appeared. Theaker *et al.* (2000) identified five main risk factors for critically ill patients developing pressure sores:

- vaspressors (e.g. noradrenaline)
- APACHE II > 12
- faecal incontinence
- anaemia
- length of stay > 2 days.

Many of these unsurprisingly overlap, in that sicker patients are likely to stay longer, have higher APACHE scores, receive inotropes and suffer more complications.

Whatever means is used, assessment should identify actual and potential problems, and be understood by all staff so that effective care can be planned and maintained.

## Prevention

Pressure on skin can be decreased either by changing position or increasing surface area over which pressure is spread. Two hourly pressure area care owes more to ritual than logic.

Many aids have been marketed, although most ICUs mainly use either *low air loss mattresses* (e.g. Trasair Statis 2002®, Nimbus®2 or 3) or *tilting/kinetic beds* (e.g. Pegasus®) – see Chapter 27. Choice of *mattress* or other aids may be restricted by

- patient's weight – with very obese patients, weight limits of aids (including hoists) should be checked before use
- pathology – e.g. head or spinal injury patients require a firm mattress to maintain spinal alignment
- cost, if equipment needs to be hired.

With the wide choice of commercial aids available, increasing levels of litigation, and professional individual accountability of nurses, *improvised aids* should be avoided.

Changes in knowledge and products are rapid. Most hospitals employ tissue viability nurses, but it is also valuable to identify a link specialist among ICU staff to

- provide information for all unit staff
- apply information to special needs and problems of ICU patients
- audit skincare
- link to wider resources (e.g. tissue viability nurse).

## Necrotising fasciitis

Necrotising fasciitis is rare (Forbes & Rankin, 2001; Gully, 2002), although incidence is increasing (Jallali, 2003). Infection usually follows minor trauma or surgery (Neal, 1994), beginning as cellulitis unresponsive to antibiotics. It may be caused by aerobic, anaerobic or (more often) mixed infections (Minnaganti *et al.*, 2000). Infection spreads rapidly (3–5 cm each hour) through connective tissue, especially extremities or the perineum (Jallali, 2003). Initially skin and muscle are spared (Gully, 2002), but progression causes toxic shock syndrome, septic inflammatory response syndrome (SIRS) and multiorgan dysfunction syndrome (MODS). Depending on how quickly and effectively it is treated, mortality ranges from 20 to 70 per cent (Forbes & Rankin, 2001; Gully, 2002).

Early stages of the disease are acutely painful (Neal, 1994). Necrotising fasciitis should be treated with aggressive surgical debridement and intravenous antibiotics, such as penicillin G and benzylpenicillin and clindomycin (Forbes & Rankin, 2001; Gully, 2002; Copson, 2003), but multiorgan dysfunction syndrome often necessitates transfer to the ICU for system support. Hyperbaric oxygen can improve oxygen delivery to tissues (Jallali, 2003) but is not available in most hospitals. Extensive infection may leave residual deformity (Hinds & Watson, 1996), and amputation may be necessary (Jallali, 2003).

Tissue necrosis causes gas production (hydrogen, methane, hydrogen sulphide, nitrogen) and putrid discharge, although purely streptococcal infections have no odour (Neal, 1994). The smell (and grey colour) of rotting flesh, distressing enough for staff, can cause profound distress to patients and visitors. Air-fresheners can help mask the smell, although chemicals should not enter exposed wounds. Gross (oedematous) swelling of flesh may make patients almost unrecognisable, so visitors should be carefully prepared.

### Implications for practice

- ICU patients are 'high risk' for pressure sore development.
- Sores develop if external pressure exceeds capillary occlusion pressure. 20–25 mmHg is usually a safe upper limit for sustained pressure. ICU patients can therefore develop sores in many places, including the backs of heads.
- Proactive nursing assessment of all skin surfaces and risk factors should be made at least once daily, identifying any special aids needed.
- No ideal assessment tool exists for the ICU, but whatever is used should be familiar to all staff.
- Improvised aids may cause harm, so are usually best avoided.
- Pressure area aids should allow tissue perfusion, so pressures should be below capillary occlusion pressure (20–25 mmHg) for part of each cycle.
- Unit link nurses for tissue viability can be a valuable resource.
- Necrotising fasciitis is a rare, but potentially devastating, infection that progresses rapidly and should be treated aggressively.

## Summary

Skin has many functions; the cost of skin breakdown can be measured in mortality, humanitarian terms (morbidity), increased length of stay in the ICU, increased financial costs and litigation.

Various scoring systems have been designed to assess skin integrity, but none are ideal for the ICU, and the best system is only as good as the staff using it. Pressure sores continue to occur in the ICU. The culture of guilt surrounding pressure sores is unhelpful to everyone; despite good nursing, sores will occur, so nurses should assess and minimise risk factors to reduce the incidence.

## Further reading

General nursing journals frequently carry articles on skincare, the *Journal of Wound Care* specialising in the topic. Most anatomy texts include detailed chapters on skin; Casey (2002) reviews anatomy. Theaker *et al.* (2000) review pressure sores from crtical care perspectives. Articles occasionally appear on necrotising faciitis, Gully (2002) being a useful nursing review. www.routledge.com/textbooks/0415373239

For clinical scenarios, clinical questions and the answers to them go to the support website at www.routledge.com/textbooks/0415373239

## Clinical scenarios

Norman Robinson is a 60-year-old gentleman who tripped on an uneven paving stone and sustained a superficial abrasion to the lateral aspect of his left knee. Within 24 hours, his leg was increasingly painful, oedematous and he was unable to extend his knee or weight bear. Two days following this fall, Mr Robinson was diagnosed with necrotising fasciitis and had aggressive surgical debridement. This involved 'degloving' his left leg and the application of skin grafts taken from his right leg. He was admitted to the ICU following surgery for mechanical ventilation and organ support. Mr Robinson is increasingly oedematous with extensive (offensive smelling) wound exudate from both legs and constant diarrhoea. He weighs 93 kg and is 1.68 m tall.

Other results include pyrexia of 38.5°C, tachycardia 115 beats/min, MAP 73 mmHg, CVP 20 mmHg and urine output greater than 60 ml/hour over the last 4 hours. Blood investigation revealed creatinine 218 $\mu$mol/litre, urea 18.4 mmol/litre, albumin 17 g/litre, platelets 61 $\times$ $10^{-9}$/litre, Hb 8.5 g/dl, WBC 14 $\times$ $10^{-9}$/litre. Microbiological examination of tissue from left leg show large presence of *Staphylococcus aureus* and Beta Haemolytic Group A *Streptococci*. Appropriate antibiotics have been prescribed.

Q.1 Identify Mr Robinson's risk factors for developing further skin breakdown.

Q.2 Consider the range of pressure relieving equipment in your clinical area, select appropriate mattress type, aids and other interventions to optimise skin integrity.

Q.3 Review wound assessment and documentation for Mr Robinson. How should his exudative wounds and skin grafts be managed to minimise other complications and promote wound healing?

# Chapter 13

# Children in adult ICUs

### Contents

| | |
|---|---|
| Introduction | 123 |
| Differences | 123 |
| Initial assessment | 124 |
| Family | 125 |
| Neurological | 125 |
| Ventilation | 125 |
| Cardiovascular | 126 |
| Fluid balance | 126 |
| Thermoregulation | 126 |
| Drugs | 127 |
| Stabilisation | 127 |
| Meningitis | 128 |
| Legal aspects | 128 |
| Implications for practice | 129 |
| Summary | 129 |
| Support groups | 130 |
| Further reading | 130 |
| Clinical scenarios | 130 |

### Fundamental knowledge

Local policies about consent & child protection

## Introduction

Paediatric intensive care is a speciality provided in the UK by regional centres. However, when children initially become critically ill they are often in their local hospital. Children are usually only admitted to the ICU if additional care to that available on paediatric wards is needed, and until retrieval teams from paediatric ICUs (PICUs) arrive to transport patients to specialist centres (DOH, 1997; Hallworth & McIntyre, 2003). The occasional emergency paediatric admission creates two main problems for staff in general (adult) ICUs:

- when children are admitted, their condition is usually at its most critical/ unstable
- admission is so infrequent, most staff in general ICUs have little or no experience of paediatric nursing.

Hazinski (1998) identifies three areas of expertise needed for nursing children in adult ICUs:

- knowing how children differ from adults (e.g. signs of distress, organ failure)
- appreciating anatomical, physiological and psychological differences
- critical care skills (knowing how to ventilate children, adjust drugs and perform resuscitation).

Neonates would be admitted to SCBU, not adult ICUs, so neonates are not discussed in this chapter. At least half of all children admitted to ICU are under two years old (Bennett, 1999), this age group having little reserve function and susceptible to critical illness, crises often develop more rapidly and acutely. This chapter therefore focuses mainly on younger children, identifying main differences between nursing critically ill adults and children, and priorities of care until paediatric retrieval services arrive. Pathologies necessitating ICU admission are often similar to those identified in other chapters. Meningitis is discussed.

## Differences

Children, especially young children, are still developing. They are less physically, psychologically and (often) emotionally developed than adults. Physical growth necessitates higher metabolic rates, increasing oxygen and nutritional demands, while increasing physiological waste. Many physiological parameters, such as heart rate and cardiac index, are therefore higher than with adults.

Most units have centralised places for storing paediatric equipment. The commercially successful Broselow®/Hinkle Paediatric Emergency System (Armstrong Medical), which contains standard emergency paediatric equipment in an easily-accessible colour-coded layout and transportable bag, is used on many units.

## Initial assessment

### Airway

Proportionally increased oxygen demand, carbon dioxide production and smaller airways make children prone to respiratory problems. For the first six months of life, children breathe through their noses (Wilkinson, 1997), so any nasal obstruction necessarily obstructs the airway. Children's tongues are relatively larger than their oropharynx, making airway obstruction more likely (Patel & Meakin, 2000). Relatively small inflammatory responses, or mucous, can obstruct airways. Paediatric endotracheal tubes, and suction equipment, are necessarily smaller than adult ones, making tubes more prone to obstruction by mucous, and removal more difficult due to smaller and more flimsy catheters. Marsh (2000) suggests normal endotrachael tube sizes for children over one year to be

$$\text{internal diameter} = \frac{\text{age} + 4}{4}$$

or approximately the diameter of the child's finger. Tibballs (2003) recommends 6FG suction catheters for neonates, 8FG for infants and small children, and 10FG for older children. Being especially prone to hypoxia, children should always be preoxygenated before suction.

### Breathing

Children have little physiological reserve, small respiratory systems and high metabolic rates, making them very susceptible to hypoxia. Proportions and function also differ between paediatric and adult airways. Davies and Hassell (2001) suggest that normal respiratory rates are:

- <1 year     30–40 breaths/minute
- 2–5 years    20–30 breaths/minute
- 5–12 years  15–20 breaths/minute
- >12 years   12–16 breaths/minute.

### Circulation

Unless born with congenital abnormalities, children usually have healthy cardiovascular systems. Cardiovascular changes are therefore usually indicate respiratory dysfunction (Davies & Hassell, 2001), such as hypoxia. Normal pulse rates per minute are

- <1 year: 120–160
- 1–3 years: 90–140
- 4–5 years: 80–110
- 6–10 years: 75–100
- 11–13 years: 60–95.

## Family

Admission to intensive care is usually emotionally traumatic for both children and parents (Teare & Smith, 2004). Casey's (1988) model emphasises the importance of involving parents.

Parents often experience guilt and anger, however illogical both may be. Even more than relatives of adult patients, they need information and emotional support. Parents with other children experience additional stress (Clarke, 2000). Involving parents in care can provide psychological comfort for the parents, and restore normality for their child (Teare & Smith, 2004).

Waiting rooms should cater for visiting siblings by providing toys, books, other activities and small chairs (Clarke & Harrison, 2001; Vint, 2005) – A&E departments often cater for visiting children better than ICUs. Ventilators and other machines can cause psychologically trauma, but imagining what they are not allowed to see may create more trauma than reality. Children and parents should be able to make informed choices about whether siblings should visit (Clarke, 2000; Vint, 2005). Providing books for children to become familiar with the ICU can help prepare them (Clarke & Harrison, 2001).

Some children are physically or mentally abused. Vague history, or bruising that is not adequately accounted for, may indicate nonaccidental injury. Suspected abuse should be reported, but is emotionally, legally and politically contentious, so should be referred to senior staff. Written records and verbal reports should remain factual.

## Neurological

Children are normally active, make good eye contact, respond to familiar voices and faces, and are active. Observing interaction with their parents therefore can indicate neurological state. Slow responses, irritability, lethargy, high-pitched or weak cries usually indicate problems. Active children may dislodge invasive equipment, so arterial cannulae are usually avoided with conscious children.

Immature vital centres, and other brain tissue, makes them prone to exaggerated responses:

- fitting
- pyrexia
- hypertension.

Neck muscles of young children are weak, and their head is disproportionately large, so children are prone to spinal-cord injury. Children are especially susceptible to meningitis.

## Ventilation

Although artificial ventilation is avoided whenever possible, children ill enough to need admission to adult ICUs usually suffer severe respiratory failure.

Until about eight years of age, airways are very narrow and relatively tortuous, so to avoid further narrowing the airway uncuffed tubes are used for intubation (Bennett, 1999; Patel & Meakin, 2000). Initially, oral tubes are usual, but once stabilised, tubes are usually changed to nasal (Duncan, 2003).

Physiologically, children normally have fast respiratory rates, so this will usually be mimicked on ventilators. Otherwise, paediatric ventilation is similar to that of adults, only with proportionally smaller volumes. Most ventilators include paediatric settings.

## Cardiovascular

Children in shock are more likely to survive if given aggressive fluid resuscitation (Morgan & O'Neill, 1998; Thomas & Carcillo, 1998). Their immature nervous systems are less sensitive to catecholamines (Wilkinson, 1997), so proportionally larger doses may be needed.

Cardiac arrest usually only occurs once physiological reserves are exhausted (Zaritsky, 1998) – usually after prolonged hypoxia. Paediatric resuscitation algorithms have a few differences from adult ones, so should be displayed prominently in bedareas where children and nursed.

## Fluid balance

Children normally have high fluid intake and high metabolism. However, immature renal function gives them less reserve to offload waste water, so may develop extreme fluid and electrolyte imbalances more rapidly than adults, needing proportionally more or less fluid, depending on needs and problems. Fluid balance should be very carefully monitored. With very young children, if not catheterised, this includes weighing nappies, wound and incontinence pads.

Children have high metabolic rates, so are especially susceptible to hypoglycaemia, and critically ill children may not have eaten for some time. Blood glucose should therefore be assessed, especially if fitting occurs (Davies & Hassell, 2001). Drug infusions are often diluted in glucose, although free water from glucose solutions can increase intracranial pressure, causing fitting.

## Thermoregulation

Very young children are prone to extremes of temperature because they have

- an immature hypothalamus
- larger body surface area in proportion to body mass
- brown fat (which insulates more effectively than white fat).

They can therefore rapidly develop pyrexial or hypothermic. Limited immunity exposes them to greater risk of infection. Temperature should therefore be monitored regularly, and problems treated promptly. Small children can rapidly develop febrile convulsions.

## Drugs

Most adult drugs are prescribed and administered dispensed in standard doses. Most paediatric drugs dosages should be individually prescribed according to patients' weight or body surface area. Weight should therefore always be recorded on admission. If children cannot be, or have not recently been, weighed, parents may know or have records – specialist community public health nurses' (formerly called 'health visitors') records. If no other source is available, weight can be estimated in children over one year of age by adding four to their age, and doubling the sum:

$$\text{weight} = (\text{age} + 4) \times 2$$

Until one year of age, 10 kg is usually a fair estimate of likely weight.

Normal paediatric doses, far smaller than adults ones, are often unfamiliar to nurses used to caring for adults, so access to paediatric formularies and a reliable quick reference guide are strongly recommended. Hepatic metabolism does not reach adult rates until about six months, so very young children often need proportionally smaller doses. However, most drugs used in the ICU achieve immediate effects so, as with adults, most doses are titrated until desired effect is achieved.

Generally less evidence exists for drug safety and efficacy with children than adults, because paediatric research creates ethical problems, so some familiar drugs are not licensed for paediatric use. For example: propofol, dubiously implicated in fatalities and other major complications such as epilepsy (Parker et al., 1992), is widely used (Murdoch & Cohen, 2000) but not recommended for ICU paediatric use.

Morphine remains the 'gold standard' opioid for children, although other standard opioids are also used. Ketamine, not an opioid, causes less cardiovascular instability, and with children seldom causes the nightmare-like hallucinations it can with adults (Dallmeyer, 2000).

Murdoch and Cohen (2000) suggest that propofol, midazolam and chloral hydrate are the most widely used paediatric sedatives in the ICU, although practice varies greatly between units. Chloral hydrate, which is given nasogastrically, has no analgesic effect. It can cause nausea, but is less likely to if diluted with water (Dallmeyer, 2000). Triclofos, a chloral hydrate derivative, causes less nausea and vomiting.

Drugs are sometimes given intraosseusly, but nurses should only use this route if competent to do so.

## Stabilisation

Ideally, paediatric nurses stay with patient, as they have paediatric expertise, such as knowing drug dosages and normal paediatric physiology; however, this is not always feasible. Early transfer to a specialist paediatric unit is usually arranged (Hallworth & McIntyre, 2003), but until paediatric retrieval teams arrive, children should be stabilised and optimised. Priorities are establishing a patent airway and intravenous cannulation (Ramnarayan et al., 2002). Regional centres usually advise, or have prewritten protocols for, standard drugs and other interventions.

Significant heat loss can occur on transfer, so children should be 'mummy wrapped' in insulating blankets, with woollen hats and gloves. This also protects vascular access and makes them easier to handle during transfer.

Most likely adverse events during transfer are

- loss of monitoring (batteries)
- loss of intravenous access
- accidental extubation
- blocked endotracheal tube
- exhaustion of oxygen (ml of oxygen required = minute volume × time of transfer in minutes)
- incomplete kit
- ventilator malfunction
- pump battery failure.

Equipment should be carefully checked before transfer

## Meningitis

Infection can cause inflammation of the meninges, or subarachnoid space (Kennedy, 2003). Viral meningitis is more common and less serious than bacterial meningitis. Bacteria usually responsible for childhood meningitis are

- *Streptococcus pneumoniae*
- *Neisseria meningitides*
- *Haemophilus influenza* type b (Hib).

Incidence peaks under one year of age, before immunity matures, with a lesser peak during adolescence (Maclennan, 2001). Meningitis can progress rapidly, death following within hours of mild non-specific febrile symptoms. Neck stiffness is often the earliest specific symptom. One in seven survivors suffer permanent disability, especially hearing loss (Peate, 2004). Prompt and appropriate treatment is therefore vital.

Meningitis is usually diagnosed by lumbar puncture – infected cerebrospinal fluid (CSF) contains protein and leucocytes. Lumbar puncture is contraindicated with raised intracranial pressure, as it may cause *tentorial herniation* ('coning'). Treatment is mainly intravenous antibiotics with aggressive system support. Meningitis usually causes photophobia, so children should be nursed in a dark room.

Meningitis is a notifiable disease, so all contacts should be traced. Antibiotics are usually given to everyone who had prolonged contact with bacterial meningitis during the previous week.

## Legal aspects

Children have different status in law to adults. Some laws specificy ages at which people can act independently of their parents, although ages differ for different laws. In the wake of the Gillick case and the 1989 Children's Act, concepts of legal 'minors' have changed from age-related to competence-related (Dimond, 2005). Nurses should clarify what rights children and others do, and do not, have. If in any doubt, advice should be sought from their Trust's legal department.

### Implications for practice

■ Children are rarely admitted to adult ICUs, but when they are, they are usually in crisis, awaiting transfer to regional PICUs. Priority is therefore to stabilise the child – establish patent airway and vascular access.
■ Respiratory failure is the most common cause for admission.
■ Primary cardiovascular disease is rare; cardiovascular failure is usually secondary to hypoxia.
■ Most units have a room or trolley with readily accessible paediatric equipment, including

   ● paediatric drug formularies
   ● paediatric resuscitation guidelines
   ● regional PICU protocols

and staff should familiarise themselves with local paediatric equipment.
■ Paediatric drug doses are almost always far smaller, usually varying with size/age. Before giving any drugs, nurses should carefully check prescriptions and amounts, seeking further advice if concerned about anything.
■ Parents usually suffer guilt and anxiety, so need information and support, and should be actively included in the child's care.
■ Waiting rooms should cater for siblings – toys, small chairs and information booklets.
■ If unsure of children's legal status, or concerned about non-accidental injury, seek advice from senior staff.
■ Meningitis usually begins with non-specific fever-like symptoms, but bacterial meningitis can be rapidly fatal. Neck stiffness is usually the earliest specific symptom.
■ Meningitis is a notifiable disease; anyone having prolonged contact with bacterial meningitis during the previous week should be given prophylactic antibiotics.

### Summary

Paediatric admissions to adult ICUs are rare, but when they occur, they are usually brief, with the aim of stabilising for transfer. Principles of nursing critically ill children are largely similar to nursing adults, with proportionally smaller volumes and sizes. Adult ICU nurses are however usually unfamiliar with these sizes, so should carefully check all prescriptions and calculations, seeking advice if they have any concerns.

Parents and siblings usually experience extreme psychological crises, needing information and support. Family should be prepared, and involved in care as much as possible.

## Support groups

Childline: 0800 1111

Meningitis Research Foundation: 080 8800 3344

National Meningitis Trust, Fern House, Bath Road, Stroud, Gloucestershire GL5 3TJ, Information line: 0891 715577; support line: 0345 538118

NSPCC Child Protection Helpline (24 hour): 0808 800 5000

Families Anonymous: 0845 1200 660; Doddington & Rollo Community Association, Charlotte Despard Avenue, Battersea, London SW11 5HD; Faxline: 020 7498 1990; e-mail: office@famanon.org.uk

## Further reading

Bennett (1999) provides a useful overview of paediatric intensive care. Various specialist books are available, including Williams and Asquith (2000), Davies and Hassell (2001) and Stack and Dobbs (2004). Clarke (2000), Clarke and Harrison (2001) and Vint (2005) have researched needs of children visiting ICUs. Specialist articles periodically appear in various nursing and medical journals. www.routledge.com/textbooks/0415373239

For clinical scenarios, clinical questions and the answers to them go to the support website at www.routledge.com/textbooks/0415373239

## Clinical scenarios

Annabel White is a healthy 16-year-old who ingested an unknown amount of alcohol at a local nightclub. On admission to the Adult ICU, Annabel is conscious but disorientated with a self-ventilating respiratory rate of 39 breaths per minute, tachycardia (164 beats per minute) with hypotension (80/40 mmHg). Blood investigations reveal metabolic acidosis and hypo-glycaemia. Annabel's parents are aware of her admission but not yet present.

Q.1 Review local hospital policies on paediatric admissions to ICU. What documentation is needed and who should be informed about Annabel's admission?

Q.2 Annabel is non compliant with interventions, for example oxygen therapy, positioning and assessment. Consider issues regarding her autonomy, legal age of competence and consent. Can Annabel refuse treatment? Who should advocate for Annabel and give consent on her behalf?

Q.3 Consider the impact of the ICU environment on Annabel and the impact of her presence on other ICU patients and staff. Outline nursing strategies which may be used to promote compliance and stabilise her condition.

Chapter 14

# Older patients in ICU

**Contents**

| | |
|---|---|
| Introduction | 132 |
| Ageing | 132 |
| Physiological effects | 133 |
| Outcome | 134 |
| Ageism | 135 |
| Implications for practice | 136 |
| Summary | 136 |
| Further reading | 136 |
| Clinical scenarios | 137 |

## Introduction

Most patients in hospital (Hubbard *et al.*, 2004) and the ICU (Adelman *et al.*, 1994) are over 65. Healthcare should be provided according to clinical need, regardless of age (DOH, 2001b). Yet limited material appears about older people in specialist literature, making them a potentially neglected majority. Comparing quantity and quality against paediatric critical care literature illustrates the relative neglect.

Age is not a disease, and diseases suffered by older people are not unique to their cohorts. Physiological ageing, multiple pathology and polypharmacy often complicate their physical needs, while negative attitudes by society, hospitals and staff may limit access to services or mar their psychological care (DOH, 2001b). Admission of old people to the ICU raises ethical questions:

- Should older patients be admitted to ICU?
- With limited resources, what proportion should be spent on older people?
- Can suffering caused by ICU admission be justified by outcome?
- Should older patients be treated differently?

Most old people are healthy, but healthy people are not admitted to the ICU. This chapter outlines effects physiological ageing can have on major body systems before focusing on wider social and attitudinal issues. The International Council of Nurses position statement on 'Nursing Care of the Elderly' (ICN, 1991) advocates that nurses should help older people maintain independence, self-care and quality of life. Such aims can be easily lost in physiological crises and technological intervention.

Although USA healthcare retains with words 'geriatric' and 'gerontology', these are generally considered pejorative in the UK – old age is not a disease, so does not need treating. The terms 'elderly' and 'elders' are often, although not always, disliked by older people, so are usually avoided in UK healthcare. Currently, the preferred UK term is 'older' person or adult. Varying terminology should be remembered when undertaking literature searches.

## Ageing

Ageing can be

- chronological (number of years lived)
- sociological (role in society, for example retirement)
- physiological (physical function).

(De Beauvoir, 1970)

Chronological ageing, often >65, is statistically simple and clear, so adopted by much medical literature, especially quantitative research, and (with qualification) by the DOH (2001b), but is usually medically arbitrary, failing to recognise each person's uniqueness and individuality. So nurses should approach each person as an individual, rather than chronological stereotype.

Ageing almost inevitably brings decline in most physiological functions although rates of decline vary between systems and individuals. *Reserve function* – the difference between actual level of function and minimum function needed for homeostasis – provides a barrier against disease. Progressive decline in reserve function increases likelihood of chronic and multiple disease in later years, such as diabetes mellitus.

Underlying chronic conditions, including chronic pain such as arthritis, are more common among older people. Arthritis may be visually apparent, but individual assessment may identify other needs, enabling nurses to avoid inflicting accidental pain.

## Physiological effects

Hypertension, reduced stroke volume and cardiac output and other *cardiovascular* changes are partly age-related (Vanhoutte, 2002), but mainly from acquired damage, especially from smoking (Padwal *et al.*, 2001; Fogarty & Lingford-Hughes, 2004). Older people may suffer from various cardiovascular diseases, including

- dysrhythmias, especially atrial fibrillation (see Chapter 22)
- coronary artery disease
- heart valve disease
- atherosclerosis
- peripheral vascular disease.

However caused, poor perfusion affects all other body systems.

Nearly all aspects of respiratory function significantly decline with age (Mick & Ackerman, 2004), and incidence of acute *respiratory* failure increases (Behrendt, 2000), although healthy older people retain sufficient reserve capacity (Watson, 2000b).

*Central nervous system* degeneration progresses throughout life, although cerebral atrophy makes older people more able to compensate for increased cerebral volumes, making them more likely to survive intracranial hypertension. Neurophysiological changes are complex, but older people are at greater risk from the three Ds:

- dementia
- delirium
- depression.

Up to half of hospitalised people over 70 develop delirium (Danter, 2003), so confusion should always be treated as acute and reversible until proven otherwise. Reality orientation can be useful, but may provoke aggression; alternative approaches, such a validation therapy (Feil, 1993), seek to empower rather than control people. But most approaches rely on verbal responses, limiting their value for intubated, sedated patients. Communication can be problematic with all ICU patients, but acute limitation may be compounded by dysphasia, hearing loss, impaired vision or impaired memory. Communication needs should therefore be individually assessed – relatives may be a valuable source for information or achieving communication.

*Renal* problems typically associated with ageing (e.g. incontinence, prostatic obstruction) are alleviated by catheterisation. Age-related decline in renal function (Chalmers, 2002) may cause abnormal biochemistry, such as elevated serum creatinine, but like most other critically-ill patients, acute renal failure is usually caused by hypovolaemia.

Age-related elastin and collagen loss, together with poorer perfusion makes older *skin* more fragile, prone to sheering pressure sores, and delays healing (Penzer & Finch, 2001). Most pressure sores occur in people, hence the weighting for age on Waterlow and other assessment scales. Pressure area aids can reduce incidence of pressure sores, but optimising endogenous factors (nutrition, perfusion) reduces risks. Reduced capillary perfusion impairs cutaneous drug absorbtion (e.g. GTN/fentanyl patches, 'essential' massage oils) and removal of metabolic waste.

*Gastrointestinal* function declines with age (Eliopoulos, 2001), but the gut's large functional reserve normally sustains adequate function (Firth & Prather, 2002). As with other critically-ill people, gut failure can precipitate sepsis and other crises.

*Liver* dysfunction is mainly pathological rather than chronological (Eliopoulos, 2001). Reduced ability to metabolise drugs may necessitate reduced doses and more careful monitoring of plasma drug levels.

Older people are more frequently *malnourished* than younger people (Devlin, 2000) due to factors such as poverty, poor mobility, maldentition, reduced gut motility, digestive problems, lack of facilities or constipation. Undernourished and obesity predisposes them to multiple risk factors, including immunocompromise which increases risks of hospital-acquired infections, and muscle weakness which delays weaning from artificial ventilation (Adams & Murphy, 2000; Dardaine *et al.*, 2001; Pearce & Duncan, 2002).

As *muscles* and bone atrophy, they are replaced by fat. Fat repels water, so older people are more prone to dehydration. As calcium metabolism declines, less is absorbed, while stored (skeletal) calcium is leached, reducing bone density, so making bones more brittle and liable to fracture. Muscle weakness contributes to delayed weaning from ventilation and prolongs rehabilitation.

## Outcome

Most studies about older ICU patients measure mortality, increasingly to hospital discharge or later. Whether old patients benefit from critical care or whether consuming limited critical care resources for the old is just are debated, depending partly on different measures and views. Esteban *et al.*'s (2004) multinational survey found higher ICU and hospital mortality among older people, but similar ventilation times. Others (e.g. Dardaine *et al.*, 2001; Somme *et al.*, 2003) found that age did not affect mortality. However, under-lying physiological function does affect outcome (Taylor *et al.*, 2002; Boumendil *et al.*, 2004), so physiological rather than chronological age-related criteria for ICU admission may be justified.

Mortality is easily measured, but quality of life, a more valuable (if more subjective) measure of outcome, does not necessarily correlate with health out-comes (Covinsky, 1999). Nierman *et al.*'s (2001) USA study found that three-quarters survived to discharge, half being discharged back to their own homes.

Chronological age alone should not determine ICU admission (Dardaine *et al.*, 2001). Overt or covert admission criteria may prevent sicker older patients being admitted (DOH, 2001b), so comparison with younger (poten-tially sicker) cohorts of ICU patients can be misleading. Outcome to hospital discharge and functional recovery is as good as with younger ICU patients (Mick & Ackerman, 2004), but lower costs of care with older people (Ely *et al.*, 1999) may reflect sicker older patients being refused admission. Conflicting research and practice makes healthcare for critically ill older adults into a covert lottery.

## Ageism

'Ageism', the 'notion that people cease to be people... by virtue of having lived a specific number of years' (Comfort, 1977: 35), may be overt (e.g. refusing serv-ices to people over a certain age (Bytheway, 1995)) or covert (e.g. attitudes).

Overt chronological age criteria for critical care admission are now rare (DOH 2001b), but evidence-based medicine and predictive scoring (e.g. APACHE (Knaus *et al.*, 1985)) can create covert ageism – APACHE II scores chronological age to account for physiological ageing, as well as scoring pathophysiologies. APACHE scores of older people are therefore disproportionately increased.

Older people may have sensory or expressive communication difficulties. While staff should optimise communication, they should be aware of insidious prejudice, stereotyping or other negative attitudes, such as speaking loudly to all old people, rather than assessing whether they have any deficit, and if so how to compensate for it.

Many older people grew up before the National Health Service existed so they remember a very different society (and social values); doctors (and nurses) were presumed to always know best. Their beliefs and values may therefore differ significantly from those of nurses caring for them; different generational values may cause misunderstandings. Nurses should empower choices, which with older people may take more encouragement.

Bereavement, social mobility and physical immobility may leave older people isolated, deprived of social supports (families, friends). Friends/family may treat the older person as a burden. Psychological isolation can become self-fulfilling, encouraging older people to adopt child-like dependant behaviour and/or appear confused.

135

## Implications for practice

■ Older patients already form about half of UK ICU admissions; numbers will probably increase, so ICU nurses should actively consider needs and quality of care.

■ Function of all body systems declines with age, but most older people are healthy. When acute ill-health necessitates ICU admission, care should anticipate recovery.

■ Reduced function, and possible multipathology, necessitates individualised, holistic care.

■ Confusion should be treated as acute and reversible, until proven otherwise.

■ Sensory or expressive communication limitations may be acute or chronic, so should be individually assessed, and individualised strategies planned to overcome limitations.

■ In-service and post-registration education should include significant focus on nursing older people in the ICU.

■ Ageism, insidious throughout society, can easily, and insidiously, influence care; reflecting on and evaluating nursing care (individually and in groups) helps identify areas for development.

## Summary

Definitions of 'old' are arbitrary, but pragmatically many ICU patients are 'old', a potentially neglected majority. Paucity of literature on older patients in the ICU makes this one of the most neglected aspects on ICU nursing.

Pathologies experienced by older people are largely those suffered by younger patients. Multiple pathologies, system dysfunction and slower metabolism, make physiological needs of older patients complex. ICU admission can also threaten psychological and social health. Nurses can humanise potentially threatening and ageist ICU environments to meet the needs of older patients.

## Further reading

Key texts about nursing older people are Norman and Redfern (1997), Redfern and Ross (1999), Heath and Schofield (1999) and Heath and Watson (1995). De Beauvoir (1970) provides highly readable and challengingly sociological perspectives. Medical studies of age-related outcome frequently appear, but otherwise literature on older people in the ICU is infrequent. Material from specialist journals, such as *Age & Ageing* and *Nursing Older People* can often be applied to the ICU. Mick and Ackerman (2004) review implications of physiological ageing for the ICU. The *National Service Framework* (DOH, 2001b) raises many concerns about general healthcare which, although not ICU-specific, are often applicable. www.routledge.com/textbooks/0415373239

For clinical scenarios, clinical questions and the answers to them go to the support website at www.routledge.com/textbooks/0415373239

## Clinical scenarios

Albert Rose is an active and independent 89-year-old who was admitted to the ICU following emergency laparotomy for perforated bowel. He has an illeostomy and two abdominal drains with a total of 2 litres blood loss in the first 4 hours. He is mechanically ventilated with an Hb of 8.2 g/dl and Hct of 29 per cent.

Q.1 Review the main age related physiological changes and expected normal values for an 89-year-old in the ICU. What are the implications of these changes in managing Mr Rose's treatments?

Q.2 Analyse the significance of Mr Rose's Hb value on his recovery. Examine the benefits and adverse effects of blood transfusion with elderly ICU patients. Should Mr Rose be transfused?

Q.3 Consider possible outcomes for Mr Rose following discharge from hospital. Formulate a strategy to promote his physical and mental recovery.

Chapter 15

# Infection control

### Contents

Introduction                                      139
Infection in the ICU                              139
Ventilator associated pneumonia (VAP)  140
Organisms                                         140
Controlling infection                             142
Implications for practice                         145
Summary                                           146
Further reading                                   146
Clinical scenarios                                146

### Fundamental knowledge

Universal precautions
Asespsis
Immunity (see Chapter 40)
Common hospital-acquired infections
Local infection control guidelines

Hospital nosocomial (hospital acquired infection – HAI) rates remain 8–10 per cent (Emmerson, 1997); one-third are preventable (Bion *et al.*, 2001), one-third are acquired in ICUs (Eggimann & Pittet, 2001). Infection can be endogenous or exogenous. Half of the patients admitted to an ICU are already colonised by micro-organisms that will cause subsequent infections (Eggimann & Pittet, 2001), and one in 20 ICU patients develop bloodstream infections (Laupland *et al.*, 2002). Endogenous infection, from organisms already harboured by patients, in the ICU usually occurs through the respiratory tract (e.g. ventilator-associated pneumonia – VAP), but can also occur through skin, especially though central venous lines (DOH, 2001c) and the gut. Exogenous infection is usually though contact (staff, procedures, equipment), but can also be airborne. Exogenous cross infection causes up to one-third of hospital acquired infections, at least half of which are preventable (Harbath *et al.*, 2003).

Bacteria that are commensals (harmless) to healthy people may become pathogens to vulnerable ICU patients. 'Infection' only occurs when people develop pathological responses to micro-organisms. Destroying commensals with antibiotics enables opportunist infection from organisms colonising (but not necessarily infecting) healthier people.

Infection control has generated much research and debate, but fewer solutions. Most ICU patients are immunocompromised, whether from pathologies (e.g. hepatic failure), treatments (immunosuppressive drugs) or age-related decline in immunity. This makes each member of staff a potential source of infection. This chapter identifies incidence, sources and effects of infection in ICU, describes some prevalent bacteria (methicillin-resistant *Staphylococcus aureus*, Pseudomonas, vancomycin resistant Enterococci), and medical/nursing treatments, emphasising prevention rather than treatment.

## Infection in the ICU

Infection requires

- a micro-organism (source)
- a reservoir (where sufficient quantities can breed)
- a means of transfer
- a susceptible host.

Micro-organisms are found in any environment which humans can inhabit. ICU patients and their environments frequently provide reservoirs for micro-organisms to reproduce. Most ICU patients are susceptible to infection. So once micro-organisms gain entry into patients (any invasive device, procedure or wound), or across barriers within the body, infection can occur.

On admission, one-fifth of ICU patients have infections (Alberti *et al.*, 2002), which are often the cause of admission. ICU nosocomial infection rates vary, but after one day nearly one-fifth of patients acquire infections

(Alberti *et al.*, 2002), and incidence continues to increase. Overall ICU nosocomial infection rates may be as high as 60 per cent (Emmerson, 1997).

The most common causes of infection in ICU are

- ventilator-associated pneumonia
- intra-abdominal infections following trauma or surgery
- bacteraemia from intravenous devices.

(Eggimann & Pittet, 2001)

Septicaemia (bloodstream infection) can be detected through blood cultures. Debate persists about indications for blood cultures, many units taking cultures if patients' temperatures exceed an identified limit – often 38–38.4°C. Such figures reflect greater likelihood of infective rather than metabolic pyrexia (see Chapter 8), but are not always reliable.

## Ventilator associated pneumonia (VAP)

Nearly all ICU patients have bacteria colonising their upper respiratory tracts (Andrews, 2000; Castre, 2001). Up to half of all ventilated patients acquire infection (Matthews & Matthews, 2000). Mortality among patients with VAP is 71 per cent, compared to 29 per cent mortality for those without (Young & Ridley, 1999).

Sixty per cent of ventilator-associated pneumonias are caused by mutliresistant organisms (Akca *et al.*, 2000), making treatment more problematic, costly and prolonged. VAP can be reduced by chest physiotherapy (Ntoumenopoulos *et al.*, 2002) and nursing patients semirecumbent (45°) (Drakulovic *et al.*, 1999).

## Organisms

Bacteria are divided between gram 'positive' or 'negative', depending whether they retain crystal violet-iodine complex stain. Gram positive organisms include

- Staphylococci (including methicillin-resistant *Staphylococcus aureus* – MRSA)
- Clostridium
- Enterococci
- Streptococci.

Gram negative organisms include

- Acinetobacter
- Enterobacter
- *Escherichia coli*
- *Helicobacter pylori*
- Klebsiellae

- Proteus
- Pseudomonas
- Serratia.

Gram negative organisms have thinner cell walls, so produce endotoxins for protection. Endotoxin stimulates inflammatory responses. Traditionally, gram negatives were hospital-acquired, while gram positives were community-acquired, but mutation of resistant gram positive organisms (e.g. MRSA, VRE) means most hospital-acquired infections are now gram positive (Humphreys, 2001). The two most prevalent organisms infecting ICU patients are *Staphylococcus aureus* (30.1 per cent) and Pseudomonas (32.1 per cent) (Vincent *et al.*, 1995), both opportunistic infections.

Gram negative organisms tend to colonise moist areas, whereas gram positives are usually transmitted by direct contact and airborne spread (Barrett, 1999). Infection control has therefore changed from concern about moist reservoirs to airborne and direct contact risks. Hand hygiene is especially more important in the era of increasingly prevalent, and virulent, gram positive organisms.

Most types of *Staphylococci aureus* remain methicillin sensitive (MSSA), but MRSA has becomes increasingly problematic, frequently colonising respiratory tracts (Theaker *et al.*, 2001). The UK has the highest incidence of MRSA in Europe – colonising nearly one-tenths of all ICU patients on admission (Thompson, 2004), and one-third of long-stay ICU patients (Theaker *et al.*, 2001). One-fifth of all Staphylococci isolated from ICUs are resistant (Eggimann & Pittet, 2001), and frequently spread from ICUs to other clinical areas (Morgan *et al.*, 2000). Screening is cost-effective enabling early treatment (Platt, 2001; Rubinovitch & Pittet, 2001), so all admissions to ICU should routinely be screened for MRSA (nose, groin and throat swabs, CSU, sputum and other relevant specimens, such as wound swabs).

MRSA usually spreads by hands of staff (Working Party Report, 1999), with up to one-quarter being carriers (Haddadin *et al.*, 2002), so using gloves significantly reduces nosocomial infection.

MRSA infection is difficult and expensive to treat. Chlorhexidine reduces surface colonisation, while many strains remain susceptible to vancomycin, teicoplanin, rifampicin and fucfusidic acid, but these more aggressive antibiotics have more potent side-effects. Concern about vancomycin-resistant Enterococci (VRE) may further limit vancomycin use. Topical tea tree oil may also be effective (Caelli *et al.*, 2000).

MRSA has developed epidemic strains (EMRSA), strains 15 and 16 being most widespread, difficult to treat, and causing nearly all UK MRSA septicaemias (Winter, 2005). Spread should be contained by

- identifying infection (routine screening of all admissions)
- collaboration with Infection Control departments
- informing wards before discharge
- thorough cleaning of bedareas and changing curtains, following discharge.

*Pseudomonas*, an opportunistic organism, causes one-tenth of hospital acquired infections (Thuong *et al.*, 2003). It especially colonises moist environments, such as washbasins (Berthelot *et al.*, 2001). Human skin colonisation is brief, but highly pathogenic (Pittet & Boyce, 2001), and colonisation of respiratory and urinary tracts frequently occurs (Bertrand *et al.*, 2001). Pseudomonas remains the single main cause of ventilator-associated pneumonia (Thuong *et al.*, 2003).

*Vancomycin resistant Enterococci* is increasing prevalent (Humphreys, 2001). Enterococci are intrinsically resistant to most antibiotics (Elliott & Lambert, 1999), and can survive on surfaces for up to seven days (Lueckenotte, 2000). Recent antibiotic research has largely been invested in developing gram positive antibiotics, however, infection control measures (especially hand hygiene and careful handling of antibiotics) remain the most important way to prevent VRE spreading. VRE has been most problematic in the USA (Michel & Gutmann, 1997) and Japan. Although currently rare in Europe, in May 2000 one outbreak occurred in Utrecht (Ridwan *et al.*, 2002), and further spread is probably only a question of time.

*Multi-resistant Coliforms* (e.g. Klebsiella, Enterobacter, Acinetobacter, *E. Coli*). Although systemic infection from these is relatively rare, sepsis from multi-resistant coliforms is difficult to treat, and effective antibiotics (e.g. colistrin) are relatively toxic. Patients infected with micro-organisms should be isolated, and Infection Control involved with their management.

*Fungal* infection and mortality among critically ill patients is rising. The most common fungal infection in the ICU is from *candida* spp. Fluconazole remains the most widely used antifungal drug. ICU patients are especially susceptible to oral and skinfold fungal infection, so maintaining hygiene significantly reduces infection rates.

## Controlling infection

Appropriate antibiotics should be prescribed by medical staff, usually on advice from microbiology. Some hospitals rotate antibiotics, to limit development of resistant micro-organisms, but this practice remains controversial. Duration of treatment with antibiotics should be identified and clearly recorded, usually on drug charts. Nurses should inform medical staff if prescriptions are due for review. Some antibiotics have narrow therapeutic ranges (e.g. gentomycin, vancomycin), so blood samples should be sent for assay levels according to local protocols, and at the appropriate time before or after antibiotic dose.

Around 20–25 per cent of ICU infections are catheter-related (Brun-Buisson, 2001). Many *invasive* procedures and treatments are unavoidable with critical illness, but each may introduce infection into immunocompromised patients. Nurses can usefully question whether some may be avoided: alternative routes for drugs may be possible. Central lines remain the single main cause of nosocomial septicaemia (Randolph, 1998), but are usually necessary for managing critical illness. Many dressings and antibiotic-impregnated devices have been marketed to reduce infection, but evidence for efficacy is generally ambiguous (Woeltje & Fraser, 1998), some increasing both infection and occlusion rates (Wright et al., 2001). Total parenteral nutrition presents especially high infection risks, so should be given through dedicated lines (DOH, 2001c). Unused cannulae (peripheral or central) create unnecessary risks, so should be removed.

Hospitals and units often provide evidence-based guidelines for replacing lines and equipment. Staff extending times beyond these or manufacturers' recommendations may be legally liable (see Chapter 48). Insertion dates of all invasive equipment should be clearly recorded.

Family and friends rarely move between patients, but *staff* can easily transfer hospital pathogens (often resistant) between patients. Minimising movement of staff between patients, use of gloves and no-touch technique significantly reduce cross-infection, but should not be considered substitutes for hand hygiene.

Moving *equipment* between patients can also spread infection. Where dedicated equipment is not practical (e.g. portable X-ray, 12-lead ECG), nurses should ensure any equipment touching patients is clean.

*Airborne* bacteria may be transmitted through

- dust
- airborne skin scales
- droplets.

Airborne infection is significantly reduced by use of in-line suction catheters (see Chapter 5). Other ways to reduce airborne infection in ICU include

- planning higher-risk procedures at times of least disturbance
- careful disposal of linen (e.g. bringing linen skips/bags to bedsides, carefully rolling linen inwards to trap skin scales)
- air-flow systems.

*Hand hygiene* remains the simplest, easiest, cheapest and most important way to reduce transient colonisation (Pittet & Boyce, 2001) and hospital-acquired infections (Woeltje & Fraser, 1998), but is often inadequately or poorly performed. Washing often misses the parts most likely to touch patients – thumbs, fingertips and backs of hands (Ayliffe et al., 2001), frequently observed with handwashing outside hospital. The RCN (2005) described good techniques. Hands should be dried thoroughly after washing as moisture, including wet alcohol, facilitates bacterial growth. Hand hygiene compliance deteriorates when workload increases, so maximising productivity in healthcare may conflict with maintaining quality care (Humphreys, 2001). Nurses should ensure all staff touching their patient have adequately washed their hands.

Alcohol rubs are generally better antimicrobials than soap and more convenient (Girou et al., 2002; Girou, 2003), although some organisms, such as C difficile, may survive alcohol rubs. Sufficient amounts should be dispensed (this varies between products), spread fully over hands and allowed to dry. Local Infection Control departments can advise on the amount and time used for products. Wearing gloves is not an alternative to hand hygiene (Pittet & Boyce, 2001).

Most Trust uniform policies stimulate that nurses should not wear wristwatches or rings on fingers (except wedding rings) as these can harbour micro-organisms.

Anyone (staff or family) visiting any patient on ICU should clean their hands before entering the unit. Alcohol rubs should be placed by each entrance to the unit, with prominent signs informing people to prevent infection by cleaning their hands.

*Aprons* reduce transmission of bacteria carried on staff clothing, while reminding staff to wash their hands (associations with 'gowning up'), so it should be worn by anyone having patient contact. Using colour codes for each bedspace encourages staff to change aprons and wash hands between patients, and makes it visually obvious if they do not. Unfortunately, increased costs of purchasing various aprons may encourage some Trusts to attempt inappropriate, and counterproductive, short-term savings.

Clothing is a potential carrier of micro-organisms – Amyes and Thomson (1995) cite one study where MRSA colonised 20 per cent of staff, but 82 per cent of their clothes. Ideally clean *uniforms* should be worn each shift, and not worn outside the unit. Washes at 71°C kill most micro-organisms (Parker, 2002), although not necessarily hepatitis B or VRE (Parker, 1999). Uniforms should be laundered at the highest temperature material will stand (65°C for at least 10 minutes, or 71°C for at least 3 minutes), then dried quickly and thoroughly (McCulloch, 1998). Uniforms should not be washed with other clothing (Callaghan, 1998) – most casual clothing cannot stand these temperature (see labels on clothing), so home washes are usually considerably cooler and seldom sterilise clothes. Hot air dryers may also be extensively contaminated with bacteria (Bruton, 1995), so home drying is probably inappropriate. Ironically, concern about professional image is prompting some Trusts to replace 'scrubs' with traditional uniforms, yet most Trusts supply insufficient uniforms and lack laundry facilities (Nye *et al.*, 2005), encouraging staff to wear uniforms for more than one day (Callaghan, 1998) and launder uniforms (inadequately) at home. Staff from other areas in direct contact with patients should be encouraged to either change into unit clothing or remove jackets/coats worn outside the unit (before washing their hands).

Critical illness necessitates contact with many staff, but *unnecessary staff* should be discouraged from visiting and movement of staff between beds minimised. Conflicts with educational needs, especially in teaching hospitals, should be evaluated against risks to patients. Units should not be used as corridors to other areas.

*Inadequate staffing* (quantity and quality) increases cross-infection (Vacca, 1999; Eggimann & Pittet, 2001; Humphreys, 2001) so managers responsible for understaffing are also responsible for risks they create (Vincent, 2003). Changing nurse:patient ratios from 1:1 to 1:2 increases central-line infection risk by 60 per cent (Brun-Buisson, 2001).

Although it is speculative and debated, gut bacterial translocation probably causes sepsis, inflammatory responses and lung injury (Harkin *et al.*, 2001; MacFie, 2004). *Selective digestive decontamination* (SDD) can prevent pathogen colonisation by routine use of selective, nonabsorbable antibiotics. Despite many favourable, if often poorly designed (van Nieuwenhoven *et al.*, 2001), trials (e.g. Silvestri *et al.*, 2001), SDD is not widely used (Bion *et al.*, 2001), has little influence on outcome (Woeltje and Fraser, 1998), and is not recommended for routine use (Ewing & Torres, 2002). Prophylactic antibiotics may encourage antibiotic resistance (Chastre, 2001).

### Implications for practice

- Hand hygiene should be carried out before and after each aspect of care, and before approaching and after leaving each bedarea.
- Alcohol handrubs should be available at each bedarea, and be used before and after any patient contact. Staff should know how much to use, and how long it takes to dry. Some infections, such as C difficile, are resistant to alcohol, necessitating handwashing.
- All taps should have elbow-operated levers at elbow height; taps should not be turned on by hand.
- Towels dispensers should provide individual paper towels that will not drape in moist sink units.
- Nursing/medical documentation should include easily accessible flow sheets of specimens sent and the results. Each entry should be dated and signed.
- Equipment (e.g. Heat Moisture Exchangers) should be changed according to manufacturer's instructions (normally daily); catheter mounts should be changed at the same time as humidifiers.
- Invasive techniques and disconnection of intravenous lines should, when possible, avoid times of dust disturbance (e.g. floor cleaning, damp dusting).
- Strict asepsis must be observed when breaking/bypassing normal non-specific immune defences, such as when handling intravenous circuit, treating open wounds, or procedures involving the trachea, stomach or jejunum.
- Using prepacked intravenous additives (e.g. potassium) reduces contamination risks.
- Clothing worn outside the ICU should be removed before approaching patients.
- Adequate laundry facilities should be provided for staff to change uniforms daily.
- Hospital infection control nurses and other specialists should be actively involved in multidisciplinary teamwork.
- Colour coding bedareas (aprons, equipment) discourages inappropriate movement between bedspaces.

## Summary

Infection incurs costs in human life, morbidity and budgets. Antibiotics and other medical treatments can reduce morbidity and mortality, but preventing infection is humanly (and financially) preferable. Problems from multiresistant organisms are likely to escalate.

Hand hygiene remains the most important way to prevent infection. Hygiene is helped by adequate and appropriate facilities, including accessible alcohol handrubs, aprons and unit guidelines/protocols. All multidisciplinary team members should be actively involved in making decisions, nurses having an especially valuable role in co-ordinating and controlling each patient's environment.

## Further reading

Articles on infection control frequently appear in specialist and general journals. Vincent (2003) reviews medical issues, while Platt (2001) and RCN (2005) discuss MRSA. Journals specialising in infection control include *Journal of Hospital Infection* and *Infection Control and Hospital Epidemiology*. The DOH has issued guidelines on principles of infection control (DOH, 2001d) and central line management (DOH, 2001c). There are many texts on microbiology and infection control, including *Ayliffe et al.* (2001). www.routledge.com/textbooks/0415373239

For clinical scenarios, clinical questions and the answers to them go to the support website at www.routledge.com/textbooks/0415373239

## Clinical scenarios

Nadeen Persad is a 32-year-old with chronic renal failure who was successfully resuscitated following cardiopulmonary arrest. She requires admission to the ICU for closer monitoring. An ICU doctor and nurse (who is 4 months pregnant) go with appropriate transfer equipment to retrieve the patient while an ICU bed is prepared for the admission. On arrival to the ward, the ICU doctor and nurse are informed that Nadeen has active pulmonary *Tuberculosis* and *Acinetobacter* in her diarrhoea.

Q.1 Consider the common transmission modes and pathogenicity of *Tuberculosis* and *Acinetobacter*. Specify the infection control precautions to be followed in order to minimise potential cross transmission of the micro-organisms to other patients and staff when transferring and admitting Nadeen to ICU.

Q.2 In addition to the prepared bed area, the ICU has two protective isolation rooms available where airflow in one room is under positive pressure and the other room is under negative pressure. Provide a rationale for which area or room Nadeen should be admitted into.

Q.3  Management of Nadeen's infections focused on three main areas:

- Containment (e.g. screening of staff, visitors).
- Prevention of cross-transmission. (Exogenous: to other patients, endogenous: other sites within Nadeen, minimising vectors etc.)
- Eradication (specific antibiotics, administration routes etc).

Design a nursing care plan for Nadeen whilst on ICU incorporating published Infection Control Guidelines, local clinical guidelines and holistic nursing approach. Integrate professional, psychosocial, psychological and physical aspects into this plan.

Chapter 16

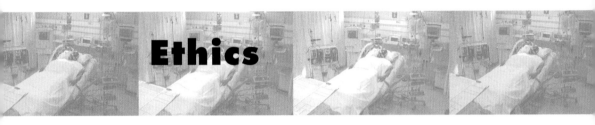

# Ethics

**Contents**

Introduction                          149
Time out 1                            149
ICU – an ethical quagmire?            150
Ethical principles                    150
Time out 2                            152
Time out 3                            152
Ethical theories                      154
Implications for practice             155
Summary                               155
Further reading                       155
Clinical scenarios                    156

**Fundamental knowledge**

Local policies (on issues identified in this chapter)

## Introduction

Professional expectations (expected norms) are clarified in NMC publications, especially the Code of Conduct (NMC, 2004). But making individual decisions about individual aspects of patient care raises options and dilemmas, which are not always resolved by codes. Ethics is about values. Applying ethics to practice helps decision-making, it does not replace it.

Beauchamp and Childress (2001) identify four ethical principles:

- autonomy
- non-maleficence
- beneficence
- justice.

Ethical principles provide a framework to explore dilemmas, so decisions should consider all four. There are many ethical theories, but three widely cited ones are:

- duty-based
- goal-based
- rights-based.

Ethical theories identify different sets of beliefs; understanding our own and others' sets of beliefs (values) helps understanding differences.

This chapter includes some legal and professional perspectives. Unlike ethics, these expectations can be enforced, so nurses should consider their individual professional (and legal) accountability.

Meanings of *ethics* and *morals* vary. Literal translation of both is 'norm' (Greek = *ethos*, Latin = *mores*), but they have diffeent connotations. Many (but not all) people interpret 'ethics' as applying to groups (e.g. nursing ethics), whereas 'morals' implies individual and personal values. These interpretaions are followed in this text, but some texts use the terms interchangeably.

### Time out 1

Using a dictionary, jot down definitions of 'ethics' and 'morals'. Consider similarities and differences between these definitions.

How close are these definitions to your own understanding of the terms?

Can ethics ever be immoral, or morals unethical? Why? Include professional ethics/morals in your consideration. National ethics/morals are supposedly represented by national law. So can laws be immoral/unethical? Why?

## ICU – an ethical quagmire?

Ethical dilemmas in ICU are caused by

- cost/resource limitations
- technology
- values.

Healthcare costs and demand continue to increase more than budgets, making rationing of resources inevitable. ICU is financially expensive (see Chapter 50), so insufficient resources to meet demand too often causes refusal of admission, postponed surgery, interhospital transfer or premature discharge. Applying economics to healthcare makes many staff uncomfortable, but while decisions should never be made solely on economic grounds, finance cannot be ignored where resources remain finite. If economic decisions are not made by those delivering care, they will be made by others.

ICU relies on *technology* to support and monitor physiological function. Breathing and heartbeat can be replaced by technology, but may prolong dying rather than prolong life. There is (arguably) a difference between living and being alive (Rachels, 1986).

Decisions may be influenced by quality of life. This much-used term is *value*-laden: what one person considers acceptable quality, another may not. Some value preserving life at all costs, while others believe 'nature' should always take its course. When faced with crises, people may change previously expressed opinions. Nurses, patients and doctors view quality of care and patient satisfaction differently (Shannon *et al.*, 2002), so should try to identify, and then respect, patients' wishes, rather than assume patients' wishes will concur with their own.

## Ethical principles

### Autonomy

Autonomy ('self-rule') is making free, informed choice. How far anyone fully 'rules' themselves is questionable. Impaired consciousness, debility and treatments (e.g. intubation) severely limit the abilities of ICU patients to rule themselves; they are disempowered. ICU staff control information, their environment and even basic physiological functions (including rest/sedation). Disempowerment can be (literally) fatal (Seligman, 1975).

The NMC (2004) states that nurses must obtain consent before giving any treatment or care. With unconscious patients this is clearly impractical, but some conscious ICU patients suffer intracranial pathologies (e.g. encephalopathy, hypoxia) or psychological problems (e.g. psychoses) that may prevent them making informed decisions. Dimond (2001) suggests nurses should use the common law power to act out of necessity in the best interests of mentally incapacitated people. Booth (2002) questions whether patients can ever be fully informed, and if not how much information is sufficient. Where possible, nurses should help people make informed decisions.

Maintaining safety sometimes necessitates physical restraint, for example to prevent self-extubation. However, force may exacerbate problems (Barr, 1996) and could lead to civil actions for assault and imprisonment (Donaldson, 1997) and criminal liability under the Offences Against the Persons Act, 1961 (Stuart, 1996), so physical restraint should only be used as a last resort (Watson, 2002). Ethical differences between physical and chemical restraints are debateable.

*Consent* by relatives for mentally competent adults has no legal validity (Dimond, 2005). Unfortunately many ICU patients cannot make informed decisions, so are vulnerable. Decisions made by others, however well-intentioned, may not always be in patients' best interests. Nurses therefore have an important role in advocating for, and protecting, their patients.

Consent for children under 18 years of age depends on age and other criteria (Dimond, 2005). If competent, very young children may (legally) make more profound decisions than older ones. Rights of children, and parents, can therefore cause complex dilemmas. The BMA (1999) suggests that while competent minors may consent to treatment, their refusal may be overturned. ICU nurses caring for children should seek current advice from their paediatric colleagues or other expert sources, such as hospitals' legal advisors.

Actions in patients' best interests may be condoned, but *nonconsensual touch* (including any nursing/medical intervention without valid consent) is technically an assault (McFadzean & Dexter, 1999). 'Best interests' may be unclear: quality of life is subjective, so if values of patients and healthcare staff differ, decisions made for unconscious patients (advocacy) may not reflect patients' best interest. Relatives' opinions, while not legally binding, may provide insight into patients' wishes, while building goodwill between relatives and staff. However, relatives' values may differ (Priestly, 1999), and extreme stress/guilt can result from believing they are making 'life or death' decisions.

ICU nurses may care for patients recruited into research studies. In the UK, approval for research involving people, including vulnerable populations, such as critically ill or unconscious patients, necessitates approval by regional ethical committees. When patients are unable to consent, usual current ethical requirements are that relatives give lack of objection, with patients being asked for retrospective consent whenever possible. The Mental Capacity Bill, currently being drafted, may make any research on incompetent patients illegal. The key document for medical research ethics, the Declaration of Helsinki, adopts deontological rather than utilitarian perspectives, stating that the well-being of research subjects should take precedence over interests of science and society (World Medical Association, 2000). Ironically, ethical rigour in research is increasingly bypassed by labelling experiments 'clinical trials'.

*Advance directives* ('living wills') state patients' wishes for specific (stated) treatments to be withheld (e.g. ventilation). Case law has established Advance Directives as legally binding in the UK (DOH, 2001e). Advance directives must necessarily anticipate situations before they occur, but wishes may have changed since writing the 'will' (although this would not affect validity of a last will and testament). Nurses finding evidence of an advance directive (possibly through discussions with relatives) should alert unit managers and the multidisciplinary team.

## Nonmaleficence

Not doing harm, fundamental to healthcare since the Hippocratic Oath, is restated in Nightingale's (1859/1980) *Notes on Nursing*, Roper *et al.*'s (1996) first (and presumably primary) activity of living and the *Code of Conduct* (NMC, 2004). In law, proven harm is more culpable than failing to do good.

Healthcare exposes patients to potential *harm*, such as fear, pain, complications and nosocomial infection. ICU patients unable to express their own wishes are vulnerable to (unintentional) harm. Benefits and risks from pulmonary artery catheters have been much debated, the UK generally viewing risks as not being justified (harmful), whereas the USA and some other countries consider them beneficial.

## Time out 2

List equipment available in your ICU. Which do you consider ordinary, and which extraordinary? How would you feel about removing equipment in the extraordinary list from dying patients? Discuss this with some colleagues.

## Time out 3

If your unit has an information book for bereaved relatives, read through it. If you consider further information should be added to it, discuss this with your unit manager. If your unit does not produce a booklet, contact the hospital's patient's officer and find what is available locally. Your local branch of CRUSE may also be able to provide information.

## Beneficence

Doing good (beneficence) underlies Clause 2 of nurses' *Code of Conduct* (NMC, 2004), but 'good' is relative and value-laden, and may cause harm. Telling the truth is often considered good, but if truth may distress confused people, others may consider 'white lies' a greater good. Relatives should be denied information that breaches duty of confidentiality, the 'good' to patients over-riding any 'good' to their relatives.

Where possible, patients should participate in decisions, but with many ICU patients this is not possible. When survival becomes doubtful, decisions of which life-supporting treatments to withdraw/withhold raises dilemmas.

Values may differ between nurses, other professions, patients and families. Nurse advocacy aims to do good, but what is 'good' remains subjective.

Harm and good can co-exist: *double effect*. If relieving pain is good, but killing is harmful, morphine can both do good (relieve pain) and harm (kill). Pope Pius XII ruled that actions (e.g. giving morphine) should be judged by primary and secondary intentions (Rachels, 1986). If the primary intention is to relieve pain, then undesirable effects of hastening death may be acceptable, whereas giving morphine with the primary intention of hastening death is active euthanasia, a criminal offence in the UK. If in any doubt about patients' comfort, pain relief should be provided (BMA, 2002).

If life is sacrosanct, then *death* becomes the greatest possible harm, but if death is preferable to continued suffering, then life support can be harmful. Harm (quality of life) is therefore individual, unpredictable and debateable. For patients, the quality of their death is important (Curtis, 1998). Where prognosis is unacceptably poor, withdrawing or withholding active treatment, including cardiopulmonary resuscitation, is humane and beneficent. Hospitals have detailed policies and guidelines for designating patients 'not for cardiopulmonary resuscitation', so readers should be familiar with their local policies.

There is no legal or moral difference between withholding and withdrawing treatment (BMA, 2002). Death of critically ill patients usually follows within hours of decisions to withdraw (Hall & Rocker, 2000), but methods of withdrawing vary between doctors, individual patients and (sometimes) according to bed demand (Ravenscroft & Bell, 2000). Most ICUs stop supplementary oxygen, inotropes and haemofiltration, but maintain ventilation. Roman Catholic theology distinguishes ordinary from extraordinary interventions (Rachels, 1986): ordinary ('natural'/'God-given') must be preserved, but extraordinary (created by humans, so unnatural) interventions may be withdrawn. Ventilators replace breathing, a natural function, so may be 'ordinary', whereas drugs (e.g. inotropes) may not. The House of Lords (1993) ruled nasogastric tubes were 'extraordinary', creating an apparent absurdity of nasogastric tubes being extraordinary, while ventilators are ordinary. When active treatment is withdrawn, palliative care should continue, including maintaining comfort and fundamental care. Each team member has to live with their own conscience, so decisions should be humane, and reflect consensus of the whole team.

Euthanasia ('good death') presumes life is no longer preferable to death, so treatment becomes harmful, 'mercy killing' (active euthanasia) or 'letting die' (passive euthanasia) becomes beneficent. Active euthanasia is illegal (murder) in the UK (and most nations), and despite some calls for its legalisation, such as Doyal's (2001) BMJ editorial, is likely to remain illegal in the UK. In Oregon, USA, where active euthanasia is legal, half of the patients who requested euthanasia changed their minds, incidence being especially high among those with symptoms of depression (Emmanuel et al., 2000). The high incidence of acute psychoses among ICU patients would make this an especially vulnerable group if euthanasia were to be legalised in the UK.

### Justice

Justice carries connotations of

- retribution/punishment
- fairness.

Denying treatment to one group of patients (e.g. cardiac surgery to current smokers) may be viewed as *punishment* for their deliberate actions. But limited resources necessitates rationing, which should attempt *fairness*. But fairness is subjective – those denied access usually consider injustice has been performed.

NHS *rationing* largely adopts the 'first come first served' principle; private healthcare tends to ration by ability to pay. But healthcare professionals normally wish to be fair, so when demand on ICU beds exceeds, decisions may be made to discharge/transfer prematurely, or set earlier time-limits on active treatments. Budgetary and political pressures may conflict with nurses' duty of care and their own values of fairness.

## Ethical theories

### Duty

Duty-based theory (deontology) develops Kant's belief that people are an end in themselves, not the means to an end. These values are reflected in nursing by respect for individuals and duty of care.

These apparently laudable aims can create dilemmas:

- Nursing is learnt through clinical practice, so patient care (means) is a learning experience (end) for the nurse.
- Nurses caring for two patients (e.g. covering breaks) may have to choose between two conflicting duties of care.
- How far does (moral) duty of care extend? Refusing admission because beds are unavailable means denying care.
- Whether nurses who have not completed care (e.g. nursing records) when shifts end should work (usually unpaid overtime) to complete their duty of care?

### Goal

Goal-based (utilitarian, consequentialist) theory supports actions that achieve desired goals – 'the end justifies the means' or 'the greatest good for the greatest number'. This could justify rationing services that do not meet the needs of the majority, and arguably underlies nearly every healthcare macro reorganisation.

At micro level, goal-based ethics is not widely used in the UK. It can disadvantage minorities simply because they are minorities. The recent Alder Hey scandal, where organs were retrieved from children without consent may have been motivated by utilitarian ethics (or may have been simple system error). For the ICU, utilitarianism could justify closure, as compared with most specialities, ICU costs per patient are disproportionately large.

## Rights

The right of one person necessarily imposes a duty on another person, so nurse advocacy may be a consequential duty of patients' rights. But rights of two different people may conflict. Many units have afternoon rest periods. While afternoon rest benefits many, some patients remain awake and bored throughout the rest period. Claiming to uphold others' rights (e.g. nurse advocacy) may be used for paternalistic or other ends.

## Implications for practice

- Ethical principles and theories provide frameworks for reflection.
- Each nurse should clarify their own values and beliefs, considering their ethical contexts, and apply ethical frameworks to help guide their practice.
- Ethical dilemmas seldom have absolute answers, but ethics can help nurses justify professional decisions, recognising that different ethical beliefs may result in differing conclusions.
- Advance directives ('living wills') are legally binding for opting out of, but not into, treatments.
- Where possible and appropriate, patient choice should be empowered.
- When paternalistic decisions are necessary, they should be guided by patients' best interests.
- Practice raises various ethical dilemmas; informal discussion can be cathartic, while ethical forums (preferably multidisciplinary) can diffuse conflict and contribute to professional (and unit) development.

## Summary

Ethics is about understanding values and justifying decision-making. The ethical principles and theories outlined in this chapter provide frameworks for considering dilemmas raised in later chapters or through practice. Various dilemmas have been (briefly) raised; each can be pursued through the wide range of texts and articles on ethics. But ethics should be used to guide practice, not stored on library shelves. Readers are therefore encouraged to consider and discuss ethical dilemmas with colleagues.

## Further reading

Useful books on ethics include Beauchamp and Childress (2001) biomedical text, Tschudin's (2003) nursing text and Draper and Scott's (2004) intensive care focused book. There are nursing and medical journals devoted to ethical issues, but other journals frequently include ethics. Dimond (2005) remains the key text on nursing and the law.

Authorities such as the World Health Organisation, Department of Health, and professional bodies, have issued important guidelines and ethical requirements, such as *The Declaration of Helsinki* (World Medical Association, 2000), and DOH (2001a, 2001b). www.routledge.com/textbooks/0415373239

For clinical scenarios, clinical questions and the answers to them go to the support website at www.routledge.com/textbooks/0415373239

## Clinical scenarios

John, a 65-year-old business man and long-term ICU patient, is dependant on invasive ventilatory support and vasoactive drugs. He is the most stable ICU patient on a day when the ICU is full and another ward patient requires admission following their successful cardiopulmonary resuscitation. A decision is made to transfer John to an ICU in another hospital in order to admit the more critically ill patient. John and his relatives refuse to be transferred.

Q.1 Which ethical principle guided the decision to transfer John?

Q.2 Can John (or his relatives) override this decision?

Q.3 Identify other ethical principles involved and any ethical conflicts (e.g. with John's autonomy, non-maleficence, consent, justice, resource distribution, Code of Professional Conduct).

Q.4 Compare your ethical understanding and moral reasoning with that of other members of the interdisciplinary team (e.g. other grades, doctors) and legal department of your hospital.

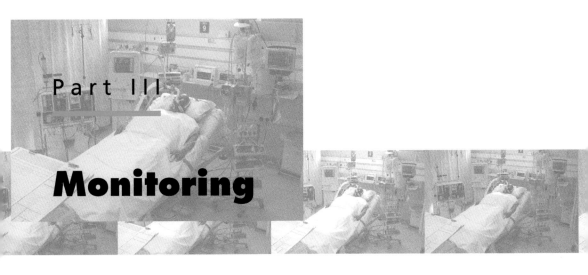

# Part III

# Monitoring

# Chapter 17

# Respiratory monitoring

## Contents

| | |
|---|---|
| Introduction | 160 |
| Visual | 160 |
| Tactile | 161 |
| Auscultation | 161 |
| Breath waveform | 163 |
| Indexed measurements | 165 |
| Pulse oximetry | 165 |
| Capnography | 167 |
| Implications for practice | 167 |
| Summary | 168 |
| Further reading | 168 |
| Clinical scenarios | 168 |

## Fundamental knowledge

Haemoglobin carriage of oxygen (see Chapter 18)
Respiratory anatomy
Normal mechanics of breathing – muscles, negative pressure
Cough reflex and physiology

## Introduction

Traditional nursing observations of respiratory rate and depth are extended in the ICU by visual and aural observation of ventilation. This Chapter assumes familiarity with simpler respiratory observations; ventilator settings are discussed in Chapter 4 and arterial blood gas analysis in Chapter 19. Lung function tests, such as spirometry and forced expiratory volume, which have little value for most ICU patients, are not discussed, but may occasionally be used when assessing patients receiving noninvasive ventilation, especially for COPD. This chapter mainly describes technological monitoring used by nurses. Means used by other professions (e.g. chest X-rays, imaging, bronchoscopy) are not discussed. Whatever the means used, all procedures should be explained to patients.

Much information is gathered from machines, which may have 'acceptable' error margins of 5–10 per cent. Isolated figures mean little. Trends should be assessed, and interpreted holistically, in the context of individual patients.

## Visual

Respiratory history is usually gained from individual handover and interdisciplinary notes – medical, nursing, physiotherapy. Additional valuable fundamental information can be gained visually:

- Skin colour and texture (and any clamminess) indicates perfusion – especially lips and tongue.
- Finger clubbing and abnormal chest shape indicate chronic problems.
- Accessory muscle use indicates respiratory distress.
- Shallow breathing may reflect reduced demand, but with tachypnoea indicates other problems – possibilities include pain or limited airflow.
- Unequal chest wall movement – causes should be investigated, but could include pneumothorax.

Other signs of respiratory problem include

- inability to complete sentences without pausing for breath
- sudden confusion – more often caused by hypoxia than nonrespiratory factors
- cyanosis – a late sign, appearing only with desturation <85–90 per cent, and not appearing with severe anaemia (<3–5 g/dl (Lumb 2000; Darovic, 2002a)).

Cough reflex (e.g. on suction) may be lost with deep unconsciousness, but most ICU patients retain some (weakened) cough reflex. Coughs may be productive or unproductive. Unproductive coughs may be caused by absence of anything in airways to clear or insufficient force. If extubated, ability to cough effectively could be assessed by peak flow – below 160 litres/minute usually indicates insufficiency. Coughing should be assessed and observations recorded.

**Table 17.1 Sputum colour – possible causes**

| Colour | Possible cause |
| --- | --- |
| Black | Tar (cigarette smoking) |
| | Old blood |
| | Coal (in ex-miners) |
| | Smoke inhalation (rescued from fires) |
| Pink | Fresh blood (Frothy pink sputum often |
| | indicates pulmonary oedema) |
| Cream, green | Infection |
| Yellow | Infection |
| | Allergy (e.g. asthma) |

Sputum should be observed for

- volume
- colour (see Table 17.1)
- consistency (e.g. frothy, tenacious, watery)
- purulence
- haemoptysis.

If specimens are required, these should be collected and sent without delay. Observations (including frequency of suction) should be recorded.

## Tactile

Movement of sputum in larger airways can create vibration on the chest wall, which may be felt by placing a flat hand palm-down across the sternum ('tactile crepitations'). Although not as reliable as auscultation, this can quickly identify need for suction, but if no vibration is felt, lungs fields should be auscultated.

## Auscultation

Breath sounds are created by air turbulence, and are useful to assess

- intubation (bilateral air entry)
- bronchial patency/bronchospasm
- secretions
- effect of suction (before and after).

Breath sounds should be assessed at the start of each shift. Stethoscopes are usually best placed over

- right and left main bronchi
- mid-lobe (usually just to the side of the nipple)
- bases of lungs (front, side or back).

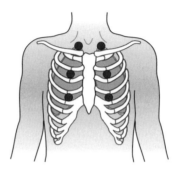

**■ *Figure 17.1* Auscultation sites for breath sounds (anterior chest wall)**

comparing sounds from both lungs (see Figure 17.1). All sounds are created in bronchioles but transmitted and dulled through lower airways. Chest (and abdominal) sounds can be deceptive, so should not be absolutely relied upon.

Sounds may be normal, abnormal, diminished or absent. Abnormal sounds may be heard on inspiration, expiration, or on both phases, so having identified abnormal sounds, nurses should listen to further breaths to identify on which phases sounds occur. Names of sounds vary between texts (Wilkins *et al.*, 2004), but normal sounds are often called:

- *bronchial*: high pitched, loud, air blowing through a tube (the trachea)
- *bronchovesicular*: medium pitch, heard at lung apices
- *vesicular*: low pitch and volume, like rustling wind, heard in most parts of lungs.

Abnormal sounds include

- *stridor*: monophonic inspiratory wheezes from severe laryngeal or tracheal obstruction
- *wheeze (rhonchi)*: obstruction of lower airways. Inspiratory wheezes indicate constant obstruction (e.g. COPD), whereas expiratory wheezes indicate bronchospasm
- *crackle (rales, crepitations)*: abnormal fluid may in airways (e.g. mucous) or interstitial spaces (e.g. pulmonary oedema)
- *pleural rub*: grating sound caused by friction between inflamed pleural surfaces from pleural disease (e.g. pneumonia, pleurisy).

Absent sound may indicate absent airflow:

- obstruction (sputum plug)
- pneumothorax

■ atelectasis
■ emphysema.

or lack of transmission to the chest wall (e.g. obesity, small tidal volume, pleural effusion, pneumothorax).
    Artefactual sounds include

■ heartbeat
■ gut movement
■ clothing
■ friction of stethoscope against equipment (e.g. cotsides)
■ chest hair (crackles)
■ airflow in special beds.

Interpreting breath sounds is a skill. Listening to healthy lungs (your own) is an essential baseline. Readers unfamiliar with listening to abnormal breath sounds should ask a respiratory physiotherapist or other expert to auscultate with them. Recordings of breath sounds (see further reading) are also valuable.

## Breath waveform

Figure 17.2 shows a normal self-ventilated breath waveform. Each breath has three active phases:

■ inspiration
■ inspiratory hold (or 'plateau')
■ expiration.

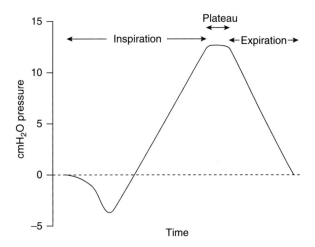

**Figure 17.2 Normal (self-ventilating) breath waveform**

A fourth phase is passive:

■  expiratory hold.

Inspiration affects, and is affected by, bronchial muscle stretch; patients with chronic obstructive pulmonary disease cannot fully dilate bronchi during short inspiratory time. Most gas exchange occurs during plateau (peak inflation pressure). Expiration is passive recoil; short expiration time of muscle spasm (asthma) causes gas trapping (and distress).

   Positive-pressure ventilation creates slightly different patterns, which can be manipulated to optimise ventilation. Waveform displays (available on most ventilators) indicate effectiveness of modes and settings (Branson, 2005), so enabling changes to

■  maximise volume while minimising peak inflation pressure
■  reduce work of breathing
■  reverse atelectasis (recruit alveoli)
■  improve lung compliance.

Waveform displays compare two variables, such as

■  flow:time
■  pressure:time
■  pressure:volume (see Figure 17.3).

Pressure:volume loops indicate compliance. Flow:time graphs show triggering below the baseline. This should then be followed by rising inspiratory flow (above the baseline). Triggers without inspiratory flow indicate wasted work of breathing. Expiratory flow on flow:time graphs normally returns below the

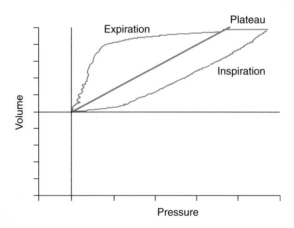

■ *Figure 17.3 Pressure:volume (hysteresis) graph*

baseline; if above, gas-trapping is occurring. Manufacturers' booklets often provide usefully illustrated guides to what is available, and readers not familiar with observing waveforms should set up a ventilator circuit with a test lung, viewing various modes, and manipulating the test lung to mimic coughs, a triggered breath and resistance.

Waveforms are affected by ventilator settings and modes. For example, pressure controlled modes make pressure waveforms peak at preset pressures, regardless of what happens in airways (e.g. sputum plug, biting tube).

## Indexed measurements

Attempts to rationalise and weaning have encouraged quantification of respiratory function, usually indexed to patient size. Two examples are Oxygen Index (OI)

$$= \frac{FiO_2 \times MAP \times 100}{PaO_2}$$

and Rapid Shallow Breathing Index (RSBi)

$$= \frac{\text{respiratory rate (f)}}{\text{tidal volume } (V_T) \text{ in litres}}$$

Advocates claim oxygen index $> 26$ or RSBi $< 100$ indicates likely successful weaning, but reliability of either measurement remains unclear.

## Pulse oximetry

Pulse oximetry indicates peripheral (capillary) saturation of haemoglobin by oxygen ($SpO_2$). In health, peripheral and arterial saturations are within 2 per cent (Jensen et al., 1998), making $SpO_2$ and $SaO_2$ practically identical.

Pulse oximetry is noninvasive and continuous, so is a useful means to monitor oxygenation. However, oximetry measures saturation of haemoglobin – the oxygen stored in the haemoglobin 'bank'. Because oxygen dissociation from haemoglobin is complex, the relationship between $SO_2$ and partial pressure of oxygen in arterial blood ($PaO_2$) varies – see the oxygen dissociation curve in Chapter 18. While most arterial oxygen is transported by haemoglobin, the little dissolved in plasma is immediately available for diffusion. As $PaO_2$ determines oxygen transfer into tissues, oximetry seldom substitutes for arterial blood gas analysis in critically ill patients.

Limitations of oximetry include

■ *poor perfusion:* pulse oximetry calculates saturation by measuring light absorption through a finger or other tissue. Only 2 per cent of total light absorption is by blood, so poor blood flow causes unreliable signals ('noisy signal'). Most oximeters in the ICU show capillary pulse waveforms (*plethysmograph* or 'pleth'), which should reflect arterial pulses. Poor waveforms indicate insufficient signal (blood supply), probably making readings spurious. Repositioning probes, or warming peripheries, may improve accuracy

■ *anaemia*: oximetry measures percentage saturation of haemoglobin, not quantity of haemoglobin, or oxygen, available. Saturation should always be interpreted relation to haemoglobin levels

■ *haemoglobinopathies*: although detecting problems with oxygen carriage, oximetry cannot identify causes; laboratory analysis and other clinical signs remain necessary to fully assess respiratory pathophysiology

■ *carbon monoxide* saturates haemoglobin, making it bright red, allowing transmission of more light across the finger. Normally little or no carbon monoxide (0–2 per cent) is either present in air or produced by the body. Carboxyhaemoglobin levels above 3 per cent cause over-reading (Jensen et al., 1998). Peripheral oximetry is unreliable with carbon monoxide poisoning (smoke inhalation, car-exhaust inhalation, faulty gas appliances, tobacco inhalation). Blood gas analysers use many more colours than oximeters, so blood gas analysis saturation is reliable with carboxyhaemoglobin

■ *hypercapnia*: oximetry does not measure carbon dioxide. Carbon dioxide can be assessed by blood gas analysis, end-tidal carbon dioxide and depth/rate of breathing

■ *shivering* prevents clear signals, so causing low, or no, readings

■ *dark colours* either on the skin (e.g. skin colour, nail varnish) or in blood (e.g. bilirubinaemia), absorb more red light, causing under-readings of 3–5 per cent (Wahr & Tremper, 1996). Trends remain constant, but patients' saturation may be slightly higher than what oximeters indicate (blood gas analyser saturation is more accurate)

■ *intravenous dyes* are usually used to show arteries (blue dyes) or veins (red dyes). Blue dyes absorb more red light, so cause oximetry under-readings, while red dyes transmit more red light, causing over-readings. Methylthioninium chloride (formerly called 'methylene blue' in the UK) is a widely used contrast. Dye half-life indicates how long dyes may affect readings. Intravenous dyes may be metabolised relatively quickly, and so cause unreliable trends due to diminishing effect

■ *external light*, if detected by the light sensor, can affect readings, red (e.g. sunlight) causing over-readings, and blue (e.g. florescent) causing under-readings. These can affect probes on ears – finger probes are contoured for fingers, not ears, and ear probes lack light shields. Shielding ear probes from light may give lower, more accurate, results

■ *low level accuracy*: accuracy below SpO$_2$ of 80 per cent remains unproven on most machines. Such dangerously low levels should necessitate urgent arterial blood gas analysis rather than esoteric discussion about accuracy

■ *burns*: a Medical Devices Agency (MDA, 2001) safety notice instructs

● tape should not be used to hold probes in place (unless recommended by manufacturers)

- probes should be checked and resited at least every four hours, or more frequently if indicated by manufacturer's recommendations or patients' circulatory status and/or skin integrity.

As readings would normally be recorded hourly, it seems sensible to change sites with each recording site used on observation charts.

## Capnography

End-tidal carbon dioxide ($PECO_2/PETCO_2$) enables continuous noninvasive breath-by-breath monitoring of expired concentrations, end-tidal approximating to residual alveoli levels. Comparing arterial and end-tidal carbon dioxide indicates dead-space. $PECO_2$ is usually <1 kPa below arterial tensions (Capovilla et al., 2000), but ratios between expired and mixed venous carbon dioxide diminish as deadspace increases (V/Q mismatch).

Capnography increases deadspace, and expired carbon dioxide seldom fully reflects alveolar concentrations or function, but where carbon dioxide causes particular concern (e.g. inverse ratio ventilation, permissive hypercapnia, head injury, high frequency ventilation and other alternative modes) it may show useful trends.

Maciel et al. (2004) found sublingual PCO2 ( $P_{sl}CO_2$) reliable.

## Implications for practice

- Information should be interpreted holistically – in the context of other relevant observations, underlying disease and treatments.
- Respiratory monitoring should meet clinical needs while minimising risks, where appropriate noninvasive or minimally invasive modes should be selected.
- ICU nurses should undertake visual, tactile and auscultatory respiratory assessment on all patients.

  - ICU nurses should recognise different breath sounds, recording and reporting any changes.
  - Cough reflex and strength should be assessed.

- Ventilator waveform display indicates airway response to ventilation, enabling optimal adjustment of settings.
- Pulse oximetry provides continuous information about haemoglobin saturation by oxygen, but does not measure

  - oxygen carrying capacity (Hb)
  - carbon dioxide

  and may be affected by other factors.
- Oximeter probes should be moved frequently, usually 1–2 hourly.

■ Poor ('damp') waveforms on pulse oximetry or capnography indicate readings are probably unreliable.

■ Spirometry and vital capacity assessment may be useful with noninvasive ventilation and extubated patients, especially if they have COPD. Low peak flow (<160 litres/minute) and vital capacity (<2.5 litres) indicate poor respiratory function and probable inability to cough effectively.

## Summary

Respiratory monitoring is fundamental to intensive care. Much can be assessed non0invasively, by listening and looking. Ventilators provide much information, especially if waveforms are displayed. Readers should take early opportunities to become familiar with available means of respiratory monitoring on their units. Whatever means is used, observations can only be as reliable as those making and interpreting the observations. ICU nurses therefore should understand the physiology and mechanics of lung function and pathophysiology. Respiratory monitoring is therefore fundamental to care underlying many of the pathologies discussed in the third section of this book.

## Further reading

Most texts describe widely used methods of monitoring. Classic texts include Lumb's (2000) respiratory physiology, and Darovic's (2002a) haemodynamic monitoring (including a chapter on respiratory assessment). Wilkins *et al.* (2004) describe lung sounds, providing a useful accompanying CD. Law (2000) provides a useful guide to assessing sputum. Articles on oximetry, such as Fox (2002) and Allen (2004) periodically appear in nursing journals.

For readers seeking information about tests not described here, useful pocket books include Dakin *et al.* (2003) on lung function tests, and Corne *et al.* (2002) or Jenkins (2005) on X-rays. www.routledge.com/textbooks/0415373239

For clinical scenarios, clinical questions and the answers to them go to the support website at www.routledge.com/textbooks/0415373239

## Clinical scenarios

Kathleen Fogarty is a 58-year-old lady who was admitted to the ICU for mechanical ventilation to support deteriorating respiratory function. The cause of her recent deterioration is unknown, but possible diagnoses include bronchospasm, basal pneumonia or aspiration of upper airway secretions.

Kathleen has a visible and widespread drug-related erythematous rash, worse at extremities and extensive oral ulcerations. Kathleen's sputum is thick, mucopurulent, yellow-green and copious. On auscultation, she has expiratory phase and late expiratory wheeze, vesicular breath sounds are diminished in apices and crackles in right base. Kathleen's $E_TCO_2$ is 6.5 kPa and $SpO_2$: 94 per cent.

Q.1 Identify and interpret Kathleen's abnormal lung sounds; explain their relevance to other results and her recent deterioration.

Q.2 Review additional investigations or monitoring required to fully assess Kathleen's respiratory function.

Q.3 Evaluate the nurse's role with respiratory monitoring in your own clinical area. Consider the range of monitoring approaches available and the nurse's role in interpreting and acting on results, troubleshooting, training and supervising.

# Chapter 18

# Gas carriage

## Contents

| | |
|---|---|
| Introduction | 171 |
| Partial pressure | 171 |
| Oxygen carriage | 172 |
| Haemoglobin | 172 |
| Oxygen dissociation curve | 173 |
| Cell respiration | 174 |
| Oxygen debt | 175 |
| Oxygen toxicity | 175 |
| Carbon dioxide transport | 175 |
| Heliox | 176 |
| Haemoglobinopathies | 177 |
| Implications for practice | 179 |
| Summary | 179 |
| Further reading | 179 |
| Support groups | 180 |
| Clinical scenarios | 180 |

## Fundamental knowledge

Pulmonary anatomy and physiology (including vasculature)
Normal respiration (including chemical + neurological
    control and mechanics of external respiration)
Deadspace
Erythropoietin and erythropoiesis
Types of anaemias (listed in Table 21.2)

## Introduction

Studying physiology and pathology necessitates reductionism, but body systems function as parts of the whole body, not in isolation. Cardiovascular and respiratory functions are particularly closely interdependent: delivering oxygen and nutrients to tissues, while removing carbon dioxide and other waste. Respiration should achieve adequate tissue oxygenation, so gas movement across lung membranes forms external respiration, gas movement between tissue cells and capillaries forms internal respiration.

This chapter explores internal respiration, identifying various factors that affect tissue perfusion and oxygenation. The structure of haemoglobin, and its effect on oxygen carriage and the oxygen saturation curve are identified. Carbon dioxide carriage and some haemoglobinopathies (carbon monoxide poisoning, sickle cell, thalassaemia) are also discussed.

Fraction of inspired oxygen ($FiO_2$) should be expressed as a fraction (or decimal). So 100 per cent oxygen = $FiO_2$ of 1.0 (not 100).

## Partial pressure

Transfer of gases across capillary membranes is determined by pressure gradients, so differences between partial pressure of intracellular and capillary oxygen levels determine tissue oxygenation. Partial pressure of arterial oxygen ($PaO_2$) therefore indicates oxygen available for diffusion to cells.

Air is approximately 21 per cent oxygen and 79 per cent nitrogen, with negligible amounts of other gases – only 0.04 per cent is carbon dioxide. Barometric, and so alveolar, pressure (at sea level) is 101.3 kPa. Total atmospheric pressure includes water vapour. At 37°C (i.e. normal alveolar temperature) water vapour exerts a constant pressure of 6.3 kPa, irrespective of total barometric pressure. Pressure of all gases is the difference between total barometric pressure and water vapour. This is then divided proportionally between the different gases (see Table 18.1).

Alveolar gas tensions are altered by rebreathing 'deadspace' gas, relatively carbon dioxide rich and oxygen poor. Physiological adult deadspace is about 150 ml, with additional pathological deadspace when alveoli are not perfused. Artificial ventilation deadspace begins at the inspiratory limb ('Y' connector)

*Table 18.1* **Partial pressures of gases at sea level (approximate)**

|  | Concentration in air (%) | Pressure in air (kPa) | Pressure in alveoli[a] (kPa) |
|---|---|---|---|
| Water vapour |  | variable[b] | 6.3 |
| Oxygen | 21 | 21.27 | 13.3 |
| Carbon dioxide | 0.03 | 0.03 | 5.3 |
| Nitrogen | 79 | 80 | 76.4 |

Notes:
[a] Warmed to 37°C, hence constant water vapour
[b] Depends on temperature

of ventilator tubing. Small breaths or large deadspace therefore lower alveolar partial pressure of oxygen ($PO_2$).

## Oxygen carriage

Oxygen is carried by blood in two ways:

- plasma (3 per cent)
- haemoglobin (97 per cent).

At normal (sea-level) atmospheric pressure 3 ml of oxygen is dissolved in every litre of blood, so an average 5 l circulation would contain 15 ml of oxygen, insufficient to maintain life. When haemoglobin oxygen carriage is prevented (e.g. carbon monoxide poisoning), increasing atmospheric pressure (hyperbaric oxygen) increases plasma carriage, enabling therapeutic levels to be achieved. Oxygen tension in plasma determines partial pressure ($PO_2$), the pressure gradient that enables transfer of oxygen to tissues.

Tissue oxygen supply is affected by

- haemoglobin level
- oxygen saturation of haemoglobin
- oxygen dissociation
- perfusion pressure.

Perfusion pressure is discussed in other chapters.

## Haemoglobin

Erythrocytes are mainly haemoglobin. Erythrocyte diameter averages 7 nanometers (nm), just smaller than capillaries (8–10 nm). This places haemoglobin, and oxygen, close to capillary walls. Unlike carbon dioxide, oxygen is not a very soluble gas, so minimising distance between haemoglobin and cells outside capillaries optimises oxygen delivery to cells.

Haemoglobin (Hb) combines haem (iron) and globin (polypeptide protein). 'Normal' levels are 14–18 g/dl for men and 12–16 g/dl for women, but while lower concentrations reduce oxygen carrying capacity, haemodilution improves perfusion (oxygen delivery), so survival from critical illness is highest when haemoglobin is 7–9 g/dl (Herbert *et al.*, 1999), although specific groups, such as older people, may benefit from higher levels (Boralessa *et al.*, 2003).

Polypeptides of normal adult haemoglobin (HbA) consist of two alpha and two beta chains: $\alpha_2 + \beta_2$. Slight biochemical differences between alpha and beta chains are insignificant for clinical nursing, but abnormalities of either chain can cause pathologies. Haemoglobin has a high affinity for oxygen. If all four limbs of the molecule carry oxygen, it is described as fully (100 per cent) saturated. Normal arterial ($SaO_2$) or capillary (peripheral – $SpO_2$) saturation is about 97 per cent.

**Table 18.2 Some factors affecting oxygen dissociation**

Curve shifts to right (increased oxygen dissociation from haemoglobin) with
■ increased temperature
■ acidosis (pH) – the Böhr effect
■ increased $CO_2$
■ increased 2,3 DPG (diphosphoglycerate).

Curve shifts to left (decreased oxygen dissociation from haemoglobin) with
■ reduced temperature
■ alkalosis
■ (some) haemoglobinopathies (e.g. HbF)
■ carbon monoxide
■ decreased $CO_2$
■ decreased 2,3 DPG (diphosphoglycerate).

While haemoglobin transports oxygen efficiently, its high affinity for oxygen limits dissociation: only 20–25 per cent of available oxygen normally unloads, making normal venous saturations ($SvO_2$) 70–75 per cent. This large venous reserve can provide oxygen without any increase in respiration rate or cardiac output. While $SaO_2$ indicates oxygen availability, the $SaO_2$–$SvO_2$ gradient indicates tissue uptake (consumption) of oxygen.

Intracellular changes in haemoglobin molecules can change ('shift') oxyhaemoglobin dissociation. Shifts to the left reduce, while shifts to the right increase, dissociation (see Table 18.2). For example, reduced dissociation with alkalosis may cause low $PaO_2$ and oxygen delivery to tissue, despite high $SpO_2$.

Foetal haemoglobin (HbF) resembles haemoglobin A, except that gamma ($\gamma$) chains replace beta and 2,3 DPG (diphosphoglycerate) concentrations are higher. Gamma chains increase affinity for oxygen, facilitating transfer from maternal blood (HbA). By 6 months of age, 96 per cent of haemoglobin is normally adult haemoglobin (HbA) (Lloyd & Lewis, 1999), but foetal haemoglobin can (abnormally) persist throughout life, predisposing its carrier to tissue hypoxia. Other haemoglobinopathies are discussed later.

Other measurements that are useful to some diseases include

■ *O2Hb*: fraction of total haemoglobin combined with oxygen
■ *MetHb* (methaemoglobin): oxidised iron ($Fe^{+++}$) in haemoglobin reduces oxygen carriage. Normally methaemoglobin is <2 per cent. Nitric oxide can cause methaemoglobin, but this is rarely used now
■ *RHb*: reduced or deoxygenated haemoglobin, usually associated with blood transfusions.

## Oxygen dissociation curve

Saturation of haemoglobin by oxygen $SO_2$ and partial pressure of oxygen ($PO_2$) measure different aspects of oxygen carriage – comparable to differences between money in bank accounts (haemoglobin – $SaO_2$) and ready cash (plasma – $PaO_2$). Because dissociation of oxygen from haemoglobin changes,

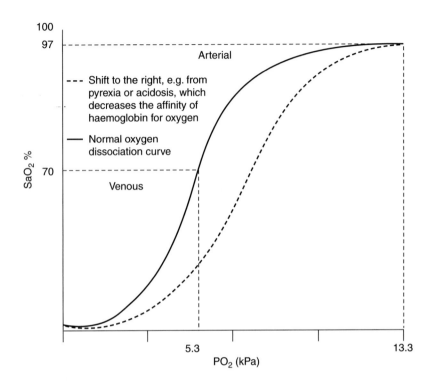

**Figure 18.1 Oxygen dissociation curve**

relationship between $SaO_2$ and $PaO_2$ varies, represented by the oxygen dissociation curve (see Figure 18.1). On the *plateau* ($SaO_2 > 95$ per cent), oxygen
readily dissociates from haemoglobin, causing marked changes in $PaO_2$ with
little/no change in $SaO_2$. Below the 'venous point' (75 per cent saturation),
$SaO_2$ falls rapidly while $PaO_2$ hardly changes.

## Cell respiration

The purpose of respiratory function is to supply tissue cells with sufficient
oxygen to enable aerobic metabolism in mitochondria. Measuring mitochondrial respiration is not practical, so cruder parameters (e.g. arterial gas tensions) are measured instead. However, measured parameters only partly
indicate delivery of oxygen to cells, and removal of carbon dioxide.

Partial pressures of oxygen progressively fall with further stages of internal
respiration: capillary pressure of 6.8 kPa gives tissue pressure of 2.7 kPa, and
mitochondrial pressure of 0.13–1.3 kPa. Conversely, intracellular carbon
dioxide tensions are higher. Relative differences in pressures create the
concentration gradient that enables diffusion across capillary and cell membranes. Reduced alveolar partial pressure (from respiratory failure) reflects
proportional reductions in tensions elsewhere, resulting in tissue hypoxia.

Supplementary oxygen increases alveolar tensions, proportionally increas' tensions elsewhere.

## Oxygen debt

In hypoxic conditions, oxygen and glycogen are withdrawn from haemoglobin and myoglobin (muscles), creating a 'debt' that is normally repaid once high oxygen demand ceases. So after completing strenuous exercise we continue to breathe deeply. Anaerobic metabolism for intracellular ATP production produces lactic acid.

Prolonged critical illness can cause cumulative oxygen debt which, with recovery, flushes toxic acids and cytokines into the circulation, causing potential reperfusion injury (see Chapter 24).

## Oxygen toxicity

Hyperoxia releases free oxygen radicals (Wilson et al., 2001), so prolonged exposure to high concentrations of oxygen can damage lung tissue. High concentration oxygen also 'washes out' nitrogen from lungs – nitrogen being an inert gas, and the majority (79 per cent) of air, distends alveoli. Increasing oxygen concentration reduces nitrogen, potentially causing atelectasis. Maximum concentrations and time are debated, but most intensivists aim to limit prolonged (>24 hours) supplementary oxygen to <60 per cent. Short periods of high concentration do not appear to cause harm. Severe hypoxia sometimes necessitates using high concentrations, so risks from tissue hypoxia should be weighted against dangers from oxygen toxicity. PEEP helps prevent atelectasis from nitrogen washout.

## Carbon dioxide transport

Air contains virtually no carbon dioxide (0.04 per cent). Metabolism produces 200 ml of carbon dioxide every minute. Carbon dioxide diffuses by concentration gradients from cells into capillary blood, and from pulmonary capillaries into alveoli. Normal concentrations of blood carbon dioxide are 48 ml/decilitre (arterial) to 52 ml/decilitre (venous). Carbon dioxide is normally the most important 'drive' for the respiratory centre in the brainstem. Carbon dioxide is also vasoactive, stimulating vasoconstriction.

Carbon dioxide carriage is relatively simple compared with oxygen carriage. It is carried in blood through three means:

- plasma
- haemoglobin
- bicarbonate.

*Plasma* – Carbon dioxide is approximately twenty times more soluble than oxygen, so is readily carried in solution by plasma.

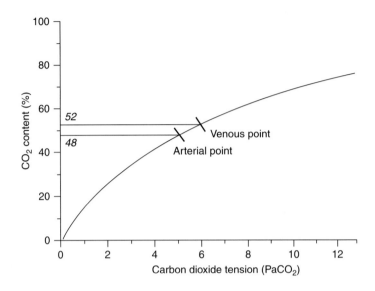

**Figure 18.2 Carbon dioxide dissociation curve**

*Haemoglobin* – A quarter of carbon dioxide is carried as carbaminoglobin. Carbon dioxide binds to globin, not haem, so unlike carbon monoxide does not displace oxygen.

*Bicarbonate* – Most (approximately three-quarters) of carbon dioxide carriage occurs as a component of plasma bicarbonate.

Diffusion of carbon dioxide occurs through simple tension gradients, making the carbon dioxide dissociation curve virtually linear (see Figure 18.2). Like the oxygen dissociation curve, carbon dioxide dissociation can move to the right or left. Rightward shifts (lowering carbon dioxide content per unit of $pCO_2$) occur with raised oxygen concentrations in blood, and is sometimes called the 'Haldane effect'.

## Heliox

Like air, heliox contains 21 per cent oxygen, but instead of nitrogen, the remainder is helium. Helium has a low density (three times less than air) so, being less affected by airway resistance, reduces work of breathing (Kass, 2003; Reuben & Harris, 2004). With airway obstruction, where work of breathing is excessive, heliox may enable adequate oxygenation. It should be given through a non-rebreathing mask so it is not diluted with room air (Kass, 2003). Benefits should occur within minutes, buying time to resolve the underlying problem (Calzia & Stahl, 2004). Its value beyond one hour is limited (Ho *et al.*, 2003). Use and availability are often limited by its relative expense, although costs of alternatives, and need for urgent intervention, may make it cost-effective.

Heliox is useful in acute severe asthma, gaining time for steroids to work (Kass & Terregino, 1999). It has also been useful with noninvasive ventilation (Jaber *et al.*, 2000), although few ventilators (invasive or noninvasive) are designed to work with heliox (Calzia & Stahl, 2004), and it may affect ventilator monitoring. An animal study found heliox increased hypercapnia and respiratory acidosis (Watremez *et al.*, 2003).

Heliox is inert, colourless, odourless and tasteless. It disperses quickly, so should not significantly affect anyone nearby. It does however affect patients' vocal cords, so they should be warned about a temporary high-pitched, squeaky voice.

## Haemoglobinopathies

Critical illness is frequently complicated by haemoglobinopathies; three are described below.

*Carbon monoxide* poisoning causes about one thousand deaths each year in the UK. There are four likely causes of carbon monoxide poisoning in patients:

- suicide attempts using car exhaust fumes – 45 per cent of cases (Harvey & Hutton, 1999)
- smoking
- faulty gas appliances
- smoke inhalation (fire victims).

Carbon monoxide is usually measured by blood gas analysers (COHb or FCOHb).

Normal concentrations of carbon monoxide in air and the body are insignificant, non-smoker levels normally being 1 per cent or less. Endogenous production can increase with some pathologies – for example, haemolytic anaemia can cause levels of 5 per cent (Blumenthal, 2001). Heavy cigarette smokers may have 15 per cent carboxyhaemoglobin (Blumenthal, 2001), while cigar smokers' levels may reach 20 per cent (Harvey & Hutton, 1999); blood donated by smokers causes bank blood to contain carboxyhaemoglobin levels of 1.1–6.9 per cent (Harvey & Hutton, 1999).

Symptoms usually begin when blood levels exceed 10 per cent, and 40 per cent carboxyhaemoglobin may prove fatal (Blumenthal, 2001). Carbon monoxide has a far greater affinity for haemoglobin (more than two hundred times) than oxygen has, so prevents oxygen carriage. Carbon monoxide causes myocardial depression – myoglobin also has greater ($\times 40$) affinity for carbon dioxide than for oxygen (Harvey & Hutton, 1999). In air, carbon monoxide's half-life is 320 minutes, but supplementary oxygen significantly reduces this: 100 per cent oxygen reduces half-life to 74 minutes (Blumenthal, 2001). Lactic acidosis should not be corrected unless extreme, as acidosis increases oxygen dissociation from haemoglobin (Blumenthal, 2001). Carbon monoxide poisoning may also be treated with hyperbaric oxygen (see Chapter 28).

177

Carbon monoxide makes pulse oximetry inaccurate, but saturations on blood gas analysers remain reliable (see Chapter 17). Blood gas analysers usually also measure carbon monoxide levels.

*Thalassaemia* ('Cooley's anaemia') is caused by defective globin genes. It is classified as alpha or beta thalassaemia, depending on which gene is affected. Thalassaemia may also be classified as major, intermedia or minor, depending on its severity. The genetic defect reduces erythrocyte life, so reducing erythrocyte concentration. The abnormal haemoglobin also releases less oxygen. Typically, people with beta thalassaemia have Mediterranean ancestry. Alpha thalassaemis is most prevalent in south-east Asia.

If Hb is below 9.5 g/dl, blood should be transfused (Blood Transfusion Task Force, 2001). Large volume and frequent transfusion can cause iron overload (Buswell, 1996), so desferrioxamine (an iron chelator) may be given to prevent hepatic failure. Splenectomies may be performed where erythrocyte destruction exceeds production, and younger patients may receive bone marrow transplant.

*Sickle cell* (HbS) is caused by glutamic acid in beta haemoglobin chains being replaced with valine residue. When hypoxic, this abnormality links chains together as stiff rods, changing erythrocyte shape from elliptical into sickle. These can occlude small capillaries, causing ischaemic pain (severe cramp), necrosis and infarction in tissue beyond occlusions. Deformed erythrocytes rupture, causing clotting and further obstruction. Cerebral and renal microcapillaries are at special risk. HbS cells have reduced lifespans, causing chronic haemolytic anaemia.

Sickle genes cause erythrocytes infected by malarial parasites to adhere to capillary walls, denying parasites the potassium they need to survive. Sickle cells providing protection from malaria, this mutation flourished in the malarial belt. However people with sickle cell disease now live worldwide.

Sickle cell crises may occur with any hypoxic stressor – exercise, altitude, surgery, anaesthetic gases or critical illness. Crises may be fatal. People with both haemoglobin chromosomes (HbS, HbS) are most at risk, people with sickle cell trait (HbS, HbA) can sickle with extreme hypoxia. Those at risk should be safeguarded by optimising oxygen (e.g. pre-oxygenating with endotracheal suction).

Crisis management should provide

- analgesia
- oxygen
- fluids
- blood (exchange) transfusion.

Sickle crisis pain is intense, requiring strong analgesia, such as morphine or diamorphine (BCSH Task Force Sickle Cell Working Party, 2003). Despite anecdotal concerns about addiction and feigning crises to obtain opioids, benefits from analgesia to those in crisis far outweigh risks from drug abuse.

Delivering oxygen to ischaemic tissues relieves ischaemic pain and prevents further injury. Target oxygen saturation should be 95 per cent (British Committee for Standards in Haematology, General Haematology Task Force by the Sickle Cell Working Party, 2003). Increasing blood volume, and reducing viscosity, with intravenous fluids optimises perfusion. Urgent exchange blood transfusion should be given to reduce HbS to below 30 per cent (Frewin *et al.*, 1998).

### Implications for practice

- Oxygen is vital for life, so adequate oxygen delivery to cells, as well as adequate oxygen carriage by haemoglobin, should be achieved.
- Oxygen dissociation from haemoglobin is affected by various factors (see Table 18.2), including pH and temperature.
- $PaO_2$ measures plasma oxygen, whereas $SaO_2$ measures oxyhaemoglobin. Variable relationships between these two can be seen from arterial blood gas analysis.
- Prolonged use of high concentration oxygen (>60 per cent for >24 hours) can cause toxic lung damage, so should be avoided if possible. Where it cannot be avoided, PEEP should be used to compensate for nitrogen washout.
- Heliox may provide adequate oxygenation despite airway obstruction, so can usefully create time for other interventions.
- Carbon monoxide poisoning should initially be treated either with hyperbaric oxygen or pure oxygen. Pulse oximetry is erroneous, but saturations from blood gas analysers remain accurate.
- Patients with thalassaemia usually need blood transfusion, with iron overload prevented by chelators. Their liver function should be closely monitored.
- Sickle cell disease can cause life-threatening crises, usually prevented by adequate oxygenation and hydration.
- Sickle cell crisis needs strong and sufficient opioid analgesia, oxygen (to achieve 95 per cent saturation), fluids and blood transfusion.

### Summary

Oxygen is primarily carried by haemoglobin ($SO_2$), but partial pressure in plasma ($PO_2$) creates the pressure gradient for transfer to tissues. Complex, changeable, relationships between $SO_2$ and $PO_2$ are shown by the oxygen dissociation curve, which may be 'shifted' to the right or left by various factors. Haemoglobinopathies also affect oxygen carriage.

### Further reading

Gas carriage is described in most anatomy and critical care texts. Herbert *et al.*'s (1999) landmark research is especially valuable reading. Articles on haemoglobinopathies appear periodically in nursing journals (such as

Newcombe, 2002; Bennett, 2005), with authoritative guidelines from the BCSH Task Force Sickle Cell Working Party (2003). Kass' (2003) heliox study is useful. www.routledge.com/textbooks/0415373239

For clinical scenarios, clinical questions and the answers to them go to the support website at www.routledge.com/textbooks/0415373239

## Support groups

The Sickle Cell Society: 54 Station Road, London, NW10 4UA; 020–8961–7795.

UK Thalassaemia Society: 19 The Broadway, London N14 6PH; 0800–7311109.

## Clinical scenarios

Nina Walker is 36 years old and was admitted to the ICU with a head injury and fractured spine at C5 from falling down stairs. The first blood gas taken was from a central vein while Nina was self-ventilating via a face mask with $FiO_2$ 0.6, in flat supine position wearing a hard collar. The second blood gas is arterial, taken 12 hours post intubation and mechanical ventilation using spontaneous mode and $FiO_2$ 0.25. Nina's respiratory rate is 16 bpm, her Hb is 9.8 g/dl and core temperature at 12 hours is lower at 35.7°C

Blood gas and electrolyte values are:

|  | On admission to ICU Central *venous* blood $FiO_2$ 0.6 Temperature 35.9°C | 12 hours later Arterial blood $FiO_2$ 0.25 Temperature 35.7°C |
|---|---|---|
| pH | 7.27 | 7.51 |
| $PaO_2$ (kPa) | 3.30 | 13.36 |
| $PaCO_2$ (kPa) | 6.84 | 3.80 |
| $HCO_3$ (mmol/l) | 21.1 | 25.3 |
| BE (mmol/l) | −2.5 | +0.3 |
| Lactate (mmol/l) | 3.3 | 1.9 |
| $SO_2$ (%) ($SvO_2/SaO_2$) | 48.5 | 97.9 |

Q.1 Using the oxygen dissociation curve (Figure 18.1) verify Nina's percentage $O_2$ saturation of haemoglobin for both blood gas results (plot the position of her $PO_2$ incorporating her Hb, temperature and other arterial blood gas values). Repeat this using the carbon dioxide dissociation curve (Figure 18.2) to calculate $CO_2$ content percentage.

Q.2 Explain any shifts in the oxygen dissociation curve and haemoglobin's affinity for $O_2$ at Nina's cellular (tissue) and alveolar membrane for both venous and arterial blood gases. How does the level of carbon dioxide in blood effect oxygen transport?

Q.3 Review alternative assessment approaches that can be used by nurses to monitor effectiveness of oxygen transport to Nina's tissues (consider and specify types of visual observation, laboratory investigations, blood oximetry values such as $O_2Hb$, COHb, HHB, MetHb, RHb).

Chapter 19

# Acid–base balance and arterial blood gas analysis

### Contents

Introduction                        183
Acid–base definitions               183
pH measurement                      183
Respiratory balance                 184
Metabolic balance                   185
Renal control                       186
Chemical buffers                    186
Acidosis                            187
Tonometry                           188
Blood gas samples                   188
Reading samples                     189
Compensation                        192
Implications for practice           192
Summary                             193
Further reading                     193
Clinical scenarios                  193

### Fundamental knowledge

Cell metabolism (oxygen consumption, carbon dioxide
production)

## Introduction

Arterial blood gas analysis provides valuable information about respiratory and metabolic function, including acid–base balance. Most analysers provide additional useful information about various metabolites and electrolytes. Therefore arterial blood gas sampling and analysis is a core skill for ICU staff. In addition to issues surrounding sampling and analysis, this chapter identifies some controversies that may make practice, and so results, different between different areas even within a single hospital.

Machines and 'normal ranges' vary between units, so using sample print-outs from your unit may be helpful. Standard UK use of kilopascals (kPa) is followed here. The USA uses mmHg; 1 kPa is approximately 7.5 mmHg.

## Acid–base definitions

An acid is a substance capable of providing hydrogen ions; a base (alkali) is capable of accepting hydrogen ions. Acidity is determined by the amount of free hydrogen ions, not total number of hydrogen ions, so strong acids (e.g. hydrochloric) release many free hydrogen ions, whereas weak acids (e.g. carbonic) release few. Acid–base balance is the power of hydrogen ions (pH) measured in moles per litre ('power' in the mathematical sense, for the negative logarithm). The power of hydrogen ions can be controlled (balanced) either through *buffering* or exchange. Hydrogen ($H^+$), a positively charged ion (cation), can be buffered by a negatively charged ion (anion), such as bicarbonate ($HCO_3^-$).

## pH measurement

Each litre of blood contains about 0.00004 millimole (or 40 nanamoles, nmol) of hydrogen (normal plasma sodium concentration is 135–145 mmol/litre). Despite these very small concentrations, hydrogen ions are highly reactive; small changes in concentration significantly affecting oxygen dissociation from haemoglobin ('Bohr effect') and enzyme activity (Shangraw, 2000). Plasma concentrations being so small, ions are measured by a negative logarithm: the pH scale.

Logarithms represent complex numbers by replacing multiplication/division of the actual number by addition and subtraction to the log. For example

$$10^1 = 10$$
$$10^2 = 10 \times 10 = 100$$
$$10^3 = 100 \times 10 = 1000$$
$$10^4 = 1000 \times 10 = 10,000$$

each addition to the power (log) causes a tenfold increase to the actual number. Bacteria and blood cells, being very numerous, are usually measured using the

183

log of 10. Negative logarithms similarly represent very small divisions by subtraction from the log:

$$10^0 = 1$$
$$10^{-1} = 0.1$$
$$10^{-2} = 0.01$$

Chemically, the pH scale ranges from 0–14, making pH 7 chemically neutral. Blood is normally slightly alkaline (pH 7.35–7.45). At pH 7.4, there are only 0.00004 millimoles of hydrogen ions per litre of blood. But because pH is a negative logarithm, changes of one pH represents tenfold changes in hydrogen ion concentration (acidity), while changing pH by 0.3 doubles or halves concentrations:

$$\text{pH } 7.7 = 20 \text{ nmol/litre H}^+$$
$$\text{pH } 7.4 = 40 \text{ nmol/litre H}^+$$
$$\text{pH } 7.1 = 80 \text{ nmol/litre H}^+$$
$$\text{pH } 6.8 = 160 \text{ nmol/litre H}^+$$

Although in pure chemistry, alkaline until pH 7.0, for body chemistry blood pH < 7.35 is acidotic, while pH > 7.45 is alkalotic.

Metabolism produces about 40–80 nmol hydrogen every day (Marshall, 2000), moving from intracellular to extracellular fluid through concentration gradients, intracellular (where hydrogen is produced) concentrations being highest (normally 7.0 (Atherton, 2003)). Interstitial and venous pH is normally 7.35 (Marieb, 2004).

Blood pH outside 7.0–7.8 is usually fatal (Marieb, 2004), although Selby and James (1995) report rare survival from pH 6.4. Arterial pH below 7.0 usually leads to coma and death, while levels above 7.8 overstimulate the nervous system, causing convulsions and respiratory arrest.

Acid–base balance is controlled through

- respiratory
- metabolic (renal function, chemical buffers)

functions.

## Respiratory balance

Carbon dioxide dissolves in water to form carbonic acid:

$$CO_3 + H_2O \leftrightarrow H_2CO_3$$

a weak (pH 6.4), unstable acid. In lungs, carbonic acid, being unstable, dissociates back into water and carbon dioxide, so normal blood levels are normally maintained by adapting ventilation (rate and depth of breathing). Carbonic

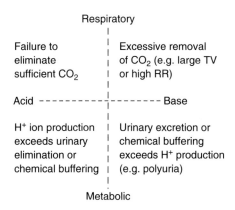

**Figure 19.1 Origin of acid–base imbalance**

acid is the main acid in blood, levels depending on carbon dioxide concentrations (PCO$_2$). Carbon dioxide is therefore considered a *potential* acid (lacking hydrogen ions, it is not really an acid), so *respiratory acidosis* is the failure to remove sufficient carbon dioxide (i.e. high PaCO$_2$) and *respiratory alkalosis* is the excessive removal of carbon dioxide (i.e. low PaCO$_2$) (Figure 19.1).

Hypercapnia stimulates respiratory centres to increase ventilation (rate and depth), removing more carbon dioxide. So although respiration cannot remove hydrogen ions, it can inhibit carbonic acid formation, restoring homeostasis. Respiratory acidosis is caused by hypoventilation. Respiratory alkalosis is caused by hyperventilation.

In health, respiratory response to acidosis is rapid, exerting up to double the effect of combined chemical buffers (Marieb, 2004). Doubling or halving alveolar ventilation can alter pH 0.2, returning life-threatening pH of 7.0 to 7.2 or 7.3 in 3–12 minutes (Guyton & Hall, 2000).

## Metabolic balance

Metabolic balance is more complex. Acids are

- ingested (e.g. wine, most crystalloid IVIs)
- produced (metabolism)

removed through the

- kidneys

and buffered by

- chemicals.

Bases (e.g. bicarbonate) are

- produced
- reabsorbed (renally)
- ingested/infused (e.g. antacids).

*Metabolic acidosis* may be from:

- hyperchoraemia or
- tissue acids (especially lactic or ketoacids)

and can be distinguished by the anion gap (see later). Hyperchloraemic acidosis usually from excessive normal saline infusion (Funk *et al.*, 2004). Ketoacids are from alternative metabolism (starvation, insulin-lack). Lactate (see later), the main cause of metabolic acidosis in ICU, indicates anaerobic metabolism, usually from perfusion failure.

Hydrogen ($H^+$) ions, an essential component of any acid, are removed by the kidney or buffered by bases. Acidosis therefore occurs if

- hydrogen production exceeds removal (excessive production; renal failure)
- buffer production is insufficient (especially, liver failure).

*Metabolic alkalosis* is caused by excessive removal/buffering of hydrogen ($H^+$) ions or excessive production/absorption of bases due to:

- polyuria
- hypokalaemia (causing excess $H^+$ in urine)
- gastric acid loss (e.g. excessive nasogastric drainage, vomiting)
- excessive buffers (e.g. colonic reabsorption from constipation).

## Renal control

Other than insignificant transdermal loss, hydrogen ions are only removed from the body in urine, actively being exchanged into glomerular filtrate when other cations (mainly sodium) are reabsorbed. The extent of active hydrogen ion excretion into urine is seen on urinalysis: normal blood (from which urine is formed) pH is 7.4, while normal urinary pH is 5.0.

Kidneys usually excrete 30–70 mmol of hydrogen ions daily, but can remove 300 mmol daily within 7–10 days. Renal failure therefore causes metabolic acidosis.

## Chemical buffers

Chemical buffers respond rapidly, within seconds, balancing hydrogen ions by binding acids to bases. They do not eliminate acids from the body.

*Bicarbonate* is the main chemical buffer of extracellular fluid, responsible for half of all chemical buffering. Hydrogen ions are essential to produce bicarbonate ($HCO_3^-$). Bicarbonate can combine with hydrogen to produce carbonic acid:

$$HCO_3^- + H^+ = H_2CO_3$$

*Phosphate* ($PO_4^{3-}$) is the least important buffer in blood, but the main urinary, interstitial and intracellular buffer.

*Plasma and intracellular proteins* Albumin is the main plasma protein, although histidine (in haemoglobin) is also a significant buffer. Hypoalbuminaemia, common in critical illness, therefore reduces metabolic buffering.

Chemical buffers are produced in many places, but especially in the liver, therefore hepatic failure causes metabolic acidosis.

## Acidosis

Acidosis (blood pH < 7.35) may be:

- respiratory = failure to excrete sufficient carbon dioxide (= high $pCO_2$)
- metabolic = failure to excrete/buffer sufficient $H^+$ ions (= base excess below −2; low $HCO_3$).

Acidosis

- increases respiratory drive
- shifts the oxygen dissociation curve to the right, increasing oxyhaemoglobin dissociation.

Treating acidosis rather than underlying causes therefore deprives hypoxic tissues of available oxygen (Winser, 2001),

- reduces blood carriage of carbon dioxide (Cavaliere *et al.*, 2002)
- is negatively inotropic, and reduces effectiveness of infused inotropes.

Acidosis is a symptom, not a disease. Many critically ill patients tolerate arterial pH significantly below 7.2 (Forsythe & Schmidt, 2000), as seen with permissive hypercapnia (see Chapter 27). Treatment should focus on underlying pathologies. Oxygen delivery to peripheries should be optimised, without increasing cell metabolism.

Bicarbonate infusions to reverse acidosis can cause many problems, including

- exacerbating intracellular acidosis (sodium bicarbonate does not transfer into cells, but does form carbon dioxide, which can transfer and form carbonic acid) (Forsythe & Schmidt, 2000)

187

■ alkalosis reduces oxygen dissociation from haemoglobin (shifts the oxygen dissociation curve to left).

Bicarbonate infusions should only be used in immediate life-threatening situations, such as pH <7.1 or cardiopulmonary resuscitation exceeding 20–25 minutes (Winser, 2001).

## Tonometry

Hypoxic tissues metabolise anaerobically, which produces many hydrogen ions. Highly vascular, gastric (intramucosal) pH (pHi) may indicate acidaemia, although so far tonometry has proved more useful for research than in practice (Hingley, 2000; Beale *et al.*, 2004). For accuracy, feed should be aspirated before measurement (Marshall & West, 2003).

## Blood gas samples

Blood gas samples can monitor respiratory function and acid–base balance, but should not be taken until 20–30 minutes after any changes to ventilation, or any interventions that affect respiratory function (Coombs, 2001). Intra-arterial blood pressure monitoring being used for most patients in adult ICUs, arterial lines provide easy access for obtaining samples for blood gas analysis. Transcutaneous gas analysis is noninvasive, but more useful for neonates than for adults. Intra-arterial electrodes enable continuous gas tension monitoring, $PiO_2$ correlating well with arterial samples ($PaO_2$) (Abraham *et al.*, 1996). However, equipment is costly, and intra-arterial monitoring has not (yet) established itself in ICU practice.

Before taking samples, sufficient fluid should be withdrawn from arterial lines to prevent *dilution from saline* flush, although lumen diameter and proximity of the sampling port usually necessitate removing only about 0.5–1 ml.

Applying *negative pressure* may cause frothing (Szaflarski, 1996) and cell damage, so minimal pressure should be used; arterial samples may fill passively from blood pressure. *Air* in samples causes falsely low readings, so should be expelled (Szaflarski, 1996). Samples should be covered (with hubs, not fingers) to prevent atmospheric gas exchange.

*Delay in analysing* causes inaccuracies, as blood cells in samples continue to metabolise: potassium and carbon dioxide levels increase, pH and oxygen fall. As ICUs usually have analysers on the unit, this rarely causes significant problems, but usually justifies interrupting routine calibrations.

*Erythrocyte sedimentation* affects many results, especially haemoglobin, so samples should be mixed continuously, using a thumb roll, not vigorous shaking (which causes haemolysis).

Continuous gas analysis is currently impractical and too costly for widespread clinical use (Ault & Stock, 2004), but future technological improvements may make this, or transcutaneous gases, practical alternatives.

## Reading samples

This chapter describes key measurements, although configurations of machines often vary greatly. Standard symbols used for some other measurements are listed in Table 19.1. 'Normal' figures may differ between texts and between machines. Analysers usually measure some electrolytes and metabolites. These are listed in Table 19.2 and discussed in Chapter 21. Having a printout from a patient you have recently cared for will be useful while reading through this section.

## Temperature

Blood gas analysers can measure samples at various temperatures. Temperature affects dissociation of gases, so $PaO_2$, $PaCO_2$, pH, base excess, and $HCO_3^-$ results differ with different temperatures – best seen by re-analysing samples at different temperatures. If no specific temperature is selected, machines default to analysing samples at 37°C.

Debate persists between correcting sample to patient temperature (pH-stat) and analysing all samples at 37°C (alpha-stat). Balance of evidence currently favours noncorrection, but consistency between staff is probably more important than theoretical rigour. Units should therefore identify which approach to adopt, ensuring all staff (including occasional agency/bank staff) follow that approach.

### Table 19.1 Some symbols commonly found on blood gas samples

F = fractional concentration in dry gas
P = pressure, or partial pressure
Q = volume of blood
A = alveolar
a = arterial
c = capillary
I = ideal

### Table 19.2 Main electrolyte + metabolite results measured by most blood gas analysers

| Electrolyte/metabolite | Normal range |
| --- | --- |
| Sodium (Na$^+$) | 135–145 mmol/litre |
| Potassium (K$^+$) | 3.5–4.5 mmol/litre |
| Calcium (Ca$^{++}$, also written Ca$^{2+}$)[a] | 1.1–1.3 mmol/litre |
| Chloride | 95–105 mmol/litre |
| Glucose | 4.1–6.1 mmol/litre |
| Lactate | <2 mmol/litre |

Note:
[a] Blood gas analysers measure ionised calcium, not total calcium; biochemistry laboratories measure total calcium
See Chapter 21 – blood results

## pH

Normal: 7.35–7.45

pH measures overall acidity or alkalinity of blood; it does not differentiate between respiratory and metabolic components. (NB Ph = *pharmacopoeia* or *phenyl*.)

## PaCO₂

Normal: 4.5–6.0 kPa

Carbon dioxide dissolves in water, forming carbonic acid (see earlier). High carbon dioxide tension (high $PaCO_2$) therefore indicates respiratory acidosis, while low carbon dioxide tension indicates respiratory alkalosis.

## PaO₂

Normal: 11.5–13.5 kPa

$PaO_2$ measures partial pressure of oxygen in plasma. *Oxygen content* ($CaO_2$) is the sum of both oxygen dissolved in plasma ($PaO_2$) and oxyhaemoglobin.

## A-a gradient

Normal: 2 kPa

Alveolar arterial (A-a) gradient indicates whether '*shunting*' is occurring. Measurement is only reliable if $FiO_2$ is entered into the analyser.

## HCO₃⁻

Normal: 23–27 mmol/litre

Bicarbonate is the main buffer in blood, so low bicarbonate indicates metabolic acidosis, while high levels indicate metabolic alkalosis. However, respiratory function affects bicarbonate levels:

$$CO_2 + H_2O \leftrightarrow H_2CO_3 \leftrightarrow HCO_3^- + H^+$$

(carbon dioxide + water forms carbonic acid, which dissociates to bicarbonate and a hydrogen radical).

Actual bicarbonate (ABC), the amount measured by the machine, therefore derives mainly from metabolic, but also partly from respiratory, function. Normally negligible, the respiratory component becomes increasingly significant with increasingly abnormal $PaCO_2$. Microchip calculation enables removal of the respiratory component to provide an (estimated) purely metabolic figure, *standardised bicarbonate* (SBC, $HCO_3^-$-std). Bicarbonate being used to assess metabolic function, SBC is more reliable than $HCO_3^-$. Readers should note and consider differences between actual and standardised figures on printouts, discussing these with unit staff.

## Base excess (BE)

Normal: ±2

Base excess measures metabolic acid–base balance, indicating moles of acid or base needed to restore one litre of blood to pH 7.4 (provided $pCO_2$ remains constant at 5.3 kPa).

Unlike pH, base excess is linear, so easier to understand. Neutral is zero, positive base excess is too much base (alkaline; metabolic alkalosis), while negative base excess is insufficient base (metabolic acidosis). Faint/absent minus signs may need to be inferred by readers from other measurements – if bicarbonate levels are low, then base excess must be negative.

Base excess is calculated from bicarbonate levels, so although base excess is viewed as a metabolic figure, carbon dioxide affects bicarbonate (above). Standardised base excess (SBE, BE-std) more accurate indicates metabolic balance.

## Saturation

Normal: 97%

Saturation indicates percentage saturation of haemoglobin by oxygen (see Chapter 17). Blood gas analysers use many colours to calculate saturation, pulse oximeters use only two, so analysers are more accurate.

## Anion gap

8–16 mmol/litre

When metabolic acidosis (low pH and low SBE) is identified, the balance between the positively charged and negatively charged ions

$$(Na^+ + K^+) - (Cl^- + HCO_3^-)$$

indicates whether acidaemia is hyperchloraemic (normal anion gap) or from metabolic acid production (raised anion gap) (Durward, 2002). Raised anion gaps therefore indicate abnormal metabolism (anaerobic, or alternative energy sources) in the ICU, usually caused by perfusion failure. Acidosis with a normal anion gap indicates electrolyte imbalance. As chloride is measured by most analysers, electrolyte imbalances are easily seen, so the additional value of anion gap measurement is questionable. Although chloride and bicarbonate are the main anions, there are smaller quantities of other ones not included in anion calculations, but affecting results, including albumin (low in most ICU patients) (Durward, 2002).

## Lactate

Normal: <2 mmol/litre

Normal metabolism produces about 0.8 mmol/kg/hour of lactate (Cooper, 2003), but anaerobic metabolism significantly increases production. Raised lactate indicates perfusion failure. Lactate is converted into lactic acid (pH 3.4), causing/increasing metabolic acidosis.

## Compensation

Homeostasis aims to keep blood pH 7.4. Overall pH of blood balances respiratory with metabolic function (see Figure 19.1). Acidosis or alkalosis from one quadrant will, with time and effective homeostatic mechanisms, compensate for an opposite excess in another to restore 'neutral' blood pH of 7.4.

When analysing samples, identify

- is pH normal (7.35–7.45)?
- respiratory acid/base balance ($pCO_2$)
- metabolic acid–base balance (bicarbonate, base excess).

If pH is normal, but respiratory and metabolic balances are abnormal and opposite, compensation is succeeding. If pH is abnormal compensation is incomplete (if metabolic and respiratory balances are opposite) or absent (if metabolic and respiratory balances are not opposite).

Most problems seen in ICU begin with acidosis – respiratory (respiratory failure) or metabolic (e.g. kidney or liver failure). Alkaloses are usually compensatory. Respiratory compensation occurs quickly (within minutes), but metabolic compensation takes hours or days to be fully effective (and to fully stop). So metabolic compensation only occurs in response to prolonged respiratory complications. Metabolic 'overshoot' may be seen in the ICU where artificial ventilation resolves the primary respiratory acidosis, but metabolism continues to compensate.

### Implications for practice

- Unit policy should identify whether to analyse samples at patient's temperature or 37°C.
- Analyse gases by identifying

  - respiratory acid–base balance ($CO_2$)
  - metabolic acid–base balance (bicarbonate, base excess)
  - whether compensation is occuring, and if so (from patients' history) which way?

- Standardised bicarbonate and base excess levels should be used rather than $HCO_3^-$ and BE figure.
- For teaching/learning, re-analysing samples at differing temperatures illustrates how temperature affects gases.
- Acidosis is usually from disease, alkalosis usually from compensation.
- Acidosis is not usually treated with bicarbonate unless immediately life-threatening (pH <7.1).

## Summary

Blood gas analysis remains one of the most valuable means of monitoring respiratory and metabolic function. ICU nurses both take and interpret arterial blood gas samples, so need to know potential sources of error (sampling, transporting), standard unit practices (e.g. whether or not to enter patients' temperature) and how to interpret results, in a logical sequence, in the context of their patient. 'Normal' figures may vary slightly, but principles remain applicable. Electrolytes and metabolites, not discussed here, are included in Chapter 21.

## Further reading

Chapters on acid–base balance are included in many physiology, ICU and clinical chemistry/biochemistry texts. Martin (1999) provides a useful book for developing interpretation skills. Articles occasionally appear (e.g. Coombs, 2001; Simpson, 2004). Potential errors from taking samples are summarised by Szaflarski (1996). www.routledge.com/textbooks/0415373239

For clinical scenarios, clinical questions and the answers to them go to the support website at www.routledge.com/textbooks/0415373239

## Clinical scenarios

Arterial blood gas analysis on admission to the ICU:

| Patient history | 36-year-old female who is unconscious from taking aspirin overdose. | 45-year-old male, known alcoholic with history of vomiting, had developed difficulty in breathing. | 62-year-old male with a history of congestive cardiac failure with 15 per cent ejection fraction, pneumonia and bilateral pleural effusions. | 75-year-old female, had a dynamic hip replacement, developed a chest infection, developed reduced respiratory function and possible pulmonary embolism. |
|---|---|---|---|---|
| FiO$_2$ | 0.6 | 0.35 | 0.28 | 0.4 |
| pH | 7.25 | 7.55 | 7.48 | 7.29 |
| PaO$_2$ (kPa) | 9.32 | 11.9 | 12.6 | 7.49 |
| PaCO$_2$ (kPa) | 8.10 | 4.6 | 3.05 | 11.05 |
| HCO$_3^-$ (mmol/litre) | 21.2 | 34.4 | 20.1 | 33.7 |

| BE (mmol/litre) | 1.9 | 6 | −6.3 | 12.4 |
|---|---|---|---|---|
| Lactate (mmol/litre) | 1.5 | 0.7 | 0.8 | 0.5 |

Q.1 Identify the acid–base status of the four blood gases (acidosis, alkalosis, respiratory, metabolic, compensated or uncompensated).

Q.2 Analyse the likely causes of the acid–base disturbances. Consider their effect on other organs/systems and how the ICU nurse can assess, anticipate and minimise any potentially adverse effects.

Q.3 Review potential sources and direction of analytical errors (e.g. air bubbles in blood sample can falsely decrease $PO_2$) which can occur with these blood gas analysis results.

Chapter 20

# Haemodynamic monitoring

**Contents**

| | |
|---|---|
| Introduction | 196 |
| Skin assessment | 196 |
| Arterial blood pressure | 196 |
| Noninvasive blood pressure measurement | 197 |
| Intra-arterial measurement | 197 |
| Central venous pressure | 199 |
| Measuring CVP | 200 |
| Dangers | 201 |
| Flow monitoring | 202 |
| Ultrasound | 207 |
| Implications for practice | 207 |
| Summary | 207 |
| Further reading | 208 |
| Clinical scenarios | 208 |

**Fundamental knowledge**

Experience of using invasive monitoring (including 'zeroing')
Cardiac physiology – atria, ventricles, valves
Cardiac cycle: systole, diastole
Relationship between cardiac electrical activity (ECG) and
output (pulse, blood pressure)
How breathing affects venous return
V/Q mismatch
Oxygen dissociation (see Chapter 18)

## Introduction

The purpose of the cardiovascular system is perfusion, supplying cells with oxygen and glucose needed for normal anaerobic metabolism (energy) and removing metabolic waste (carbon dioxide, metabolic acids, water). Without perfusion, cells die. Haemodynamic monitoring therefore aims to indicate perfusion. Generally, more invasive modes provide more information, but create more problems/risks. Options chosen therefore depend on balancing benefits against burdens. Monitoring equipment is diagnostic, not therapeutic, so once risks outweigh benefits or maximum time limits are reached, they should be removed.

This chapter describes more frequently used modes, with some noninvasive options, to extend knowledge rather than develop psychomotor skills. Electrocardiography (ECGs) is discussed in Chapter 22. Formulae such as the Fick equation are not included for derived measurement, as microchip technology has replaced need for nurses to calculate them.

'Normal' figures are cited here as a guide, but many assume 'average' 70 kg patients and individuals can have wide healthy variations, so ideally measurements should be compared with pre-morbid baselines. Consistency between measurements, and measurers, is therefore important.

## Skin assessment

Pale, discoloured, cyanosed or clammy skin indicates poor perfusion (whether from hypovolaemia, vascular disease or excessive vasoconstriction). Although noninvasive and easily visible, skin discolouration may be acute or chronic, and has limited value in critical illness.

*Capillary refill* indicates peripheral perfusion. Capillary refill is assessed by pressing on a finger pad or nailbed for 5 seconds. On releasing pressure, initial blanching should vanish within 2 seconds (Ahern & Philpot, 2002). Delayed capillary refill indicates peripheral perfusion failure, from hypotension, hypovolaemia or excessive peripheral vascular resistance, but should not be used to imply perfusion of main organs (Pamba & Maitland, 2004). Peripheral vasodilatation (e.g. from SIRS) causes peripheral pooling: central hypotension, warm/'flushed' extremities and rapid capillary refill.

## Arterial blood pressure

This is the pressure exerted on arterial walls. Pressure is determined by flow and resistance. Flow is affected by driving force (cardiac output, or left ventricular ejection) and viscosity. Resistance (afterload) is both vascular (constriction, atherosclerosis) and interstitial (e.g. oedema). Capillary bloodflow ('microcirculation') is reduced if blood viscosity increases (see Chapter 21).

Diastolic pressure is the pressure exerted on the arterial wall during the resting phase of the cardiac cycle. Abnormally low diastolic pressure (<80 mmHg) indicates either hypovolaemia or vasodilatation. Once CVP is optimised with fluids, vasopressors (e.g. noradrenaline) may be needed.

Systolic – maximum perfusion, pressure is momentary, but perfusion continues variably throughout the whole pulse cycle. Average pressure across the whole pulse cycle, including diastole, therefore indicates average perfusion pressure. Average pressure is calculated by monitors as mean arterial pressure (MAP). The widely cited formula of MAP = diastole + ⅓(systole − diastole) is only accurate if diastolic time is two-thirds of the cycle (Darovic, 2002b), so monitors are more accurate than paper calculations of MAP.

Of the three pressures, MAP is least affected by differences between arteries or artefact, such as damp traces (Darovic, 2002b; Safar *et al.*, 2003), so with poor arterial traces, MAP usually remains reliable. MAP is normally 70–105 mmHg; lower figures indicating questionable perfusion of vital organs, and higher figures indicating hypertension and hyperdynamic states.

Pulse pressure, the pressure created by each pulse (systolic minus diastolic), indicates vessel response to pulse. Stereotypical normal pulse pressure is:

$$120 - 80 = 40 \text{ mmHg}$$

High (wide) pulse pressures usually indicate vascular disease, such as atherosclerosis (Haider *et al.*, 2003), while low (narrow) pulse pressures usually indicate arterial hypovolaemia, which may be caused by

- systemic hypovolaemia
- poor cardiac output
- excessive vasodilatation (e.g. SIRS).

Other haemodynamic monitoring (e.g. CVP) may indicate likely causes.

## Noninvasive blood pressure measurement

Cuff pressure monitoring provides adequate information for most hospitalised patients, but greater frequency and accuracy is usually needed in the ICU. Bladder width should be 80 per cent of arm circumference (Beevers *et al.*, 2001). Smaller cuffs over-read, while larger cuffs under-read.

## Intra-arterial measurement

Direct (invasive) arterial pressure monitoring provides

- continuous measurement
- visual display
- access to arterial blood for sampling.

Noninvasive blood pressure is 'dampened' by tissues between arteries and skin surfaces. Intra-arterial measurement should be more accurate, often being 5–20 mmHg above noninvasive pressure measurements.

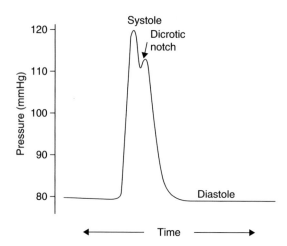

**Figure 20.1 Arterial trace**

Pulse waveform (see Figure 20.1) indicates cardiac function. The area beneath the wave indicates pulse volume, with a normal sharp upstroke indicating healthy left-ventricular function. Shallower upstrokes therefore indicate poor left ventricular outflow (e.g. left ventricular function, aortic stenosis). Upstrokes should normally be uninterrupted, but extensive systemic vasodilatation and low systemic vascular resistance (e.g. SIRS) can cause an anacrotic notch on upstrokes, with widening of the dicrotic notch. After the peak, there should be a small second peak on descent – the dicrotic notch, when the aortic valve closes. Poorly defined or absent diacrotic notches indicate aortic valve incompetence. Breathing can cause 'arterial swing'. Rises in late inspiration indicate cardiac overload, while falls in early expiration indicate hypovolaemia.

Disconnection, or significant oozing around arterial cannulae, can cause rapid blood loss, so security of connections should be checked, sites covered by transparent bio-occlusive dressings and (if possible) placed where easily observed. Waveform display should be continuously monitored, with alarms normally set to give early warning of problems such as hypertension, hypotension and disconnection. Although rare, arterial lines can occlude arteries, care should include checking colour, warmth and capillary refill of extremities beyond cannulae.

Errors can be caused by

- transducer level (should be at heart level; small changes in height cause large errors in measurement)
- occlusion – patency should be maintained with continuous infusion (normally at 300 mmHg) with sodium chloride 0.9%. Traditionally, heparin (usually 1000 iu) was added to 500 ml of saline, but benefits of heparin seem slight, and it may cause HITTS (see Chapter 26), so most units now use normal saline without heparin (Garretson, 2005).

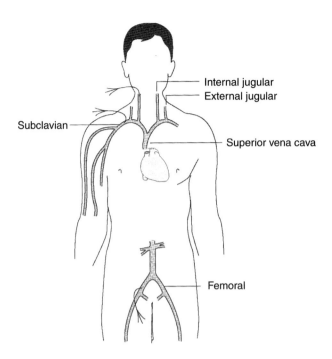

Subclavian

Internal jugular
External jugular

Superior vena cava

Femoral

**■ *Figure 20.2* Main central venous cannulation sites**

■ drugs – no drug should be given through arterial lines (bolus concentrations can be toxic), so lines and all connections/taps should be clearly labelled and identified (e.g. using red bungs).

### Central venous pressure

Central venous pressure (CVP) directly measures pressure in the vena cava (usually, superior), so is determined by

■ blood volume returning to the heart ('filling pressure' or 'preload')
■ function of the right atrium and ventricle
■ intrathoracic pressure.

Ideally, pressure should be measured from the distal (tip) lumen, with no other infusions running simultaneously through that lumen. When distal lumens are unavailable, differences from other lumens are usually insignificant.

Low CVP usually indicates fluid loss (e.g. haemorrhage, excessive diuresis, gross extravasation). Various factors can cause high CVP:

■ hypervolaemia (e.g. excessive fluid infusion, renal failure)
■ cardiac failure (e.g. right ventricular failure, pulmonary embolism, mitral valve failure/regurgitation, tamponade)

199

- increased intrathoracic pressure (e.g. positive pressure ventilation, PEEP/CPAP)
- lumen occlusion/obstruction (e.g. cannula against vein wall; thrombus)
- high blood viscosity (rare, but possible following massive blood transfusion)
- artefact (e.g. fluids infusing through transduced lumen).

If causes of high pressure are not obvious, nurses should seek advice. Very high pressures (>18) may indicate pulmonary oedema.

## Measuring CVP

Ideally, central venous pressure is measured supine from midaxilla (phlebostatic axis: intersection of lines from midsternal fourth intercostal space and midaxilla) and in the ICU recorded in millimetres of mercury. Because most ICU patients are now nursed semirecumbent, CVP is frequently measured in other positions. Pressure falls as positioning becomes more upright, so position should be recorded with CVP, and changes in position should be considered when assessing trends. Measurements taken when patients are lying on their side are unreliable.

Normal supine midaxillary measurements in self-ventilating patients is 0 to +8 mmHg (mean +4 mmHg). Normal range increases with positive intrathorasic pressure (by 3–5 cmH$_2$O) and with PEEP/CPAP. Transducers should be 'zeroed' at midaxilla level – open the port from the monitor to air and press calibration. Marking midaxilla on skin or fixing transducers to one position helps maintain consistency between measurements.

Central venous pressure being far lower than arterial, waveforms are more difficult to analyse, but should show three phases: 'a' (with 'x' descent), 'c' and

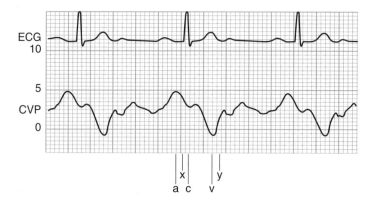

**Figure 20.3 CVP waveform**

'v' (with 'y' descent) (see Figure 20.3):

a: initiated by right atrial contraction (so absent with atrial fibrillation)
x: pressure falls with atrial relaxation
c: initiated by right ventricular contraction and tricuspid valve closure, so should follow the QRS wave on ECGs
v: initiated with right atrial filling (so corresponds with T waves on ECGs)
y: pressure falls with tricuspid valve opening (ventricular filling).

Breathing causes 'respiratory swing':

- rising with positive pressure ventilator breaths (increased intrathoracic pressure)
- falling with self-ventilating breaths (negative pressure).

Ideally, pressure should be measured between breaths, although many units monitor the mean.

Where transducer monitoring is not available, manometers can measure CVP. Mercury being neurotoxic, manometers use isotonic fluids (e.g. 5% glucose). Readings are therefore in centimetres of water ($cmH_2O$) rather than millimetres of mercury (mmHg):

$$1 \ cmH_2O = 0.74 \ mmHg$$
$$1.36 \ cmH_2O = 1 \ mmHg$$

Differences, negligible with low pressures, accumulate with higher ones.

## Dangers

Inserting central lines can puncture any surrounding tissue (lung puncture = pneumothorax, arteries, myocardium). Nurses assisting during insertion should observe patients and monitors (ECG, airway pressures), reporting any concerns. Once inserted, lines should be stitched and position checked by X-ray before use.

Once inserted, problems include:

*Infection*, usually from skin commensals (Safdar & Maki, 2004), occurrs in 4–18 per cent of patients (Elliott *et al.*, 1994). Rates are higher with femoral lines (Brun-Buisson, 2001; Waldmann & Barnes, 2004). Sites should be covered with transparent semi-permeable dressings (Brun-Buisson, 2001; Pratt *et al.*, 2001).

*Dysrhythmias* can have many causes, including myocardial irritation from catheters entering the heart. The ECG should be continuously monitored and any unexplained dysrhythmias reported and recorded.

*Drugs* may need to be given centrally because

- rapid effect is necessary
- drugs would be insufficiently diluted in peripheral veins, causing thrombophlebitis/necrosis (hypotonic, hypertonic, too acidic or alkaline)
- peripheral flow is poor/absent (shock).

Drugs given centrally can have rapid effects, so patients and monitors should be closely observed during and after administration. Nurses should observe lines during drug administration, and flush lines thoroughly afterwards and between drugs to avoid precipitation/interaction (furosemide precipitates with many drugs). Central lines deadspace is usually 1 ml (Cooper & Cramp, 2003).

Central vein *thromboses* may release emboli, causing pulmonary embolism. Obstructed flow may indicate thrombi or extravasation, so forcing fluid/drugs through obstructed lines may dislodge emboli or force fluid into interstitial spaces. The RCN (2003b) recommend flushing blocked catheters with 10 ml normal saline. Lumens which remain obstructed should be labelled, reported and not used. Alternatively, obstructions can be removed with

■ urokinase
■ percussive technique.

(Stewart, 2001)

Urokinase, like other thrombolytics, could cause severe side effects such as haemorrhage and anaphylaxis, although so far no complications have been reported from the small amounts needed to unblock catheters (Polderman & Girbes, 2002). The percussive technique described by Stewart uses 1 ml of normal saline in a 10 ml syringe; after pulling back, the plunger is allowed to snap back. Stewart claims 94 per cent success rate, with no reported complication. However, his practice-based report is supported by only six (mostly old) references, so nurses should remember their individual accountability before adopting this technique.

Air emboli of 50–100 ml are fatal (Polderman & Girbes, 2002). The small bubbles often seen in intravenous lines are not harmful, but (self-ventilating) negative intrathoracic pressure of 4 cmH$_2$O could draw 90 ml of air in one second through an 18 gauge needle (Polderman & Girbes, 2002). Central lines should, whenever possible, be easily visible and checked regularly, especially with self-ventilating patients. Nurses should regularly check whether all connections are secure.

Central lines should be removed with patients positioned head-down, so any accidental air emboli should rise to pedal rather than cerebral circulation. Self-ventilating patients should breathe out and hold their breath (out) during removal, so intrathoracic pressure equals atmospheric pressure.

## Flow monitoring (cardiac output studies)

CVP measures cardiac preload, but monitoring flow through the heart provides more information about the heart and vascular function. Direct and derived measurements, with commonly used abbreviations, are described below, with normal ranges summarised in Table 20.1. Most measurements are derived, relying on information such as

■ haemoglobin
■ central venous pressure.

**Table 20.1 Normal flow monitoring parameters (not all parameters are available on all machines)**

| | |
|---|---|
| CI | 2.5–4.2 litres/minute/m² |
| CO | 4–8 litres/minute |
| CVP (self ventilating) | 0 to +8 mmHg (right atrial level) |
| DO₂ | 900–1100 litres/minute |
| DO₂I | 520–720 mililitres/minute/m² |
| EVLW | 5–7 ml/kg (3500–4000 ml for 70 kg) |
| LCWI | 3.4–4.2 kg·m/m² |
| LVSWI | 50–60 gm·m/m² |
| PAP | 10–20 mmHg |
| PPV | <10 per cent |
| PVR | <250 dynes/second/cm⁵ |
| PVRI | 255–285 dynes/second/cm⁵/cm² |
| RCW | 0.54–0.66 km·m/m² |
| RVSWI | 7.9–9.7 gm·m/m² |
| SSV | <10 per cent |
| SV | about 70 ml at rest (range 60–120 ml) |
| SVI | 35–70 ml/beat/m² |
| SvO₂ | 75 per cent |
| SVR | 800–1200 dynes/second/cm⁵ |
| SVRI | 2000–24000 dynes/second/cm⁵/m² |
| VO₂ | 200–290 litres/minute |
| VO₂I | 100–180 mlitres/minute/m² |

Many are indexed to

- height and
- weight

thus avoiding problems of many 'normal' figures assuming 'average' weight of 70 kg. Indexing output to body surface area (m²) makes figures comparable between different (non-average) patients, so they are generally used. But, like other derived measurements, incorrect data fed into machines causes incorrect results.

*Pulmonary artery catheters* (PAC, also called pulmonary artery floatation catheters – PAFC and 'Swan Ganz') were the first widely used means to directly measure cardiac function. Various less invasive alternatives are now available (see later). Many studies, including the (unpublished) UK PACMan trial, show no benefit, rather often harm from PAFCs, so few UK units now use them. Any reader encountering one should only use it if they are competent to do so; many older ICU texts describe PAFCs. Some measurements below are only available with PAFCs.

Less invasive means include:

- *PiCCO* – Peripherally Inserted Continuous Cardiac Output
- *LidCo®* – Lithium Derived Cardiac Output
- transoesophageal *doppler.*

All three analyse pulse waveform (contour) to derive measurements. Many studies, such as Chaney and Derdak (2002), confirm PiCCO and LidCO® are as reliable as PAFCs. Lithium measurements used for LidCO may be unreliable if paralysing agents are used. Doppler cardiac output studies may (Dark & Singer, 2004) or may not (Bettex et al., 2004) be reliable, but are not widely used in the UK, possibly because many systems can only be used for 12 hours.

Noninvasive means include

■ thoracic electrical bioimpedance
■ partial carbon dioxide rebreathing.

*Thoracic electrical bioimpedance* (TEB) uses ECG-like electrodes, measuring differences in thoracic resistance (bioimpedance) to high-frequency, very low-magnitude electrical currents. Aortic flow supplies less than 1 per cent of thoracic bioimpedance, so high signal-to-noise ratio may cause significant inaccuracies. Whole-body electrical bioimpedance is accurate (Cotter et al., 2004), but TEB has only limited value (Raaijmakers et al., 1999), and is less accurate with diseases such as ARDS that cause significant fluid shifts (Chaney & Derdak, 2002). Thoracic bioimpedence monitoring has not been widely adopted in UK ICUs.

*Partial carbon dioxide rebreathing* causes patients to periodically rebreathe (carbon dioxide-rich) gas. Capnography then measures differences between breathing and non-rebreathing carbon dioxide tensions. As acid–base buffering keeps venous carbon dioxide tensions essentially constant, differences in arterial carbon dioxide reflect cardiac output. Both animal and human studies show good correlation with thermodilution measurements. Readings are available at three minute cycles. However capnography relies on constant respiratory rate to tidal volume ratio, so use of partial carbon dioxide rebreathing to measure cardiac output is confined to ventilated patients (without triggering). It should not be used if rebreathing carbon dioxide may cause problems.

*Cardiac output* (CO)
Normal: 4–8 litres/minute
*Cardiac index* (CI)
Normal: 2.5–4.2 litres/minute/m²
To meet increased cardiac demand most ICU patients have pathologically high cardiac outputs. Inotropes further increase output. Due to differences in both cardiac output and body surface area, children's cardiac index is high and decreases with age. Myocardial dysfunction, left ventricular failure, and mediators may inhibit output.

*Stroke volume* (SV)
Normal: about 70 ml at rest (range 60–120 ml)
*Stroke volume index* (SVI)
Normal: 35–70 ml/beat/m².

Stroke volume is the amount of blood ejected with each contraction of the heart, so HR × SV = CO. Stroke volume relies on adequate preload and muscle contractility so if it is poor, preload (CVP) should be optimised with fluids before using inotropes. Like cardiac output, stroke volume can be indexed: stroke volume index (SVI) or stroke index (SI).

*Systemic vascular resistance* (SVR)
*Systemic vascular reistance index* (SVRI)
Normal SVR: 800–1200 dynes/second/cm$^5$
    SVRI: 2000–24000 dynes/second/cm$^5$/m$^2$.
Systemic vascular resistance ('afterload') is the resistance met by cardiac output from blood vessels. Blood pressure is the sum of HR × SV × SVR. Excessive vasodilatation (distributive shock, such as SIRS) reduces SVR. SVR monitoring is therefore useful for inotrope/vasopressor therapy.

*Left cardiac work* (LCW)
*Left cardiac work index* (LCWI)
Normal LCWI: 3.4–4.2 kg/m/m$^2$
*Left ventricular stroke work* (LVSW)
*Left ventricular stroke work index* (LVSWI)
Normal LVSWI: 50–60 gm/m/m$^2$.
Managing severe left ventricular failure is a delicate balance between maintaining adequate cardiac output and myocardial oxygenation. Insufficient work deprives the brain of oxygen. Excessive work deprives the myocardium of oxygen. Measuring left ventricular work enables calculation of muscle strength (contractility) and more careful titration of therapies.

*Right cardiac work* (RCW)
*Right cardiac work index* (RCWI)
*Right ventricular stroke work* (RVSW)
*Right ventricular stroke work index* (RVSWI)
Normal RCW: 0.54–0.66 km/m/m$^2$
    RVSWI: 7.9–9.7 gm/m/m$^2$.
Measuring right ventricular function assists management with right heart failure.

Pulmonary artery pressure
Normal: $\frac{8-15}{15-25}$ mmHg
Pulmonary vascular resistance/pulmonary vascular resistance index
Normal: PVR <250 dynes/second/cm$^5$
    PVRI 255–285 dynes/second/cm$^5$/cm$^2$.
Pulmonary hypertension may be caused by ARDS, pulmonary oedema, pulmonary embolism and other pathologies. Pulmonary hypotension with high central venous pressure indicates right-sided heart disease, such as tricuspid valve stenosis/regurgitation or right ventricular infarction (usually inferior myocardial infarction) or septal defects (rare in adults).

Venous saturation/mixed venous saturation ($SvO_2$)

Normal: 65–75 per cent.

Venous saturation measures oxyhaemoglobin in venous blood, and so what remains after dissociation within capillaries. When compared with arterial oxygen saturation, venous saturation therefore indicates tissue oxygen demand and uptake, and can be used to derive oxygen delivery and oxygen consumption.

In health, approximately one-quarter of available oxygen is consumed, so higher $SvO_2$ indicates failure of oxygen delivery to tissue cells from reduced

■   oxygen dissociation from haemoglobin (e.g. hypothermia)
■   tissue uptake.

Low $SvO_2$ indicates high oxygen demand.

PAFCs can measure mixed venous saturation – saturation of blood in the pulmonary artery, indicating total systemic oxygen consumption. Because PAFCs are seldom used in the UK, venous saturation is usually from central lines in the superior vena cava ($ScvO_2$). Although not identical, the two may (Rivers et al., 2001a; Dickens, 2004) or may not (Chawala et al., 2004) show comparable trends – views appear to reflect prevailing national attitudes to PAFCs. Venous samples should be clearly labelled – if mistaken for arterial, inappropriate treatments may be commenced. Monitoring saturation from central lines in the inferior vena cava is seldom useful, as this would only indicate oxygen demand/uptake in the legs.

*Delivery of oxygen ($DO_2$)*
*Delivery of oxygen index ($DO_2I$)*
Normal: $DO_2$ 900–1100 l/minute
        $DO_2I$ 520–720 ml/minute/m².
This indicates whether oxygen reached its target – the tissues.

*Consumption of oxygen ($VO_2$)*
*Consumption of oxygen index ($VO_2I$)*
Normal: $VO_2$ 200–290 litres/minute
        $VO_2I$ 100–180 ml/minute/m².
Oxygen is needed by all cells, so delivery has little value unless tissues extract it.

*Stroke volume variation (SSV)*
Normal: <10 per cent.
Stroke volume varies with changes in intrathoracic pressure (breathing). In health variations are small, but hypovolaemia increases variations. SVV >10 per cent indicates need for fluids. Hypotension with SVV <10 per cent is usually an indication for inotropic support.

Pulse pressure variation (PPV) is similar to SSV, and similarly is normally <10 per cent.

*Extra vascular lung water (EVLW)*
Normal: 5–7 ml/kg (3500–4000 ml for 70 kg)

Aggressive fluid management may cause pulmonary oedema, progressing to ARDS. Calculating EVLW therefore enables optimisation of fluid management (Holm *et al.*, 2000; Sakka *et al.*, 2002) and inotrope therapy (Salukhe & Wyncoll, 2002).

## Ultrasound

Ultrasound enables visualisation and measurement of the heart and bloodflow through central vessels, so is valuable for medical diagnosis. Among the most frequent measurements from cardiac ultrasound is *ejection fraction*. The average healthy adult left ventricle can hold about 130 ml of blood, but only ejects 70–90 ml. The volume ejected can therefore be expressed as a fraction, or more often percentage, of total ventricular volume. A normal healthy ejection fraction is 0.6–0.75 or 60–70 per cent. Smaller ejection fraction usually indicates extensive left ventricular damage, usually from myocardial infarction.

## Implications for practice

- Skin colour, warmth and capillary refill indicate peripheral perfusion.
- Diastolic blood pressure and pulse pressure indicate systemic vascular resistance.
- Mean arterial pressure (MAP) indicates perfusion pressure.
- Intra-arterial blood pressure monitoring is usually more accurate than noninvasive measurement, provided arterial traces do not look dampened.
- The diacritic notch on arterial traces shows aortic valve closure.
- Low CVP indicates hypovolaemia; high CVP may be from fluid overload, cardiac failure, positive intrathoracic pressure, user error or catheter obstruction.
- Indexed measurements are adjusted to body surface area (m²), so are usually used.
- SvO$_2$ (compared with SaO$_2$) indicates oxygen uptake.
- SVR enables optimisation of vasopressors.
- SVV and EVLW enable optimisation of fluid therapy.
- Nurses using less familiar equipment should remember their individual and professional accountability, only using equipment if competent to do so, and within manufacturers' instructions.

## Summary

Haemodynamic monitoring necessarily forms a major aspect of intensive care nursing. Means described here can provide much information to guide therapy. All modes, especially invasive ones, have complications, so should only be used if benefits outweigh problems. Nurses should actively assess and, where possible, initiate appropriate monitoring, remembering their individual accountability when using equipment. Equipment should only be used by staff competent to do so, and within manufacturers' guidelines and time limits.

## Further reading

Valuable recent medical reviews include Chaney and Derdak (2002) and Polderman and Girbes (2002). Beevers *et al.* (2001) are authorities on hypertension. Cooper and Cramp's (2003) pocketbook is valuable for managing critically and acutely ill patients. Garretson (2005) reviews arterial catheters and nursing care. Hett and Jonas (2004) describe less invasive modes of cardiac flow monitoring.

## Clinical scenarios

Mrs Ellen Harrison, 62 years old, is admitted to the ICU with a chest infection and possible sepsis. She is sedated, mechanically ventilated with intravenous infusions of noradrenaline at 0.4 mcg/kg/min and milrinone at 248 ng/kg/min. Mrs Harrison is 1.75 m tall and weights 75 kg (body surface area of 1.90 m²). A pulmonary artery catheter is floated to provide additional information and tract responses to drug infusions.
    Her haemodynamic profile reveals:

| | | |
|---|---|---|
| BP | 140/50 mmHg (MAP 80 mmHg) | |
| HR | 112 bpm | |
| Rhythm | Sinus tachycardia with self-terminating runs of unifocal ventricular ectopics | |
| CVP | 16 mmHg | |
| CO | 5.6 litres/minute | CI 2.9 litres/minute/m² |
| SV | 61 ml | SVI 32 ml/beat/m² |
| SVR | 744 dynes/second/cm⁵ | SVRI 1416 dynes/second/cm⁵/m² |
| PVR | 157 dynes/second/cm⁵ | PVRI 300 dynes/second/cm⁵/m² |
| LVSWI | 23 gm/m/m² | |
| RVSWI | 4 gm/m/m² | |
| PAP | 38/20 mmHg (mean PAP = 27 mmHg) | |
| PCWP | 14 mmHg | |
| SvO2 | 81 per cent | |

Q.1 (a) Identify nursing interventions that can assist in preventing complications associated with PA catheters.

(b) Why is a chest X-ray performed after the insertion of a PA catheter?

(c) Note symptoms which may indicate pulmonary infarction.

Q.2 Compare Mrs Harrison's haemodynamic values to normal parameters. Reflect on likely cause and implications of abnormal results, for example, on Mrs Harrison's perfusion and oxygen delivery; will she be warm, cool, dilated, constricted.

Q.3 Consider the clinical implications of Mrs Harrison's haemodynamic values and how they may guide changes in her vasoactive drug infusions rates. Devise a plan of care to include rationales for choice of prescribed drugs and/or fluid therapies and haemodynamic goals.

# Chapter 21

# Blood results

## Contents

| | |
|---|---|
| Introduction | 210 |
| Haematology | 210 |
| Albumin and total protein | 215 |
| Biochemistry | 216 |
| Implications for practice | 220 |
| Summary | 221 |
| Further reading | 221 |
| Clinical scenarios | 221 |

## Introduction

Blood is a major transport mechanism for the body, so what is in blood reflects body activity. ICU nurses usually download results from desktop computers, so recognising abnormal values and knowing what to do about them enables early and appropriate interventions. This chapter outlines main haematology and biochemistry results. Liver function tests, including albumin, are outlined in Chapter 42 and cardiac markers (troponin, myoglobin, CK) are included in Chapter 30.

Although results are discussed individually below, low levels may be caused by

- dilution
- loss
- failure of supply or production

while high levels may be from

- dehydration (haemoconcentration)
- excessive intake/production
- failure to metabolise or remove (e.g. hepatic or renal dysfunction).

Dilution (from large volume intravenous infusion) and haemoconcentration (from excessive drainage or fluid shifts) are not identified specifically below, but should always be considered as possible causes of high (haemoconcentration) or low (haemodilution) results.

Sampling errors may cause erroneous results such as

- venepuncturing limbs where IVIs are running
- insufficient blood
- incorrect bottles
- incorrect inversion times for bottles (resulting in insufficient mixing of additives)
- incorrect labelling

so results appearing inconsistent with patients' clinical state should be checked.

Many treatments of abnormalities are identified, but other treatments are possible. Treatments identified are those normally used in the ICU, so are not necessarily appropriate in other settings.

## Haematology

There are three types of blood cells:

- erythrocytes (red blood cells – RBCs)
- leucocytes (white cells)
- platelets

**Table 21.1 Erythrocyte results**

| | | |
|---|---|---|
| RBC | males | $4.5–6.5 \times 10^{-12}$/litre |
| | females | $3.9–5.6 \times 10^{-12}$/litre |
| Hb | males | 13.4–17 5 g/dl |
| | females | 11.5–17 5 g/dl |
| PCV /Hct | males | 40–52% |
| | females | 36–48% |
| MCV (mean cell volume) | | $80–95 \ \mu m^{-3}$ |
| MCD | | $6.7–7.7 \ \mu m$ |
| MCHC (mean corpuscular haemoglobin concentration) | | 32–35 g/dl |
| MCH (mean corpuscular haemoglobin) | | 28–32/g |

so, a full blood count includes

■ haemoglobin (oxygen carriage)
■ white cell count (WCC – immunity), with specific types of white cells also counted
■ platelets and other clotting measurements.

All blood cells are produced by bone marrow, so diseases or treatments that cause bone marrow suppression affect counts of all cells. Various tests that can be performed on erythrocytes (summarised in Table 21.1), but haemoglobin is the main one used in the ICU. Haemoglobin is also measured by blood gas analysers.

### Haemoglobin (Hb)

Normal: 13–18 g/dl (men) and 11.5–16.5 g/dl (women).

Polycythaemia (raised levels) is usually an adaptive response to chronic hypoxia. People living at very high altitudes are often polycythaemic, but in the UK it is usually a response to chronic lung, or sometimes cardiac, disease.

Critical illness usually causes low levels from

■ blood loss
■ dilution
■ reduced erythropoeisis
■ reduced erythrocyte lifespan, with sepsis (McLellan et al., 2003)

and sometimes anaemia (see Table 21.2) or other causes, including iatrongenic.

Haemoglobin transports most oxygen in arterial blood, so low haemoglobin reduces oxygen carrying capacity. Oxygen delivery to cells is a paradox between oxygen carriage (erythrocytes) with oxygen delivery (plasma). Blood is plasma and cells; plasma is mainly (90–95 per cent) water, and most blood

### Table 21.2 Some types of anaemia

*iron deficiency*: the most common cause of anaemia. In the ICU this is usually due to blood loss, impaired erythrocyte production and reduced erythrocyte lifespan. With rapid blood loss (e.g. trauma, surgery), plasma is replaced within 1–3 days, but erythrocytes take 3–6 weeks to return to normal numbers, so haemoglobin concentration (grams per decilitre) will be low between these two times. Impaired renal production reduces erythroposeises, while sepsis reduces erythrocyte life

*microcytic*: chronic blood loss exhausts iron stores, so although erythrocytes numbers may be normal, they contain relatively little haemoglobin and are small

*aplastic*: bone marrow dysfunction (e.g. from chemotherapy or radiation) prevents erythrocyte formation

*megablostaic*: lack of vitamin B12, folic acid or intrinsic factor delays erythropoesis, resulting in large, misshapen erythrocytes

*haemolytic*: erythrocytes are prematurely destroyed. In the ICU, this frequently occurs with sepsis. Elsewhere, abnormalities, often genetic, cause abnormal fragility, resulting in premature haemolysis. So despite large numbers being formed, their lifespan in short, resulting in low erythrocyte and haemoglobin levels.

cells (99 per cent) are erythrocytes. Higher haemoglobin concentrations therefore make blood thicker, while lower levels make it more dilute. Dilute blood flows more easily through capillaries, from which tissue cells receive oxygen. So dilute blood carries less oxygen but delivers it more effectively. Moderate anaemia improves survival from critical illness, survival being highest with Hb 7–9 g/dl (Herbert *et al.*, 1999).

Blood counts may also identify reticulocytes. Recticulocytes are immature erythrocytes, released prematurely from bone marrow. When released, erythrocytes lose their nucleus, so premature released cells remain immature, less able to carry oxygen. Normal reticulocyte counts are 0.5–1.5 per cent for men and 0.5–2.5 per cent for women (Mahon & Hattersley, 2002). Excessive release of reticulocytes is usually caused by increased demand, such as chronic hypoxic states, or exogenous erythropoetin.

Because most blood cells are erythrocytes, paced cell volume (PCV), also called haematocrit (Hct), also indicates erythrocytes, as a percentage of total volume.

*Treatment:* low Hb (<7 g/dl) can be treated by blood transfusion.

## White cell count

Normal: $5–10 \times 10^3$/microlitre.

Leucocytes form part of the immune system, so raised levels usually indicate infection. Counts may be raised by excessive immune responses. Immunodeficiency inhibits this response, and severe sepsis destroys large numbers (see Chapter 33), so infection cannot be excluded if counts are normal or low.

Low counts (leucopaenia) can be treated with granulocyte colony stimulating factor (GCSF), but this takes about one week to work, so although it is useful for oncology, it has little value in critical illness.

**Table 21.3 Normal white cell counts**

| White cell type | $\times 10^9$/litre | per mm$^3$ | % |
|---|---|---|---|
| Neutrophils (polymorphs) | 2.5–7.5 | 2500–7500 | 50–70 |
| Basophils | <0.2 | <200 | ≤3 |
| Eosinophils | 0.04–0.44 | 40–400 | ≤5 |
| Lymphocytes | 1.5–4.0 | 1500–4000 | ≤12–50 |
| Monocytes | 0.2–0.8 | 200–800 | 3–15 |

Note: (UK uses $\times 10^9$/litre)

There are two main groups of leucocytes:

■ granulocytes
■ agranulocytes

identified by whether or not cell membranes contain granules. Granulocytes tackle acute infections, whereas agranulocytes fight long-term chronic problems. Both main groups have further sub-types of cells. Normal counts are identified in Table 21.3.

Within hours of release, leucocytes migrate from blood into tissues where they remain unless mobilised back into the bloodstream by infection – hence rapid rises in WCC with infection.

*Treatment:* usually, underlying causes are treated – e.g. infection with antibiotics. Low neutrophil count may be an indication for protective isolation (reverse barrier nursing).

### Granulocytes

There are three types of granulocytes:

■ neutrophils (polymorphoneuclear, so 'polymorphs')
■ basophils
■ eosinophils

identified by laboratory staining.

Most leucocytes (50–70 per cent) are neutrophils. Neutrophils are the first and main defence against infection, destroying bacteria by phagocytosis, resulting in pus. With infection, neutrophil count rises before other types of leucocytes.

Basophils promote inflammatory responses, so are normally associated with healing, allergic responses or persistent problems. Basophils are mainly responsible for releasing the inflammatory mediators from mast cells – histamine, leucotrienes and proteases (Minors, 2004) that often complicate critical illness.

Eosinophils are mainly anti-parasitic and involved in allergic reactions (Minors, 2004).

213

### Agranulocytes

There are two types of agranulocytes:

- lymphocytes – T and B
- monocytes.

Most (four-fifths) lymphocytes are *T-lymphocytes*, which recognise and kill infected cells. Antigen recognition causes enlargement and differentiation into

- *killer cells* (also called cytolytic, cytotoxic, T8 or CD8), which attach themselves to invading cells where they are activated, secreting lympho-toxins, cytokines and interferon, which kill or prevent replication of cells;
- *helper cells* (also called T4 or CD4), which assist B-lymphocytes increase antibody production. Most helper cells contain the CD4 marker, and so are labelled CD+ (CD = cluster designation);
- *memory cells*, which memorise antigens;
- *supressor (or regulatory) cells*, which limit damage to the body's own tissue (Guyton & Hall, 2000). Not all texts identify this fourth group of T-lymphocytes.

*B-lymphocytes* produce antibodies and release immunoglobulins to neutralise toxins and viral activity, promoting bacterial lysis and phagocytosis. Of the five immunoglobulins, three (*IgA, IgG, IgM*) are mainly carried by intravas-cular B-lmyphoctes. Each group of immunoglobulins has further subclasses (e.g. Ig has four, labelled $Ig^1$, $Ig^2$, $Ig^3$, $Ig^4$).

*IgA*, relatively unimportant for systemic humoral immunity, is found mainly in mucus membranes: mucus, saliva, tears, sweat and breast milk.

*IgD* only trace amounts are found in serum (Feldkamp, 2003), primarily on plasma membranes of B-lymphocytes.

*IgE* attaches itself to antigen cell membranes of basophils and mast cells of connective tissue, initiating leucocyte destruction or damage. Leucocyte damage releases intracellular vasoactive mediators, including histamine. Unless antigens are present, serum contains only trace amounts of IgE (Feldkamp, 2003).

*IgG*, the main immunoglobulin in blood, is a major mediator of allergic reactions. IgG readily enters tissues, coating micro-organisms prior to phagocytosis.

*IgM* is the first immunoglobulin released during primary immune response to antigens.

*Monocytes* migrate from blood into tissues, where they can mature into macrophages ('big eaters'). Counting macrophages is impractical, as they are in interstitial spaces, but precursor monocytes can be measured in blood.

### Platelets (thrombocytes)

Normal: 150–400 × 10⁹/litre.

Formed in the bone marrow, platelets circulate in the bloodstream for about 10 days. Normally kept inactive by endovascular chemicals (e.g. prostacyclin), they are activated by platelet activating factor (release by endothelium of damaged blood vessels) to assist with clotting.

Platelet counts are often low in critical illness, from

- loss from bleeding
- impaired production
- anti-platelet drugs (e.g. aspirin, clopidogrel).

However, impaired blood flow and immobility exposes ICU patients to high risk of deep vein thrombosis (DVT), and pulmonary embolism (PE). Most ICU patients are therefore prescribed prophylactic anticoagulants, titrated against clotting studies.

*Treatment*: platelets can be transfused if indicated.

### Albumin and total protein

Normal: albumin 35–50 g/litre
total protein (TP): 60–80 g/litre.

Plasma proteins create most of the *colloid osmotic pressure* that retains normal plasma volume within the bloodstream. Low plasma protein levels therefore causes excessive extravasation, hypovolaemia and oedema. Proteins also

- bind drug
- transport substances (e.g. bilirubin)
- are antioxidants.

So plasma protein, especially albumin, deficiency causes hypovolaemia, oedema and many other complications. Although there are many plasma proteins, more than half of total protein concentration is albumin, and albumin exerts three-quarters of plasma protein colloid osmotic pressure.

The liver produces plasma proteins from dietary protein. Malnutrition and liver hypofunction therefore cause hypoalbuminaemia. Normal albumin half-life is 18–20 days (Maloney *et al.*, 2002). ICU patients usually have significantly reduced plasma protein levels, reductions usually worsening with severity of disease.

*Treatment*: exogenous albumin has only transient effects. Patients should be fed early, enabling the liver to produce albumin.

### Clotting studies

Normal APTT: 25–35 seconds
PT: 10–12 seconds
INR: normal 0.9–1.1.

In addition to platelet count, clotting is usually measured by:

- activated partial thromboplastin time (APTT – replaced partial thromboplastin time – PTT)
- prothromin time (PT); also called activated prothromin time (APT)
- international normalised ratio (INR).

D-dimers are discussed separately below. Other possible studies (not discussed further) include

- bleeding time (BT): normally 3–10 minutes, which measures platelet plug formation
- thrombin time (TT): normally 12 seconds, which tests fibrinogen conversion to fibrin
- fibrinogen: normal 1.8–5.4 g/litre.

APTT and PT are measured against a control, which is often (but not always) 1. INR measurement includes the control, so is simpler, and is usually the preferred test.

*Treatment*: with anticoagulant therapy INR should normally be kept between 2.0–2.3 (BCSH, 1998). Outside these levels, anticoagulant dose should be adjusted.

## D-dimers

Normal: <250 nanograms/ml (μg/litre), sometimes reported as 'negative'.

D-dimers are fibrin degradation products. Fibrinolysis (clot breakdown) releases fibrin from clots, releasing fibrin degradation products (FDPs). In health, only small amounts of FDPs and D-dimers circulate in blood, but excessive fibrinolysis generates excessive levels. D-dimers can originate from any clot breakdown, but as cardiac markers would be tested if myocardial infarction were suspected, elevated D-dimers are likely to indicate either deep vein thrombosis or pulmonary emboli. If D-dimers are negative, DVT can be excluded (Wells *et al.*, 2003; British Thoracic Society, 2003), but positive/ elevated results may be caused by renal failure (Kelly *et al.*, 2002), so D-dimers on their own are insufficient to confirm diagnosis of PE (Rathbun *et al.*, 2004).

*Treatment:* treat the disease – e.g. with intravenous heparin.

## Biochemistry

C-reactive protein indicates inflammation, is widely used, and so is discussed first. Important urea and electrolyte (U + E) results, and the ones discussed here, are

- sodium
- potassium

- chloride
- glucose
- phosphate
- magnesium
- calcium
- urea
- creatinine.

Most electrolyte deficiencies can be treated by electrolyte supplements, through various routes. Many intravenous electrolytes should be infused through central lines.

### C-reactive protein

Normal: CRP = 0–10 mg/ml.

C-reactive protein (CRP) is an acute phase protein, released with systemic inflammation (Venugopal *et al.*, 2002; Tousoulis *et al.*, 2003; Lobo *et al.*, 2003). Causes of inflammation are inferred from individual patient contexts. In the ICU, CRP, with other results, usually infers sepsis/SIRS (see Chapter 33) (Póvoa, 2002; Warren *et al.*, 2002).

*Treatment*: treat the disease – e.g. SIRS with system support.

### Sodium (Na⁺)

Normal: 135–145 mmol/litre.

Sodium is the main intravascular cation. Abnormal levels usually indicate hydration status. Hyponatraemia can be caused by excessive sodium loss (vomiting, diarrhoea, sweating), but in ICU patients is usually caused by fluid shifting from intracellular (where sodium concentration is normally 14 mmol/litre) to intravascular spaces, causing dilution. Severe hyponatraemia ($<120$) may cause encephalopathy.

*Treatment*: hyponatrameia is treated by giving sodium, usually as normal saline, relying on the kidney to remove excess water while conserving salt. Hypernatraemia usually indicates dehydration, rehydration being achieved with water, usually as 5% glucose.

### Potassium (K⁺)

Normal: 3.5–4.5 mmol/litre.

Potassium is used for cardiac conduction; hypokalaemia impairs conduction, so can provoke bradycardia and escape dysrhythmias, while hyperkalaemia can cause trachydysrhythmias. With patients at risk of cardiac dysfunction (most ICU patients) it is safer to maintain levels at 4–5 mmol/litre, slightly higher than normal physiological levels.

Most (90 per cent) potassium loss is renal, so blood potassium levels usually follow urine output: polyuria causes hypokalaemia, while oliguria causes hyperkalaemia. Intracellular fluid contains far higher potassium concentrations (140–50 mmol/litre), so extensive cell damage (such as major trauma) or large fluid shifts can also cause hyperkalaemia. Haemolyis causes potassium leak from damaged blood cells, so haemolysed samples indicate high potassium.

*Treatment*: life-threatening hyperkalaemia (>6 mmol/litre) should be urgently treated with intravenous glucose and insulin infusion, which transfers potassium into intracellular fluid. Concurrent intravenous calcium (gluconate or chloride) stabilises cardiac conduction. Less severe hyperkalaemia (5–6 mmol/litre) may be treated with calcium resonium, given orally if the gut is functional and the patient able to take it, or rectally if not (Humphreys, 2002). If hyperkalaemia is caused by fluid shifts, patients should be aggressively rehydrated.

A few small paediatric studies, such as Kemper *et al.* (1996), used salbutamol to transport potassium into cells, but this practice seems questionable.

Hypokalaemia is treated with potassium supplements. Strong potassium concentrations (such as 40 mmol in 100 ml) are often infused in the ICU, but must be given through a central line, as peripheral infusion is very painful and likely to cause severe thrombophlebitis. Strong potassium concentrations should only be used in critical care areas (NPSA, 2002) where continuous ECG monitoring, potassium analysers and high staffing levels are available.

### Chloride (Cl⁻)

Normal: 95–105 mmol/litre.

As the main extracellular anion, hyperchloraemia can cause metabolic acidosis (see anion gap, Chapter 19). Normal saline fluids are hyperchloraemic (154 mmol/litre chloride), so excessive infusion of intravenous saline can cause hyperchloraemic acidaemia. Hyperchloraemia can also impair mental function and cause abdominal discomfort, headaches, nausea and vomiting.

*Treatment*: hyperchloraemia is usually from excessive saline infusions, which should be discontinued.

### Glucose ($C_6H_{12}O_6$)

Normal: 4.4–6.1 mmol/litre.

Glucose is the main source of intracellular energy (see Chapter 24), needing insulin to transport it into cells. Insulin deficiency or resistance therefore causes hyperglycaemia. In critically ill patients, the stress response and various drugs (e.g. corticosteroids, adrenaline) reduce insulin production and increase insulin resistance. Even moderate hyperglycaemia aggravates immunocompromise (Torpy & Chrousos, 1997). Maintaining normoglycaemia reduces mortality from critical illness (Van Den Berghe *et al.*, 2001),

*Treatment*: hypoglycaemia is treated by giving glucose. Hyperglycaemia in the ICU is usually treated with insulin infusions (see Chapter 46).

## Phosphate ($PO_4^{3-}$)

Normal: 0.8–1.45 mmol/litre.
   Most (85 per cent) phosphate is in bones. Elsewhere, phosphate

- produces ATP (cell energy)
- produces 2,3 DPG (assists oxygen dissociation from haemoglobin)
- buffers acids (phosphate is the main intracellular buffer)
- reduces free fatty acids.

Hyperphophosphaemia, rare in the ICU except when patients have chronic renal failure, stimulates parathyroid hormone production, so may cause calcium imbalance, and so dysrhythmias.
   Hypophosphataemia often occurs, causing potential

- muscle weakness, including respiratory muscles (which may delay weaning)
- intracellular acidosis
- intracellular hypoxia.

*Treatment*: hypophophataemia is usually treated by phosphate infusion (often 50 mmol over 24 hours). Oral supplements are also available.

## Magnesium ($Mg^{++}$) or ($Mg^{2+}$)

Normal: 0.75–1.0 mmol/litre.
   Magnesium ('nature's tranquilliser') stabilises cell membranes, reducing conduction. Blood magnesium, only 1 per cent of total body magnesium,

- vasodilates
- delays atrioventricular cardiac conduction.

Hypomagnesiumaemia, usually from malnutrition or excessive diuresis, occurs in many ICU patients (Dubé & Granry, 2003), and may cause tachy-dysrhythmias (Abbott *et al.*, 2003; Dubé & Granry, 2003) and other problems. Hypermagnesiumaemia (>3 mmol/litre) may cause cardiac and/or respiratory arrest.
*Treatment*: Various magnesium supplements (and concentrations) are available.

## Calcium ($Ca^{++}$) or ($Ca^{2+}$)

Normal: total calcium 2.25–2.75 mmol/litre; ionised levels 1.1–1.3 mmol/litre.
   Like magnesium, only 1 per cent of body calcium is in blood, but blood calcium facilitates

- cardiac conduction
- muscle cell contraction
- cell function
- clotting.

About half blood calcium is normally protein-bound, and half free (*ionised*, or unbound). Laboratories normally measure total blood calcium, but gas analysers normally measure ionised calcium. Only free (unbound) calcium is active.

Protein binding is affected by various factors, including

■ plasma protein concentration (mainly albumin)
■ pH – acidosis releases more calcium from protein, so increasing ionised levels.

With abnormal blood protein levels, laboratories may 'correct' calcium levels to reflect the amount of physiologically active (ionised) levels.

Hypocalcaemia may be caused by

■ sepsis
■ renal dysfunction
■ heparin therapy

and other diseases and treatments.

*Treatment*: Hypocalcaemia is treated with calcium supplements.

### Urea

Normal: 3–9 mmol/litre.

Urea is a nitrogenous waste product of (any) protein metabolism, and is normally cleared in urine. High urea and creatinine usually indicates renal failure, but if uraemia disproportionately exceeds creatinine (ratio is usually approximately 1:20) excessive protein metabolism is more likely, especially from digestion of blood following gastrointestinal bleeds.

*Treatment*: raised urea (and creatinine) indicate renal failure. Support, possibly including renal replacement therapy, should be considered.

### Creatinine

Normal: female 50–90 micromol/litre, male 70–120 micromol/litre.

Creatinine, a waste product of muscle metabolism (hence gender differences), is normally cleared in urine. With renal failure, levels usually rise steadily 50–100 micromol/day (Skinner & Watson, 1997), so function should be assessed through trends from a series of samples.

*Treatment*: as urea.

### Implications for practice

■ Blood results reflect body activity.
■ Samples should be taken and labelled carefully to avoid erroneous results or delay.
■ Low results are caused by: dilution, loss or failure of supply/to produce.

- High levels are caused by: dehydration (haemoconcentration), excessive intake/production or failure to clear.
- Optimum Hb for critically ill patients is 7–9 g/dl.
- Persistent hyponatraemia and hyperkalaemia is often caused by fluid moving from intracellular to intravascular compartments.
- Severe hyponatraemia (<120 mmol/litre) may cause encephalopathy.
- Maintaining normoglycaemia (4.4–6.1 mmol/litre) increases survival from critical illness.
- Nurses should identify and report normal results.

## Summary

Blood is the transport system of the body, so abnormal results indicate problems, but may also cause further complications. Nurses usually download results before medical staff, so understanding main results and how abnormalities should be managed enables earlier treatment.

## Further reading

Higgins (2000) provides an accessible book about laboratory investigations. Journals intended primarily for medical students occasionally publish articles overviewing interpretation of blood results (such as Ackrill & France, 2002). Van Den Berghe (2001) and Herbert *et al.* (1999) significantly changed practice. www.routledge.com/textbooks/0415373239

For Clinical Scenarios, Clinical questions and the answers to them go to the support website at www.routledge.com/textbooks/0415373239

## Clinical scenarios

Henry Duff is a 68-year-old known diabetic. He was admitted two days ago with bleeding gastric ulcers and has frequent episodes of melaena. He is self ventilating on 28% oxygen via nasal cannulae, with a respiratory rate between 18–28 breaths/min. He has an intravenous infusion of Omeprazole (80 mg over 10 hours) in progress. Henry appears to be hallucinating, reports visual disturbances, is confused and at times agitated with the following blood results.

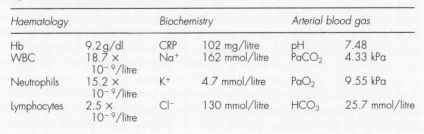

| Haematology | | Biochemistry | | Arterial blood gas | |
|---|---|---|---|---|---|
| Hb | 9.2 g/dl | CRP | 102 mg/litre | pH | 7.48 |
| WBC | 18.7 × 10$^{-9}$/litre | Na$^+$ | 162 mmol/litre | PaCO$_2$ | 4.33 kPa |
| Neutrophils | 15.2 × 10$^{-9}$/litre | K$^+$ | 4.7 mmol/litre | PaO$_2$ | 9.55 kPa |
| Lymphocytes | 2.5 × 10$^{-9}$/litre | Cl$^-$ | 130 mmol/litre | HCO$_3$ | 25.7 mmol/litre |

| Platelets | 234 × 10$^{-9}$/litre | HCO$_3$ | 25 mmol/litre | Base excess | 1.1 mmol/litre |
|-----------|-----------------------|---------|---------------|-------------|----------------|
| MCV | 90 μm$^3$ | Glucose | 10.5 mmol/litre | Lactate | 1.5 mmol/litre |
| | | PO$_4$$^{-3}$ | 0.74 mmol/litre | | |
| INR | 1.2 | Mg$^{2+}$ | 0.72 mmol/litre | | |
| APTT ratio | 1.58 | Ca$^{2+}$ | 2.38 mmol/litre | | |
| | | Urea | 18.6 mmol/litre | | |
| | | Creatinine | 136 μmol/litre | | |
| | | Bilirubin | 36 mmol/litre | | |
| | | ALT | 38 iu/litre | | |
| | | Alk Phos | 129 iu/litre | | |
| | | Albumin | 16 g/litre | | |
| | | Gamma GT | 132 iu/litre | | |

Q.1  Interpret Henry's blood results and note the clinical significance of abnormal values. Consider which of the abnormal blood results is caused by Henry's pathophysiology, and which may be caused by sampling errors.

Q.2  Explain the potential causes of Henry's hypernatreamia. Identify interventions and therapies that should be implemented to resolve abnormality.

Q.3  Review other blood tests which could aid the assessment process for Henry's condition, and provide a rationale for these suggestions.

# Chapter 22

# ECGs and dysrhythmias

## Contents

| | |
|---|---|
| Introduction | 224 |
| Basic principles of elecrocardiography | 225 |
| Lead changes | 227 |
| Atrial kick | 227 |
| ST abnormalities | 227 |
| U waves | 229 |
| Action potential | 229 |
| General treatments | 230 |
| Atrial/junctional dysrhythmias | 231 |
| Atrioventricular blocks | 238 |
| Bundle branch block | 240 |
| Ventricular dysrhythmias | 240 |
| Asystole | 244 |
| Pulseless electrical activity (PEA) | 245 |
| Implications for practice | 245 |
| Summary | 246 |
| Further reading | 246 |
| Clinical questions | 246 |

## Fundamental knowledge

Myocardial physiology – automaticity, conductivity, rhythmicity

Normal limb electrode placement

Normal cardiac conduction (SA node, AV node, Bundle of His, Purkinje fibres)

Physiology of normal sinus rhythm
Current resuscitation council guidelines
Experience of using continuous ECG monitoring and
taking 12 lead ECGs

## Introduction

Some dysrhythmias are immediately life threatening. If not immediately life threatening, dysrhythmias usually compromise cardiac function (reduced stroke volume, increased tachycardia and myocardial hypoxia) and are usually symptoms of some problem. Dysrhythmias may be acute or chronic. Chronic dysrhythmias (atrial fibrillation being especially common) should be controlled, but can rarely be reversed. Most acute dysrythmias should be actively reversed if possible, with close haemodynamic monitoring and support where reversal is not possible.

Although ICU nurses seldom see the range of dysrhythmias encountered in coronary care units, ECG monitoring is standard, so nurses should be able to

■ identify dysrhythmias
■ identify likely causes from patients' histories
■ know usual management and treatment for commonly-occurring dysrhythmias.

As with almost all problems, early intervention reduces complication and improves survival and outcome, so ICU nurses should develop expertise in this fundamental aspect of critical care monitoring.

This chapter briefly revises normal cardiac conduction. Action potential is then described, to explain effects of both electrolytes and some drugs on cardiac impulses. Some commonly used drugs are mentioned, but practices vary, so users should consult Summary of Product Characteristics (SPC) or pharmacopaedias for detailed information on drugs.

Normal conduction begins in the sino-atrial node, passing through atrial muscle to the atrioventricular node, then passing from the atrioventricular node through the ventricular conduction pathway and into ventricular myocytes. There are therefore three key stages in normal cardiac conduction and the ECG:

■ atrial (P wave)
■ atrioventricular node (PR interval)
■ ventricular (QRS complex, ST segment, T wave).

Dyrhythmias can originate in any part of the heart. This chapter discusses dysrhythmias in sequence: atrial, atrioventricular, ventricular.

The etymologically more accurate 'dysrhythmia', rather than the more popular 'arrhythmia', is used here as, except for asystole, rhythms are problematic rather than absent. Being for ICU nurses caring for patients with acute physiological crises, this chapter focuses on acute rather than chronic problems.

## Basic principles of electrocardiography

An ECG is a graph of myocardial electrical activity, representing three dimensional events in two. This section summarises basic principles for revision. Any parts unfamiliar to readers should be revised further before proceeding (e.g. from Hampton, 2003a).

- ECG graph paper, unlike standard mathematical graph paper has only 25 (5 × 5) small squares in each large square
- each small square is 1 mm
- horizontal axis represents time
- ECGs are normally recorded at 25 mm/second
- recorded at 25 mm/second, one large square = 0.2 seconds, one small square = 0.04 seconds
- vertical axes represent voltage; a calibration square (normally 10 mm = 1 mv = 2 large squares) should appear at the beginning or end of ECGs
- normal sinus rhythm (Figure 22.1) is labelled PQRST
- P = atrial *depolarization*
- QRS = ventricular depolarisation
- T = ventricular *repolarisation*
- SA and AV nodes have both sympathetic and parasympathetic nerve fibres, so are affected by brainstem control and vagal stimulation
- electrical conduction is normally rapidly followed by related muscle contraction, except PEA (see later)
- limb electrodes are normally colour-coded:
  - red = right arm
  - yellow = left arm
  - black/green = left leg
- electrical 'pictures' remain unchanged anywhere along limbs, or on a line between the limb joint and heart, so electrodes may be placed anywhere along the picture line
- limb leads examine electrical activity along a vertical plane. The electrodes on the right arm, left arm and left leg (forming 'Einthoven's triangle') create the following limb leads:

      lead I = right arm to left arm (bipolar)
      lead II = right arm to left leg (bipolar)
      lead III = left arm to left leg (bipolar)
      aVR = augmented Vector Right (arm; unipolar)
      aVL = augmented Vector Left (arm; unipolar)
      aVF = augmented Vector Foot (left leg; unipolar)

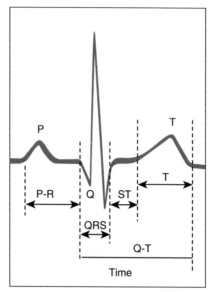

Normal wave form

■ *Figure 22.1 Normal sinus rhythm*

■ chest leads examine electrical activity along a horizontal plane, from right atrium, through right ventricle, septum, left ventricle, to left atrium (Figure 22.2):

   C (or V) 1 (red): 4th intercostal space, to right of (patient's) sternum
   C2 (yellow): 4th intercostal space, left of sternum
   C3 (green): between C2 and C4
   C4 (brown): 5th intercostal space, midclavicular line
   C5 (black): between C4 and C6
   C6 (purple): 5th intercostal space, mid axilla

nb: breast tissue (fat is a poor conductor), wounds or invasive equipment may necessitate slight approximations

■ normal times: P wave = 0.1 seconds (2.5 small squares)
         PR interval* = 0.12–0.2 seconds (3–5 small squares)
         QRS = 0.06–0.12 seconds (1½–3 small squares)
         T wave = 0.16 seconds (4 small squares)
         QT interval = < 1/2 preceding R–R interval, maximum 0.4 seconds (2 large squares)

* measure PR intervals from beginning of the P wave to the start of the QRS

■ sinus rhythm = technically, any rhythm origination from the sinoatrial node, although in practice the term is often used to describe regular rhythms of 60–100 bpm originating from the SA node.

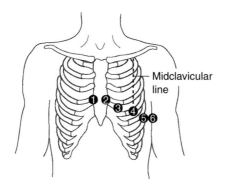

Midclavicular
line

■ *Figure 22.2* **Chest lead placement**

Table 22.1 Provides a framework for ECG interpretation.

## Lead changes

Each lead views cardiac conduction differently, changes being more prominent
in leads which best view areas of ischaemic/infarcted myocardium:

- anterior : C1–C4
- lateral: I, aVL, C4–C6
- anterior lateral: I, aVL, C4–C6
- anterior septal: C1–C3
- inferior: II, III, aVF
- apex: C5, C6
- septum C2, C3.

Usual lead placement does not view posterior myocardium clearly, but posterior infarction is best seen in C1 and C2.

## Atrial kick

Atrioventricular dyssynchrony, which occurs with any rhythm where atrial
contraction does not precede ventricular contraction (almost all dysrhythmias
originating below the atrium) causes loss of 'atrial kick', reducing stroke
volume by one-fifth (Falk, 2001). Unless compensatory tachycardia occurs,
reduced stroke volume causes hypotension.

## ST abnormalities

From the S wave, ECG complexes should return almost vertically to the isoelectric
line, with a gap then occurring before the T wave (ventricular repolarisation). Any
ST elevation or depression should be noted and, if new, reported.

### Table 22.1 Framework for ECG interpretation

*Recording the ECG*
Are electrodes correctly placed (red = right arm, yellow = left arm, green/black = left leg)?
Is there a clear baseline (isoelectric line)?

*Regularity*
Is the rhythm regular?
If not, is it

- ■  regularly irregular (is there a pattern?)
- ■  irregularly irregular (no pattern).

*P wave*
Does the P wave appear before the QRS?
Is there one P wave for every QRS?
Is the shape normal?
Are P waves missing?

*PR interval*
Is the PR interval 3–5 small squares?

*QRS complex*
Is QRS width within 3 small squares?
Is the QRS positive or negative?
Is the axis normal?
Does it look normal?

*ST segment*
Does the isoelectric line return between the S and the T?
If not, is it

- ■  elevated (>1 mm above isoelectric line)
- ■  depressed (<0.5 mm below isoelectric line)?

*T wave*
Does the T wave look normal?
Is the QT interval <1/2 preceding R–R interval, and maximum 0.4 seconds

*Tachycardia (>100/minute)*
narrow complex (usually with P waves) = atrial (supraventricular)
wide complex (without P wave) = ventricular.

ST elevation (1 mm in chest leads, 2 mm in limb leads) in two or more consecutive leads usually indicates acute myocardial infarction. Classification of *acute coronary syndromes* into

- ■  ST elevation myocardial infarction (STEMI)
- ■  non ST elevation myocardial infarction (NSTEMI) and
- ■  unstable coronary syndromes

is discussed in Chapter 30. Chest pain, together with either ST elevation or a new left bundle branch block, is sufficient indication for urgent thrombolysis.

ST elevation can also be caused by other problems, including pericarditis, hyperkalaemia and pulmonary embolism (Wang *et al.*, 2003).

Causes of ST depression include digoxin, ischaemia, ventricular hypertrophy and hypokalaemia.

## U waves

U waves are often absent, but if present appear like a second, smaller T wave, and are often difficult to detect. U waves often appear in healthy people, especially athletes (Meek & Morris, 2002), so are not usually pathological, but may indicate electrolyte abnormality, especially hyperkalaemia (Slovis & Jenkins, 2002) or hypercalcaemia (Meek & Morris, 2002).

## Action potential

While interstitial and intravascular concentrations of sodium and potassium are similar (normally $Na^+$ 135–45, $K^+$ 3.5–4.5), intracellular concentrations are approximately opposite (normally $Na^+$ 14, $K^+$ 120–40). This maintains resting muscle cell membrane potential (or charge) at approximately minus 70–90 millivolts (mv).

Sequential opening of various channels in myocyte membranes changes cation (sodium, calcium and potassium) concentrations, making this charge progressively less negative, and eventually positive (about +30 mv), before restoring the resting negative charge. When electrical charge changes, cells are electrically excitable, so able to initiate or conduct impulses. Changing

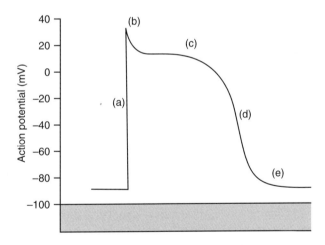

(a) Rapid depolarisation: influx via fast sodium channel (phase 0).
(b) Fast calcium channel open (phase 1).
(c) Plateau: slow calcium channel open (phase 2).
(d) Rapid depolarisation: potassium channel open (phase 3).
(e) Resting phase (phase 4).

**Figure 22.3 Action potential**

229

electrical charge of myocyte membranes therefore create the potential for action, shown graphically in Figure 22.3.

Action potential is divided into *phases*, numbered 0–4 (see Figure 22.3).

*phase 0* (upstroke) is the *fast sodium* channel opening, allowing rapid influx of extracelluar sodium ions into sodium-poor intracellular fluid, causing rapid depolarisation.

*phase 1* (spike) is the *fast* or transient *calcium* opening briefly, allowing calcium influx. This gives action potential graphs their characteristic peak.

*phase 2* is the 'plateau' (or absolute refractory period), caused by the *slow* or long lasting *calcium* channel opening. This prevents cardiac muscle responding to further stimulus, ensuring co-ordinated action, and so strength of contraction. Hypercalcaemia therefore increases contractility – excitability can be reduced with calcium channel blockers.

*phase 3* is when the *potassium* channel opens, allowing potassium efflux and rapid repolarisation.

*phase 4* is the 'resting' or depolarisation phase. Slow passive potassium leak restores negative resting membrane charge. Catecholamines shorten, while vagal stimulation prolongs, this phase.

## General treatments

*Myocardial hypoxia* is often present, so oxygen is usually a first-line treatment.

*Underlying causes* (e.g. hypokalaemia) of dysrhythmias should be resolved, but asymptomatic dysrhythmias seldom require treatment. However, usual symptoms (e.g. pain, dyspnoea, syncope) may remain unrecognised in semiconscious ventilated patients. Cardiac rhythm affects blood pressure:

$$\text{blood pressure} = \text{heart rate} \times \text{stroke volume} \times \text{systemic vascular resistance}$$

so haemodynamic compromise necessitates action.

Most *drugs* used either suppress myocardial automaticity or change conduction through the AV node (some increasing, others decreasing). Bradycardic dysrhythmias may need positive *chronotropes* (e.g. atropine). Tachycardic dysrhythmias are often caused by overexcitability of conduction pathways. Atrioventricular node conduction can be reduced with digoxin (cardiac glycoside). Ventricular conduction may be blocked with

■ β-blockers (esmolol, sotalol, propanolol), which inhibit beta receptors (see Chapter 35)
■ calcium channel blockers (e.g. diltiazem) increase refractory periods of action potentials, so slow ventricular conduction. Verapamil should not be given after β-blockers or digoxin.

Antidysrhythmic drugs ('Vaughan Williams classification' – see Table 22.2) are classed according to effect on action potential.

**Table 22.2** Antidysrhythmic drug classification (Vaughan Williams), after Bennett (2002)

*Class I drugs*
drugs: IA: quinidine, procainamide, disopyramide, pirmenol
  increase duration of action potential; affecting atria and ventricles
IB: lidocaine, mexiletine, tocainide
  shorten duration of action potential; affect only ventricles
IC: flecainide, propafenone, encainide
  less effective, but affect atria and ventricles
action: inhibit sodium channel

*Class II drugs*
drugs: beta-blockers, bretylium
action: reduce rate of pacemaker discharge

*Class III drugs*
drugs: amiodarone, sotalol, dofetilide, bretylium
action: prolongs action potential

*Class IV drugs*
drugs: verapamil, diltiazem
action: calcium antagonists

Poor flow (e.g. atrial stasis) can cause thrombus formation, necessitating anticoagulants. Poor cardiac output may necessitate positive inotropes (see Chapter 35).

If drugs fail, electrical interventions can convert unstable tachydysrhythmias (*cardioversion*) or resolve symptomatic bradycardia (*pacing*). Cardioversion resembles emergency defibrillation, usually using lower energy (Joules), with conscious patients usually electively sedated beforehand.

Vagal stimulation (e.g. carotid massage, orbital pressure) temporarily slows down one-quarter of supraventricular tachycardias (Walker, 2003a), so can help diagnosis and buy time for further treatment, but will not affect rhythms originating below the atrioventricular node. Carotid massage can also cause complications, so should only be performed by those who know how to use it.

Monitors are neither an end in themselves, nor substitutes for observing patients, but a means to provide information which should be evaluated in context of the whole person.

## Atrial/junctional dysrhythmias

### Sinus arrhythmia (Figure 22.4)

Sinus arrhythmia occurs in a few young, usually athletic, people. Inspiration increases intrathoracic pressure sufficiently to cause parasympathetic (vagal) stimulation, slowing sinoatrial rate. Expiration restores the faster rate. Variations between complexes (e.g. R–R interval) exceed 0.16 seconds, but rate usually remains only 4–6 bpm apart. High ventilator tidal volumes may cause sinus arrhythmia. Unless problematic (rare), it should not be treated.

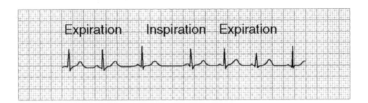

■ *Figure 22.4 Sinus arrhythmia*

### Sinus bradycardia

Although any sinus rate below 60 bpm is technically sinus bradycardia, most adults remain asymptomatic with higher bradycardic rates, increased ventricular filling compensating for reduced rate to maintain cardiac output. Significant problems usually only develop with rates below 50.

Sinus bradycardia may be caused by

■ excessive parasympathetic stimulation (e.g. metoclopramide, severe pain/anxiety, CNS depressants)
■ conduction delays (ischaemic/infarcted myocardium, digoxin, calcium channel blockers, β-blockers)
■ hypoxia
■ hypothermia
■ raised intracranial pressures
■ antihypertensives
■ some endocrine states (e.g. hyperthyroidism, myxoedema).

Treatment: sinus bradycardia is only treated if symptomatic (e.g. dizziness, dyspnoea, hypotension, chest pain). Obvious causes should be removed, so oxygen should be optimised. Children are especially susceptible to hypoxic bradycardia, so should urgently be given oxygen, unless there are other obvious causes for bradycardia.

Drugs include

■ anticholinergics (atropine) block parasympathetic stimulation
■ sympathomimetics – stimulating sympathetic nerves (adrenaline).

If problematic, such as causing hypotension, severe refractory sinus bradycardia may necessitate pacing (temporary or permanent).

### Sinus tachycardia

Tachycardia is any sinus rate >100/minute. Although normal in young children, tachycardia is abnormal with adults. Mild tachycardia is usually compensatory for increased oxygen demand (e.g. pyrexia, hypovolaemia, sepsis). It can also be from stimulants, such as positive chronotropic drugs – most positive inotropes have positive chronotropic effects. Faster tachycardias (>140/minute) may be compensatory, caused by stimulants, or dysrhythmic in origin, such as from ectopic atrial pacemakers.

Tachycardia reduces ventricular filling, stroke volume and myocardial oxygenation time, while increasing myocardial work. Rates >140/minute usually require treatment.

Treatment: as supraventricular tachycardia (later).

### Atrial tachycardia (Figure 22.5)

Atrial tachycardia is tachycardia originating in the atria, from ectopic pacemakers. Technically any tachycardia originating above ventricles is supraventricular, but 'supraventricular tachycardia' usually implies very fast (> 160/minute) rates. Such rapid tachycardia severely compromises cardiac output and myocardial oxygenation, necessitating urgent treatment.

With very fast rates differentiating supraventricular from ventricular tachycardia, atrial flutter and other dysrhythmias can be difficult. Slowing rates with carotid massage may help diagnosis, and gain time for drug therapy.

Treatment: Drugs used include

- amiodarone
- digoxin
- procainamide, disopyramide
- β-blockers
- calcium channel blockers.

If drugs fail, cardioversion may reverse supraventricular tachycardia.

### Sick sinus syndrome

Sick sinus syndrome (i.e. sinoatrial node sickness) causes intermittent bradycardia and escape rhythms. Escape rhythms are often atrial tachycardias, causing 'tachy-brady syndrome'.

Treatment: If problems persist, pacing can replace sinoatrial function.

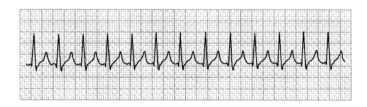

### Figure 22.5 Atrial (supraventricular) tachycardia

### *Ectopics*

Ectopics may originate from

- atrial
- junctional
- ventricular

sites (foci). Impulses may be

- *premature* (before expected impulses) or
- *escape* (expected complexes are absent, so ectopic impulses 'escape' into gaps).

Premature complexes indicate overexcitability. Escape ectopics indicate failed conduction. Likely causes of overexcitability or failed conduction include

- damaged conduction pathways (infarction, oedema, hypoxia)
- drugs/stimulants
- electrolyte imbalance (especially potassium; also calcium, magnesium)
- acidosis.

Treatment: Occasional ectopics seldom need treating, but underlying causes should (if possible) be resolved. Potassium imbalance is the most likely single cause, so serum potassium is usually maintained at 4–5 mmol/litre. Calcium imbalance can also cause ectopics.

Frequent premature ectopics should be treated before they progress to dysrythmias. Escape ectopics provide a pulse that would otherwise be missed, so are 'a friend in need' and should never be treated. Drugs used vary with focus and cause (see later).

### *Atrial ectopics (Figure 22.6)*

Atrial ectopics may be idiopathic or due to atrial stretch (e.g. chronic pulmonary disease, valve disease, MI). Conduction and succeeding QRS complexes are normal, but P waves usually look abnormal, and may be hidden in preceding T waves. Treatment is usually initiated when there are more than six atrial ectopics per minute.

Treatment: Premature atrial ectopics may be treated with

- digoxin
- calcium channel blockers.

Escape ectopics should not usually be treated, but the cause of sinoatrial failure should be identified and treated.

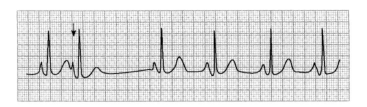

■ *Figure 22.6* **Premature atrial ectopic**

## Atrial fibrillation (AF) (Figure 22.7)

AF may be acute or chronic. Chronic AF is the most common dysrhythmia, especially in older people. Critical illness may provoke acute AF.

Impulses from multiple atrial foci cause erratic, uncoordinated atrial muscle contraction ('quivering'). Atrial activity being uncoordinated, there are no P waves, but atrial 'quivering' (fibrillation or 'f' waves) may (or may not) cause wavy baselines to the ECG. The abbreviation 'AF' implies atrial fibrillation, not atrial flutter (later).

Many (400–600/minute) weak and irregular impulses reach the atrioventricular node. Few of these are conducted by the atrioventricular node, conduction depending on strength and frequency of atrial impulses. Provided ventricular pathways are intact, conduction from the AV node is normal (normal QRS complexes and T waves). Ventricular response may be fast ('fast AF'), normal or slow ('slow AF'), but is irregularly irregular. Loss of 'atrial kick' significantly reduces stroke volume.

*Treatment*: Chronic AF is usually controlled with

■ digoxin

Thrombi, from atrial stasis, increase risk of stroke sixfold (Hart *et al.*, 2003), so should be prevented with

■ anticoagulants (e.g. warfarin, although in ICU DVT prophylaxis may suffice). Both digoxin and warfarin have narrow therapeutic ranges, so

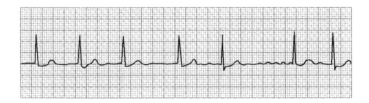

■ *Figure 22.7* **Atrial fibrillation**

235

blood levels should be checked. Asymptomatic chronic atrial fibrillation ('controlled AF') with near-normal ventricular response (<100) should not need further treatment. Uncontrolled chronic AF may respond to increasing digoxin, cardioversion or pulmonary vein ablation (Alchaghouri, 2004). Acute atrial fibrillation may be treated with

- amiodarone (Falk, 2001)
- digoxin
- flecainide (Alchaghouri, 2004)
- other drugs to block A–V node conduction (e.g. β-blockers, calcium channel blockers) (Falk, 2001)
- cardioversion.

Unless AF is immediately life threatening, cardioversion (whether for acute or chronic AF) should only be performed after adequate anticoagulation (Wakai & O'Neill, 2003).

### Atrial flutter (Figure 22.8)

Atrial flutter is usually from re-entry of impulses into the right atrium, creating regular, but rapid, waves with distinctive saw tooth shapes ('F' waves), often at rates of 300/minute. AV node conduction imposes a regular block. 4:1 AV block with atrial rates of 300 creates ventricular responses of 75/minute. But blocks can change suddenly, usually to even numbers. Sudden changes to 2:1 or 8:1 cause life threatening tachycardia or bradycardia.

Treatment: Cardioversion is usually the preferred treatment. If cardioversion fails, drugs may block conduction or reduce atrial rates:

- calcium blockers
- digoxin
- β-blockers
- anticoagulants
- flecanide
- digoxin.

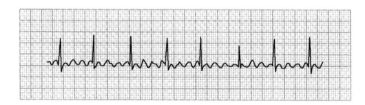

**Figure 22.8 Atrial flutter**

'Overpacing' can also be used – setting a faster rate on an external pacemaker. Where pacing wires are already inserted, such as following cardiac surgery, this may be the preferred option.

### Wolff–Parkinson–White syndrome (WPW) (Figure 22.9)

WPW is caused by a rare congenital abnormality. An abnormal atrioventricular conduction pathway, the Bundle of Kent, bypasses the AV node. With two atrioventricular pathways, impulses can enter through one and return through the other, refiring atria ('circus' movement), causing sudden, gross, lifethreatening tachycardia. Circus movement widens bases of QRS complexes ('delta' waves).

There are two types of WPW: A and B. With type A (more common), aberrant pathways are on the left, causing tall R waves. Type B, with pathways on the right, cause deep S waves. Type does not affect treatment.

*Treatment*: β-blockers, disopyramide, flecainide or amiodarone may reduce lifethreatening tachycardia. Drugs to avoid include digoxin, adenosine and verapamil, all of which may increase conduction. Cardioversion may restore stability, but ideally aberrant pathways are destroyed by catheter radiofrequency ablation.

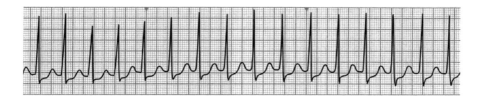

■ *Figure 22.9* Wolff–Parkinson–White syndrome

### Junctional (or 'nodal') rhythm (Figure 22.10)

Junctional rhythm describes impulses originating in the AV node or atrioventricular junction. Intrinsic pacemaker rates slow as conduction pathways

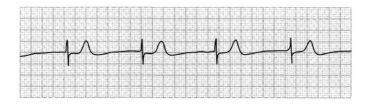

■ *Figure 22.10* Nodal/junctional rhythm

237

progress ('lower is slower'). Higher impulses normally overpace, so lower impulses only escape when higher impulses fail. Intrinsic junctional rate is usually 40–60, although acceleration can occur.

Irritation (oedema, mechanical – e.g. central lines in the right atrium) may cause junctional ectopics. Oedema from cardiac surgery often causes transient junctional rhythms (hence epicardial pacing wires). P waves are not normally seen as, although atrial conduction occurs, it is retrograde (inverted P waves) and occurs simultaneously with ventricular conduction (QRS).

Treatment: Junctional rates are often sufficient to support life, but should be closely monitored. If bradycardia becomes symptomatic, treat as above (atropine, pacing).

## Atrioventricular blocks

Any conduction pathway may be blocked by:

- infarction
- oedema
- ischaemia.

If oedema or ischaemia resolve, blocks usually disappear. Infarction usually causes permanent block. Blocks may occur at the atrioventricular node (first, second or third degree) or in one of the bundle branches.

### First degree block (Figure 22.11)

First degree block delayed atrioventricular node conduction, prolongs PR intervals beyond 0.2 seconds (5 small squares). Despite delay, every impulse is conducted, so a QRS complex follows each P wave. Chronic first degree block is usually from age-related enlargement of the atrioventricular node, and rarely causes problems. Acute block may be caused by digoxin toxicity, β-blockers, calcium channel blockers, AV node infarction/ischaemia/oedema or endocarditis.

Treatment: Acute block should be monitored, but only treated if bradycardia causes problems. Chronotropic drugs (e.g. atropine) or pacing can resolve symptomatic bradycardia.

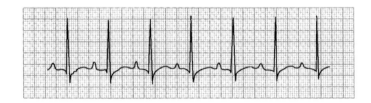

■ *Figure 22.11* First degree block

## Second degree block

Second degree block or incomplete heart block, occurs when only some P waves are conducted, usually causing slow ventricular rates. There are two types of second degree block:

Type 1: progressive lengthening of PR intervals until an atrial impulse is unconducted (P without a QRS complex), caused by impaired atrioventricular node conduction (Figure 22.12).

Type 2: constant PR intervals, with regular unconducted P waves (e.g. 2:1; see Figure 22.13). Second degree heart block Type 2 is less common but more serious than Type 1, as it is more likely to progress into 3rd degree block or asystole (Jevon, 2003).

Type 1 is still often called Wenkeback or (less often) Mobitz Type 1, while Type 2 is often called Mobitz or Mobitz Type 2.

Treatment: Oxygen should be optimised. Drugs used include

■ atropine.

If symptoms persist pacing may be needed.

## Third degree block (Figure 22.14)

Complete heart block, causes complete atrioventricular dissociation. P waves are regular (unless AF is also present), but unrelated to QRS complexes, and some P waves may be 'lost' in QRS or T waves. Ventricular pacemakers cause

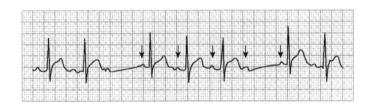

■ *Figure 22.12* Second degree block (Type 1)

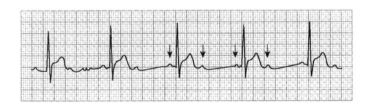

■ *Figure 22.13* Second degree block (Type 2)

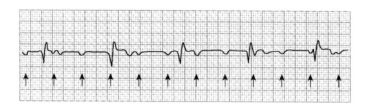

■ *Figure 22.14* **Third degree block**

wide, regular but slow QRS complexes – often 30/minute. Cardiac output and blood pressure are compromised.

Treatment: Unless transient, pacing is almost invariably needed. Until pacing is commenced, oxygen should be optimised.

## Bundle branch block (Figure 22.15)

This occurs when conduction through one of the branches, or one or more of the left hemibranches, of the bundle of His is blocked. This creates two QRS complexes – a normal one from the intact branch, and a widened ventricular-shaped complex from impulses travelling around the blocked branch. This RSR, or biphasic QRS, wave creates the characteristic M or W shapes on ECGs.

New left bundle block, together with chest pain, indicates myocardial infarction, is classified as a STEMI (ST wave elevated myocardial infarction), and should be treated with urgent thrombolysis.

Although seen on limb leads, differentiation of right from left bundle block is clearest on chest leads. Left bundle branch block causes a W in early, and an M in late leads; right bundle branch block reverses this picture (mnemonics: MaRRoW and WiLLiaM).

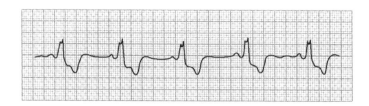

■ *Figure 22.15* **Bundle branch block**

## Ventricular dysrhythmias

Ventricular impulses originate in ventricular muscle, so travel from muscle fibre to muscle fibre rather than through conduction pathways. This makes their progress relatively slow, giving them a typically wide QRS complexes.

Persistent dysrhythmias are likely to recur, so are often treated by implantable defibrillators. Few models give any warning, so patients suddenly experience a defibrillation shock. Not surprisingly, some patients experience psychiatric problems.

### Ventricular ectopics (Figure 22.16)

This originates from ventricular foci outside normal conduction pathways, so lack P waves, and are conducted (slowly) from muscle fibre to muscle fibre. Taking longer, this creates their characteristically wide (>3 small squares) and bizarre shape on ECGs. Ectopics originating near the ventricular apex are conducted downwards, giving positive complexes; those originating near the base have retrograde conduction through ventricular muscle, giving negative complexes. T waves are discordant – in the opposite direction to QRS waves. Complexes from a single focus ('unifocal') look alike; ectopics with different shapes originate from different foci ('multifocal'). A sequence of three or more ectopics is sometimes called a *salvo*.

Treatment: Isolated ectopics are insignificant, but frequent ectopics suggest conduction problems (escape) or overexcitability (premature). Underlying causes (electrolytes, hypoxia) should be resolved. Premature ventricular ectopics may be reversed by overpacing.

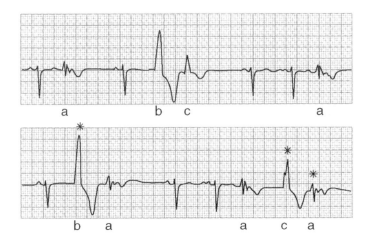

**Figure 22.16 Multifocal ventricular ectopics**

### Bigeminy and trigeminy (Figure 22.17)

These are sinister extensions of ventricular ectopics, occurring regularly. Bigeminy is one ventricular ectopic every other complex; trigeminy is one

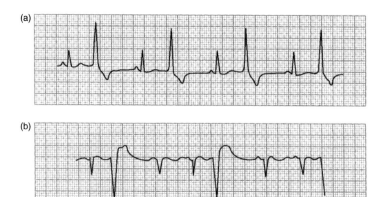

**Figure 22.17 Bigeminy and trigeminy**

ventricular ectopic every third complex. Ectopics are usually unifocal, usually from hypoxia or digoxin toxicity.

Treatment: Trigeminy is not usually treated, but provided underlying causes are resolved, bigeminy can be treated with

- disopyramide
- lidocaine (formerly 'lignocaine' in UK).

### Ventricular tachycardia (Figure 22.18)

This a regular rhythm, with unifocal rapid impulses originating from an ectopic focus in ventricular muscle, usually caused by ischaemia. Asymptomatic VT rarely persists, either reverting or progressing after a few minutes. Rates are often 200–50, inadequate ventricular filling time causing poor stroke volumes and systemic hypotension. Increased myocardial work-load with inadequate oxygen supply makes ventricular tachycardia progress rapidly into ventricular fibrillation and cardiac arrest.

Treatment: Ventricular tachycardia is an arrest situation requiring urgent resuscitation and defibrillation. Current resuscitation guidelines should be followed.

Precordial thumps remain controversial, as they may convert ventricular tachycardia into less easily treated rhythms. Current European recommendations include a single precordial thump 'if appropriate' (European Resuscitation Council, 2001). With conscious patients, coughing can mimic thumps.

Implantable defibrillators may be inserted for long-term management.

*Accelerated idioventricular rhythm*, sometimes called 'slow VT' or 'ventricular escape rhythm', typically occurs following myocardial infarction. Ventricular

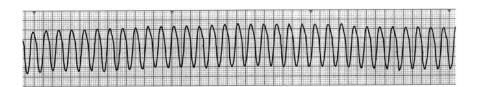

■ *Figure 22.18* Ventricular tachycardia

rate is usually below 120/minute (Houghton & Gray, 2003), so does not normally require treatment. However, this rhythm should be closely monitored, as more sinister rhythms may develop.

### Torsades de pointes (Figure 22.19)

A rare type of multifocal ventricular tachycardia, causes ECG traces to twist around isoelectric baselines. Rates are often 200–50. If prolonged or untreated it leads to ventricular fibrillation.

Torsades de pointes may be caused by drugs (e.g. amiodarone, vancomycin, soltolol), severe electrolyte imbalance (especially hypokalaemia, hypomagnesaemia), subarachnoid haemorrhage, myocardial infarction, angina, bradycardia, sinoatrial block or congenital abnormality.

Treatment: Electrolyte imbalances or underlying causes should be treated. Drugs include

■ magnesium.

(Kaye & O'Sullivan, 2002)

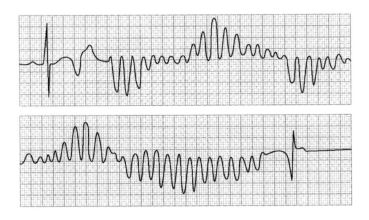

■ *Figure 22.19* Torsades de pointes

If drugs fail, temporary atrial or ventricular pacing or cardiopulmonary resuscitation may be necessary.

### Ventricular fibrillation (VF) (Figure 22.20)

This is almost invariably fatal in 2–3 minutes. Patients are usually unconscious, with no pulse or blood pressure. VF may be coarse or fine; fine ventricular fibrillation may appear like asystole, so increasing gain on ECGs shows whether 'f' waves are present.

Treatment: Ventricular fibrillation is an arrest situation, treated with debribrillation, following current Resuscitation Council guidelines.

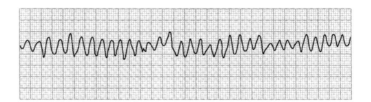

**Figure 22.20 Ventricular fibrillation**

## Asystole (= ventricular standstill)

Asystole, literally absence of systole, appears as an uninterrupted isoelectric line, although progression from dysrhythmias to asystole may persist for considerable time ('dying' heart), with occasional irregular atrial or ventricular complexes.

Absence of any cardiac function is an arrest situation, but resuscitation rarely succeeds. Before initiating arrest calls, staff should take 10 seconds to asses patients (pulse, ECG): absence of complexes on ECGs may be caused by

- disconnection
- failed electrodes (e.g. drying of gel)
- fine VF.

If patients appear moribund, electrodes are intact, and increasing size ('gain') of ECGs still shows asystole, then initiate cardiac massage and an arrest call.

Treatment: Cardiac massage is essential to maintain effective circulation. Defibrillation should not be attempted with asystole – there is no rhythm to defibrillate. Drugs include

- adrenaline (1 mg)
- atropine (3 mg).

If P waves are present, external or transvenous pacing may be used.

## Pulseless electrical activity (PEA)

PEA results in whatever electrical activity is seen on the screen not being translated into a pulse and arterial blood pressure trace. ECG traces are usually abnormal, often showing tachycardia and with low amplitude complexes.

Causes of electromechanical dissociation can be summarised as '4Hs and 4Ts':

■ Hypoxia
■ Hypovolaemia
■ Hyper/hypokalaemia
■ Hypothermia
■ Tension pneumothorax
■ Tamponade
■ Toxic/therapeutic disturbances (drug overdose)
■ Thromboemboli (e.g. PE, MI).

Causes are often obvious from patients' histories.

Treatment: Pulseless electrical activity is an arrest situation, so an arrest call should be initiated, and Resuscitation Council guidelines followed. Underlying causes should also be corrected, otherwise PEA usually recurs.

## Implications for practice

■ Most dysrhythmias are only treated if problematic.
■ Almost all non-sinus rhythms cause loss of 'atrial kick', and so smaller stroke volumes.
■ Chest pain, together with either ST elevation (1 mm in chest leads, 2 mm in limb leads) in two or more consecutive leads or a new left bundle branch block indicates acute myocardial infarction.
■ Ectopics may originate from any part of the heart. Atrial ectopics have abnormal P waves, but normal QRS. Junctional ectopics have no P wave, but normal QRS. Ventricular ectopics have no P wave, and wide and bizarre QRS.
■ Isolated ectopics are insignificant, but frequent premature ectopics indicate over-excitability. Escape ectopics are 'a friend in need' so should not be treated. However, causes of failed conduction should be resolved.
■ Myocardial hypoxia and electrolyte imbalances cause many dysrhythmias.
■ Current Resuscitation Council guidelines should be displayed on units in easily visible areas for staff caring for patients.
■ Nurses should know current Resuscitation Council guidelines, where emergency drugs and equipment are stored and how to summon help urgently.

245

## Summary

Critical illness exposes ICU patients to various symptomatic dysrhythmias, so ICU patients are usually continuously monitored; ICU nurses should therefore be able to recognise common dysrhythmias and initiate appropriate action. The ICU staff should already be familiar with basic electrocardiography, so this chapter has discussed dysrhythmias most likely to be seen in ICU, together with standard treatments. Staff should be familiar with current Resuscitation Council guidelines.

## Further reading

Current Resuscitation Council guidelines should be familiar and available; new guidelines were published in 2005, after completion of this text. There are many books about ECG interpretation. Hampton (2003a) provides a useful overview, with supplementary detail in Hampton (2003b) and examples for practice in Hampton (2003c). Houghton and Gray (2003) is also useful. www.routledge.com/textbooks/0415373239

For clinical scenarios, clinical questions and the answers to them go to the support website at www.routledge.com/textbooks/0415373239

## Clinical questions

Q.1 Describe how you would perform a 12-lead ECG on an ICU patient who is awake. Include how you would explain procedure, position patient and apply electrodes to ensure an accurate and optimal ECG tracing.

Q.2 For continuous bedside ECG monitoring in ICU, which lead (e.g. I, II, III, aVF, aVR, C1) is usually chosen for waveform analysis? Justify your choice in relation cardiac physiology and note expected waveform.

Q.3 Reflect on situations where external carotid massage has been performed for tachycardia. Appraise desired effects, limitations, safety issues and nurse accountability. What other strategies can be used to reduce life threatening tachycardia in emergency situations?

# Chapter 23

# Neurological monitoring

## Contents

| | |
|---|---|
| Introduction | 248 |
| Intracranial pressure | 248 |
| Cerebral blood flow | 249 |
| Cerebral oedema | 251 |
| Glasgow Coma Scale (GCS) | 251 |
| Pupil size and response | 252 |
| Limb assessment | 253 |
| Jugular venous bulb saturation | 254 |
| ICP measurement | 254 |
| Implications for practice | 255 |
| Summary | 256 |
| Further reading | 256 |
| Clinical scenarios | 256 |

## Fundamental knowledge

Intracranial anatomy

Cerebral blood supply – carotid arteries, Circle of Willis

Cerebral autoregulation and the effect of hypo/hyper-capnia on cerebral arteries

Brain stem tests, 12 cranial nerves and physiology of vital centres

Sedation (see Chapter 6)

## Introduction

Many ICU patients have acutely altered neurological function, whether from chemical sedation, disease of other organs/systems or specific neurological disease/damage. Some ICUs specialise in neurosurgery or neuromedicine, but most units receive patients with head injuries and cranial pathologies. Many conditions, such as meningitis, hepatic failure, can increase intracranial pressure, causing both acute confusion and physiological complications. Assessing and monitoring neurological function is therefore important for all ICU patients.

There are two main parts to the body's nervous system – central and peripheral. The central nervous system is the brain and spinal cord. Peripheral nerves link the spinal cord to all other organs and tissues. Either, or both, parts of the nervous system may be dysfunctional, and therefore assessment should measure whichever part of the nervous system is a cause for concern.

The simplest way to assess neurological function is whether someone is responding appropriately and in their normal manner. Unfortunately diseases and treatments prevent normal responses in many ICU patients, but with conscious patients their actions and communication (non-verbal as well as verbal) should be assessed. Other noninvasive assessments can indicate

- consciousness (GCS)
- cranial nerve function (pupil responses, gag, cough, facial movements)
- spinal nerve function (limb movement).

The value of various invasive modes remains debated, so it is often limited to neurological centres, but some options are included here. Whatever way neurological function is assessed, it should be understood by staff and beneficial to patients. Assessments recorded and reported should remain factual and any limiting factors are to be noted with the report. For example, intubated patients cannot make a verbal response, and pupil size or muscle strength may be evaluated differently by different observers. Where treatments, such as intubation, prevent assessment, this should be recorded. Where assessors are uncertain about their evaluation, they should seek a second opinion and avoid the temptation to follow any previously charted observations.

## Intracranial pressure

Most of the total adult intracranial volume (average 1.7 ml) is brain tissue, the remaining 300 ml normally being equally divided between blood and cerebrospinal fluid – CSF (Hickey, 2003b). Because the skull is rigid and filled to capacity with essentially noncompressible contents (the *Monro-Kellie hypothesis*), increasing one component necessarily compresses others. Small and transient increases of intracranial contents may be compensated for (*compliance*) by displacing blood and CSF into the spinal column, so coughing, straining or sneezing do not usually cause problems. But sustained pressure, once compliance is exhausted, inevitably causes intracranial hypertension

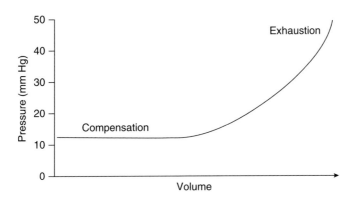

**Figure 23.1 Pressure/volume curve**

(see Figure 23.1). Any pressure on the vital centres of the brain stem may affect vital signs, so in addition, any assessment of intracranial pressure (e.g. Glasgow Coma Scale, intracranial pressure monitoring) should be evaluated in the context of vital signs, especially pulse and blood pressure.

Normal adult intracranial pressure is 0–15 mmHg. But increased intracranial contents, such as cerebral oedema or bleeding, increases intracranial pressure, causing neurological dysfunction. Two-fifths of patients losing consciousness following head injuries develop raised intracranial pressure (Odell, 1996).

Sustained intracranial pressures of 20–30 mmHg may cause injury. Cerebral autoregulation fails when ICP exceeds 40 mmHg (Hickey, 2003b). Sustained intracranial pressure over 60 mmHg causes ischaemic brain damage and is usually fatal (Bahouth & Yarbrough, 2005). Progressive cellular damage (see Chapter 24) causes

- release of vasoactive chemicals (e.g. histamine, serotonin)
- hyperkalaemia
- intracellular oedema and cell death
- increased capillary permeability, reducing colloid osmotic pressure

creating a vicious cycle of intracranial hypertension and tissue injury (see Figure 23.2).

## Cerebral blood flow

Like perfusion elsewhere, the single main factor affecting cerebral blood flow is mean arterial pressure. However, brain cells rely on a constant supply of oxygen and glucose, so without perfusion, damage and death to brain cells is rapid. Cerebral perfusion pressure (CPP) is also limited by the inability of the skull to expand, and so CPP is the difference between mean arterial pressure

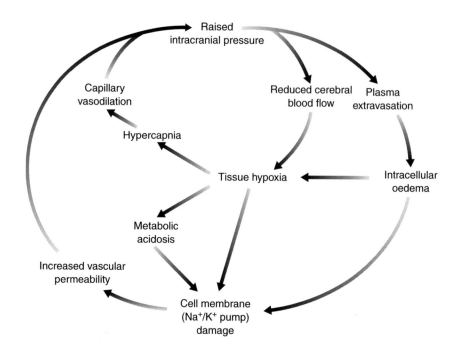

**Figure 23.2 Intracranial hypertension and tissue injury: a vicious circle**

(MAP) and intracranial pressure:

$$CPP = MAP - ICP$$

Many monitors can calculate CPP from ICP. It can also be estimated by non-invasive transcranial doppler (Edouard *et al.*, 2005).

In health, autoregulation maintains relatively constant cerebral bloodflow, but cerebral damage can cause autoregulation to fail, resulting in excessively high or low CPP. CPP should be high enough to fully perfuse the brain, without increasing intracranial pressure – generally 65–70 mmHg (Werner & Engelhard, 2000), although with traumatic brain injury target CPP is 60 mmHg (Robertson, 2001). Initial symptoms of insufficient or excessive CPP may include acute confusion and fitting, but sustained high or low CPP is likely to cause cerebrovascular accidents (CVAs – strokes).

Cerebral oxygenation is also influenced by oxygen carriage (e.g. hypoxia, anaemia). So management of intracranial hypertension should consider total trends and factors affecting cerebral demand and supply, rather than focusing on single measurements or parameters.

## Cerebral oedema

Cerebral oedema may be

- interstitial
- intracellular
- vasogenic.

Interstitial and intracellular oedema formation is discussed in Chapter 34. Most cerebral oedema is vasogenic: blood/brain barrier disruption increases capillary permeability, causing fluid and protein leak, with progressive electrolyte imbalances. Steroids should not be used for treating cerebral oedema (Hickey, 2003b).

## Glasgow Coma Scale (GCS)

Normal: 14–15.

The Glasgow Coma Scale is a widely known, tried and trusted means of assessing level of consciousness by evaluating eye, verbal and motor responses. It does not require special equipment; most staff will be familiar with using it, and it is a reliable predictor of neurological outcome. It does not measure peripheral nerve function or effectiveness of chemical sedatives, and although it does not measure pupil reaction or cardiovascular function, these are both affected by brainstem function, so neurological observation charts almost always include these as well.

Absence of any response of any component scores 1, making the minimum overall score 3. Maximum total score is 15 points (eye 4 + verbal 5 + motor 6), indicating a fully awake, alert and responsive person. A score of 14 is considered normal. Intubation prevents verbal response, so this should be clearly recorded ('T' usually being charted for verbal response).

Scores below 14 indicate impaired consciousness:

13 = mild impairment
9–12 = moderate impairment
3–8 = severe impairment (coma).

Scores of 8 or below indicate high risk of airway obstruction from impaired consciousness, so intubation is usually indicated. Assessment should include distinguishing purposeful from reflex responses – e.g. eyes opening spontaneously may be a reflex.

Although overall score adds three components together, scores for each component should also be recorded (e.g. GCS = 9, E = 2, V = 3, M4), eye responses being less reliable for predicting outcome than verbal and motor responses (Teoh et al., 2000). GCS is used to assess level of consciousness, so if consciousness is poor (from whatever cause), allowance should not be made for possible contributing factors such as drugs or alcohol. Nurses being used to identify possible concerns, any concerns should be reported, and if consensus about scores is lacking, it is safest to score low.

Assessment includes response to pain. Inflicting pain conflicts with fundamental values of nursing so should only be done when therapeutic benefits outweigh humanitarian considerations. Response to painful stimuli may already have been observed, such as localising irritation from oxygen masks or endotracheal tubes/suction. Inflicting pain may also cause physiological harm such as increasing intracranial pressure and stress responses. As peripheral stimuli may elicit spinal reflex responses of guarding or withdrawal, central stimuli should be used to assess consciousness (Cree, 2003). Central stimuli include

- supraorbital pressure (running a finger along the bony ridge at the top of the eye)
- trapezium squeeze (pinching trapezius muscle, between head and shoulders)
- sternal rub (grinding the sternum with knuckles) and Lower (2003) adds
- mandibular pressure – pushing upwards and inwards on the angle of the patient's jaw for maximum 30 seconds (Waterhouse, 2005).

Peripheral stimuli, such as nail bed pressure, can elicit central responses (Lower, 2003), such as grimacing or peripheral reflexes (see later).

Different stimuli may be appropriate for different patients and situations. Painful stimuli should not be inflicted if patients respond to clear commands (Cree, 2003; Dougherty & Lister, 2004). The trapezium squeeze should not be used if patients have neck injury, although the opposite shoulder to one-sided injury should be considered. Supraorbital pressure should be avoided with skull fractures. Sternal rub should not be used repeatedly as bruising and skin damage can be caused, and cervical spine injury may be below the lesion and so fail to elicit a response. Mandibular pressure is more difficult and may dislocate the jaw so is usually the least useful stimulus. If response from one stimulus is unclear, other stimuli should be attempted.

Neurological crises may occur rapidly; secondary damage occurring before intermittent measurement (e.g. Glasgow Coma Scale) detects deterioration (Price, 1998). Frequency of GCS monitoring varies greatly. The National Institute for Clinical Excellence (2003) recommends half hourly assessment for two hours or until GCS reaches 15; then hourly for four hours, returning to half hourly with any deterioration. However, these guidelines are designed for Accident and Emergency departments (Waterhouse, 2005). ICUs should monitor patients according to individual risk factors. GCS, or other level-of-consciousness testing, should be assessed each shift, and where it is a cause for concern will usually assess GCS at least hourly.

## Pupil size and response

Normal: PERTL; normal size varies with light level.

Normally, pupils constrict in light and dilate in darkness. Pupil response is best assessed in a darkened area (if possible) to dilate the pupils. Both eyes should be assessed for

- pupil size
- whether both pupils are equal (PE).

Eyelids may need to be gently raised. A bright light (e.g. pentorch) should then be moved from the corner to the centre of the eye, assessing

- how briskly pupils react to light (RTL).

Pupil size is usually illustrated on neurological observation charts. One-fifth of people have unequal pupils (Patil & Dowd, 2000), so minor inequalities are normal (Waterhouse, 2005). Dilated, fixed or (significantly) unequal pupils are usually a late sign of intracranial hypertension (Waterhouse, 2005). Pupil reaction is controlled by occulomotor nerve (cranial nerve III) and is normally brisk, so sluggish responses indicate either brainstem damage or cranial nerve III dysfunction. Drugs affecting pupils include atropine eyedops (dilate) and opioids (pinpoint constriction).

If gross periorbital oedema prevents pupil assessment, 'C' should be recorded on charts (Waterhouse, 2005).

## Limb assessment

Normal: equal + strong.

Limb movement requires both peripheral nerve and muscle function. Peripheral motor nerves may respond to either

- painful peripheral stimuli, transmitted through sensory nerves and causing spinal reflexes, or
- central nervous stimuli (response to commands).

Both legs and both arms should be tested together, by

- asking patients to lift their limbs
- holding feet/hands and asking patients to push you away
- asking patients to grip your hands
- if unable to move limbs, test ability to localise sensation – initially light sensations such as touch, but if these elicit no response, painful peripheral stimuli may be needed (e.g. fingernail pressure).

Assessment should evaluate

- strength (strong, medium, weak)
- co-ordination
- any unilateral weakness.

Many people are slightly stronger on their dominant side, and for GCS assessment the stronger motor response should be scored, but significant weakness on one side may indicate a stroke or other problem so should be noted and reported.

If not over-ridden by central nervous control, peripheral stimuli should cause guarding/defensive spinal reflexes such as *flexion* (withdrawal). Central nervous system damage may cause abnormal peripheral responses such as *extension* (pushing towards the stimulus) or *decorticate* posture (limbs flexed rigidly outwards).

## Jugular venous bulb saturation (SjO₂)

Normal: 60–65 per cent.

Jugular vein catheterisation (using retrograde insertion of a CVP-like catheter with oximeter) enables oxygen saturation and content measurement; on X-ray the tip should rest at border of the first cervical spine. Probes can also be introduced through ICP microtransducer burrholes (Kiening *et al.*, 1996). Like mixed venous saturation, jugular bulb saturation ($SjO_2$) indicates global cerebral oxygen delivery, provided arterial saturation is normal.

Low levels are often artefactual but may indicate cerebral hypoperfusion. High, and rising, $SjO_2$ often indicates increased cerebral blood flow, and very high levels (>85 per cent) usually indicate imminent death.

Although $SjO_2$ can monitor total (global) cerebral oxygenation, it cannot identify where ischaemia or bleeds are occurring (Clay, 2000). $SjO_2$ is rarely measured outside specialist neurological ICUs.

## ICP measurement

Normal: 0–15 mmHg.

Intraventricular catheters, usually fibreoptic, can be connected to most ICU monitors. Intracranial Pressure should be measured at the Foramen of Monro (see Figure 23.3), the mean usually being recorded. Arterial pulses affect intracranial pressure, creating waves that should have three peaks (Hickey, 2003b) (see Figure 23.4):

■ P1 – *percussion wave*: sharply peaked, with fairly constant amplitude.
■ P2 – *tidal wave*: shape and amplitude is more variable, but like an arterial waveform ends on the dicrotic notch. P2 indicates cerebral compliance (Germon *et al.*, 1994).
■ P3 – *dicrotic wave*: immediately follows the dicrotic notch.

Like other pressure monitoring waves, dampened shape indicates unreliable measurement. Probes are normally reliable but once inserted cannot be recalibrated. Suspected inaccuracy (doubtful waveforms) can be tested by lowering the patient's head, which should increase pressure, and so waveform amplitude.

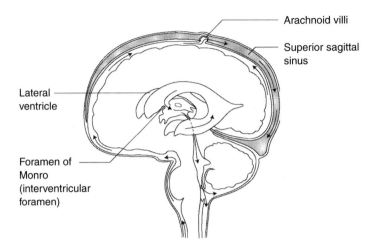

**Figure 23.3 Cross-section of the cranium showing Foramen of Monro**

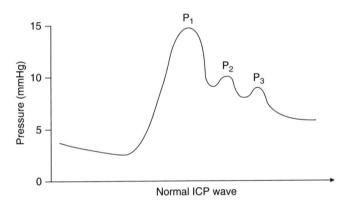

**Figure 23.4 Normal ICP waveform**

Lundberg classified three patterns of waveforms, labelled A, B and C (Chitnavis & Polkey, 1998), but their clinical value is questionable (Germon *et al.*, 1994) so they are not included here.

**Implications for practice**

- Nearly all units receive patients with head injuries so need some means to assess and monitor neurological status.
- Because the skull is rigid, any increase in contents (bleed, oedema) increases intracranial pressure, impairing cerebral perfusion.

- Where specialised neurological monitoring is unavailable, intracranial pressure can be assessed using

  - Glasgow Coma Scale (with pupil responses)
  - spinal reflexes
  - blood tests (glucose, electrolytes, gases)
  - mean arterial pressure

- the Glasgow Coma Scale is familiar and reliable for assessing level of consciousness
- ICP should be 0–15 mmHg, but transient rises are insignificant
- CPP should be sufficient to perfuse the brain, without increased intracranial pressure – 60 mmHg is usually aimed for
- continuous display is valuable for evaluating effects of all aspects of care
- patient care should be viewed holistically, so observations should be related to their overall effect.

## Summary

Intracranial hypertension can occur in many ICU patients; monitoring neurological status (outside neurological ICUs) often relies on the Glasgow Coma Scale, assessing level of consciousness rather than cerebral perfusion. More invasive methods of assessment inevitably incur greater risks but may provide more useful information to guide treatment. As with monitoring any aspect of patient care, benefits and burdens of each approach should be individualised to patients and justified by the extent to which they usefully guide treatments and care given. Management of patients with intracranial hypertension is discussed in Chapter 37.

## Further reading

The Marsden Manual provides useful, authoritative guidelines on Glasgow Coma Scale assessment. The NICE guidelines are A&E focussed so of limited value for ICU. Specialist journals include *Journal of Neuroscience Nursing, Annals of Neurology* and the *Journal of Neurology, Neurosurgery and Psychology*. Waterhouse (2005) provides a useful overview of noninvasive neurological assessment. Ravi and Morgan (2003) review intracranial pressure monitoring. www.routledge.com/textbooks/0415373239

For clinical scenarios, clinical questions and the answers to them go to the support website at www.routledge.com/textbooks/0415373239

## Clinical scenarios

Mr Michael Roberts is a 54-year-old who was admitted to the ICU unconscious. He sustained a head injury from a fall down stairs at home and was found by his partner. Mr Roberts is a known insulin dependent diabetic who drinks approximately 8 units of alcohol a day and has epilepsy. On examination Mr Roberts had a large scalp haematoma over the right parietal region, another over his right eye and bruising to his right elbow.

Mr Roberts's initial results:
Glasgow Coma Scale (GCS) 6 (E1, V1, M4)
All limbs flexing spontaneously without any stimuli
Both pupils' response to light is sluggish, equal size at 4 mm

| | |
|---|---|
| Respiration rate | 26 breaths/minute, audible gurgling breath sounds |
| $SpO_2$ | 100% on 15 litres of oxygen |
| BP | 232/120 mmHg |
| HR | 100 bpm |
| Capillary refill | <2 seconds with warm peripheries |

Mr Roberts was intubated and sent for a head CT scan which revealed a large right subdural haematoma with midline shift (9 mm) to the left side of his brain, widespread subarrachnoid haemorrhage, fracture to right parietal skull and several focal intracerebral contusions. He underwent emergency craniotomy for evacuation of subdural haematoma and insertion of ICP bolt. He was invasively ventilated, sedated with propofol and fentanyl infusions.

Mr Roberts's post operative results:
GCS 4 (E1, V1, M2)
Right pupil not assessed as eye closed from local swelling, left pupil sized at 2 mm and sluggish response to light.

| | |
|---|---|
| ICP | 35 mmHg |
| BP | 132/65 mmHg |
| HR | 68 bpm |
| Capillary refill | <2 seconds |
| Central temperature | 34.4°C |
| Blood sugar | 14.0 mmol/litre |

Q.1 Explain why the GCS is used in Mr Roberts's initial and post operative neurological assessment and what his score represents. Consider how accuracy can be ensured, the frequency of assessment and the most appropriate type of stimuli for Mr Roberts.

Q.2 Calculate Mr Roberts Cerebral Perfusion Pressure (CPP = MAP − ICP) and explore its physiological implications (i.e. to cerebral perfusion and autoregulation, effect on other body systems especially those controlled by the autonomic nervous system). What is the likely cause and significance of his temperature and blood sugar results?

Q.3 Review complications and risks associated with ICP monitoring, consider how these may be managed with Mr Roberts.

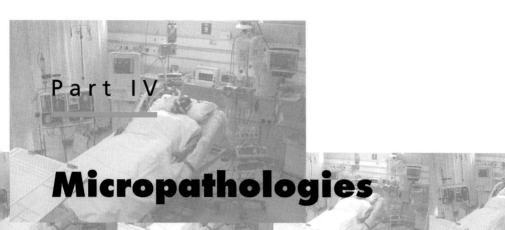

Part IV

# Micropathologies

Chapter 24

# Cellular pathology

## Contents

Introduction                        262
Cell membrane                       262
Mitochondria                        263
Intracellular ions                  263
Cell death                          264
Inflammatory response               264
Chemical mediators                  265
Cytokines                           265
Acute phase proteins                265
Radicals                            266
Implications for practice           266
Summary                             267
Further reading                     267
Clinical scenarios                  267

## Fundamental knowledge

Oxygen delivery to cells
Glycolysis

## Introduction

Focus on visible macrophysiology (systems and organs) has increasingly been replaced by recognition that disease processes originate primarily at micro-physiological levels; organ/system failure follows widespread cell failure. Cell function relies on chemical reactions, which require both oxygen and energy. Absence of oxygen and energy sources (mainly blood glucose) therefore quickly leads to cell damage and failure. Inflammation is cell-tissue's homeo-static response to protect itself, but exaggerated and inappropriate inflamma-tory responses cause life-threatening disease such as systemic inflammatory response syndrome (SIRS – see Chapter 33). Restoring oxygen and energy supplies to failing cells may enable cell survival, reversing critical illness.

There are hundreds of chemicals that a healthy body produces to help main-tain homeostasis but which, in ill-health, can contribute to or cause critical illness. A few of the most significant chemicals are identified in this chapter which therefore outlines pathological mechanisms underlying most critical illnesses. Readers may find sections in this chapter more useful as reference points for later use. This chapter begins with brief revision of cell physiology. If unfamiliar, this should be supplemented from anatomy texts.

## Cell membrane

The cell membrane separates the internal structures of the cell from its exter-nal environment. Although some passive movement of fluid and solutes does occur across cell membranes, most movement is actively regulated by various pumps and channels in cell membranes. Probably the best-known pump is the sodium–potassium pump, but many others exist including calcium channels mentioned in Chapter 22 (ECGs). Calcium channel blockers that manipulate this channel are cardiac and vascular cells. Active movement through these

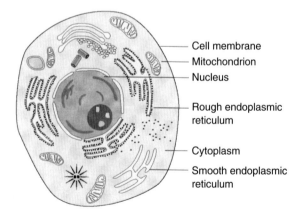

Cell membrane
Mitochondrion
Nucleus

Rough endoplasmic reticulum

Cytoplasm

Smooth endoplasmic reticulum

*Figure 24.1 Cell structure*

pumps and channels maintains normal, healthy intracellular environments. Cell failure, discussed below, affects all parts of the cell, including the cell membrane. Therefore cell failure results in increasingly abnormal intracellular environments and, if not reversed, progresses to *necrosis*.

Cell membranes are a single layer of phospholipid, interspersed with proteins and cholesterol. This phospholipid creates an oil-like film which is both flexible and self-sealing. Some passive movement of substances occurs through cell membranes, but most movement is actively regulated by various 'pumps' (e.g. chloride, glucose) in the membrane. These pumps maintain significant differences between the intracellular and extracellular environments.

### Mitochondria

Mitochondria produce adenosine triphosphate (ATP) the type of energy which cells use. *ATP is normally mainly produced from metabolism of glucose and oxygen* (Krebs' cycle):

$$C_6H_{12}O_6 + 6O_2 \rightarrow 36 \text{ ATP} + \text{waste}$$

With normal aerobic metabolism, each gram of glucose produces 38 ATP molecules but in anaerobic conditions produces only two ATP molecules (Nathan & Singer, 1999) and 2 mmol of lactic acid (Nunn, 1996). So metabolism during hypoperfusion (shock) is inefficient, causing accumulation of toxic waste (acids and carbon dioxide) and lactic acid (metabolic acidosis). Widespread cell dysfunction causes accumulation of oxygen radicals, which accelerate cell (and organ) dysfunction. Cells with high metabolic rates (including cardiac and brain cells) are especially vulnerable to hypoxic damage (Clay *et al.*, 2001).

### Intracellular ions

Intracellular sodium and potassium concentrations ($K^+$ = 120–140 and $Na^+$ = about 14 mmol/litre, reversing extracellular fluid concentrations) are maintained by the *sodium–potassium pump* in cell membranes. Electrolytes movement across membrane creates *action potential* (see Chapter 22) needed for muscle movement.

Water diffuses passively out of the cell (from sodium's osmotic pull). Cell membrane damage allows potassium efflux, causing potential hyperkalaemia and sodium influx, creating intracellular oedema. Intracellular oedema causes further cell damage.

Like sodium, intracellular levels of calcium are low. Cell damage, which may be caused by hypoxia and poor perfusion, results in failure of the cell membrane, an efflux of potassium from the cell and an influx of sodium and calcium into the cell.

High levels of calcium are toxic to cells, accumulating in the energy-producing mitochondria and damaging organelles (Hunter & Chien, 1999).

263

## Cell death

Cells may die either through *apoptosis* (cell shrinkage) or *necrosis* (cell swelling). Apoptosis is the normal way for cells to die; necrosis is pathological.

In healthy adults about 10 billion cells die each day (Renehan *et al.*, 2001), normal cell death being regulated by apoptosis. Apoptosis begins by cells detaching from adjacent cells. DNA is digested and cytopaslm shrinks. Organelles and other intracellular contents are released encased in buds of membrane. This prevents inflammatory responses. The shrunken cell and the buds are finally phagocytosed by macrophages (Kam & Ferch, 2000; Hotchkiss *et al.*, 2002).

Necrosis is an inflammatory process. Lack of adenosine triphosphate (cell energy) causes pumps in cell membranes to fail (Kam & Ferch, 2000). This causes an influx of sodium, followed by water, while preventing escape of intracellular water so causing intracellular oedema and further membrane damage. Damaged membranes allow pro-inflammatory mediators, including tumour necrosis factor alpha (TNF$\alpha$) to escape from cells. Inflammatory mediators attract neutrophils, macrophages, lysosomal enzymes and proteases into surrounding tissue (Kam & Ferch, 2000; Hotchkiss *et al.*, 2002), initiating inflammation. Cell necrosis is the cause of many pathologies seen in ICU so underlies discussion in many subsequent chapters.

## Inflammatory response

This homeostatic mechanism forms part of non-specific immunity. Damaged tissue releases pro-inflammatory cytokines (especially TNF$\alpha$ and interleukin 1), which provoke endothelium release of vasoactive chemicals, including histamine (vasodilator) and leucotrienes (increase capillary permeability). Increased blood flow and leakier capillaries enable leucocytes and other defences to migrate into infected tissue and destroy invading bacteria. When confined to an area of local damage, this homeostatic response promotes healing; but when extensive inflammatory responses occur, extensive vasodilatation and massive capillary leak cause life-threatening systemic inflammatory response syndrome (SIRS – see Chapter 33).

Inflammatory responses release many chemical vasoactive mediators, including

- tumour necrosis factor alpha (TNF$\alpha$)
- interleukins
- arachidonic acids
- prostaglandins (prostacyclin, thromboxane)
- nitric oxide.

They normally maintain homeostatis, but inappropriate or extensive circulating concentrations causes many symptoms and complications. TNF$\alpha$ and interleukin 1 initiate the cytocyne cascade and, among other effects, cause pyrexia, by resetting the hypothalamic set-point for temperature.

## Chemical mediators

Critical illness is largely caused by inappropriate and excessive homeostastic responses to lesser insults. Vasoactive mediators relax smooth arteriole muscle, causing vasodilatation, and increase capillary permeability, causing oedema. Vasodilatation and oedema together cause profound hypotension – shock, SIRS. There are many chemical mediators, many released either by vascular endothelium or the immune system. Some of the most significant are

- cytokines
- histamine
- arachidonic acid metabolites (*leucotrienes*, prostaglandins, *thromboxane A$_2$*, *eicosanoids*)
- nitric oxide
- complement cascade.

Most have similar, interdependent effects (pro-inflammatory, procoagulopathic and cytotoxic) causing progressive multiorgan dysfunction.

## Cytokines

Cytokines ('cell killers') are released mainly from leucocytes. Tumour necrosis factor alpha (TNFα, also called cachectin) is usually the first cytokine to be released and initiates the cytokine cascade. TNFα stimulates growth of new surface receptors (adhesion molecules) on vascular endothelial cells, enabling leucocyte adhesion, accumulation and phagocytosis (Abbas *et al.*, 1994). TNFα

- depresses cardiac function (negatively inotropic)
- initiates immune responses (including pyrexia)
- promotes clotting

so causes hypotension, pyrexia and thrombi. Chlorpromazine has been used to reduce production and circulating levels of TNFα (Jansen *et al.*, 1998) but has not been widely adopted.

*Interleukins* are a diverse group of chemicals, with varying effects and many pathenogenic. They have been implicated in various autoimmune disorders (Raeburn *et al.*, 2002). Interleukins 1, 6 and 8 are major mediators of critical illnesses.

## Acute phase proteins

Infection initiates early release of proteins, including *fibrinogen, alpha-1 protinase inhibitor, C-reactive protein* (CRP – see Chapter 21) and *serum amyloid associated protein* to assist phagocytosis.

## Radicals

Any biochemical reaction can release free radicals (e.g. micro-organism lysis by neutrophils, Kreb's cycle). Free radicals are molecules with one or more unpaired electron in their outer orbit; this makes them inherently unstable, reacting readily with other molecules to pair with the free electron. Reaction of two radicals eliminates both, but reactions between radicals and nonradicals produce a further radical. Reactivity is indiscriminate, so although their lifespan lasts only microseconds, chain reactions may be thousands of events long, causing the autocatalysis underlying most critical illnesses.

Pierce *et al.* (2004) suggest two free radicals are significant:

- nitrogen oxygen species (NOS)
- reactive oxygen species (ROS).

ROS, also called oxygen free radicals or oxygen radicals, are formed during reduction of oxygen to water and have been implicated in hundreds of diseases (Pierce *et al.*, 2004). Oxygen radical reactions form toxic radices such as superoxide, hydrogen peroxide ($H_2O_2$) and hydroxyl (Mak & Newton, 2001). Hydrogen peroxide is highly reactive, damaging cell membranes and DNA (Pierce *et al.*, 2004).

Oxygen metabolism occurs intracellularly, inevitably releasing some radicals. The few radicals normally produced are destroyed by antioxidants such as vitamin E, vitamin C and albumin. Massive production of oxygen free radicals overwhelms endogenous antioxidant defences. Despite many studies, antioxidant therapy has few benefits; Haji-Michael (2000) argues that only selenium and glutamine have proven benefits. Neutrophil activation increases oxygen free radical production.

Hypoxic vascular epithelium releases endogenous *nitric oxide*, a vasodilator. Increasing blood flow delivers more oxygen to the hypoxic tissue. Nitric oxide release is stimulated by nitrates, such as glyceryl trinitrate and isosorbide dinitrate. Excessive nitric oxide production causes massive vasodilatation, one factor causing SIRS.

*Reperfusion injury* is almost inevitable when tissues are reperfused. During perfusion failure, anaerobic metabolism from alternative energy sources releases many toxic mediators which accumulate in tissues that are not perfused. Reperfusion flushes large numbers of these toxic mediators into systemic circulation. Among the symptoms these can cause during reperfusion are myocardial depression and dysrhythmias.

### Implications for practice

- Most critical pathologies originate at microcellular rather than macrosystem level; understanding these processes enables nurses to understand pathologies and treatments covered in most other chapters (e.g. pressure sores, oxygen toxicity, fluid and electrolyte balance).

- Cells need energy and oxygen. Microcirculatory resuscitation requires
  - oxygen delivery to cells (tissue perfusion)
  - nutrition
  - ventilation.
- High $FiO_2$ (above 0.5–0.6) is potentially toxic so should not be used for more than a few hours.
- Reperfusion injury can cause secondary damage, so recovery requires close observation of effects (e.g. dysrhythmias) and prompt intervention.

## Summary

Cell function is complex, and knowledge of cell function and potential medical interventions is rapidly increasing. Understanding cell dysfunction is a useful basis for understanding pathophysiologies described in the remainder of this section. The microscopic nature of cell function and dysfunction make these less easy to understand the function and dysfunction of major organs. This chapter has therefore given an overview of cellular pathology and some of the more significant mediators.

Most critical illnesses originate and progress at cellular level; macroscopic symptoms are accumulations of microscopic problems. Treatments should therefore focus on underlying mechanisms of disease rather than more easily observed effects. Understanding these microscopic mechanisms enables nurses to monitor and assess effects of treatments.

Abnormal figures (e.g. disordered arterial blood gases) may be tolerated to assist cell recovery (e.g. permissive hypercapnia – see Chapter 27).

## Further reading

Current attempts to target problems from cell dysfunction prompt frequent articles in medical and scientific journals. Fewer articles have appeared in nursing journals, but Pierce *et al.* (2004) and Scheibmeir *et al.* (2005) provide recent summaries. Normal cell physiology can be revised from a recent and appropriate anatomy text such as Marieb (2004). www.routledge.com/textbooks/0415373239

For clinical scenarios, clinical questions and the answers to them go to the support website at www.routledge.com/textbooks/0415373239

## Clinical scenarios

David Roberts, 33 years old with a history of poorly controlled asthma, is admitted to the ICU following a respiratory arrest. On endotracheal suction his sputum is thick mucopurulent and arterial blood gases indicate severe respiratory acidosis.

His blood results include abnormalities in white blood cells and other blood results:

| | |
|---|---|
| WBC | $27.3 \times 10^{-9}$/litre |
| Platelets | $277 \times 10^{-9}$/litre |
| Neutrophils | $23.4 \times 10^{-9}$/litre |
| Eosinophils | $1.6 \times 10^{-9}$/litre |
| Basinophils | $0.8 \times 10^{-9}$/litre |
| Monocytes | $0.7 \times 10^{-9}$/litre |
| Lymphocytes | $0.7 \times 10^{-9}$/litre |
| | |
| Hb | 7.6 g/litre |
| CRP | 372 mg/litre |

Arterial blood gas

| | |
|---|---|
| pH | 7.26 |
| $PaCO_2$ | 8.08 kPa |
| $PaO_2$ | 8.78 kPa |
| $HCO_3$ | 24.2 mmol/litre |
| Base excess | 0.1 mmol/litre |
| Lactate | 2.3 mmol/litre |

Q.1 Draw and label a diagram of the typical eucaryotic cell. Include structures (and make brief notes on their functions) such as nucleus, cytoplasm, cytoskeleton, microtubules, endoplasmic reticulum, Golgi complex, ribosomes, mitochondria, lysosomes, cell surface (or surface membrane) with its various structures and components (e.g. desmosomes, tight junctions, gap junctions, antibody response and hormone binding sites).

Q.2 Analyse David's WBC differential results; does it indicate inflammatory response or infection? (e.g. consider functions of each cell type, cells increase in response bacteria or have digestive function which respond to allergens.)

Q.3 David develops systemic hypotension and acute lung injury. Review the cellular processes which caused this from his respiratory condition (e.g. effect of hypoxia and hypercarbia on cellular function, mitochondrial ATP production, cell membrane potential, mediators triggered, function and systemic effects of these mediators, causes of capillary permeability, role of basophils, implications of associated histamine release).

Chapter 21 identifies normal reference ranges.

Chapter 25

# Immunity and immunodeficiency

## Contents

Introduction                     270
Immunity                         270
HIV                              271
Ethical and health issues        274
Implications for practice         275
Summary                          275
Support groups                   276
Further reading                  276
Clinical scenarios               276

## Fundamental knowledge

Physiology of normal immunity

## Introduction

Immunity enables us to resist many potential pathogens, but most ICU patients are immunocompromised. This chapter describes normal immunity, illustrating dysfunction through Human Immunosuppressive Virus (HIV) and Acquired Immune Deficiency Syndrome (AIDS).

## Immunity

Classifications of immunity derive from historical schools of immunology, which increasingly recognised that different modes of immunity existed concurrently. Immunity may be

■ nonspecific (innate)
■ specific (adaptive).

Nonspecific immunity is any defence mechanism not targeting specific micro-organisms. Much human nonspecific immunity is present at birth. Specific immunity is necessarily acquired through exposure to various organisms or antibody vaccination.

Immunity may also be classified as cell mediated and humoral. Cell-mediated immunity causes T-lymphocytes to respond to (nonspecific) protein by producing various cytokines; humoral immunity is mediated by antibodies (B-lymphocytes) in the blood so is antigen-specific.

### Nonspecific immunity

Many body systems include defence mechanisms against foreign material, all potentially compromised by critical illness and treatments (e.g. intubation, steroids). Examples of nonspecific immunity include

■ stickiness of mucous membrane and cilia (trapping airway particles smaller than 2 micrometres)
■ body 'flushes' (tears, saliva), many including antibacterial lysozyme
■ sebrum (from sebaceous glands) preventing bacteemrial colonisation of skin
■ acidity/alkalinity of gastrointestinal tract
■ pyrexia (see Chapter 8)
■ inflammatory response – increases and activates phagocyte and *complements*
■ interferon – inhibits viral replication and enhances action of killer cells
■ lactoferrin – binds iron (needed by microbes for growth)
■ release of the steroid hormone cortisol (hydrocortisone) from the adrenal glands and the glucocorticoid hormone cortisone from the liver.

Nonspecific chemical defences inhibit bacteria and viruses but place stress on the body: inflammation can become pathological (e.g. SIRS – see Chapter 33), while graft versus host disease (GvHD – see Chapter 44) threatens viability of transplanted tissue (foreign protein), necessitating immunosuppressant drugs.

## Specific immunity

Specific immunity involves recognition of a specific antibody by antigens. In response to antibodies, antigens then initiate a cascade of defensive mechanisms to destroy the antibody. In health, antigen–antibody responses provide valuable defence, but excessive or inappropriate responses can cause

- allergy
- anaphylaxis

or if the body's own tissue is identified as the antigen,

- autoimmunity.

Specific immunity involves two types of lymphocytes: T and B (see Chapter 21). Antigen recognition by T-lymphocytes usually precedes B-lymphocyte production.

## Immunodeficiency

Failure of the immune system is usually secondary to either autoimmune pathologies (e.g. HIV, leukaemia, hepatic failure) or drug-induced (e.g. steroids, cyclosporin A, chemotherapy). The immune system can also be overwhelmed by infection or complex surgery/invasive treatment, exposing patients to opportunistic infections (e.g. MRSA) that may colonise, but not infect, healthier people (e.g. staff).

Older people (most ICU patients) have decreased immunity due to reduced T-cell function (Schwacha & Chaudry, 2000) and other factors.

## Steroids

Despite variable use over many decades to treat various conditions, steroid therapy remains controversial, tending to treat symptoms (inflammation) rather than causes. Symptom treatment may be justified when 'cures' prove evasive.

## HIV

Two human immunosuppressive viruses (HIV) have been identified: HIV-1 and HIV-2. HIV-1, prevalent in the West, is primarily described here. HIV-2, predominant in Africa, is structurally different from HIV-1 and may be less virulent (Lever, 2001) but causes similar symptoms. Worldwide, rates of HIV infection are increasing, especially in developing countries (Woodman, 1999).

Auto Immune Dysfunction Syndrome (AIDS) only occurs with symptoms from opportunistic infection; HIV + people who remain symptom-free are colonised, but not infected. So while HIV can lead to AIDS, it is not the same as AIDS. Half of HIV carriers will probably develop full AIDS within 9–11 years (Mann, 1999), although a few early carriers remain AIDS-free.

While HIV is rightly seen as a major threat to modern healthcare, hepatitis B causes more disease and death than HIV.

## The virus

HIV was first reported in 1981; this virus quickly created levels of fear and stigma unknown since syphilis epidemics. Hysteria was heightened by it being a sexually transmitted disease and early association with homosexuals and (to a lesser extent) intravenous drug users, even though worldwide most HIV is transmitted heterosexually.

In the West, infection among 'high risk' groups has declined, although needle sharing still causes about one-tenth of all UK HIV+ infections (Bennett & Baker, 2001). Infection rates have increased among heterosexual non-drug users. UK incidence varies greatly but tends to be highest in large inner-city areas.

HIV primarily attacks CD4 (T helper) lymphocytes so causes progressive problems from immunodeficiency. Once inside host cells, HIV transmits genetic information as a single RNA strand. Using the enzyme reverse transcriptase, it then replicates RNA into a DNA copy (hence 'retrovirus'). This clumsy arrangement is complicated by inaccuracies of enzyme replication, causing on average one mutation each replication cycle (Wainberg, 1999).

The virus may avoid detection because

- *seroconversion* takes some weeks to occur
- *HIV-2* may evade tests relying on antibody detection
- *HIV-1 subtype O* (a West African subgroup) may remain undetected by either HIV-1 or HIV-2 tests (Loussert- Ajaka *et al.*, 1994). So HIV negative results do not necessarily confirm absence of the virus. Subgroups have also emerged which are more resistant to anti-retroviral drugs (Boden *et al.*, 1999).

Initially, the virus replicates rapidly: $10^9$–$10^{10}$ daily, but after seroconversion, viral titre drops dramatically (Leigh Brown, 1999).

In 1993 the USA's Centre for Disease Control extended definitions of AIDS to include all severely immunocompromised patients (CD4 counts below $200 \times 10^6$ per litre). This definition is not accepted in the UK or Europe (Bennett & Baker, 2001), causing possible discrepancies with statistical comparisons.

Autoimmune dysfunction exposes patients to opportunistic infections:

- respiratory
- gastrointestinal
- central nervous system

although newer antiretroviral drugs have reduced incidence of opportunistic infections (Wolff & O'Donnell, 2001). Anxieties and stigma surround HIV and AIDS often increase psychological needs of patients and families and friends.

*Respiratory* failure remains the main cause of ICU admission (Morris *et al.*, 2002). Most respiratory infections are caused by the organism *Pneumocystis jirovici* (formerly called Pneumocystis Carinii Pneumonia, and still called PCP) (Thomas & Limper, 2004), usually occurring when CD4 counts fall below 200 cells/mm$^3$ (Avidan *et al.*, 2000). While this remains the single main cause of AIDS-related admission to the ICU, incidence of PCP has reduced (Morris *et al.*, 2002), and nearly half of HIV + patients on ICUs are admitted for non-respiratory reasons (Gill *et al.*, 1999). Pneumocystis forms cysts in alveoli and interstitial lung tissue, which often progress to *ARDS*. Tuberculosis (TB) infection increasingly complicates AIDS, especially in inner-city areas (Rayner, 2004), a problem aggravated by development of resistant strains (Djuretic *et al.*, 2002).

PCP causes pyrexia, a nonproductive cough and respiratory failure. Whether artificial ventilation is justified for PCP remains debated, but should partly depend on short-term prognosis. NIV may support respiratory failure without the trauma of intubation, although even this raises dilemmas of whether life or death is being prolonged.

*Gastrointestinal* dysfunction includes malnourishment and increased motility. Many patients are malnourished (with weight loss) on admission, from prolonged illness and reluctance to eat or drink due to breathlessness. Malnourishment further impairs immunity and healing, while increased motility from both disease and drugs causes diarrhoea, vomiting and nausea. Malnutrition and muscle wasting increase mortality. Nutrition should therefore be a priority. Vitamin supplements may be needed, as deficiency from malnutrition is likely. Antiemetics and antidiarroheal drugs can restore comfort and dignity. Mouthcare provides comfort and helps prevent opportunist infection.

*Central nervous system* damage and encephalitis are usually seen at postmortem. Many patients suffer both cognitive and behavioural changes such as memory loss, apathy and poor concentration. Dementia occurs in up to two-thirds of people with AIDS (Abbas *et al.*, 1994); Gill *et al.* (1999) found the mean age of HIV+ patients on ICU was 38 years, not an age-group usually associated with dementia. Cognitive changes can be especially distressful for families and friends.

*Psychological* stressors include

- stigma surrounding HIV/AIDS
- anxieties about dying.

Psychological distress needs human care and interaction, spending time with people and allowing them to express their needs. Isolation may reinforce stigmatisation or provide valuable privacy for patients and their families/ friends.

## Drug treatments

Frequent viral mutations frustrate development of ideal anti-HIV drugs. Development of more effective drugs, and use of combination therapy, have reduced incidence of AIDS-defining illnesses (such as PCP) (Mocroft *et al.*, 2000), survival rates increasing from 49 to 71 per cent between 1991 and 2001 (Morris *et al.*, 2002; Narasinghan *et al.*, 2004).

Drugs may be used to

- inhibit viral replication
- relieve symptoms
- treat/prevent complications.

Antiretroviral drugs are generally very toxic, causing many adverse effects. The three main groups of antiviral drugs are:

- nucleoside analogue reverse transcripate intibitors (NRTIs) – e.g. didanosin, lamivudine, stavudine, zalcitabine, zidovudine
- non-nucleoside analogue reverse transcripate intibitors (NNRTIs)
- *protease inhibitors* (PIs), which make virus particles immature and so non-infectious (Bennett & Baker, 2001) – e.g. indinavir, ritonavir.

*Co-trimoxazole* remains the standard treatment for PCP (Vilar & Wilkins, 1998), although other drugs such as *Pentamadine* (intravenous, nebulised) may be used instead. Pentamidine has more toxic effects, including hypo/ hyper-glycaemia, dysrhythmias and renal failure (Vilar & Wilkins, 1998).

## Ethical and health issues

HIV and AIDS have raised more ethical dilemmas and issues than any other disease in recent years. HIV tests, even when negative, may threaten insurance and mortgage policies and employment prospects. Technically, any nonconsensual touch is (legally) assault.

Relatives may discover diagnosis of HIV/AIDS from death certificates, having been unaware, and perhaps disapproving, of the deceased's lifestyle. This can cause additional distress following bereavement. But nurses' duties of confidentiality to their patients are absolute (apart from specific legal requirements), extending beyond death of patients.

Dilemmas raised through clinical practice can usefully be discussed among unit teams, contributing to professional growth of all involved. Goffman (1963) and Sontag (1989) raise provocative insights. Support agencies are identified below.

HIV and AIDS are not included in the *Public Health (Control of Diseases) Act 1984* (Dimond, 2005), probably due to historical accident of this act being drafted before AIDS became a significant problem in the UK. HIV and AIDS are not therefore notifiable diseases.

Although complacency should be avoided, risk from occupational exposure is small. Five healthcare workers have died from occupational exposure to HIV in England, Wales and Northern Ireland, with a further 11 deaths from occupational exposure abroad (Evans *et al.*, 2001). In comparison, Evans *et al.* (2001) identified 151 deaths from hepatitis B between 1997 and 2000. However, nurses fail to appreciate risks of infection from needle stick injury (Leliopoulou *et al.*, 1999). All body fluids from all patients are potentially hazardous; Gill *et al.*'s (1999) study found that 27 per cent of HIV+ patients in ICUs were undiagnosed on admission.

## Implications for practice

- Many ICU pathologies and treatments impair immunity, so high standards of infection control are needed to protect patients from opportunistic infections.
- Patients with AIDS admitted to the ICU usually need respiratory support, usually because of PCP. Appropriateness of interventions, such as whether to limit support to NIV, should be based on short-term prognosis and (where possible) patients' wishes.
- People with HIV/AIDS may experience prejudice and stigma. Nurses have a duty of care to all their patients and should promote positive attitudes among other staff.
- AIDS often causes various gastrointestinal symptoms. Nurses should assess nutritional needs and bowel function, feeding early and providing appropriate care and support.
- HIV+ patients and their families may need additional psychological support; involving specialist agencies may be beneficial.
- Unit discussions (ethical forums, case review) can stimulate useful debate for professional development.

## Summary

Most patients in the ICU are immunocompromised. Treatments and interventions increase infection risks, but proactive infection control can reduce risks from nosocomial infection.

HIV and AIDS have created medical and ethical challenges to healthcare. The unique role of nurses in the ICU team enable them to challenge and resolve stigmas and negative attitudes to meet the psychological and physiological needs of their patients.

## Support groups

| | |
|---|---|
| National AIDS helpline | 0800 012–322 |
| Terrence Higgins Trust | 0845 1221–200 |
| Body Positive | 800–566–6599 |

## Further reading

Immunology is discussed in most physiology and microbiology texts. Pratt (2003) provides an excellent text on HIV and nursing, while Bennett and Baker (2001) is a useful review, although neither is specifically ICU focussed.

Ethical dilemmas raise issues from wider contexts; Goffman's (1963) classic work on stigma (written before HIV was identified) and Sontag's (1989) outstanding investigative journalism offer valuable sociological insights, raising many ethical issues. Extreme reactions to the stigma of a fictional killer virus are effectively illustrated in the film *Outbreak* (Warner Brothers, 1995). Many experiential accounts exist, such as Gunn's (1992) poetry chronicalling deaths of friends from AIDS. www.routledge.com/textbooks/0415373239

For clinical scenarios, clinical questions and the answers to them go to the support website at www.routledge.com/textbooks/0415373239

## Clinical scenarios

Vanessa Warring, a 27-year-old single mother of two small children, was admitted to intensive care for ventilatory support following rapidly deteriorating respiratory function from right lung pneumonia. Vanessa refused consent for a HIV test pre-intubation. Microbiology results confirmed presence of *Pneumocystis* pneumonia (PCP). Her CD4 count on admission was <20 cells/mm$^3$. Over the next 10 days, Vanessa continued to deteriorate despite therapy, she became colonised with several opportunistic organisms and it was obvious that she was dying. Her children were being cared for by a social worker.

Q.1 Explain the differences in immune response between HIV positive and HIV negative people on exposure to *Pneumocystis jiroveci*. (Why is an HIV positive person more likely to develop PCP?). List other opportunistic organisms, and their source, which are likely to infect Vanessa.

Q.2 Analyse the interventions available to support Vanessa's system; include the value and limitations of these interventions (e.g. protective isolation, drug therapies of antibiotics, antiviral, antifungal, nutrition, psychological support, therapeutic relationships).

Q.3 Consider the ethical and legal issues associated with this situation. Should Vanessa's children be tested for HIV? Who should make this decision and how would this be justified?

Chapter 26

# Disseminated intravascular coagulation (DIC)

## Contents

Introduction                        278
Pathophysiology                     278
Progression                         279
Signs                               279
Treatment                           280
Related pathologies                 281
Nursing care                        282
Deep vein thromboses                282
Implications for practice           283
Summary                             283
Further reading                     283
Clinical scenarios                  284

## Fundamental knowledge

Normal clotting – intrinsic, extrinsic and common
    coagulation pathways

## Introduction

Disseminated intravascular coagulation (DIC) is secondary to other pathologies and has been variously called 'consumptive coagulopathy' and 'defibrination syndrome'. DIC is uncontrolled systemic activation of coagulation, just as *SIRS* is uncontrolled systemic activation of inflammatory homeostatic responses.

Haemostasis has four phases:

1   smooth muscle contraction (vasoconstriction; myogenic reflex)
2   formation of platelet plugs
3   formation of fibrin clot (blood clotting/coagulation), followed by retraction of fibrin clots
4   fibrinolysis.

Pathophysiology and treatments are described, together with three related syndromes:

■   haemolytic uraemic syndrome (HUS)
■   thrombotic thrombocytopenia purpura (TTP)
■   heparin-induced thrombocytopaenia and thrombosis syndrome (HITTS).

Venous stasis from immobility and procoagulant pathologies predispose nearly all ICU patients to risk of deep vein thromboses (DVT) which are the single main cause of pulmonary emboli. DVT prophylaxis, which is usually 'routine' for all ICU patients, is also discussed in this chapter.

## Pathophysiology

DIC is inappropriate systemic activation of coagulation (Levi & ten Cate, 1999). Endothelial damage, often from gram negative bacteria, activates the intrinsic clotting cascade. Pro-inflammatory mediates are released, resulting in further hypotension and increased vascular permeability. Proteolysis releases fibrin degradation products (FDPs), which cause further capillary obstruction and anticoagulation. The hepatic reticulo-endothelial system, which normally clears FDPs, becomes overwhelmed by excessive degradation productions or impaired liver function. Other circulating mediators of cellular injury, such as cytokines (e.g. IL-1, IL-6, TNFα) and antigen-antibody complexes, further complicate DIC, causing interstitial oedema and hypovolaemia.

Although gram negative bacteria cause most cases of DIC, other possible triggers include

■   viruses (especially varicella, hepatitis, CMV)
■   trauma
■   vascular disorders (aortic aneurysm)
■   severe burns
■   obstetric complications (amniotic fluid embolus, abruptio placentae)
■   hepatic failure (low-grade DIC)

- cancer
- reaction to toxins (snake venom, drugs, amphetamines)
- immunological disorders (severe allergic reactions, haemolytic transfusion reaction, transplant rejections).

(Hambley, 1995; Levi & ten Cate, 1999)

DIC is best diagnosed through D-dimer and FDP tests (Yu *et al.*, 2000).

## Progression

DIC causes four main complications:

- hypotension
- microvascular obstruction and necrosis
- haemolysis
- haemorrhage.

Stagnation of capillary flow from prolonged hypotension and systemic arteriovenous shunting causes

- metabolic acidosis
- tissue and cell ischaemia
- intracapillary thrombosis.

Procoagulant material from cell injury enters the systemic circulation, activating widespread inappropriate clotting. Proteolysis stimulates further coagulation and fibrinolysis, causing intravascular formation of fibrin (Levi & ten Cate, 1999). Excessive fibrin deposits consume clotting factors (hence 'consumptive coagulopathy') and cause inappropriate clotting. Fibrin meshes

- obstruct blood flow (especially to arterioles, capillaries and venules) causing capillary ischaemia and tissue necrosis
- haemolyse the erythrocytes that do manage to penetrate the fibrin mesh
- trap platelets (hence low platelet counts).

Consumption of clotting factors leaves insufficient supply for homeostasis, so patients bleed readily (typically from invasive cannulae and trauma, such as endotracheal suction). DIC progresses rapidly, often occurring within a few hours of the initiating cause.

## Signs

Early symptoms of DIC are typically nonspecific, such as

- mild cerebral dysfunction (e.g. confusion)
- dyspnoea

- mild hypoxia
- petechial bleeding (especially trunk)
- skin rashes
- purpura
- spontaneous mucocutaneous bleeding
- minor renal dysfunction.

As DIC progresses, symptoms become more severe. DIC prolongs *clotting times*, with high levels of FDPs such as D-dimers and reduced levels of antithrombin and many clotting factors, especially fibrinogen, platelets, antithrombin. Patients bleed from multiple sites, including arterial and venous cannulae.

*Skin* symptoms are easily visible; subdermal haemorrhages cause purpura, the skin may appear cyanotic, mottled or cool, and in latter stages gangrene may develop.

Vascular fibrin deposits form throughout the cardiovascular system, progressive *organ failure* follows:

- lungs: especially *ARDS*, pulmonary emboli and pulmonary hypertension
- kidneys (intrarenal failure)
- liver
- cerebral: microthrombi may cause confusion or cerebrovascular accidents; unconsciousness may mask neurological symptoms.

Highly vascular surface membrane are especially prone to haemorrhage. Bleeding may occur from traumatic endotracheal suction, further complicating respiratory function. The gastrointestinal tract is especially susceptible to haemorrhage, so gastric drainage/aspirate and stools should be assessed for blood (including occult and melaena). If patients are not being fed enterally, stomach decompression (free nasogastric drainage) reduces stomach stretch and acid accumulation, so helps prevent haemorrhage.

## Treatment

DIC is always secondary to an underlying problem, so resolving underlying causes is a priority (Levi & ten Cate, 1999):

- controlling inflammation
- system support, including oxygenation and nutrition.

Clotting factors should be replaced: platelet transfusion, especially fresh frozen plasma and cryoprecipitate (Green, 2003). Fresh blood and fibrinogen may also be used. Levi & ten Cate (1999) recommend only giving platelets if counts are low. Longer-term management should include restoring endogenous haemostasis (including through nutrition) to resolve underlying problems. Vitamin K may also be given. Concentrates of coagulation factors should be avoided, as they may contain traces of activated clotting factors, and DIC usually causes deficiency of all factors (Levi & ten Cate, 1999). Antifibrin should be avoided, as DIC usually causes insufficient fibrinolysis, so further inhibition of fibrinolysis is inappropriate (Levi & ten Cate, 1999).

Platelet infusions should be handled carefully, as turbulence (e.g. shaking) damages platelets, and given quickly through dedicated administration sets. Used blood giving sets should not be used for FFP and other clotting factors, as anticoagulant used with blood may adhere to plastic and neutralise FFP.

Severe acidosis may be actively reversed. System failure often necessitates support (e.g. ventilation, inotropes, haemofiltration). Various other symptoms may also require treatment (e.g. antibiotics and cytoprotective drugs to prevent gastric bleeding). Activated Protein C (ACP – see Chapter 33) can reverse DIC (Levi & ten Cate, 1999; Toh & Dennis, 2003).

Heparin, once used to release clotting factors from microthrombi, is usually counter-productive, inhibiting the anti-inflammatory effects of antithrombin (Warren et al., 2001). Levi and ten Cate (1999) recommend using heparin both for thrombolysis and to prevent DVT formation, but Green (2003) suggests that heparin may be useful as tertiary treatment, but should only be given on the advice of a haematologist. Antithrombin may (Opal et al., 2002) or may not (Warren et al., 2002) be effective for *DIC* caused by sepsis. Other possible treatments include Activated Protein C (Xigris), Tranexamic acid and aprotinin.

## Related pathologies

Haemolytic uraemic syndrome (HUS) is a rare disorder, similar to DIC but localised to kidneys, caused by fibrin deposits in renal capillaries. Parker (1997) suggests that HUS is the paediatric counterpart to TTP, but other authors apply HUS to adults. Pathology and causes of HUS are unclear, but often associated with bacterial or viral infections (especially *E. coli*), oral contraceptives, ciclosporin A or complement abnormalities (Friedman, 1992). Unless treated with urgent plasma exchange is almost invariably fatal (Short et al., 2001).

Thrombotic thrombocytopenia purpura (TTP), also rare, is traditionally considered a separate syndrome from HUS, but has similar symptoms, pathophysiology and treatments (Short et al., 2001), extending to systemic and central nervous system involvement. Symptoms typically include purpura, neurological deficits, multifocal neuropsychiatric disturbances and renal failure. TTP is usually treated by plasmapheresis and supportive therapies. Platelets may exacerbate TTP, so should not be transfused unless there is life-threatening haemorrhage (British Society for Standards in Haematology, Blood Transfusion Task Force, 2003).

Heparin-induced thrombocytopenia and thrombosis syndrome (HITTS; HIT) is caused by heparin therapy, especially unfractioned rather than low molecular weight heparin (Warkentin, 2003). Like DIC, HITTS can become fulminant, causing major organ infarction (e.g. myocardial, cerebral). Platelets may cause acute arterial thrombosis so should not be given (British Society for Standards in Haematology, Blood Transfusion Task Force, 2003). Unfraction heparin is now rarely used.

## Nursing care

Bleeding can occur anywhere, internally or externally. Nurses should therefore

■ observe skin for bruising, petechial or purpuric haemorrhages
■ observe any invasive sites for oozing/bleeding (e.g. intravenous cannulae, drains, wounds)
■ observe and test any body fluids for blood (nasogastric aspirate, vomit, stools, urine).

Daily urinalysis may also reveal protein. Any abnormal findings should be reported.

Although DIC is a medical problem, and treatments will be medically prescribed, nursing care can significantly reduce complications from trauma, sepsis and bleeding. Many nursing interventions may provoke haemorrhage:

■ endotracheal suction
■ turning
■ cuff blood pressure measurement
■ enemas
■ rectal/vaginal examinations
■ plasters/tape
■ shaving
■ mouthcare.

Some interventions may be necessary, although alternative approaches should be considered. For example, as wet shaves are likely to cause bleeding; electric shavers may be safer. Similarly, foam sticks are less traumatic than tooth-brushes. Lubrication of skin and lips (e.g. with white petroleum jelly) helps prevent cracking. Invasive cannulae and procedures should be minimised to reduce risks of haemorrhage.

Small bleeds which may be physiologically insignificant can cause great dis-tress, and possible fainting. Visitors should be warned about the possible sight of blood, escorted to the bedside and observed until staff are satisfied about their safety. If patients sense their relatives are distressed, they may themselves become distressed, aggravating their disease.

## Deep vein thromboses

Risk of thromboembolism is significantly increased with bedrest. ICU patients are often at especially high risk of developing deep vein thrombosis (DVT), as systemic inflammatory responses cause hypercoaguability. ICU incidence ranges between rates 22–80 per cent (Attia et al., 2001), incidence increasing with age (Jacobs, 2003). Pulmonary emboli are almost invariably from DVTs (British Thoracic Society, 2003). DVT delays hospital discharge by an average of one week (Parnaby, 2004).

Development of DVT is significantly reduced with subcutaneous low molecular weight heparin (Attia *et al.*, 2001; Jacobs, 2003) and knee-length anti-thrombotic stockings ('TEDs')™ (Attia *et al.*, 2001; Howard *et al.*, 2004; Morris & Woodcock, 2004; Parnaby, 2004; Prandoni *et al.*, 2004). Unless there are specific contraindications, such as excessively prolonged clotting, all patients in ICU should have

■ daily subcutaneous low molecular weight heparin
■ daily clotting screens (target INR 2–3 (BCSH, 1998))
■ knee-length anti-thrombotic stockings
■ twice daily removal and remeasuring of stockings twice daily.

### Implications for practice

■ Patients should be closely observed/monitored for complications in all body systems.
■ Nurses should minimise interventions that will cause trauma/bleeding.
■ Visitors should be warned of the possibility of seeing blood, and should be escorted and observed until safe.
■ Unless specifically contraindicated, all ICU patients should receive DVT prophylaxis (anticoagulants, TEDs™).

### Summary

DIC is a complication caused by a variety of pathological processes. Early treatments with anticoagulants have been largely superseded by more conservative (temporary) approaches of replacing clotting factors and treating symptoms to buy time while the underlying pathology is treated.

Nursing care should focus on avoiding complications of trauma, while minimising anxiety to both patients and relatives.

Patients in the ICU are at especially high risk of developing deep vein thromboses often due to prolonged immobility and pro-coagulant diseases and syndromes. DVT prophylaxis is, and should be, routine for all ICU patients, unless there are specific contra-indications. Prophylaxis generally includes daily subcutaneous injection of low molecular weight heparin, knee-length anti-thrombotic stockings and daily clotting screens.

### Further reading

Management of DIC has changed significantly over recent decades, so old material should be actively avoided. Levi and ten Cate (1999) provide the best recent medical review, but Green (2003) and Bastacky and Lee (2001) are also useful.

The British Society for Standards in Haematology, Blood Transfusion Task Force (2003) offers details and definitive guidance for platelet transfusions.

DVTs remain problematic in many specialities, generating articles in various journals. Morris and Woodcock (2004) is a useful medical review. www.routledge.com/textbooks/0415373239

For clinical scenarios, clinical questions and the answers to them go to the support website at www.routledge.com/textbooks/0415373239

## Clinical scenarios

Gary Williams is a 56-year-old Afro Caribbean admitted with a coagulopathy of unknown cause. Initial investigations revealed deranged clotting, 15–20 ml/h of cloudy urine with casts, fever (37.7°C), tachypneoic (44 breaths/minute), tachycardic (124 beats per minute) with hypotension (84/58 mmHg) and severe metabolic acidosis. He has blood shot eyes and rectal bleeding.

Gary's blood investigations values include:   Laboratory reference range:

| | | |
|---|---|---|
| INR | 1.5 | 0.8–1.1 |
| APTT ratio | 3.78 | 0.85–1.15 |
| Thrombin time (seconds) | 21 | 11–16 |
| Fibrinogen (g/litre) | 1.5 | 2–4 |
| D-Dimer (mg/litre) | 8.48 | 0.0–0.3 |
| Platelets ($10^{-9}$/litre) | 26 | 150–450 |
| Hb (g/dl) | 7.8 | 13.0–17.0 |
| WBC ($10^{-9}$/litre) | 23.1 | 4.0–11.0 |
| Neutrophils ($10^{-9}$/litre) | 22.4 | 1.7–8.0 |
| Lymphocytes ($10^{-9}$/litre) | 0.7 | 1.0–4.0 |
| Monocytes ($10^{-9}$/litre) | 0.1 | 0.24–1.1 |
| HCT | 0.24 | 0.41–0.52 |
| RBC ($10^{-12}$/litre) | 2.91 | 4.5–6.0 |
| Urea (mmol/litre) | 12.9 | 3–9 |
| Creatinine ($\mu$mol/litre) | 517 | 70–114 (Male) |
| Creatine kinase (U/litre) | 15571 | 30–210 |
| Sensitive CRP (mg/litre) | 244.8 | 0–8.0 |
| Troponin T ($\mu$g/litre) | 0.02 | 0–0.05 |

Q.1 Interpret Gary's blood results and note the clinical significance of abnormal values. Consider which blood results are related to intrinsic activation and those which are related to extrinsic activation of blood coagulation.

Q.2 Review which coagulation disorder is most likely to be associated with Gary's symptoms, vital observations and blood results (e.g. HUS, DIC or other). Consider primary cause (e.g. sepsis, rhabdomyolysis) and how diagnosis may be confirmed.

Q.3 Three units of blood, cryoprecipitate, fresh frozen plasma and platelets are prescribed. Outline the rationale for this treatment and nursing approaches which can maximise their therapeutic benefits (e.g. specify methods, routes and order of administration, storage, temperature, minimising bleeding points and/or further fibrinolysis, evaluating effectiveness).

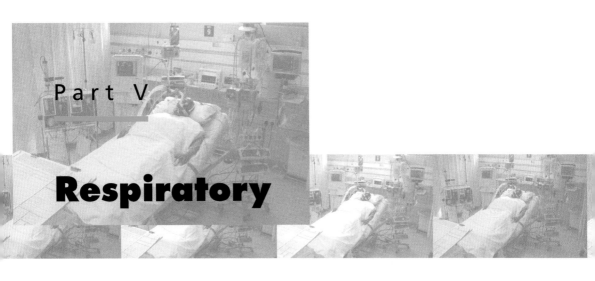

Part V

# Respiratory

Chapter 27

# Acute respiratory distress syndrome (ARDS)

**Contents**

Introduction                                  288
Pathology                                     288
Treatment                                     289
Ventilation                                   289
Positioning                                   290
Reducing pulmonary hypertension               293
Inflammatory response                         293
Fluid management                             293
Psychological support                        293
Cardiac management                           294
Implications for practice                    294
Summary                                      294
Further reading                              295
Clinical scenarios                           295

**Fundamental knowledge**

Respiratory anatomy and physiology – alveoli, pulmonary
   blood flow
V/Q mismatch; pulmonary shunting

## Introduction

ARDS, frequently progressing into multi-system failure, is a major cause of ICU admission. This chapter concentrates on pathophysiology and medical interventions and treatments. Much nursing time is devoted to assisting doctors (monitoring, giving prescribed treatments) so nurses need to understand pathology and treatments. Prolonged stay and poor prognosis may increase psychological needs of ICU patients and families.

Improved management has increased survival over the last decade (Brower *et al.*, 2001), but mortality remains high – 35–65 per cent (Ranieri *et al.*, 1999; Belligan, 2002; Hughes *et al.*, 2003). Outcome is unpredictable either at onset or when oxygenation is worst (Valta *et al.*, 1999). ARDS is usually caused by infection, multiorgan dysfunction syndrome (MODS) or ventilator-induced lung injury (Tidswell, 2001). Many victims are young, and one year afterwards survivors have poor quality of life, including respiratory limitations (Orme *et al.*, 2003), muscle wasting and weakness (Herridge *et al.*, 2003).

ARDS is defined as:

- acute injury to the lung with a $PaO_2/FiO_2$ ratio below 200 mmHg or <27 kPa, regardless of PEEP
- bilateral chest infiltrates on X-ray
- pulmonary capillary wedge pressure below 18 mmHg.

(Bernard et al., 1994a,b)

Problems created by ARDS have encouraged attempts with many treatments, none of which is without problems or criticism. However, the most promising treatments for reducing ARDS mortality focus on reducing the inflammatory response and MODS (Esteban *et al.*, 2000).

## Pathology

Early descriptions of ARDS usually identified two stages – exudative, followed by proliferative. Increasingly these stages have been seen as over-lapping, forming a continuum. ARDS is like SIRS, only confined to the lungs, causing coagulation, fibrinolysis and extravascular fibrin deposition (Idell, 2003). Inflammatory responses increase capillary permeability, so fibrin and other plasma proteins leak into and fill interstitial spaces (Bellingham, 1999). Increasingly, neutrophils follow (Deby-Dupont & Lamyl, 1999), releasing cytokines and oxygen free radicals (Quinlan & Evans, 2000). Oxygen free radicals (see Chapter 24), cause widespread cell damage, including haemorrhage (Deby-Dupont & Lamy, 1999) and hylaine membrane formation (Salmon & Garrard, 1999).

These cause

- significantly reduced functional residual capacity
- reduced (self-ventilating) tidal volume

■  high airway pressure (from reduced volume)

■  pulmonary 'shunting' (V/Q <0.8).

If high airway pressure persists, barotrauma and volutrauma cause progressive damage (see Chapter 4).

Exudation destroys alveolar basement membrane, replacing normal Type I alveolar cells, which produce surfactant, with Type II (Bellingham, 1999). Total lung collagen can double in two weeks (Bellingham, 1999) making lung tissue rigid, reducing compliance, increasing alveolar deadspace and accelerating respiratory failure (Artigas et al., 1998; Bellingham, 1999). Other problems include

■  emphysema-like lesions (Gattinoni et al., 1994)
■  capillary microembolism
■  pulmonary hypertension
■  cardiac output, initially high, falls as compensation fails
■  microcysts developing, especially in dependant lung tissue (Salmon & Garrard, 1999)
■  pneumothorax (Salmon & Garrard, 1999).

## Treatment

Treatment focuses on preventing further ventilator-induced injury, recruiting alveoli and supporting failing systems by

■  limiting $FiO_2$ below 0.65
■  optimising PEEP (10–15)
■  limiting peak inflation pressure (maximum 30–35 cmH$_2$O end expiratory pressure)
■  maximising mean inflation pressure (optimising gas exchange).

(Artigas et al., 1998)

## Ventilation

Mechanical ventilation can cause or aggravate acute lung injury (Ranieri et al., 1999). Trauma from large tidal volumes is called 'volutrauma' (sometimes called 'volotrauma'). Using smaller tidal volumes and accepting abnormally high arterial carbon dioxide tensions (*permissive hypercapnia*) to limit peak airway pressure can help alveoli recover. Reducing pre-set tidal volume (TV) from 12 to 6 ml/kg reduces mortality (by 22 per cent) and duration of ventilation (Acute Respiratory Distress Syndrome Network, 2000; Brower et al., 2001). However Brochard et al. (1998) found no benefits to reducing tidal volume provided plateau pressures were below 35 cmH$_2$O.

Permissive hypercapnia may create life-threatening respiratory acidosis, so should be used cautiously or avoided with:

- raised intracranial pressure
- anoxic brain injury (e.g. following MI)
- severe ischaemic heart disease
- hypotension
- dysrhythmias.

Panaceas for ARDS remain elusive and care should be individualised to each patient: low tidal volume ventilation is not appropriate for every ARDS patient (Ricard *et al.*, 2003). Hypercapnia being a respiratory stimulant, neuromuscular blockage may be needed.

*Pressure limited/controlled/regulated ventilation* limits peak inflation pressure, so limits further volutrauma and reduces the risk of pneumothorax (Valta *et al.*, 1999). Gas exchange can be optimised by increasing mean airway pressure and manipulating other aspects of ventilation, such as I:E ratio.

Alveolar recruitment is only likely to occur when *PEEP* exceeds 10 cmH$_2$O, but high PEEP (15 cmH$_2$O) causes pulmonary oedema (Ricard *et al.*, 2003), so levels of 10–15 are recommended (Artigas *et al.*, 1998), with levels being individualised to each patient (Rouby *et al.*, 2002). Preferences between increasing PEEP above 15 and extending inspiratory time (e.g. inverse ratio ventilation) remain controversial (Artigas *et al.*, 1998).

Nurses detecting increases in central venous and pulmonary pressures (indicative of pulmonary oedema) should alert medical staff. Nursing patients with their head elevated reduces cerebral oedema formation.

*Inverse ratio ventilation* increases mean (but not peak) airway pressure: prolonging inspiratory time increases alveolar recruitment, while shorter expiratory phases prevent alveolar collapse. But inverse ratio ventilation can cause air-trapping (auto-PEEP) and is usually distressing, requiring additional sedation and causing further hypotension.

*Lung rest* may limit or reverse damage (Gattinoni *et al.*, 1993) and high frequency oscillation significantly reduces ARDS mortality (Derak *et al.*, 2002). Liquid ventilation also shows promise (Haitsma & Lachmann, 2002). These modes are discussed further in Chapter 29.

Exogenous *surfactant* is ineffective for ARDS (Brackenbury *et al.*, 2001; Spragg *et al.*, 2003).

The vasopressor *almitine* has been used to shunt bloodflow from closed to open alveoli.

## Positioning

Horizontal positioning encourages oesophageal reflux, potentially causing aspiration and ventilator-associated pneumonia (Baktoft, 2001). This may necessitate reducing enteral feed volumes, which will prolong tissue repair, although increasing feed volumes between prone positioning could ensure adequate nutrition is supplied (Seaton-Mills, 2000) Angling the whole bed with the head up reduces reflex.

More lung tissue lies posteriorly. With ARDS, lung weight can double, causing alveolar compression and atelectasis when patients are nursed supine (Young, 1999). Nursing prone helps reverse this process.

Tidswell (2001) lists contraindications to proning as:

■ raised intracranial pressure
■ unstable head/spine injury
■ facial fractures/surgery
■ other (e.g. abdominal distension).

Studies consistently show improvements in oxygenation, reduced shunting, oxygen requirements and ventilator associated pneumonia (Brower *et al.*, 2001; Venet *et al.*, 2001; Pelosi *et al.*, 2002; Guerin *et al.*, 2004). This should increase survival, but does not appear to (Guerin *et al.*, 2004), perhaps because proning is only effective if instigated sufficiently early – usually within a few hours of ARDS developing (Breiburg *et al.*, 2000; Nakos *et al.*, 2000). Predicting who will benefit from proning is therefore difficult (Brower *et al.*, 2001).

Nursing complications of prone positioning are listed in Table 27.1.

Evidence for how long to prone, when to initiate it or when to discontinue is weak (Brower *et al.*, 2001). Recommended duration of prone positioning varies from 30 minutes to McAuley *et al.*'s (2002) 18 hours and Brower *et al.*'s (2001) twenty or more hours. Tidswell (2001) suggests some patients may benefit from 56 consecutive hours and recommends 12–20 hours per day for most patients. Vollman's (1997) 4–6 hours (drawn from literature review and substantial practice) is recommended until systematic evaluation provides more concrete guidelines.

Proning is labour-intensive. Turning takes 15–20 minutes and requires at least four nurses to turn the patient and one doctor to manage the airway

## Table 27.1 Complications of prone positioning

■ Pressure sores, especially on the thorax, head, iliac crest, breast and knee
■ Benefits do not last
■ Oesophageal reflux and vomiting
■ Safety of limbs
■ Extubation and line disconnection
■ Need for more sedation
■ Airway obstruction requiring suction
■ Facial and orbital oedema
■ Increased need for sedation and muscle relaxants
■ Transient desaturation
■ Hypotension
■ Dysrhythmias
■ Need for sufficient staff – up to 6
■ Difficult to resuscitate

(Tidswell, 2001). Sufficient staff should be gathered to move the patient safely, and position changes only once it has been clearly planned, with every member of the team clear about their role. Harcombe (2004) recommends

- pre-oxygenation before turning
- placing ECG electrodes on the back
- supporting genitalia on a pillow.

Limbs should be placed in a 'swimmer's' position.

L'Her *et al.* (2002) report development of pressure sores from proning, although Baktoft (2001) suggests proned patients developed fewer sores. During prone positioning the patient's head is at especial risk from prolonged pressure on a few areas, especially if saliva accumulates on pillows. Absorbent padding should be placed under the face to collect saliva (McCormick & Blackwood, 2001). Tidswell (2001) found abrasions frequently occurred. Prone positioning might also expose the eyes to direct pressure and trauma from pillows (see Chapter 11). Eyes should be taped or padded to prevent corneal abrasions (McCormick & Blackwood, 2001). Head positions may need to be changed more frequently than whole-body positions: MacDonald and Armstrong (2000) Harcombe (2004) recommend changing head position 2–3 hourly. Baktoft (2001) and Harcombe (2004) recommend repositioning limbs every two hours. Facial, periorbital and conjunctival oedema frequency collect (Breiburg *et al.*, 2000), but resolve once supine (Baktoft, 2001).

Ideally, resuscitation should be performed supine. As reversing the patient's position safely may cause a delay, compressions can be initiated in prone position. Once sufficient staff have gathered to safely turn the patient, prone positioning can then be reversed. Fortunately arrests in the prone position are very rare (MacDonald & Armstrong, 2000).

Kinetic therapy can mobilise bronchial secretions (Welch, 2002), reduce extravascular lung water (Bein *et al.*, 2000) and ventilator-associated pneumonia (Kennedy, 2004). Kinetic therapy needs to tilt at least 40° (Kennedy, 2004; Rance, 2005), and maybe 80–90° (McLean, 2001), for 18 hours/day (McLean, 2001; Kennedy, 2004). Problems of kinetic therapy include

- tachycardia
- hypotension
- desaturation
- diarrhoea
- discomfort and severe anxiety, necessitating sedation
- claustrophobia
- accommodating very large (in height or weight) patients
- wound dehiscence
- need for heavy sedation to tolerate the movement
- transportation (e.g. scanning).

(McLean, 2001; Welch, 2002; Kennedy, 2004)

## Reducing pulmonary hypertension

Intra-alveolar damage increases pulmonary vascular resistance, causing pulmonary hypertension. Systemic vasodilators, such as glyceryl trinitrate (GTN) may cause problematic hypotension, but nebulised prostacyclin, such as epoprostenol or phosphodiesterase inhibitors (Sildenafil), dilate pulmonary vessels without significant systemic hypotension. However, coagulopathies and frequent complicating ARDS may be aggravated by prostacyclin.

Shortage of both donor organs and centres performing lung transplants, and the rapid progression of ARDS, prevents lung transplantation from being a viable option.

## Inflammatory response

Limiting inflammatory responses should limit progression of the pathology. Steroids inhibit complement-induced leucocyte aggregation and reduce capillary permeability, so may reduce lung injury (Meduri *et al.*, 1998), but most studies fail to show any benefit from steroids (Artigas *et al.*, 1998; Brower *et al.*, 2001). Antioxidants (e.g. glutathione, selenium) may (Brandstetter *et al.*, 1997), or may not (Brower *et al.*, 2001) be useful. Ketoconazole has been used to inhibit thromboxane.

## Fluid management

Fluid management in ARDS necessitates balancing problems from pulmonary oedema against perfusion needs. Increased pulmonary permeability and pulmonary hypertension create excessive interstitial fluid (oedema); plasma albumin displaced into tissues creates an osmotic pull, accentuating tissue oedema and hypovolaemia. Fluid management therefore becomes a delicate balance of providing adequate total body hydration and intravascular volume for perfusion without increasing oedema. Myocardial dysfunction frequently occurs, compounding pulmonary (and systemic) hypovolaemia, so central venous pressure (see Chapter 20) becomes an inaccurate guide to ventricular filling. Measuring extravascular lung water (EVLW – see Chapter 20) has refined fluid management.

Intravascular volume being the likely main priority and colloids with long half-lifes (see Chapter 34) increase colloid osmotic pressure, improving perfusion and potentially reducing oedema. Early nutrition provides protein for endogenous albumin production, minimises muscle wasting and promotes immunity. Once commenced, nutrition should be adequate to meet metabolic needs (see Chapter 9).

## Psychological support

Recovery being prolonged, patients with ARDS may remain in ICU for weeks, exposing patients and family to prolonged anxiety and stress which may exhaust their coping mechanisms. Nurses can valuably offer care and support:

■ accommodation and facilities
■ enabling visiting whenever possible without causing sensory overload to patients or guilt to relatives
■ being approachable and available.

Prolonged stays can enable close rapport between families and staff, but can become stressful for both; both bedside nurses and nurse managers need to recognise distress. Families may seek hope where little exists, placing excessive trust/reliance/expectations on individual members of staff. As well as being a symptom of denial, this can be particularly stressful for staff.

One year after discharge most patients still suffer some residual cognitive impairment (Hopkins *et al.*, 1999), so patients and families should be warned about this.

## Cardiac management

Right ventricular workload will be increased by both pathology and treatments. Cardiac management is a careful balance, attempting to meet systemic oxygen demand without causing excessive cardiac workloads. Inotropes may be used to increase cardiac output, with vasodilators to reduce afterload (thereby increasing perfusion).

### Implications for practice

■ Ventilation is a delicate balance between optimising oxygenation and preventing further damage; nursing observations provide important information to guide medical management.
■ Prone position remains controversial, and can neither be completely recommended nor rejected, but if used, should be commenced early (during the oedematous stage of ARDS).
■ Flow monitoring, especially EVLW, may be needed to guide fluid management.
■ Fluid management should optimise perfusion while avoiding fluid overload; colloids, especially those exerting high colloid osmotic pressure, are especially useful.
■ Early and continuing nutrition promotes early recovery.
■ Prolonged stay and poor prognosis place psychological stressors on relatives and staff; these stressors should be acknowledged; interventions should support everyone through an especially stressful time.

## Summary

ARDS is the pulmonary manifestation of inflammatory responses. Like SIRS, it is largely a creation of the ICU's success. It causes many ICU admissions, and complicates progress of many more. Mortality remains high, and although some medical developments appear promising, panaceas remain elusive. The mainstay of treatment is system support. Prolonged ICU stay can place families, friends and nursing staff under considerable stress.

### Further reading

Much has been written on ARDS, mainly in medical journals. Evans *et al.* (2002) is a comprehensive and authoritative monograph on ARDS. Brower *et al.* (2001) provides a recent overview, as will most current textbooks. Artigas *et al.* (1998) identify controversies and areas for future research. Acute Respiratory Distress Syndrome Network (2000) discusses optimal ventilation. Breiburg *et al.* (2000) and Harcombe (2004) provide comprehensive reviews of prone positioning. Kennedy's (2004) research with kinetic therapy provides useful insights. www.routledge.com/textbooks/0415373239

For clinical scenarios, clinical questions and the answers to them go to the support website at www.routledge.com/textbooks/0415373239

### Clinical scenarios

Ann O'Reilly, a 45-year-old mother of six children who weighs 104 kg was admitted to hospital for elective ligation of fallopian tubes using fiberoptic surgery. Initially Mrs O'Reilly was making a good recovery on the ward, but on the fourth postoperative day she presented with severe shortness of breath, fever and abdominal pains. Investigations revealed perforated bowel. Ann became septic, developed ARDS and was transferred to the ICU for invasive ventilation and organ support.

In the ICU, pressure-controlled inverse ratio ventilation was commenced:
PEEP 10 cmH$_2$O
Pressure control 30 cmH$_2$O
FiO$_2$ of 0.8 (80% inspired oxygen)
Rate 16 per minute
Tidal volumes 600 ml
I:E ratio of 2:1

Arterial blood gases on these settings were:
pH            7.25
PaO$_2$        6.53 kPa
PaCO$_2$       8.47 kPa
HCO$_3^-$      16 mmol/litre
Base excess   $-5.8$ mmol/litre

Q.1  List the physiological processes, investigations and signs which led to Ann being diagnosed with ARDS.

Q.2 It is decided to place Ann in the prone position in an effort to improve her alveolar gas exchange. Analyse the rationale underpinning this approach and resources required to implement this in your own clinical area.

Q.3 Ann's gas exchange improves, allowing reduction in $FiO_2$ to 0.6 (60%). Appraise potential adverse effects of prone positioning with Ann and propose nursing strategies to minimise or prevent occurrence (e.g. abdominal wound healing, pressure areas, breast, eye, mouth care and psychological effect on Ann and her family).

Chapter 28

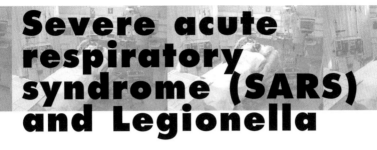

# Severe acute respiratory syndrome (SARS) and Legionella

## Contents

| | |
|---|---|
| Introduction | 298 |
| Severe acute respiratory syndrome | 298 |
| Legionnaire's disease | 301 |
| Implications for practice | 302 |
| Summary | 302 |
| Further reading | 303 |
| Clinical scenarios | 303 |

## Fundamental knowledge

Community acquired infections and their transmission
Pathology of pneumonia
Source isolation precautions

## Introduction

Sophisticated technology and treatments can now cure many diseases that were, until fairly recently, fatal. But emergence of new or mutated micro-organisms has challenged medical and ethical boundaries while attracting extensive, and often disproportionate, media attention. This chapter discusses two micro-organisms that have caused epidemics of severe community-acquired pneumonia in recent years: severe acute respiratory syndrome (SARS) and Legionnaire's disease.

Severe pneumonia usually necessitates intubation and artificial ventilation. Further management focuses largely on

1   identifying and treating micro-organisms
2   prevent further spread
3   supporting other failing systems.

However, diseases such as SARS and Legionnaire's often cause disproportionate fears among patients (if conscious), relatives and staff. This chapter is intended to help readers provide information to others.

Public fear of SARS has raised media reports and discussion of other problem 'new' infections, including avian influenza virus. Recent history suggests that further problem infections from cross-species and genetic mutations, especially viral, are likely to develop and spread rapidly. Experience from SARS suggests that any epidemic may necessitate sudden expansion of ICU facilities, supported by integrated communication of all services through a 'virtual war room' (Booth & Stewart, 2005), with information and support being provided to staff as well as visitors (Tolomiczenko et al., 2005).

## Severe acute respiratory syndrome

SARS is caused by a new virus of the coronaviridae family (SARS-CoV). Infection was first reported in China in November 2002, spreading so rapidly that by March 2003 the World Health Organisation issued a global alert. The main outbreaks occurred in Hong Kong and Canada, although by June 2003, infection had spread to 30 countries, infecting 8241 and killing 784 people (Fowler et al., 2003).

### Infection

Infection appears to be caused by close contact, especially through droplet spread (Ramsay & Gomersall, 2003), although other suspected possible means include water, clothing, hands, contaminated food and excreta (Zhong & Zeng, 2003).

The virus usually incubates in 2–7 days (Manocha et al., 2003), but can take up to two weeks (Lapinsky & Granton, 2004), causing epithelial and macrophages proliferation in the lungs (Nicholls *et al.*, 2003), and initiating a cytokine cascade. Extent of cytokine response determines severity of the disease (Nicholls *et al.*, 2003). Infection in children is relatively mild (Hon *et al.*, 2003), but older people are more often infected and more likely to die (Hon *et al.*, 2003).

## Symptoms

Initial symptoms are usually those of infective pyrexia, including chills and rigors (Ramsay & Gomersall, 2003). Within 24 hours temperature usually exceeds 38°C (Tsang & Lam, 2003).

Respiratory symptoms usually follow within 3–7 days (Tsang & Lam, 2003), including shortness of breath (Ramsay & Gomersall, 2003), and usually a non-productive cough (Tsang & Lam, 2003). Upper airway symptoms (rhinnorhoea, nasal obstruction, sneezing, sore throat, hoarseness) rarely occur (Tsang & Lam, 2003).

Other reported symptoms include malaise and diarrhoea (Peiris *et al.*, 2003; Ramsay & Gomersall, 2003).

About one-quarter of cases progress to severe respiratory failure (Fowler *et al.*, 2003; Lew *et al.*, 2003). Of these, half will need invasive ventilation (Ramsay & Gomersall, 2003), about half of whom are currently likely to die (Ramsay & Gomersall, 2003), although future medical progress might reduce mortality.

## Diagnosis

Chest X-ray typically shows unilateral and (mainly) peripheral consolidation (Lee *et al.*, 2003), with patchy infiltrates progressing from basal regions to much of the lungs (Ramsay & Gomersall, 2003). Pneumonia is visible on X-ray in 7–10 days and most patients develop lymphopaenia (CDC, 2002). Computerised tomography (CT) of lungs shows 'ground glass' appearance, with patchy peripheral consolidation (Ramsay & Gomersall, 2003). Blood creatine kinase (CK) and lactate dehydrogenase (LDH) are raised (Ramsay & Gomersall, 2003), although few UK hospitals have facilities for testing LDH. White cell count (WCC) and platelets may be low or normal (Ramsay & Gomersall, 2003). Specimens for antibody SARS-CoV tests include:

- nasal and throat swabs
- sputum
- blood
- stools (minimum 10 ml).

Specimens should also be tested for the respiratory pathogens influenza A and B and respiratory syncytial virus. Pleural effusions rarely occur (Ramsay & Gomersall, 2003).

### Prevention

Rapid spread of an initially unidentified infection exposed people to infection, especially close contacts of the original families (Manocha *et al.*, 2003), people in the hospital (Booth *et al.*, 2003) and healthcare workers (Manocha *et al.*, 2003; Lapinsky & Granton, 2004), necessitating emphasis on protecting those in contact with patients.

As SARS is spread through droplets, risk of spread is increased with coughing and sputum clearance, so nebulisers, high-flow/venturi (fixed performance) oxygen masks, noninvasive ventilation, bronchoscopy and other high-risk procedures should be avoided if possible (Li *et al.*, 2003; Manocha *et al.*, 2003; Ramsay & Gomersall, 2003).

Other patients, staff and visitors should be protected by source isolation, including:

- isolation rooms, preferable with negative pressure
- if patients are not intubated, staff and visitors should wear high-efficiency masks, such as the N-95 respirator, to prevent air-droplet and airborne acquisition (File & Tsang, 2005)
- contact precautions, including hat, long-sleeved fluid-repellent waterproof double gown, gloves, hat and overshoes
- non-reusable goggles or face shield.

As soon as SARS, or any other highly contagious infection, is suspected, patients should be transferred into source isolation precautions.

Infection control specialists should be actively involved, and can advise on whether equipment is appropriate. With better knowledge of the disease, future epidemics may be contained more effectively.

### Treatment

Drug regimes typically include

- antibiotics to cover standard community-acquired pneumonia (Ramsay & Gomersall, 2003)
- ribavirin (Manocha *et al.*, 2003; Ramsay & Gomersall, 2003)
- steroids – 1 mg/kg/day prednisolone (Ramsay & Gomersall, 2003)
- immunoglobulin (Ramsay & Gomersall, 2003)
- convalescent serum from recovering patients (Ramsay & Gomersall, 2003).

Plasmapheresis may remove cytokines and other mediators (Ramsay & Gomersall, 2003) (see Chapter 40).

Because SARS is such a new disease, future progress is likely to be initially rapid and significant, so management and treatment of future outbreaks may differ.

**Outcome**

Worldwide, one in 10 cases die (Manocha *et al.*, 2003; Zhong & Zeng, 2003), although mortality in the Canadian outbreaks was one in 20 (Booth *et al.*, 2003). However, ICU mortality was one in three (Manocha *et al.*, 2003). Most deaths occured among older people (Donnelly *et al.*, 2003; Ramsay & Gomersall, 2003).

Although it is too early to know the long-term effects of SARS, follow-up of patients has already identified psychological problems and avascular necrosis of large joints (Chan & Ng, 2005).

# Legionnaire's disease

*Legionella pneumophilia* is usually a community-acquired infection that can cause atypical pneumonia. Infection was first identified in 1976, among delegates to the American Legion convention at a Philadelphia hotel, and has since been responsible for sporadic outbreaks worldwide. Each year approximately 300 cases of Legionella infection are diagnosed in the UK (Harper, 2004), causing about 3 per cent of UK hospital admissions for community-acquired pneumonia (Lim *et al.*, 2001), but it is one of the main causes of severe community-acquired pneumonia necessitating ICU admission (the others being *Streptococcus pneumoniae*, *Haemophilus influenzae*, and Gram-negative enteric rods) (de Castro & Torres, 2003; Blasi, 2004).

Being a waterborne organism, many infections are caused through breathing in aerosol droplets from water-cooling towers (Brown *et al.*, 1999). Some outbreaks outside the UK have been spread from hospital water supplies (Stout & Yu, 2003). In the UK 15 per cent of infections occur within hospitals (Harper, 2004). Being a weak pathogen, immunocompromised and older people are at greatest risk (Gould, 2003), although it can infect previously healthy people.

Atypical pneumonia means that lower respiratory tract infections do not cause lobar consolidation (Hindiyeh & Carroll, 2000). If atypical pneumonia is identified, proximity to infected water, or foreign travel could indicate *Legionella* infection. Most centres can test urine for Legionella, and blood cultures should be sent. Testing for *Legionella* should be specified, as few laboratories otherwise test for it. Empiric antibiotics should be commenced – erythromycin or (increasingly) azithromycin are usually used, but clarithromycin cefuroxime, rifampicin, co-trimoxazole, tetracycline, or doxycycline are also useful, especially in combination.

Severe pneumonia often causes sepsis, SIRS and multi-system failure, so following identification and antibiotic therapy, treatment focuses on system support, especially artificial ventilation. Microbiology services should be urgently involved, both for advice and to report and follow-up contacts. Overall mortality from Legionella ranges between 10–15 per cent (Gould, 2003), but due to increased severity of both infection and complication, one-third of patients with Legionella admitted to the ICU will die (Gacouin *et al.*, 2002).

Risks of spread through hospital water supplies have encouraged development of products such as disposable shower heads and water filters.

## Implications for practice

- Respiratory infections are usually spread by droplet infection.
- Preventing spread of any infection is important, but where knowledge of how to cure micro-organisms, such as the SARS coronavirus, is limited, isolation to protect others is usually necessary, preferably in rooms with negative airflow systems.
- Staff exposed to SARS Co-V patients should have disposable protective equipment against droplet and contact infection (gloves, dust mist particulate, masks, goggles, long-sleeved water-repellent double gowns, hat and overshoes).
- With SARS Co-V, open respiratory treatments, such as noninvasive ventilation, nebulisers, or high-flow oxygen masks should, where possible, be avoided.
- Patients with atypical pneumonia needing ICU admission should have urine tested for *Legionella* and *pneumococcal urinary antigen*; request forms should specifically state these tests, as they are not routinely tested by most laboratories.
- Hospital water supplies can spread *Legionella* infection, so Estates Departments should be contacted if there is any concern.
- Risk of transmission to staff is high, so Infection Control and Occupational Health departments should be involved to provide advice and monitoring.

## Summary

Legionnaire's disease and SARS are two recent, and often fatal, respiratory infections that appear to disproportionately affect older and immunocompromised people. Initial limited knowledge of how to treat SARS Co-V, together with public fear, encouraged emphasis on the containing spread. While containment is important for any potentially fatal respiratory infection, history of treating AIDS victims suggests that progress in medical knowledge and treatment will enable more proactive, patient-centred approaches in future. Many of the current approaches to SARS described in this chapter may be superseded in the fairly near future. However, like the HIV virus, possible viral mutation also makes the continuing effectiveness of current, or future, treatments unpredictable.

Legionella is a relatively rare cause of community acquired pneumonia, but is one of the four most frequent community-acquired pneumonias necessitating ICU admission.

## Further reading

The Canadian and Hong Kong SARS outbreaks prompted many medical case reports and reviews, including Booth *et al.* (2003), Fowler *et al.* (2003), Manocha *et al.* (2003), Nicholls *et al.* (2003), Tsang and Lam (2003) and Zhong and Zeng (2003). Few nursing articles have appeared on SARS, Marthaler *et al.* (2003) being one of the few.

Stout and Yu (1997) is a thorough medical review of Legionnaire's disease, while Gould (2003) offers nursing perspectives. www.routledge.com/textbooks/ 0415373239

For clinical scenarios, clinical questions and the answers to them go to the support website at www.routledge.com/textbooks/0415373239

## Clinical scenarios

Mr Bishop is a 43-year-old gentleman who works as an air conditioner maintenance engineer. He recently returned from a month-long holiday abroad and has since developed a fever and respiratory infection. He was admitted to the ICU for respiratory support with a diagnosis of atypical pneumonia and *Legionnella pneumophilia* or SARS-CoV as the suspected causative organism.

Q.1 Identify investigations, tests and other sources of information which could confirm Mr Bishop's diagnosis. State which specimens should be collected, their frequency and type of test used to detect suspected infection.

Q.2 Mr Bishop needs to be transferred to a suitable unit equipped with protective isolation rooms and correct ventilation air flow. Review the resources and procedures required in order to contain causative organism, avoid contamination of others, particularly health care workers. Consider which corridors and lifts should be used and how the route through the hospitals to and from the transfer ambulance will be kept clear of people. Outline the decontamination strategy for ambulance and transfer personnel.

Q.3 Review national and local hospital guidance on managing a patient who has suspected or confirmed SARS-CoV. Note the location and geography of negative pressure isolation rooms with critical care facilities, infection control policies for containment and screening of SARS-CoV. Specify types of protection clothing, masks, education and skills required for health care staff and visitors, reporting outbreaks, cleaning regimes and decontamination strategies.

Chapter 29

# Alternative ventilatory modes

## Contents

Introduction                                           305
ECMO                                                   305
ECMO variants                                          306
High frequency ventilation                             306
High frequency oscillatory ventilation
    (HFOV)                                             307
High frequency percussive ventilation   308
High frequency jet ventilation          308
Liquid ventilation                                     308
Hyperbaric oxygen                                      309
Implications for practice                              310
Summary                                                311
Further reading                                        311
Clinical scenarios                                     311

## Fundamental knowledge

Alveolar physiology, gas exchange and pulmonary function
Surfactant production and physiology
V/Q mismatch

304

## Introduction

Conventional ventilators remain the mainstay of ICU respiratory support, but there are some significantly different methods of ventilation which are occasionally used, usually as 'rescue therapies' when disease (usually ARDS) deteriorates despite optimal conventional ventilation. Modes discussed in this chapter are

- extracorporeal membrane oxygenators (ECMO)
- extracorporeal carbon dioxide removal (ECCO$_2$R)
- intravenous oxygenators (IVOX)
- high frequency ventilation (HFV), especially oscillatory (HFOV) and jet (HFJV)
- liquid ventilation (perfluorocarbon – *PFC*)
- hyperbaric oxygenation

although availability is often confined to specialist units.
   Alveolar recovery is optimised if

- inflated sufficiently to prevent further atelectasis
- movement is minimised (low tidal volumes, to minimise volutrauma)
- overdistension (high peak inflation pressures – barotrauma) is avoided.

Many modes discussed here achieve these aims, assisting alveolar recovery.
   Some modes are neither new nor established. Evidence on these is often sparse and dated, usually reflecting paediatric practice.
   Most modes provide comparable oxygenation to conventional modes, but may provide lung protection. Many achieve better carbon dioxide clearance than conventional ventilation, so reducing respiratory drive. This may enable reduction of sedatives, and so side-effects. Hypocapnia may cause respiratory alkalosis (see Chapter 18).

## ECMO

Extracorporeal membrane oxygenation (ECMO), initially developed as 'bypass' for open-heart surgery (see Chapter 31), can replace or augment conventional ventilation.
   Neonatal survival with ECMO support remains consistently high – 88 per cent (Bartlett *et al.*, 2000). Older children fare less well – 70 per cent (Bartlett *et al.*, 2000). Adults generally fare worst – 56 per cent, and lower with cardiac failure (Bartlett *et al.*, 2000), although Hemmila *et al.* (2004) found ECMO improved survival from ARDS.
   Like haemofiltration, ECMO pumps blood extracorporeally through a semipermeable membrane, usually at 70–120 ml/kg/minute (Caron & Berlandi, 1997). Circuits can be venoarterial (V-A) or venovenous (V-V). Venoarterial circuits (usually from right jugular vein to right common carotid artery) expose

the patient to greater risk from fatal emboli, so are rarely used with adults. Venovenous (usually right internal jugular vein to femoral vein) are usually used for adults (Bartlett *et al.*, 2000), but require adequate cardiac function, so venoarterial circuits may be used if patients have cardiac failure (Bartlett *et al.*, 2000).

Conventional lung ventilation using low rate and volumes is usually maintained during ECMO to prevent atelectasis.

*Complications* of ECMO include

- *respiratory alkalosis*: supplementary carbon dioxide (e.g. carbogen – 5 per cent carbon dioxide, 95 per cent oxygen) may be needed (Caron & Berlandi, 1997)
- *coagulopathies/DIC*: circuits cause physical trauma to platelets (as with haemofiltration), compounding problems from anticoagulants and underlying pathologies; platelet and erythrocyte damage is reduced with transmembrane pressures below 300 mmHg (Caron & Berlandi, 1997)
- *cost*: from equipment, staff and extending life (or death) of very sick patients. Firmin and Killer (1999) suggest that 80 per cent of patient workload is from attending to circuits, compared to 20 per cent on nursing care of patients.

## ECMO variants

Extracorporeal Carbon Dioxide Removal ($ECCO_2R$) uses modified ECMO with low blood flow (20–30 per cent of cardiac output) to remove carbon dioxide. Supplementary oxygen will be needed, but $ECCO_2R$ allows significant reduction in mechanical ventilation (Conrad *et al.*, 2001). $ECCO_2R$ and ECMO have similar complications, although $ECCO_2R$ is less invasive.

Intravenous oxygenators (IVOX) resemble miniature ECMO membranes, inserted percutaneously. Pure oxygen is passed through the fibres, which provides supplementary (not complete) oxygenation. Carbon dioxide removal is more efficient. IVOX shares most complications of ECMO. Additional complications include

- *internal placement* which makes monitoring, adjustment and control more difficult than ECMO
- *thrombus formation*
- *oxygen toxicity*: although not reported in literature, prolonged exposure of endothelial cells to pure oxygen with IVOX presumably causes the same complications as pure oxygen from conventional ventilation (see Chapter 18).

## High frequency ventilation

High frequency ventilation (HFV) includes various infrequently used modes, which have largely failed to establish a place in practice. Frequent but small tidal volumes prevent alveoli closure, so may prevent ventilator-associated lung injury (Carney *et al.*, 2005). High frequency jet ventilation (HFJV) and high frequency oscillatory ventilation (HFOV) are used in some ICUs.

Complications of most high frequency modes include

- *safety*: chest wall movement and air entry are barely perceptible and spirometry is impractical, and some ventilators have few alarms. Blood gas analysis and pulse oximetry are among the few remaining means of monitoring
- *variable tidal/minute volumes* are difficult to measure (Krishnan & Brower, 2000)
- *gas trapping/shunting*
- *peak intra-alveolar pressures* are higher than measurable peak airway pressure. Excessive pressure may impair perfusion, so increasing mean airway pressure may exacerbate V/Q mismatch
- *humidification*: early problems have largely been overcome by pump-controlled instillation of fluid (Pierce, 1995) and specialised humidifiers (e.g. high temperature vaporizers (ACCP, 1993)). However, nurses should actively assess effectiveness of humidification, reporting and recording problems.
- *noise* like CPAP, high frequency modes are usually noisy, provoking stress responses, inhibiting sleep and contributing to sensory overload
- *limited evidence*.

## High frequency oscillatory ventilation (HFOV)

Adding oscillation (5–10 Hz) to modified CPAP circuits or near-conventional ventilators achieves a form of high frequency ventilation that can significantly reduce mortality from ARDS (Derak *et al.*, 2002; David *et al.*, 2003). Oscillation of alveolar air creates an active expiratory phase, reducing gas-trapping and improving carbon dioxide clearance. Carbon dioxide clearance can be increased either by increasing the power of the diaphragm or reducing the frequency. CPAP recruits alveoli and improves oxygenation. Both CPAP and fast respiratory rates (150–600 breaths each minute) keep alveoli open.

Usually a rescue therapy, FiO$_2$ is usually commenced at 1.0, with mean peak airway pressure slightly above the patient's previous setting (usually 3 cmH$_2$O) (Macintosh & Britto, 2000). As with other high frequency modes, tidal volumes are small (10–15 ml), so only slight chest and abdominal wall movement ('wiggle') is seen. Amplitude of oscillation (delta P, $\Delta$P) is increased until this movement reaches the groin or upper thighs (usual adult frequency 3–8 Hz). Mean pressure and oxygen are titrated down as oxygenation allows. Carbon dioxide removal can be increased by increasing amplitude, decreasing frequency, or creating a cuff leak – usually 5–7 cmH$_2$O (Higgins *et al.*, 2005).

Lungs should be auscultated, but low tidal volumes prevent clear air entry sounds. 'Wiggle' should be monitored – change indicating altered lung compliance or airway resistance. Suction causes alveolar deflation, and possible atelectasis, so should only be performed if specifically indicated, and if possible avoided completely for the first 12 hours. On chest X-rays at most eight pairs of ribs should be visible; if more appear, lungs are overdistended.

307

Neonatal use has demonstrated alveolar recruitment and maximisation of alveolar lung volume (Bouchut *et al.*, 2004). It may increase risk of intraventricular haemorrhage (Keogh & Cordingley, 2002), although Bouchut *et al.* (2004) found no difference in cardiac output, organ perfusion, central venous pressure or cerebral perfusion between HFOV and conventional ventilation.

Fort *et al.*'s (1997) preliminary study with ARDS patients found HFOV achieved higher mean airway pressures (improved gas exchange) with lower peak pressure (less barotrauma) and reduced (potentially toxic) oxygen levels than conventional ventilators.

## High frequency percussive ventilation

This mode delivers 200–900 pneumatic percussive beats/minute superimposed on traditional large tidal volumes (Hynes-Gay & MacDonald, 2001) to mobilise secretions (Velmahos *et al.*, 1999). Alternating traditional ventilation between high frequency breaths releases pressure, and so limits complications from breath stacking (Velmahos *et al.*, 1999). To allow air to escape, the ETT cuff is partially deflated (Velmahos *et al.*, 1999).

## High frequency jet ventilation

HFJV (or 'jet') uses tidal volumes of 1–5 ml/kg – with most adults, approximately the same volume as physiological deadspace. Small tidal volumes may reduce lung injury, especially if patients have bronchopleural fistulae (Krishnan & Brower, 2000). Rates of 100–300 are usually used (Keogh & Cordingley, 2002). HFJV can be delivered through minitracheostomy (Allison, 1994), preventing many complications of intubation.

Carbon dioxide clearance is efficient. Pulmonary secretions are mobilised, presumably due to constant chest wall 'quivering' resembling physiotherapy, so increasing alveolar surface area and gas exchange. However, there is insufficient evidence of benefits for most units to justify costs of buying equipment and training staff for the small number of patients who might benefit (Krishnan & Brower, 2000).

## Liquid ventilation

Liquid ventilation with perfluorocarbon (PFC) is now being used in some adult ICUs to treat ARDS. Perflurocarbons are very efficient oxygen carriers, dissolving 17 times more oxygen than water (Brower *et al.*, 2001). Up to 50 ml of oxygen can be dissolved in every 100 ml of perfluorocarbon (Greenough, 1996) (plasma carries 3 ml per 100 ml). Unlike haemoglobin, perflurocarbons do not bind oxygen; so more oxygen is delivered across the fluid-filled airways (Remy *et al.*, 1999). Carbon dioxide, which is more soluble than oxygen, is four times more soluble in perfluorocarbon than in water (Greenough, 1996). Perfluorocarbon is also anti-inflammatory, improving macrophage responses and creating fewer oxygen free radicals (Lange *et al.*, 2000; Haitsma & Lachmann, 2002).

Partial liquid ventilation can be achieved using conventional ventilators, although perfluorocarbon lost through evaporation should be replaced. Pressure-controlled ventilation should be used to prevent over-distension (Haitsma & Lachmann, 2002).

Whether ventilation is partial or complete, perfluorocarbon (heavier than water) should be trickled down to fill dependent alveoli, preventing alveolar collapse (Dirkes *et al.*, 1996) – 'liquid PEEP'. Each day, after endotracheal suction, fresh perfluorocarbon is instilled over a couple of hours, until a meniscus is seen within the endotracheal tube (Kallas, 1998). During instillation, patients should lie supine and be ventilated with pure oxygen (Kallas, 1998). Once instilled, liquid maintains patency of alveoli, but with partial liquid ventilation the meniscus should be checked hourly and topped up to prevent atelectasis reforming (Schlicher, 2001; Haitsma & Lachmann, 2002). Because the lower airways are filled with liquid rather than air, breath sounds will change to fine rales and rhonchi and bubbling may be heard; if these sounds are not present, a pneumothorax has probably occurred (Schlicher, 2001).

Mucus, sputum and other lung fluids are lighter than perfluorocarbon, so should float to the surface where they can be removed. As this is most likely to occur soon after instillation, debris needs frequent removal during the first few hours (Schlicher, 2001). Mucous plugs can be formed, probably caused by mobilising mucous from distal to proximal areas of the lungs (Haitsma & Lachmann, 2002). A sudden fall in oxygen saturation indicates airway obstruction from sputum plugs (Schlicher, 2001). Following suction, perfluorocarbon fluid level should be topped up and volume instilled recorded. Secretions and fluid removed should be measured and recorded.

*Complications* of liquid ventilation include

■ *long-term effects unknown*: monkeys killed three years after one hour's treatment had analysable amounts of perfluorocarbon in lung and fat tissue (Greenough, 1996). Perfluorocarbon appears to be inert (Remy *et al.*, 1999), but animal studies do not always reflect human experience
■ *pneumothorax* is more likely to occur (Haitsma & Lachmann, 2002)
■ *increased intrathoracic pressure*: instilling intrathoracic fluid should logically increase intrathoracic pressure and reduce cardiac output, but this does not seem to occur
■ *increased pulmonary vascular resistance* (Greenough, 1996).

## Hyperbaric oxygen

Ratios between gases in air remain constant; if temperature remains constant, water content (volume) of humidified air also remains constant. So changes in atmospheric pressure alter the volume of each gas that can be dissolved in plasma. At sea-level atmospheric pressure (approximately one bar) only small volumes of oxygen are dissolved in plasma (3 ml oxygen per 100 ml blood). If haemoglobin carriage is prevented (e.g. carbon monoxide poisoning) tissues rely on plasma carriage.

Twenty-one per cent oxygen at 2.8 bar (= 18 metres depth of water) increases oxygen pressure from 21 to 284 kPa, providing sufficient plasma carriage to meet normal metabolism (Pitkin *et al.*, 1997). Hyperbaric oxygen of 3 bar reduces half-life of carbon monoxide from 320 minutes in room air and 74 minutes with 100 per cent oxygen to 23 minutes (Blumenthal, 2001).

Hyperbaric chambers can be *single patient* or *rooms* into which staff and equipment can enter. Hyperbaric pressure can be discontinued once haemoglobin oxygen carriage is available (at most, usually a few hours).

*Complications* of hyperbaric oxygen include

- *evidence*: is largely limited to enthusiastic anecdotes rather than controlled trials
- *high atmospheric pressures*: causes barotrauma to ears, sinuses and lungs, tonic-clonic seizures and impairs vision (Oh, 2003)
- *monitoring*: oxygen not being carried by haemoglobin, pulse oximetry values has no value
- *infusions*: pressure may cause pump inaccuracy (Dohgomori *et al.*, 2002), and tubing should be pressure-resistant (Bailey *et al.*, 2004)
- *access*: single-person chambers may prevent equipment (including ventilators) being used, while transfer of equipment (e.g. emergency equipment) between normal and hyperbaric pressures may be restricted or delayed. This may affect: ventilation, inotropes and other infusions/mechanical support
- *scarcity*: few units have hyperbaric chambers, necessitating long-distance transfer of hypoxic patients.

Hyperbaric oxygen may provide support, enabling short-term survival; however it does not reduce the incidence of neurological complications following carbon monoxide poisoning (Scheinkestel *et al.*, 1999).

## Implications for practice

- Modes discussed in this chapter are rarely seen outside specialist units; where used, staff should take every opportunity to become familiar with their use.
- These modes are usually 'rescue therapies', so individual complications of each mode are compounded by complications of severe pathophysiologies; nursing care should be actively planned to optimise safety for each patient.
- Visitors and patients may be anxious about use of rarer modes, or frightened by particular aspects (e.g. liquid ventilation = 'drowning'), so should be reassured.
- Monitoring facilities are often limited with unconventional modes, so nurses should optimise remaining facilities (e.g. pulse oximetry, blood gases), which may need to be measured more frequently.
- Highly invasive modes (e.g. ECMO) may cause haemorrhage; cannulae should (where possible) be easily visible.
- Sensory disruption from noise should be minimized.

## Summary

Modes discussed in this chapter are rarely used, but may offer significant benefits to some patients. ICUs not using these modes may transfer patients to units which do. This chapter provides an introduction to these modes for staff unfamiliar with them or new to units where they are used. More experienced users will wish to pursue supplementary material.

Whenever rarer modes/treatments are used the potential for unidentified complications is increased. Therefore the decision to use (or suggest) alternatives modes should be tempered by considerations of patient safety:

- How will the patient benefit?
- What are the known complications?
- What is the likely risk from unidentified complications (research base)?
- Do staff on the unit have the competence to use the mode safely?

Where unusual equipment is used, staff should take every reasonable opportunity to become familiar with it, but remember the focus of nursing should be the patient, not the machine.

## Further reading

Most clinical literature on these modes is found in medical journals. There is often little recent literature on modes that are neither new nor established, but as equipment may have evolved little, older literature remains largely valid. Kallas (1998) discusses various modes. Bartlett *et al.* (2000) review ECMO, while Derak *et al.* (2002) review HFOV. Bailey *et al.* (2004) summarises hyperbaric oxygen therapy. Haitsma and Lachmann's (2002) chapter discusses liquid ventilation. www.routledge.com/textbooks/0415373239

For clinical scenarios, clinical questions and the answers to them go to the support website at www.routledge.com/textbooks/0415373239

## Clinical scenarios

Mrs Margaret Sheppard is a 60-year-old known asthmatic who was admitted to a respiratory ward with community-acquired pneumonia. Her respiratory function continued to deteriorate over nine days. She was then admitted to ICU with a diagnosis of ARDS, intubated and commenced on High Frequency Oscillatory Ventilation (HFOV) to assist her breathing. The HFOV parameters were set as:

| | |
|---|---|
| mPaw (Mean Airway Pressure) | 35.3 cmH$_2$O |
| FiO$_2$ | 1.0 (100% O$_2$) |
| Bias flow | 20 litres/minute |

Frequency                          5.0 Hz
Amplitude (Delta P)                82 cmH$_2$O
Inspiratory time                   30%

Q.1  Explain the functions and settings used, and identify other respiratory observations/assessments required to be performed with patients receiving HFOV.

Q.2  Mrs Sheppard becomes increasingly hypercarbic (rising PaCO$_2$). Explain what parameters should be adjusted and the mechanism to reduce her CO$_2$ level.

Q.3  If the oscillator piston stops functioning, what actions should be taken? List the emergency equipment needed.

Q.4  Analyse potential complications of HFOV and strategies used to minimise these.

Q.5  Consider the criteria used to wean Mrs Sheppard and when the HFOV should be discontinued or changed to conventional ventilation.

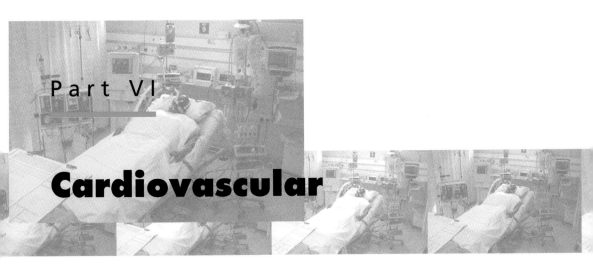

# Part VI

# Cardiovascular

# Chapter 30

# Acute coronary syndromes

## Contents

| | |
|---|---|
| Introduction | 316 |
| Myocardial oxygen supply | 317 |
| Atherosclerosis | 317 |
| Pathology | 318 |
| Cardiac markers | 319 |
| Treatments | 319 |
| Thrombolysis | 321 |
| NSTEMI | 322 |
| Other drugs | 322 |
| Percutaneous repair | 323 |
| Angiogenesis | 323 |
| Rest | 323 |
| Psychological stress | 323 |
| Prognosis | 324 |
| Health promotion | 324 |
| Implications for practice | 324 |
| Summary | 325 |
| Further reading | 325 |
| Clinical scenarios | 325 |

## Fundamental knowledge

Coronary arteries – structure and location
Coagulation cascade + thromboxane $A_2$
Renin-angiotensin mechanism

## Introduction

Heart disease remains the leading cause of death in Western industrialised societies, with UK mortality remaining among the highest in the world (DOH, 1999), so the Department of Health (DOH 2000c) issued aggressive targets of

- call to needle time 60 minutes
- door to needle time 20 minutes (since April 2003)

for people suffering from myocardial infarction.

Often confusing and conflicting classification of myocardial infarction has been simplified by the classification of *Acute Coronary Syndromes*.

*STEMI*:

- ST elevation (+/− Q waves) in two or more consecutive leads (1 mm in chest leads, 2 mm in limb leads)
- new bundle branch block
- troponin positive

*NSTEMI*:
The ECG may be normal or show various abnormalities, such as

- transient or aborted ST elevation
- ST depression
- T wave inversion

but troponin is positive.

*Unstable angina*
Various ECG abnormalities may occur, but

- ST depression (0.5 mm below isoelectric line)
- transient ST elevation
- T wave inversion

commonly occur. Troponin is negative. Patients are however at risk of infracting and developing cardiogenic shock.

Patients with uncomplicated infarctions are unlikely to be admitted to ICU, but infarction may occur in patients already on the unit, or additional complications, such as renal failure, may necessitate admission. This chapter identifies underlying pathophysiology and treatments (especially thrombolysis).

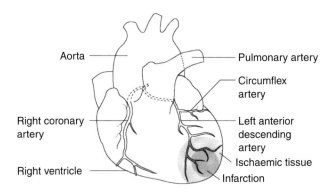

**Figure 30.1** **Coronary arteries, with inferior myocardial infarction**

## Myocardial oxygen supply

Five per cent of cardiac output enters the two coronary arteries (*right* and *left*) from the aorta. The left artery divides into the *left anterior descending* and *circumflex*. At rest, myocardium normally extracts nearly all available oxygen, and as myocytes rely on aerobic respiration, leaving little reserve for oxygen debt.

When myocardial oxygen demand exceeds supply, ischaemia results. Ischaemia is transient; if reversed (reducing oxygen demand, increasing oxygen supply, or both), the myocardium recovers; unreversed ischaemia progresses to irreversible cell damage and death.

Coronary artery disease often begins in childhood, and steadily progresses through life (Nissen, 2002). Symptoms (angina) usually only occur once coronary arteries are three quarters occluded. This leaves little physiological reserve between the onset of symptoms and ischaemic tissue death. Symptoms, such as angina, often precede infarction by less than 30 minutes, and one-fifth of infarctions are 'silent' – not preceded by any warning. Survivors often suffer residual cardiac disease.

## Atherosclerosis

Lipids, especially cholesterol and low density lipoproteins, and calcium penetrate tunica intima, forming a thickening of the tunica intima (Woolf, 2000) and plaque. This provokes an inflammatory reaction, macrophages infiltrating and enlarging the necrotic core (Klodgie *et al.*, 2003). Damage to the tunica intima and the inflammatory response releases vasoactive chemicals, including cytokines (Boersma *et al.*, 2003) and triggers of clotting such as platelet activating factor.

317

C-reactive protein (CRP – see Chapter 21) is an acute phase protein released with systemic inflammation. Although released with many other conditions, CRP is often measured to confirm suspected acute coronary syndromes (Ridker *et al.*, 2001; Kemp *et al.*, 2004).

## Pathology

Contraction ceases before ischaemic muscle dies, so there is a vital interval between cardiac arrest and myocardial death when interventions have a reasonable chance of success.

Antman *et al.*'s (2000) risk scoring system to guide use of thrombolysis in myocardial infartion (TIMI; see Table 30.1) has been used to monitor cardiac care. The score identifies seven risk factors:

- age 65 or older
- at least 3 factors for CAD
- prior coronary artery stenosis of 50 per cent or more
- at least two episodes of angina in the last 24 hours
- use of aspirin in the last seven days
- elevated serum cardiac markers.

Mortality increases with the number of risk factors present:

Although mild drinking appears to be cardio-protective (Lorgeril *et al.*, 2002), heavy drinking causes atherosclerosis. Maximum benefit is gained from limiting alcohol to 1 unit/day (women) or 2 units/day (men) (Riley, 2002). Alcohol consumption may be under-reported, so nurses can usefully provide patients/families with information to discourage excessive consumption.

Circadian rhythm causes blood to become thicker, platelets more active and fibrinolytic activity to decline during the morning (Tanaka *et al.*, 2004). This makes plaque rupture and myocardial infarction more likely to occur during the morning, especially during winter (Arntz *et al.*, 2000; Soo *et al.*, 2000; Tanaka *et al.*, 2004). Vigorous early morning stimulation (such as early bed-baths) is best avoided with all at-risk patients.

### Table 30.1 TIMI risk score (Antman *et al.*, 2000)

| Number of risk factors | Mortality risk (%) |
| --- | --- |
| 0/1 | 4.7 |
| 2 | 8.3 |
| 3 | 13.2 |
| 4 | 19.9 |
| 5 | 26.2 |
| 6/7 | 40.9 |

## Cardiac markers

Injured cells release chemicals. Identifying and measuring these chemicals enables diagnosis of cell damage. The most useful chemical markers to identify mark cardiac damage are troponin (T or I) and myoglobin, although creatine kinase (CK) and its isoenzymes are sometimes still measured.

*Troponin* is found in striated muscle (Kucher & Goldhaber, 2003). There are three types of troponin: C, I and T. Troponin I and T can be detected in blood with 4–6 hours of infarction (Albarran, 1998) and, being protein-bound may be detected up to 14 days following infarction (Jowett & Thompson, 2003). Troponin is the recommended test for suspected myocardial infarction (Joint European Society of Cardiology/American College of Cardiology Committee, 2000). Negative results may occur if infarction is less than 4–6 hours old, so with negative results troponin should be retested 12 hours after the time of suspected infarction (not the time of the first test), as troponin will by then be present if infarction has occurred. There is currently no accepted normal range for troponin (Dawson & Edbrooke, 2000), and range depends on individual assays, but levels exceeding 0.1 microgram/litre usually indicate infarction, higher levels indicating greater damage. Troponin levels can therefore be used to identify low, medium and high risk.

Mild rises in blood troponin may be caused by pulmonary embolism (Douketis *et al.*, 2002; Kucher & Goldhaber, 2003), pericarditis (Bonnefoy *et al.*, 2000), renal failure (Aviles *et al.*, 2002) and any other damage to myocardium.

*Myoglobin* (see Chapter 39) is released following muscle damage, including myocardial infarction. Normal serum myoglobin is below 85 nanograms/millilitre, but serum levels rise significantly within 30–60 minutes following myocardial infarction (Williams *et al.*, 2005).

*Creatine kinase* levels rise quickly following a myocardial infarction, peaking in about 24 hours, but returning to normal within 2–4 days. CK is also released from brain and skeletal muscle. Release of creatine kinase by other muscles can mislead diagnosis, so CK measurement is no longer recommended (Joint European Society of Cardiology/American College of Cardiology Committee, 2000). It remains useful for the 4–14 day interval after infarction where troponin would remain elevated and a second infarction is suspected (Kemp *et al.*, 2004).

CK has three isoenzymes, which can differentiate the source of serum CK: MM (skeletal muscle), MB (heart), BB (brain). With availability of troponin tests, most laboratories no longer test isoenzymes.

## Treatments

Immediate treatment for myocardial infarction follows the mnemonic MONA:

- Morphine
- Oxygen (high concentration)

- Nitroglycerine (GTN; isoket™)
- Aspirin (300 mg).

(Tough, 2004)

Subsequent treatments also discussed include

- thrombolysis
- other drugs
- percutaneous coronary interventions
- percutaenous coronary angioplasty
- angiogenesis.

Cardiac surgery is discussed in Chapter 31.

### Morphine

Ischaemic myocardium, like other muscle, causes cramp (angina). Pain stimulates the sympathetic nervous system, causing coronary vasoconstriction and further ischaemia. Infarction causes severe 'crushing' pain (Tough, 2004). Prompt and powerful analgesia is both a humanitarian and physiological necessity. Morphine remains the 'gold standard' opioid.

### Oxygen

Anerobic metabolism releases many cytokines (see Chapter 24). Simultaneously, homeostatic responses trigger tachycardia, increasing oxygen demand while further reducing oxygen supply. Infarcts are therefore more likely to extend if myocardium remains hypoxic. Optimising oxygen delivery reduces imbalance between oxygen demand and oxygen supply.

### Nitrates

Nitrates (e.g. isosorbide mono-/di-nitrate, glyceryl trinitrate) dilate coronary arteries, which increases oxygen supply, and reduce preload, which decreases myocardial work and oxygen demand. Isosorbide dinitrate can be given sublinguially, enabling ready access and quick absorption.

### Aspirin

A single dose of 300 mg aspirin can reduce or prevent infarction. Patients may already take one aspirin tablet each day, unaware that normal cardiac doses are 75–150 mg/day, and not 300 mg. Like colleagues elsewhere, ICU nurses should ensure that patients and significant others understand the prescribed dose.

Clopidogrel is an alternative to aspirin (Clopidogrel in Unstable Angina to Prevent Recurrent Events Trial Investigators, 2001).

## Thrombolysis

Thombolytic drugs ('clot busters') are indicated where patients experience chest pain together with either ST elevation or a new bundle branch block (Jowett & Thompson, 2003). Current door-to-needle target time for thrombolytics is 20 minutes (DOH, 2000c). Complications of thrombolysis include revasculariation dysrhythmias and bleeding.

Reperfusion of any ischaemic tissue flushes cytokines, oxygen radicals and other toxic chemicals (see Chapter 24) into myocardial circulation, causing myocardial stunning (Grech *et al.*, 1995). Myocardial stunning (asytole) is often followed by brief ventricular tachycardia or other dysrhythmias. Dysrhythmias are usually benign, but should be monitored and recorded. Persistent life-threatening dysrhythmias should be treated.

Thrombolytics and anticoagulants unavoidably create risks of bleeding. Intracranial and subarachnois haemorrhages may be fatal or cause a CVA. Bleeding can also occur elsewhere – especially the gut, lungs and genitourinary tract, the nose and around cannulae or other invasive equipment. Intramuscular injections should be avoided, and patients observed for signs of bleeding, including altered neurological state and haematuria.

*Stretopkinase*, the cheapest thrombolytic drug, is widely used in the UK. It activates plasminogen into plasmin, causing lysis.

Streptokinase is derived from streptococci, so may cause anaphylaxis. Although streptokinase-induced anaphylaxis is very rare, it may prove fatal, so streptokinase is considered a once-in-a-lifetime drug. The antidote for streptokinase is tranexamic acid. Patients, and close relatives, should be made aware that they must never have a second dose and given relevant information sheets; this should be recorded in nursing notes. Many patients choose to wear medi-alert bracelets, as subsequent myocardial infarction may cause unconsciousness.

*Tissue plasminogen activator (t-PA)*, also called recombinant tissue plasminogen activator (rt-PA) and alteplase, is an endogenous vascular epithelium enzyme which activates plasminogen bound to fibrin, so limiting systemic effects. Because it is more expensive than streptokinase, rt-PA is usually only given if specifically indicated, such as

- patients who have previously received streptokinase
- high risk patients.

*Urokinase* is only used for ocular thrombolysis and arteriovenous shunts.

*Third generation thrombolytics*, marketed during the 1990s, are usually modified or mutant t-PA, so achieve similar results, but having longer half-lifes can be given as one or more boluses (Verstraete, 2000). The most widely used in the UK are currently *reteplase* (Rapilysin®) and *tenecteplase* (Metalyse®).

321

## NSTEMI

Myocardial infarction without ST segment elevation or new left bundle branch block (NSTEMI) is more difficult to manage, partly because suspected infarction usually necessitates confirmation by cardiac marker analysis, and partly because NSEMI usually indicates more extensive plaque damage (Jones, 2003). Angiography is therefore essential to identify whether percutaneous repair is feasible – percutaneous repair being contraindicated if lesions are extremely tortuous, calcified or located in a bend (Bertrand *et al.*, 2002).

## Other drugs

*Beta-blockers* (drugs ending in -olol) inhibit beta stimulation of the heart, and are the best drug for treating overt coronary artery disease (Cruickshank, 2000). Beta receptors (which are stimulated by positives inotropes such as dobutamine) increase both heart rate and stroke volume, which increases myocardial workload (oxygen consumption) while reducing diastolic time (myocardial oxygen delivery). Beta-blockers therefore reduce myocardial work.

*Ace-inhibitors* inhibit angiotensin converting enzyme. Angiotensin contricts far more than noradrenaline, so inhibiting the enzyme necessary for its activation prevents hypertension.

*Antioxidants*, such as vitamin E, may prevent atherosclerosis (Chengi & Katz, 2000), but most studies have shown no cardiovascular benefits from antioxidants (Heart Protection Study Collaborative Group, 2002a; Hodis *et al.*, 2002)

*Calcium channel blockers* (e.g. nifedipine, amlopidine, verapamil, diltiazem) regulate the calcium channel of action potential, the first 'gateway' to open (see Chapter 22). This reduces myocardial excitability and vasodilates arteries.

*Statins* are the most effective lipid lowering drug, reducing low density lipoproteins and cholesterol (Gotto, 2001; Sanmuganathan, 2001; Heart Protection Study Collaborative Group, 2002b; Jensen *et al.*, 2004) and are also antioxidant (Shishehbor *et al.*, 2003), thereby reducing coronary heart disease mortality (Holme, 2000; Aronow *et al.*, 2001; Packer *et al.*, 2001). Statin therapy is recommended when total cholesterol exceeds 5.0 mmol/litre, or LDL cholesterol exceeds 3 mmol/litre (Foulkes, 2001; Sanmuganathan, 2001), but is also beneficial when lipids are low but CRP raised (Ridker *et al.*, 2001). Used for long-term treatment, they are unlikely to be commenced in ICU, but patients already on statin therapy should resume their treatment as soon as practical.

As most cholesterol synthesis occurs overnight, most statins should be given at night (McLoughin, 2004). Statins are mainly metabolised in the liver, where cholesterol synthesis mainly occurs, so it should be avoided with active liver disease or high alcohol intake (McLoughin, 2004).

## Percutaneous repair

Percutaneous interventions improve outcome and reduce hospital stay and costs compared with open heart surgery (Weaver *et al.*, 2000; Hlatky *et al.*, 2004) or thrombolysis (McClelland *et al.*, 2005). Where it is immediately available, percutaneous interventions increase survival from myocardial infarction (and cerebrovascular accidents) compared with thrombolysis (Weaver *et al.*, 2000).

Percutaneous cardiac interventions (PCI) include

- percutaneous transluminal coronary angioplasty (PTCA)
- percutaneous transluminal coronary rotational artherectomy
- directional coronary atherectomy
- laser atherectomy
- intracoronary stenting.

Percutaneous coronary angioplasty uses a balloon-tipped catheter to dilate stenosed arteries. The balloon diameter is usually about 1 mm. Endothelial damage from angioplasty can leave a flap of intima, which may cause sudden occlusion (Brady & Buller, 1996); abrupt vessel closure during or following angioplasty occurs in 4–8 per cent of patients (Windecker & Meier, 2000), necessitating urgent graft surgery. Implanting coronary stents widens the lumen, reducing severity of restenosis (Brady & Buller, 1996).

## Angiogenesis

Stem cells can be transplanted (via an angiography/angioplasty approach) to form new collateral circulation (Fujita & Tambara, 2004). Collateral circulation however may not be capable of significant further growth, and even if it is, collateral vessels are usually tortuous and fragile, so provide a poor alternative to many other treatment options available. Transplanting myocardium (*cardiomyoplasty*) is currently at the stage of animal study rather than clinical use (Lee & Makkar, 2004).

## Rest

Individualised mobilisation, as early as patients' conditions allow, promotes recovery. Adequate sleep (quality as well as quantity) facilitates physical and psychological healing (see Chapter 3), so planned care should minimise interventions overnight and allow rest periods during the day. Relaxation and other stress-reduction techniques (e.g. guided imagery, biofeedback) may also be beneficial.

## Psychological stress

Physical or psychological stress stimulates catecholamine release (see Chapter 1), which causes vasoconstriction, hypertension and other detrimental effects. While the stress response can be life-preserving for healthy people faced by

323

physical danger in the community, negative emotions and the stress response can be life-threatening to people with coronary heart disease (Todaro *et al.*, 2003).

## Prognosis

In the immediate post-infarction period, newly infarcted myocardium is surrounded by oedematous, ischaemic tissue (see Figure 30.1), causing volatile ECG changes following infarction. Oedema may subside, enabling reperfusion and recovery, or progress to further infarction.

## Health promotion

Patients and families are often receptive to health information following infarction and should be offered advice to reduce risks of further attacks. The British Heart Foundation produce a range of useful booklets that are available in most hospitals. Walking or vigorous exercise is cardioprotective (Manson *et al.*, 2002), although exercise levels should be built up gradually to prevent acute ischaemia from sudden over-exertion.

Many people with coronary heart disease are overweight (Montaye *et al.*, 2000), so may benefit from referral to dieticians. Poly-unsaturated fatty acids (PUFAs; see Chapter 9) are cardioprotective (Harper & Jacobson, 2001; Hu *et al.*, 2002). PUFAs may be found in fish and fish oil (especially herrings, mackerel, pilchards, salmon, sardines) (Daniels, 2002), rapeseed oil (Daniels, 2002), soya, leeks and walnuts (Harper & Jacobson, 2001). Fresh (not canned) fruit and vegetables provide antioxidants and help reduce hypertension (Daniels, 2002; John *et al.*, 2002), especially green leafy vegetables and vitamin-C rich fruits (Joshipura *et al.*, 2001).

Cholesterol control is vital, but most cholesterol is produced by the body rather than being consumed in food, so although cholesterol intake should be limited, abstinence is not a substitute for statins.

## Implications for practice

- Hypoxic myocardium needs oxygen.
- Tropins are the best marker for myocardial infarction.
- New STEMI should be treated by urgeny thrombolysis.
- NSTEMI should be managed by angiography, possibly proceeding to percutaneous coronary interventions or open heart surgery.
- Infarction risk is greatest between 06.00–10.00, so avoid early morning strenuous stimulation (e.g. bedbaths) with all patients (unless requested by the patient).
- Pain relief is important both for humanitarian reasons and to prevent further stress responses; opioid analgesics are usually needed, and their efficacy should be assessed.
- Rest is important for healing, so should be actively planned, and effectiveness assessed.

## Summary

UK reductions in infarction rates are disappointing both in relation to Health of the Nation targets and reductions in most other countries. However, in-hospital prognosis following infarction is improving, partly from effective use of thrombolytic therapy. The incidence of patients with uncomplicated myocardial infarctions being admitted to ICUs will vary, but usually ICU admission will be when infarctions complicate other pathologies or progress to prolonged cardiac failure. Nursing care of patients with myocardial infarctions should focus preventing further damage.

## Further reading

Hatchett and Thompson (2002) and Jowett and Thompson (2003) are key books on cardiac nursing. The DOH national framework (2000c) remains the key policy document. Articles on cardiology frequently appear in both nursing and medical journals. Bertrand *et al.* (2002) provide comprehensive guidelines for managing NSTEMI and Unstable Angina, while Kemp *et al.* (2004) describe biochemical markers.

Tough (2005) and Verstraete (2000) review thrombolysis. Jones (2003) summarises acute coronary syndromes, Tough (2004) describes assessing chest pain and Daniels (2002) offers dietary advice for health promotion. www. routledge.com/textbooks/0415373239

For clinical scenarios, clinical questions and the answers to them go to the support website at www.routledge.com/textbooks/0415373239

## Clinical scenarios

Mr Howard Gray is a 52-year-old insurance broker with a history of angina. He was admitted to the ICU four hours after he had woken up in the early morning with 'crushing' chest pain, unrelieved by sublingual nitro-glycerine and with worsening dyspnoea.

His ECG shows wide Q waves (area of necrosis) in leads $V_2$-$V_6$, and ST elevation (area of injury) in leads I, aVL & $V_2$-$V_6$, with ST depression in II, III and aVF, no T wave inversion (peripheral area of ischaemia) noted.

HR 128 bpm
BP 80/45 mmHg (MAP 57 mmHg)
12 hour Troponin T level 0.63 µg/litre

Q.1 Using a diagram of the surface of the heart and Mr Gray's ECG changes, identify which part of his myocardium is damaged and note the main coronary arteries that supply this area. List other cardiac markers used to assess myocardial damage.

Q.2 Mr Gray is given thrombolytic therapy. Review your role in administering and monitoring the effectiveness of this therapy (note frequency and type of investigation/assessment, identification of potential adverse effects).

Q.3 Evaluate the advice, information and follow up services offered to patients like Mr Gray by your clinical practice area. What role does the ICU nurse have in relation to health promotion, advice and cardiac rehabilitation following infarction?

# Chapter 31

# Cardiac surgery

## Contents

Introduction                                    328
Open heart surgery                              328
Minimally invasive cardiac surgery              329
Valve surgery                                   330
Coronary artery bypass grafts                   330
Heart failure                                   331
Transplants                                     332
Postoperative nursing                           333
Implications for practice                       341
Summary                                         341
Further reading                                 342
Clinical scenarios                              342

## Fundamental knowledge

Cardiac anatomy – arteries and valves
Coronary artery disease
Angioplasty (see Chapter 30)

## Introduction

Coronary artery and valve disease (see Chapter 30) remain major causes of UK mortality, especially among older people. When drug therapies cannot support cardiac failure, surgery may be needed either to repair or replace damaged tissue. Cardiac surgery significantly improves quality of life (Hunt *et al.*, 2000), older people gaining similar benefits to younger ones, although often taking longer to recover (Conaway *et al.*, 2003). Recent advances in cardiac surgery have made surgery a viable option for more 'high risk' patients and procedures. While beneficial for patients, this can create apparently poor statistical comparisons against previous outcomes.

This chapter describes open heart surgery, minimally invasive (percutaneous, or closed) alternatives, means to support failing hearts (intra-aortic balloon pumps, ventricular assist devices) and transplant surgery. Much nursing care follows from actual and potential problems created by surgical procedures; this chapter begins by briefly describing intraoperative procedures.

'Bypass' can variously mean:

1   blood pump oxygenators, or cardiopulmonary *bypass* (CPB; also called ECMO – see Chapter 29) which replaces cardiac and lung function during surgery
2   surgery which grafts vessels to *bypass* occlusion in coronary arteries.

In this chapter, 'bypass' refers to grafts; in practice, contexts often clarify intended meanings.

## Open heart surgery

Open heart surgery necessitates opening the thorax by sternotomy. Traditionally the aorta and vena cavae were cross-clamped, isolating the heart and lungs from the circulation. Circulation was then maintained with a cardiopulmonary bypass pump, while the heart was arrested with cardioplegia (see later) or slowed with beta-blockers (usually to about 40 bpm).

However, cardiopulmonary bypass may cause:

- neurological complications, including strokes and delirium (Heames *et al.*, 2002; Lorenz & Coyte, 2002; Zamvar *et al.*, 2002; Lytle & Sabik, 2004)
- lung damage, including atelectasis (Fisher *et al.*, 2002)
- inflammatory responses (Fisher *et al.*, 2002; Heames *et al.*, 2002; Munro, 2003; Paparella *et al.*, 2004).
- renal failure (Khan *et al.*, 2001)
- blood cell damage, causing anaemia and prolonged clotting (Fisher *et al.*, 2002; Lorenz & Coyte, 2002; Paparella *et al.*, 2004).

Although bypass pump designs have improved, most open-heart surgery is now '*off-pump*' coronary artery bypass – OPCAB. Cardiac motion can be minimised with suction, to enable surgery. Khat *et al.* (2004) studies suggest graft patency (measured at 3 months) is reduced with off-pump surgery, but most studies show reduced

- neurological impairment
- inflammatory responses
- respiratory distress
- renal failure
- sternal infections/complications
- morbidity
- ICU and hospital stay
- costs.

(Khan *et al.*, 2001; Abu-Omar & Taggart, 2002; Heames *et al.*, 2002; van Dijk *et al.*, 2002; Zamvar *et al.*, 2002; Al-Ruzzeh *et al.*, 2003; Ascione *et al.*, 2004; Berson *et al.*, 2004).

Currently, off-pump surgery is impractical for valve repair/replacement, deep vessels and very small conduits, or patients who are very haemodynamic unstable or in cardiogenic shock.

*Cardioplegia*, a potassium-rich (typically 15–30 mmol/l (Fisher *et al.*, 2002)) crystalloid used to arrest myocardium and so reduce metabolic oxygen demand, can cause postoperative dysrhythmias. Traditionally, cold cardioplegia (4–10°C) was used to reduce metabolism, but 'warm' (normothermic) cardioplegia is generally considered more cardioprotective so is usually used.

*Hypothermia* (core temperature of 28–32°C) reduces metabolic oxygen demand and causes peripheral vasoconstriction (reducing venous capacity). Complications of hypothermia are identified in this chapter. Many centres have abandoned inducing peripoperative hypothermia. To prevent hypervolaemia, two units of blood are usually removed for postoperative *autologous* transfusion. Postoperative rewarming causes vasodilatation, necessitating fluid monitoring and replacement.

*Sternotomies* are closed with permanent wire loops (usually five, visible on X-rays).

## Minimally invasive cardiac surgery

Minimally invasive surgery, using thoractomy or laproscopic approaches, reduces mortality and complications (Mihaljevic *et al.*, 2004), speeds recovery (Gunn *et al.*, 2003; Shirai *et al.*, 2004) and can be performed under epidural anaesthetic (Kessler *et al.*, 2001). *Minimally invasive direct coronary artery bypass grafting* is often abbreviated as MIDCAB.

Transmyocardial laser revascularisation may be used together with open heart surgery or angioplasty (Trehan *et al.*, 1998), but percutaneous transmyocardial laser revascularisation is generally only used when extensive coronary artery disease makes open-heart surgery or angioplasty impractical (Oesterie *et al.*, 2000). Further percutaneous coronary interventions (PCIs) are discussed in Chapter 30.

Complication rates are low (Morgan & Campanella, 1998). Minimally invasive saphenous vein harvest significantly reduces postoperative pain (Horvath *et al.*, 1998). Bleeding may occur, so chest drains are inserted. Being less invasive, postoperative respiratory failure is less likely so artificial ventilation is seldom needed postoperatively.

## Valve surgery

Mitral valve disease, typically a late complication of rheumatic fever, has decreased in Western countries, but ageing populations have caused increasing incidence of age-related aortic stenosis (Blackburn & Bookless, 2002).

Diseased valves can be repaired or replaced. Replacement valves are either

- biological (human cadaver, xenografts – porcine, bovine, baboon)
- prosthetic.

Biological valves are less thrombogenicic, so do not require life-long anti-coagulation therapy, but are more likely to degenerate; one-third of porcine valves fail within 11 years (Chikwe *et al.*, 2004). Most (>85 per cent) mitral valve replacements in UK now use mechanical valves (Chikwe *et al.*, 2004).

Percutaneous valvuloplasty achieves better results than open surgical replacement (Vahanian & Palacios, 2004). However percutaneous aortic valve implantation remains largely experimental (Vahanian & Palacios, 2004).

Valve surgery is more complex than bypass grafts, so has higher mortality (Fisher *et al.*, 2002). Postoperative risks of valve surgery (open or percutaneous), include

- tamponade
- infarction
- emboli
- dysrhythmias (from oedema and manipulation)
- chest pain.

(Lamerton & Albarran, 1997)

## Coronary artery bypass grafts

Occluded coronary arteries can be bypassed by grafts to restore myocardial blood supply. Autoharvest avoids complications of rejection. The saphenous vein is the easiest large vein to remove, but atherosclerosis is less likely to occur with arterial grafts (Fisher *et al.*, 2002). The most commonly grafted arteries are the internal mammary artery (*IMA*, especially left – LIMA) and increasingly radial artery (Chowdhury *et al.*, 2004; Zacharias *et al.*, 2004). Synthetic and animal grafts have also been used.

Early mortality rates from cardiac surgery are low – about 2–3 per cent (Livesey, 2002; Bridgewater *et al.*, 2004; Rathore, 2004), and long-term survival is high – 95 per cent at one year, 75 per cent at 10 years and 60 per cent at 15 years (Livesey, 2002).

Ten year patency and survival is longer for IMA (90 per cent) than vein (60 per cent) grafts (Goodwin & Dunning, 2000). Postoperative complications include

■ pain (parietal pleural incision, used for IMA harvest, disrupts richly innervated tissue)
■ spasm (arterial muscle), causing angina-like pain and more bleeding from anastomoses.

Bilateral IMA grafts cause sternal devascularisation, so increasing sternal wound complications, and are therefore rarely used (Goodwin & Dunning, 2000).

### Heart failure

Intra-aortic balloon pumps (IABPs) and ventricular assist devices (VADs) maintain perfusion in heart failure (Hausmann *et al.*, 2002), so can 'buy time' for transplantation, surgery or postoperative recovery (Hollenberg *et al.*, 1999). While enabling survival, highly invasive devices expose severely immunocompromised patients to risks from infection and thromboembolism.

Balloon inflation in the upper descending aorta (see Figure 31.1) is synchronised with diastole, displacing (usually) 40 ml of blood both upward (coronary and cerebral arteries, improving myocardial and cerebral perfusion)

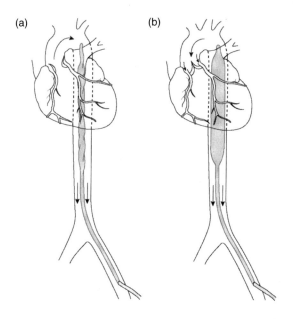

■ *Figure 31.1* **Intra-aortic balloon pump – inflated (a) and deflated (b)**

331

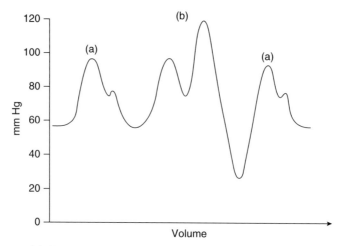

(a) Unassisted arterial pressure
(b) Augmented pressure with inflation increasing
    pressure after closure of the aortic valve creating
    a second pressure wave after the dicrotic notch

**Figure 31.2 Arterial pressure trace showing augmented pressure from use of an intra-aortic balloon pump**

and downward (increasing systemic pressure, perfusion and preload, shown by augmented pressure on arterial blood pressure traces – see Figure 31.2).
    Problems of IABP include complications of femoral artery cannulation

- rapid haemorrhage
- difficulty observing the site
- infection.

Balloon rupture (rare) or gas diffusion through the balloon exposes gas used to aortic blood so soluble gases (e.g. helium) are used. Gas cylinders maintain constant pressures to compensate for leaks. Alarms should sound before reserve gas in cylinders is exhausted, but nurses should still check cylinder volume and know how to replace them.
    VADs can be dual-chamber (see Figure 31.3), but single chamber left ventricular assist devices (LVADs) are usually used (Westaby, 2001).

## Transplants

Heart and heart/lung transplant can resolve endstage cardiac failure. Insufficient supply and preoperative mortality has encouraged interest in *xenograft* (including genetically engineered) and artificial alternatives, despite continuing problems with each alternative.

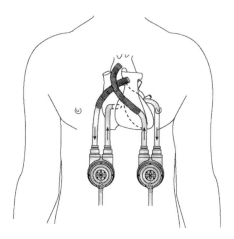

■ *Figure 31.3* **Ventricular assist devices (left and right)**

## Postoperative nursing

In addition to needs of any postoperative patient, cardiac surgery creates specialised needs. Complications vary, partly with procedures – normothermic and off-pump surgery avoids some problems. Common postoperative complications include

- pain (including that from sternal and saphenous would)
- respiratory failure and chest infection
- neurological dysfunction
- multiple and various dysrhythmias
- hypothermia and hypervolaemia
- initial polyuria causing hypokalaemia
- haemodilution
- anxiety.

Infection is a potential problem, but postoperative infection can usually be prevented through infection control and active care. Surgeons usually prescribe prophylactic antibiotics. Nurses should follow infection control guidelines and observe and report any signs of infection. Preventative care is identified in various sections below.

### Preparation

Any surgery is likely to be daunting for patients, but longstanding heart disease and traditional emotional connotations of the heart can heighten anxieties of patients undergoing cardiac surgery. Recovery is improved through preoperative information (Hayward, 1975); patients (and families) find preoperative visits useful (Lynn-McHale *et al.*, 1997).

Most patients undergoing cardiac surgery have only single organ failure, so recovery is usually rapid, most patients being transferred to stepdown units the following day. Seeing and helping patients progress rapidly can be very rewarding for nurses. Emphasis should therefore focus on normalisation, promoting homeostasis and encouraging patients to resume normal activities of living.

## Ventilation

Many centres extubate at the end of surgery, or very soon after, avoiding complications from intubation and artificial ventilation. Traditionally, postoperative ventilation was routinely used until normothermia and homeostasis were restored. Fluid shifts, hypovolaemia, infusion of large volumes of intravenous fluids and myocardial surgery (forming oedema and dysrhythmias from irritation) make cardiovascular status volatile in the immediate postoperative period. Respiratory mechanics can be impaired for up to seven hours after the operation (Ranieri *et al.*, 1999). Artificial ventilation therefore ensures adequate ventilation and oxygenation while cardiovascular stability and pulmonary blood flow are restored. Extubation exposes patients to risks from atelectasis and hypoventilation, while pain or fear of pain cause reluctance to breathe.

*Hypoventilation* and *impaired cough* may be caused by

- pain
- fear
- impaired respiratory centre function
- pleural effusion.

With adequate analgesia cover, patients should be encouraged to breathe deeply and cough. Good pain management and patient education can prevent many complications. Sternal instability, suffered by one-sixth of patients undergoing CABGs via median sternotomy (El-Ansary *et al.*, 2000a), can cause 'clicking' sounds. Although not painful, external stabilisation with hands or a single-patient-use support, such as a 'cough lock', helps deep breathing and coughing. Incentive spirometry is often useful.

Exudative pleural effusions occur in half of patients (Light *et al.*, 2002). Brims *et al.* (2004) drained on an average one litre of fluid in each patient, so improving oxygenation.

If there are no other complications, patients are likely to be extubated either at the end of surgery or within a few hours of admission to ICU or recovery areas.

## Glycaemic control

Since Van Den Berghe *et al.*'s (2001) finding, mainly with patients following cardiac surgery, that maintaining normoglycaemia reduced mortality, many centres routinely infuse 50% glucose (e.g. 20 ml/hour) until patients can eat or be fed nasogastrically. Most protocols use insulin infusions (50 iu actrapid in 50 ml saline) to maintain blood glucose between 4.5–6.1 mmol/litre.

### Hypertension/hypotension

Initial hypertension from hypothermic vasoconstriction may damage anastomoses, causing bleeding. Medical staff usually indicate upper limits for systolic pressure, frequently 100–120 mmHg, prescribing vasodilators (e.g. glyceryl trinitrate – GTN). Persistent hypertension unresponsive to nitrates indicates neurological damage.

Hypotension is usually due to

- hypovolaemia on rewarming
- myocardial dysfunction.

Fluid is replaced to maintain CVP. Hypotension despite adequate CVP indicates myocardial dysfunction; inotropic support may be needed to maintain tissue perfusion.

### Bleeding

Significant bleeding usually occurs from:

- anastomoses
- coagulopathies.

Cardiac surgery triggers both the intrinsic clotting pathway (contact between blood and the nonendothelial lining of the bypass machine) and the extrinsic pathway (tissue damage) (Dietrich, 2000).

Any sutures can prove incompetent, but aortic (from CPB) and myocardial sutures are exposed to high pressure and heartbeat/pulse movement. Arterial spasm with IMA grafts usually cause more bleeding. Pericardial bleeding may cause rapid *tamponade*. Two/three drains are inserted:

- pericardial
- mediastinal
- pleural (if pleura injured).

On arrival, volumes in each drain should be marked. Drainage, usually recorded hourly, should gradually reduce, becoming more serous. Sudden cessation may indicate thrombus obstruction, with likely tamponade; if patency of drains cannot be re-established, report this urgently, as emergency thoracotomy may be needed.

335

Coagulopathies are multifactorial (e.g. heparinsation using CPB), being monitored through full blood count and clotting studies. Haemostasis may require

- platelets/FFP
- protamine sulphate (reverses heparin)
- vitamin K
- Aprotinin (Trasylol®) (plasmin and kallikrein inactivator) (Sedrakyan et al., 2004; Smith & Shah, 2004)
- tranexamic acid (Pinosky et al., 1997).

## Fluid balance

Postoperatively, patients may have large negative fluid balances from

- fluid shifts (vasoactive mediators, low colloid osmotic pressure)
- forced diuresis.

Reversing hypothermia causes vasodilatation, necessitating large volumes of fluid. Total body hydration is normally maintained with continuous low-volume crystalloid infusion (e.g. 5% glucose), but to maintain blood volume, so most fluids infused are colloids (see Chapter 34).

Fluid charts may be divided between colloids (colloidal infusions against blood loss) and crystalloids (crystalloid infusion against urine output). Colloid replacement is given to maintain central venous pressure (e.g. above 10 mmHg); 'driving' central venous pressure hastens peripheral perfusion and so rewarming. Blood is often transfused if haemoglobin falls below 10 g/dl (haematocrit below 33 per cent). Haemodilution with colloids usually necessitates blood supplements, so patients should already have units crossmatched.

## Temperature

If hypothermic, gradual rewarming should bring central within 2°C of peripheral (pedal) temperature (avoid measuring pedal temperature on limbs from which saphenous veins are harvested). Warming hastens homeostasis and may prevent shivering (shivering increases metabolic rate, so increasing oxygen consumption and metabolic acidosis).

## Acid/base balance

Anaerobic metabolism from hypoperfusion causes metabolic acidosis. Acidosis is negatively inotropic, can cause dysrhythmias and reduces oxygen dissociation from haemoglobin. Although acidosis is closely monitored through blood gas analysis it is not usually necessary to treat acidosis following cardiac surgery.

## Dysrhythmias

Various dysrhythmias (often multifocal) often occur following cardiac (especially valve) surgery. Resolution is usually spontaneous and relatively quick. Causes include:

- chronic cardiomyopathy
- oedema (from surgery, disrupting conduction pathways)
- acidosis
- electrolyte imbalance
- hypoxia/ischaemia
- mechanical irritation (e.g. drain/pacing wire removal)
- hypothermia.

Only symptomatic and problematic dysrhythmias normally need treatment (drugs, pacing or resuscitation).

*Atrial fibrillation* frequently occurs postoperatively (McMurry & Hogue, 2004), especially if hypothermic bypass was used perioperatively (Adams *et al.*, 2000). Amiodarone is an effective treatment for acute postoperative atrial fibrillation (Kern, 2004).

Other postoperative dysrythmias include *bradycardias*, *blocks*, *junctional* and *tachydysrhythmias* frequently occur. Persistent blocks often require pacing, hence perioperative placement of epicardial wires. Epicardial wires are unipolar, a negative pole being created by inserting a subcutaneous needle. Pacing wires usually remain in place until dysrhythmias become unlikely (usually 5–10 days).

Myocardial infarction may necessitate emergency thoracotomy/sternotomy and internal massage/defibrillation (although limited infarction may cause little more than minor ECG changes, and not require resuscitation). Staff should therefore know where thoracotomy packs are situated. Internal defibrillation avoids transthoracic bioimpedance, so uses lower voltage (e.g. 20–50 J).

## Electrolyte imbalance

Other than potassium, imbalances rarely require treatment. Causes include:

- *fluid shifts* from vasoactive mediators
- *hyperkalaemia* from cell membrane damage
- *hypokalaemia* from forced diuresis; also cell recovery returning potassium to intracellular fluid
- *hormones* (e.g. aldosterone, ADH).

Hypokalaemia necessitates frequent potassium supplements, usually diluted in small volumes of maintenance crystalloid fluid to maintain plasma concentrations of 4.0–4.5 mmol/litre. Hyperkalaemia may necessitate insulin and glucose infusion (which can cause later rebound hyperkalaemia).

Most (70 per cent) patients are hypomagnesemic after bypass surgery (Gries *et al.*, 1999), which contributes to

- increased dysrhythmias
- platelet aggregation.

Currently it is not routine to administer magnesium supplements postoperatively.

### Renal function

Following initial polyuria, patients may become oliguric from

- reperfusion vasodilation
- increased circulating ADH (stress response).

Driving central venous pressure protects renal perfusion. Supplementary diuretics may be used, but some patients later require haemofiltration (see Chapter 40).

Urinary catheters can normally be removed the day after surgery.

Prolonged peri- and postoperative hypotension can precipitate acute tubular necrosis, so renal function should be closely monitored and supported.

### Pain control

Pain control is central to intensive care nursing; absence of pain is desirable for both humanitarian and physiological reasons (see Chapter 7); poor pain control may prolong recovery, circulating catecholamines impairing myocardial perfusion. Early postoperative pain usually needs opiate infusion, possibly supplemented by nonsteroidal anti-inflammatories.

Although Kuperberg and Grubbs (1997) found patients were satisfied with their analgesia, many other studies suggest postoperative pain control remains poor, nurses underestimating pain (Valdix & Puntillo, 1995; Cottle, 1997; Ferguson *et al.*, 1997). Pain is individual so should be individually assessed rather than stereotyped by operations performed. Thoracic nociceptor innervation being relatively sparse, patients often experience relatively less pain from thoracic than saphenous incisions (Fisher *et al.*, 2002), although arterial graft spasm (e.g. IMA) can cause angina, and IMA harvest disrupts richly innervated tissue. Nitrates (e.g. GTN) dilate arteries, reducing spasm pain and tension on newly grafted vessels. Saphenous vein harvest necessitates a long incision, stimulating many nociceptors so causes much pain (Horvath *et al.*, 1998).

*Types* of pain experienced following cardiac surgery include

- bone pain (sharp/throbbing)
- visceral pain
- muscle pain (harvest site)

- cardiac/angina pain
- neurogenic pain
- psychogenic pain (anxiety)
- sudden/spasm.

Continuous analgesia may alleviate underlying/continuous pain (including anxiety-related pain), but nurses should observe for breakthrough (sudden/spasm) pain which may need bolus analgesia or nitrates. Once conscious, many patients benefit from patient controlled analgesia (PCA).

Early postoperative extubation removes the need for sedation. For intubated patients, sedation usually provides comfort. Intubation, and so chemical sedation, is usually limited to a few hours, so rapidly cleared drugs (e.g. Propofol) are usually used. Hypotensive effects of Propofol can compound hypovolaemia.

### *Neurological complications*

Potentially fatal thrombi (and emboli) may be caused by

- cardiopulmonary bypass
- air emboli
- thrombotic vegetations (chronic preoperative atrial fibrillation, infective endocarditis).

Neurological deficits can cause

- impaired peripheral nerve function
- cerebral/cognitive deficits
- uncontrollable hypertension (injury to vital centres).

Cognitive deficits following cardiac surgery affect 80 per cent of patients within a few days following surgery and persists in one-third of patients (Arrowsmith *et al.*, 2000).

Cerebrovascular accidents (CVAs – strokes) occur in 3–5 per cent (10 per cent in people aged over 70), but subtle neurological and cognitive changes frequently occur (Yates & Alston, 2000). Neurological assessment is therefore a priority. CVAs may remain undetected until patients show deficits or fail to wake normally. Nurses suspecting abnormal neurological recovery should seek urgent assistance.

### *Psychological considerations*

The heart, more than any other body organ, carries emotional connotations for most people – people 'love with their heart'. Heart disease therefore conjures fear. Many patients undergoing cardiac surgery experience preoperative depression and anxiety (Yates & Alston, 2000). Psychological distress is compounded by psychological stressors of ICU (see Chapter 3). Baris *et al.*'s (1995) small-scale study found that most patients experience transient neuropsychological dysfunction following graft surgery. Postoperatively, mood is often labile, euphoria (induced by opiates and survival) being followed (day 2–4) by reactive depression.

Stress provokes tachycardia, hypertension and hyperglycaemia (see Chapter 3), all impairing recovery in patients least able to tolerate such insults. Providing information, achieving optimum pain control, relieving anxieties and minimising sensory imbalance are therefore important aspects of holistic nursing care.

### Skin care

Wound breakdown or skin ulceration may occur from poor perfusion, peri- or postoperative immobility and other factors. On regaining consciousness, pain and anxiety often make patients reluctant to move.

Wound dressings are usually removed within 24 hours, then left exposed unless oozing. Debilitation and poor cardiac output may delay wound healing. Sternal wound dehiscence is rare (3 per cent) but can prove fatal (Kuo & Butchart, 1995), especially following IMA grafts (which can reduce sternal blood supply by up to 90 per cent); complete sternal dehiscence necessitates surgical intervention.

Perfusion of graft sites (especially radial artery grafts; also arteriovenous shunts) should be protected, so pressure (e.g. blood pressure cuff, tourniquet) should be avoided.

### Normalisation

Nurses can experience considerable satisfaction from assisting rapid postoperative recovery following cardiac surgery. Normalisation should be encouraged. Families and friends should be encouraged to visit, as they would on a surgical ward. The day following surgery, patients may enjoy breakfast before transfer.

Early mobilisation should be encouraged, musculo-skeletal complications and pulmonary emboli being the main causes of delayed discharge (Johnson & McMahan, 1997). Mobilisation may begin in ICU with active exercises. IMA grafts may cause more musculo-skeletal complications than saphenous grafts (El-Ansary *et al.*, 2000b).

### Transplantation issues

Severing of sympathetic and parasympathetic pathways causes loss of vagal tone, resulting in resting heart rates of about 100 beats/minute. Denervation also (usually) prevents angina, increasing risk of silent infarction, but partial renervation does occur (Cox, 2002), 12 per cent of patients experiencing pain (Tsui & Large, 1998).

Loss of sympathetic tone impairs cardiac response to increased metabolic demands, making atropine ineffective.

Surgery preserves recipients' right atrium, which can cause P waves (one intrinsic, one graft). Although not pathologically significant, reasons for the presence of two P waves should be explained to patients, families and junior nurses.

## Implications for practice

- Care of patients following cardiac surgery has much in common with care of other postoperative patients but requires continuing full individual assessment.
- Long-standing cardiovascular disease and acute responses to cardiac surgery necessitate close monitoring and system support – especially ECG and blood pressure.
- Persistent problematic dysrhythmias may necessitate temporary pacing – epicardial wires are usually inserted perioperatively.
- Cardiac drains should be measured on arrival and excessive or sudden cessation of drainage reported.
- Nurses should know where thoracotomy packs are kept, what they contain and what will be expected of them in the event of emergency thoracotomy.
- Patients should be encouraged to take deep breaths and cough periodically, especially following extubation.
- Neurological events may prove fatal, so neurological state should be assessed as soon as possible after surgery and any concerns reported.
- Physical and psychological pain cause various complications; patients should receive adequate analgesia, its effect being monitored by frequent assessment.
- Nursing care should focus on normalisation.
- Preoperative visits and information can significantly reduce stress, but psychological care of both patients and their families remains a nursing priority.
- Relatively rapid recovery requires nurses to spend much time on technical roles of assessing, observing and administering drugs, but the human elements of care should be simultaneously maintained.
- Disease and interventions with the heart often cause greater anxiety than with other organs, so patients should be reassured and supported psychologically.

## Summary

Most patients undergoing cardiac surgery are admitted to ICU following treatment for single system failure so usually recover rapidly. This can be both rewarding and time-consuming for nurses. Many possible postoperative complications result from the necessities of intraoperative procedures;

increasing percutaneous surgery may significantly reduce numbers of open heart operations.

## Further reading

Material on cardiac surgery often dates quickly. There are a number of specialist journals, and many articles appear in medical journals. Benefits of off-pump surgery are outlined by Abu-Omar and Taggart (2002) and Khan *et al.* (2004). Gunn *et al.* (2003) and Vahanian and Palacios (2004) discuss percutaneous surgery. Neurolgocial issues are explored by van Dijk *et al.* (2002) and Zamvar *et al.* (2002). www.routledge.com/textbooks/0415373239

For clinical scenarios, clinical questions and the answers to them go to the support website at www.routledge.com/textbooks/0415373239

## Clinical scenarios

Johnny Doyle is a 57-year-old man with a history of angina, hypertension, insulin dependant diabetes and weighs 110 kg. He was admitted to ICU following off-pump coronary artery bypass grafts × 2 using saphenous vein and left IMA to right ascending vein. Mr Doyle's blood sugar is 7.5 mmol/l and managed by an intravenous infusion of 50% glucose at 20 ml/hour and insulin infusion running at 8 iu/hour.

Q.1 Describe Mr Doyle's preoperative preparation and explain relevance to ICU care (e.g. type of investigations, patient information, pre-admission visits, diabetes control).

Q.2 Examine the nursing priorities and identify potential complications in the first 24 hours post CABG surgery for Mr Doyle.

Q.3 Mr Doyle develops dehiscence of his sternal wound and can feel his sternum moving on deep breaths and coughing. Review causative factors for this complication and propose a plan of care to stabilise sternum, promote healing and recovery (evaluate various treatments approaches, pharmacological/surgical interventions, approaches used to stabilise sternum, blood sugar control).

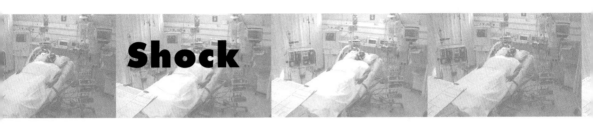

# Chapter 32

# Shock

## Contents

Introduction                        344
Stages                              345
Perfusion failure                   346
System failure                      347
Types of shock                      348
Implications for practice           351
Summary                             351
Further reading                     352
Clinical scenarios                  352

## Fundamental knowledge

Cellular pathology (see Chapter 24)

Cardiac anatomy, including the mitral valve and pericardium

Autonomic nervous system – sympathetic and parasympathetic
    regulation, especially the vagus nerve

Baroreceptors and chemoreceptors

Renin-angiotensin-aldosterone mechanism

Normal inflammatory responses (increased capillary
    permeability, leucocyte migration, vasoactive
    mediators release)

## Introduction

In health, normotension is maintained by matching blood volume to blood vessel capacity. This is achieved through autonomic reflexes and endocrine responses.

1   Hypotension is sensed by *baroreceptors* in major arteries, which activate the *hypothalamic–pituitary–adrenal (HPA) axis* (the stress response – fight or flight). More adrenocorticotrophic hormone (ACTH) is released by the pituitary gland, which stimulates adrenal production of adrenaline and noradrenaline, causing vasoconstriction. HPA axis activation also increases glucocorticoid secretion (O'Connor *et al.*, 2000).

2   Intrarenal hypotension initiates the *renin–angiotensin–aldosterone* mechanism:

renin (released by kidney)
activates angiotensinogen, (in liver)

↓

angiotensin 1
mild vasoconstriction; changed by *angiotensin converting enzyme* in (lungs) to:

↓

angiotensin 2
powerful vasoconstrictor – eight times more powerful than noradrenaline;
also increases adrenal production of

↓

aldosterone (adrenal gland)
increases renal sodium reabsorption

3   The pituitary gland releases more *antidiuretic hormone*, increasing renal water reabsorption.

So, (1) reduces blood vessel capacity, (2) mainly reduces blood vessel capacity, while (3) together with increased aldosterone production (2) increases blood volume.

Adjusting these opposite responses enables the body to compensate for problems. Shock, inadequate bloodflow to tissues or perfusion failure, occurs when compensatory mechanisms are exhausted or fail. Life-threatening hypotension may be caused by

 loss of blood volume
 increased blood vessel capacity

or both. Because compensation usually occurs, hypotension is a relatively late sign. Earlier key signs occurring during compensation are

■ tachycardia
■ tachypnoea.

Identifying these signs before hypotension occurs enables earlier intervention and may prevent avoidable complications.

There are four types of shock:

■ cardiogenic
■ obstructive
■ hypovolaemic
■ distributive.

Some of these types can be caused by different pathologies. This chapter provides an overview of effects of shock, symptoms and main treatments. Sepsis, septic shock and systemic inflammatory response syndrome (SIRS), the most common types of shock in ICU, are discussed in Chapter 33. The first three types of shock (cardiogenic, obstructive and hypovolaemic) are then discussed. Some causes of distributive shock are discussed, but the main type seen in ICU is the septic shock and the SIRS continuum, discussed in Chapter 33.

This chapter suggests likely signs and symptoms to help readers identify shock. Figures cites are a guide, and not absolute; symptoms are typical, but are not exhaustive.

## Stages

Shock is often classified into four stages, reflecting its progression and homeostatic responses:

■ *Initial* (Hypodynamic): poor cardiac output causes systemic hypoperfusion. Cells resort to anaerobic metabolism. Lactic acid begins to rise (>1.7 mmol/litre). Pulse oximetry may fail to detect a pulse.
■ *Compensation* (Hyperdynamic): neuroendocrine responses increase circulating catecholamine levels causing

  ● tachycardia
  ● increased stroke volume (palpitations)
  ● tachypnoea
  ● oliguria.

Other signs at this stage usually include

  ● dilated pupils, which still responsive to light
  ● confusion, lethargy or agitation
  ● clammy/moist skin.

■ *Progression* (Hypotensive): compensation fails (although tachycardia usually increases), causing hypotension. Arteriolar and precapillary sphincters constrict, trapping blood in capillaries. This activates inflammatory responses, including histamine release from mast cells, creating oedema. Signs include

- hypotension
- increasing tachycardia (>150 bpm)
- hyperkalaemia (from cell damage – see Chapter 24)
- worsening metabolic acidosis
- myocardia ischaemia (ECG changes)
- severely impaired consciousness
- cold/cyanotic skin
- progressive multi-organ failure.

Death often occurs at this stage, but shock may progress to a final stage:

■ *Refractory* (Irreversible): symptomatic multiorgan failure, with no response to any treatments and death becoming inevitable within a few hours.

Early detection and appropriate treatment of shock may prevent progression, reduce complications and improve outcome.

## Perfusion failure

Perfusion may fail due to

- insufficient circulating volume
- inadequate cardiac output
- excessive peripheral vasodilatation.

However caused, perfusion failure deprives cells of glucose and oxygen. Tissue cells need energy – adenosine triphosphate (ATP), which is produced in their mitochondria. Without glucose and oxygen, mitochondria metabolise alternative energy sources (body stores – fat and muscle protein), and metabolism becomes anaerobic. Both anaerobic metabolism and metabolism of alternative energy sources are inefficient, producing relatively little energy and large amounts of waste, including lactate. Without perfusion, waste products of metabolism (carbon dioxide, water and metabolic acids) are not removed, creating an increasingly hostile, acidic internal and external environment which, together with reduced energy production, progressively destroys cells. Shock therefore starves tissue cells of the oxygen and glucose they need for normal, healthy (aerobic) metabolism.

Anaerobic metabolism of alternative energy sources produces little energy but much waste, including metabolic acids (especially lactate, which forms lactic acid). Shock therefore causes metabolic acidosis:

- pH <7.35, with base excess <2.0
- lactate >2 mmol/litre.

As cells progressively fail, intracellular contents progressively leak into blood. Normal intracellular and intravascular concentrations of many substances being very different (see Chapter 24), causes many abnormalities, especially

■ hyperkalaemia.

Progressive cell failure in organs causes progressive organ failure. Early symptoms of shock should therefore be aggressively treated with urgent microcirculatory resuscitation (oxygen and fluids) to prevent organ failure.

## System failure

*Cardiovascular.* In health, hypoperfusion triggers neuroendocrine compensatory responses (described earlier):

■ hypothalamic-pituitary-adrenal axis
■ renin-angiotensin-aldosterone mechanism
■ anti-diuretic hormone release.

Complex pathologies (present in most ICU patients) cause imbalance and failure of compensatory and autoregulation mechanisms. Reduced cardiac output reduces myocardial hypoxia, which usually triggers tachycardia. Tachycardia increases myocardial oxygen consumption, but reduces ventricular filling time and myocardial oxygenation time, so it may make myocardium more ischaemic, provoking dysrhythmias and infarction.

*Respiratory.* Metabolic acidosis from systemic hypoperfusion stimulates tachypnoea. Pulmonary hypoperfusion increases pathological deadspace and V/Q mismatch. Severe shock therefore increases work of breathing without improving tissue oxygenation (Wheeler & Bernard, 1999). Ischaemic surfactant-producing cells in alveoli fail to produce surfactant, while increased capillary permeability causes pulmonary oedema, progressing to *ARDS* (once called 'shock lung').

*Renal.* Prolonged renal ischaemia (prerenal failure) causes acute tubular necrosis (see Chapter 39), which increases toxic levels of active metabolites (e.g. urea contributes to confusion/coma).

*Hepatic.* The liver has a very high metabolic rate, so is particularly susceptible to ischaemic damage, although symptoms often appear later than with other major organs. The liver has many functions (metabolic, digestive, immune, homeostatic), so hepatic dysfunction causes many problems, including bilirubinaemia and (eventually) jaundice-delayed clotting immunocompromise causing opportunistic infections, including sepsis.

*Pancreas.* Serum amylase and lipase become elevated. Pancreatic cell death releases myocardial depressant factor, further exacerbating shock.

## Types of shock

*Cardiogenic* shock is caused by failure of the heart to pump sufficient blood into the aorta, usually from

■   myocardial infarction ('coronary cardiogenic shock').

More than half of survivors from myocardial infarction die within one month from cardiogenic shock (Lindholm *et al.*, 2003). Among the patients undergoing open heart surgery, 2–6 per cent develop cardiogenic shock (Hausmann *et al.*, 2004). Other causes of cardiogenic shock include

■   valve disease, especially mitral regurgitation
■   congenital defects

and various other cardiac problems, collectively called 'non-coronary cardiogenic shock'.

Cardiogenic shock follows extensive left ventricular damage. Left ventricular dysfunction causes systemic hypotension, myocardial hypoperfusion and hypoxia and pulmonary congestion (pulmonary oedema). Compensatory tachycardia may increase myocardial oxygen supply, but also increases consumption. Extensive left ventricular damage is rapidly fatal.

Treatment attempts to increase systemic perfusion pressure while limiting myocardial hypoxia. Inotropes may be necessary to increase cardiac output, but increases myocardial workload. Intra-aortic balloon pumps (IABP) and ventricular assist devices (VAD) have other ways to maintain perfusion and are discussed in Chapter 31.

Mortality from cardiogenic shock remains high: 50–80 per cent (Hollenberg *et al.*, 1999). Survivors often develop congestive cardiac failure, necessitating cardiac surgery. Nitric oxide synthase inhibitor can reduce mortality by more than half (Cotter *et al.*, 2003).

*Obstructive* shock is caused by any obstruction to blood flow through the heart:

■   raised intrathoracic pressure (positive pressure ventilation, PEEP)
■   obstructed intrapulmonary flow (ARDS, pulmonary emboli, pneumo/haemothorax)
■   tamponade.

*Tamponade* is direct continuous compression of the heart, usually caused by pericardial haemorrhage. Accumulation forces myocardium inward, reducing intraventricular space and stroke volume.

Tamponade can be slow or quick. Rapid tamponade (usually from cardiac surgery or trauma) is an emergency, usually causing imminent cardiac arrest once compensatory tachycardia and vasoconstriction fail. Tamponade should be suspected with sudden

- CVP (or jugular venous pressure) increase
- hypotension and
- cessation of cardiac drainage.

These signs may be masked or absent by hypovolaemia; other indications include

- dysrhythmias and low voltage ECG trace
- pulsus parodoxus
- muffled apex heart sounds, due to transmission of the sounds through fluid
- mediastinal widening (on X-ray)
- pericardial fluid accumulation (shown by echocardiography).

Rapid tamponade necessitates urgent needle aspiration of pericardial fluid, seldom allowing time for diagnostic tests, the needle usually remaining in place until drainage is below 50 ml/day (Spodick, 2003). Following pericardial aspiration, patients should be closely monitored for further accumulation (ECG, CVP, drainage).

*Hypovolaemic* (haemorrhagic) shock, the type occurring most frequently in hospital patients, is caused by a rapid and large loss of blood volume, resulting in reduced blood flow and tissue perfusion. Hypovolaemia may be caused by

- acute haemorrhage (trauma, surgery, gastrointestinal bleeding)
- other excessive fluid loss (e.g. diabetic ketoacidosis)
- insufficient fluid replacement if patients have difficulty drinking or are nil-by-mouth.

With compensation, people may survive loss of two-fifths of blood volume, but without compensation, losing one-fifth of blood volume over 30 minutes may be fatal (Guyton & Hall, 2000). When compensation fails, venous return falls (low CVP), inevitably reducing stroke volume. Compensatory tachycardia may restore blood pressure, but increased myocardial oxygen consumption can cause ischaemia, dysrhythmias and infarction.

Hypovolaemic shock should be treated, or (even better) prevented, by giving adequate fluid. When acute volume loss is uncomplicated by other disease, crystalloid fluid may be adequate. However, rapid infusion of crystalloids into critically ill patients usually provides only transient benefits, and can cause pulmonary and systemic oedema – see Chapter 34. To minimise risks from hypovolaemic shock, some ICUs routinely infuse gelatins before transferring patients by ambulance (acceleration and deceleration exaggerate blood pressure in hypovolaemia).

*Distributive shock* occurs when normal vasoregulation fails. Normally only one quarter of capillaries are open at any time (Deroy, 2000). Bloodflow into capillaries is controlled by capillary sphincters. Excessive peripheral vasodilatation increases blood vessel capacity, so existing blood volume is maldistributed with excessive volume pooling in peripheral circulation at the expense of central blood volume and pressure.

The most frequent cause of distributive shock seen in the ICU is sepsis/SIRS, discussed in Chapter 33. Other types of distributive shock include

- neurogenic/spinal
- anaphylaxis
- toxic shock syndrome.

*Neurogenic/spinal* shock is caused when injury, oedema or disease of the spinal cord above the thorax interrupts autonomic sympathetic nerve control. Sympathetic tone, which increases heart rate and vasoconstriction is impaired. Paradoxically, vagal (parasympathetic) regulation, which reduces both heart rate and vasoconstriction, usually remains intact. Problems above cervical vertebra five may cause respiratory failure, necessitating artificial ventilation.

Failure of autonomic response usually makes inotropes ineffective. Flow monitoring can identify whether vasopressures are effective. Volume replacement, mainly with colloids, can compensate for increased blood vessel capacity. Unresponsive sudden hypotension usually indicates a stroke which, with critical illness may prove fatal, so medical assistance should be urgently summoned.

Nurses should assess patients' neurological status and closely monitor effectiveness of treatments.

*Anaphylactic* shock is caused by T-lymphocytes (immune system) recognising an antigen and so initiating an antigen–antibody reaction. This stimulates proinflammatory responses, releasing a range of chemical mediators from mast cells, which

- vasodilate (e.g. interleukins, prostaglandins)
- increase capillary pore permeability (e.g. histamine)
- trigger clotting (e.g. platelet activating factor).

Increased capillary and other blood vessel capacity, and increased capillary leak (reduced blood volume) rapidly causes hypovolaemia, triggering tachycardia. Smooth muscle constriction in the larynx and bronchioles rapidly causes severe respiratory distress.

Anaphylaxis typically occurs with second doses of drugs, but 'first doses' may not be danger-free – previous exposure to antigens (e.g. drugs) may be unrecorded.

Anaphylactic shock is an emergency, treated with adrenaline to restore circulating blood pressure (McLean-Tooke *et al.*, 2003). Volume expanders, oxygen and other system supports may be needed.

Allergic reactions release granules from mast cells, so can be diagnosed by testing for granules specific to mast cells. Where serum histamine peaks within a few minutes and declines within a quarter of an hour, tryptase takes one hour to rise, but remains elevated for 4–6 hours.

*Toxic shock syndrome* is a rare form of sepsis, caused by a strain of *Staphylococcus aureus* (Willis, 1997). There are very few cases each year in the UK – Michie and Shah (2003) suggest 2–5, while Willis (1997) suggests 40. Toxic shock syndrome is usually caused by poor tampon hygiene, but can be from any skin-surface staphylococci invading the body. Necrotising fasciitis (see Chapter 12) causes toxic shock syndrome. The rarity of toxic shock syndrome may delay recognition when it occurs, especially if unconscious women who are admitted to ICU have tampons in place.

*Septic Shock* and *SIRS* are the most frequently seen causes of shock in ICU, often causing *multi-organ dysfunction syndrome* (MODS) and death. These are discussed further in Chapter 33.

### Implications for practice

- Shock is a problem of inadequate tissue perfusion at microcirculatory level, so treatments should target microcirculatory resuscitation – primarily oxygen (aim $SaO_2$ >94 per cent and fluid therapy (in ICU, usually colloids) to an adequate CVP – usually 10 cmH$_2$O (+PEEP).
- Oxygen delivery can be calculated through flow monitoring, or assessed by comparing $SaO_2$ with $ScvO_2$ (see Chapter 20).
- Once CVP is optimised, cardiac output can be increased with inotropes.
- Unreversed shock will cause renal failure. Diuretics do not solve pre-renal failure, but can be fatal with hypovolaemia.
- Sudden shock may be caused by tamponade, especially following cardiac surgery. If cardiac chest drains are present, patency should be restored. Otherwise, needle aspiration by medical staff may be necessary.
- Most ICU patients are immunosupressed and shock increases vulnerability. Maintaining a normal metabolic environment (normal pH, normoglycaemia) and good infection control significantly reduces risks of sepsis.

### Summary

Many pathologies can cause shock. But however caused, shock results in inadequate perfusion to tissues which, if not reversed, will cause progressive cell damage. Cells with high metabolic rates, such as cardiac and brain cells, are especially susceptible to perfusion failure. Once sufficient cells in an organ fail, the organ will fail to function adequately.

Priorities of care therefore focus on microcirculatory (capillary) resuscitation:

- oxygen
- fluids
- system support.

Underlying causes of shock should, where possible, be treated.

Close monitoring and observation by ICU nurses, with an understanding of probable mechanisms of shock, enables prompt treatment. Nurses have an especially valuable preventative role in promoting infection control and nutrition.

## Further reading

Shock is covered in most medical and nursing texts. Reviews about particular types of shock, such as Hollenberg *et al.* (1999) and Edwards (2001), appear periodically in medical and nursing literature. www.routledge.com/textbooks/0415373239

For clinical scenarios, clinical questions and the answers to them go to the support website at www.routledge.com/textbooks/0415373239

## Clinical scenarios

Mr Reece Owen is a 71-year-old gentleman with COPD. He was originally admitted to hospital with acute exacerbation of COPD. Despite respiratory support and antibiotic therapy his physical condition deteriorated. He became confused with a low GCS, unstable ECG and was transferred to ICU for flow monitoring, intubation and mechanical ventilation (PSIMV, PEEP of 8 $cmH_2O$, $FiO_2$ 0.4).

Observations on admission include;

| | |
|---|---|
| Temperature | 34.5°C |
| Heart rate | 135 bpm |
| Rhythm | Sinus tachycardia with multi focal ventricular ectopics |
| BP | 106/55 mmHg |
| CVP | 24 mmHg |
| CO | 4.72 litres/minute |
| CI | 2.55 litres/minute/m² |
| SV | 35 ml |
| SVI | 19 ml/beat/m² |
| SVR | 1000 dynes/second/cm⁵ |
| SVRI | 1850 dynes/second/cm⁵/m² |
| $ScvO_2$ | 68% |
| SVV | 21% |

Blood results

| Haematology | | Biochemistry | | Arterial blood gas |
|---|---|---|---|---|
| Hb | 9.2 g/dl | CRP | 129 mg/litre | pH 7.13 |
| WBC | $25.5 \times 10^{-9}$/litre | $Na^+$ | 142 mmol/litre | $PaCO_2$ 7.13 kPa |
| Neutrophils | $23.5 \times 10^{-9}$/litre | $K^+$ | 4.9 mmol/litre | $PaO_2$ 14.67 kPa |
| Lymphocytes | $0.2 \times 10^{-9}$/litre | $Cl^-$ | 110 mmol/litre | $HCO_3$ 16.3 mmol/litre |
| Platelets | $334 \times 10^{-9}$/litre | $HCO_3$ | 18 mmol/litre | Base Ex −10.1 mmol/litre |

| Haematology | | Biochemistry | | Arterial blood gas | |
| --- | --- | --- | --- | --- | --- |
| MCV | 86 μm³ | Glucose | 10.5 mmol/litre | Lactate | 1.5 mmol/litre |
| | Urea | 14.2 mmol/litre | | | |
| INR | 1.5 | Creatinine | 251 μmol/litre | | |
| APTT ratio | >5.0 | Albumin | 11 g/litre | | |
| TT | >100 secs | Troponin T | 0.13 μg/litre | | |

Q1. Identify the most likely cause and type of shock that Mr Owen may be experiencing. What other investigations might confirm this.

Q2. Explain the physiology underlying Mr Owen's abnormal results. Comment on his organ and tissue perfusion.

Q3. Consider interventions and devise a plan of care aimed at optimising cardiac index, tissue oxygenation and metabolic environment for Mr Owen.

*Same patient is used in scenario for Chapter 33.*

Chapter 33

# Sepsis, SIRS and MODS

**Contents**

Introduction 355
Sepsis 355
SIRS – classification 355
Systemic inflammation 356
MODS 357
Treatments 357
Reperfusion injury 359
Implications for practice 359
Summary 360
Further reading 360
Clinical scenarios 360

**Fundamental knowledge**

Vascular anatomy – function of tunica intima
Cellular pathology (see Chapter 24), especially
    inflammatory response
Shock (see Chapter 32)
Immunity (see Chapter 25)

## Introduction

Systemic Inflammatory Response Syndrome (SIRS), often leading to Multi-Organ Dysfunction Syndrome (MODS) remains the main cause of admission to most ICUs. Inappropriate and excessive inflammatory responses throughout the cardiovascular system may be triggered by micro-organisms (septic shock) or from non-infective causes. Inflammatory responses release vasoactive mediators, causing gross vasodilatation and increased capillary permeability ('capillary leak'), resulting in distributive shock, hypovolaemia, profound hypotension and, if not reversed, progressive organ failure. If two or more organs fail, MODS exists, prognosis becoming progressively worse.

Treatment and support of individual organs and systems follows those described in previous chapters, so are not repeated here. This chapter instead summarises progressive pathology, prognosis and issues specific to the syndrome, rather than individual aspects discussed elsewhere. Mechanisms of reperfusion injury, which can complicate recovery, are discussed.

## Sepsis

Sepsis is an identified bloodstream infection. Severe sepsis and extensive bloodstream infection provokes a systemic inflammatory response syndrome. Endotoxin, released by gram-negative bacteria, depresses myocardial function by 40 per cent (Parrillo, 2001). Inflammatory responses also release other myocardial depressant factors. Septic shock therefore forms part of the continuum from a trigger to SIRS:

$$\text{sepsis} \rightarrow \text{severe sepsis} \rightarrow \text{SIRS} \rightarrow \text{MODS}$$

However, with identified infection, septic shock can be treated by targeting the infection with appropriate antibiotics/microbials, *in addition* to system support for SIRS.

Severe sepsis, whether the cause of, or opportunistic to immunocompromise caused by systemic inflammatory responses, causes up to 15 per cent of ICU admissions (Manns *et al.*, 2002), up to one-half of patients dying (Annane *et al.*, 2004). Although sepsis is usually caused by gram-negative organisms, incidence of gram-positive sepsis, such as MRSA, has increased. Viruses or fungi, especially *Candida*, cause one-tenth of cases (Cohen *et al.*, 2004).

## SIRS – classification

Less than half of patients with sepsis-like symptoms have identifiable infections (Wort & Evans, 1999), but have non-infective triggers for systemic inflammatory responses, such as trauma (Faist & Kim, 1998) and severe pancreatitis (Murphy *et al.*, 2002). SIRS therefore focuses on the problem (the systemic inflammatory response) rather than the trigger. Managing SIRS should, however, include both system support (the response) and resolve any treatable trigger.

Problems cascade from individual responses, so the individual must have a *predisposition* to the response. This is unpredictable until it occurs. Some *insult* triggers the *response*, which causes *organ dysfunction* (Levy *et al.*, 2003). SIRS was defined as two or more of

- temperature >38 °C or <36 °C
- heart rate <90
- respiratory rate >20 or $PaCO_2$ <4.3 kPa
- leucocyte count >12,000 cells/mm$_3$, <4,000, or containing >10 per cent immature neutrophils.

(ACCP/SCCM, 1992; Bone *et al.*, 1992)

While these features are typical of SIRS, and this definition enabled early identification of and intervention for patients at risk, many patients on most wards have at least two of these criteria and yet do not need ICU admission. Levy *et al.* (2003) consider the 1992 criteria too non-specific, and therefore suggests alternative criteria for SIRS being some of

- infection – documented or suspected
- general – temperature, heart rate, respiratory rate, mental state, hyperglycaemia
- inflammatory – high/low white cell count, raised CRP, calcitonin
- haemodynamic – hypotension (BP <90 mmHg, MAP <60 mmHg), cardiac index >3.5, organ dysfunction, oliguria
- perfusion – raised lactate and others signs.

'Some' indicates at least two criteria should be present, but these criteria are even more vague than the earlier ones. Extensive inflammatory responses is often clinically obvious, but confirmed by various abnormal blood results, including raised C-reactive protein (CRP) (Lobo *et al.*, 2003) and white cell count (WCC) (see Chapter 21).

## Systemic inflammation

Tunica intima forms an active part of the cardiovascular system, releasing many vasoactive chemicals, including many involved in inflammatory responses. Inflammation is a homeostatic response, to protect against infection. When local responses occur throughout the cardiovascular system, this response becomes pathenogenic. Tunica intima releases chemicals which

- vasodilate
- increase capillary pore permeability
- trigger clotting.

As blood vessel capacity increases and blood volume reduces, perfusion to all organs and systems is compromised. The pro-coagulant state, combined with hypoperfusion, facilitates thrombus formation (Mavrommatis *et al.*, 2000; Warren *et al.*, 2002), which may progress to disseminated intravascular coagulation (see Chapter 26). Neutrophil activation, by tunica intima, increases oxygen consumption, releasing superoxide radicals (Molnar & Shearer, 1999), which are negatively inotropic.

SIRS therefore creates a downward spiral of

- hypotension
- hypovolaemia
- general hypoxia
- disseminated intravascular coagulation
- free radicals formation
- leucocyte activation
- erythrocyte damage
- increased blood viscosity
- oedema.

## MODS

Mutli-Organ Dysfunction Syndrome; sometimes called 'multi-organ failure' – MOF) is usually the refractory stage of SIRS/septic shock. The sequence of organ failure varies, but often starts with respiratory failure, a major cause of ICU admission. Low-grade liver failure is often under-recognised in ICU (see Chapter 42), so symptoms such as coagulopathies (including DIC), hypofibrinogenaemia and hypoalbuminaemia may not be noticed until progression to later stages. Cardiac and coronary artery diseases are endemic in Western society; many patients admitted to ICU have underlying cardiac failure. Mediators released during critical illness provoke cardiovascular failure. Systemic hypotension and hypoperfusion leads to hepatic and respiratory failure and renal failure, often (but not always) in that order.

There is no single treatment for MODS, but system support is attempted around each problem. A problem facing all systems is microcirculatory hypoperfusion, so tissue perfusion should be optimised, assessing needs through cardiac output study monitoring, and resuscitating with (colloid) fluids to achieve desired delivery and consumption of oxygen at tissue level ($DO_2$, $VO_2$).

Infection often causes MODS, but MODS also aggravates immunocompromise. This vicious circle makes infection control particularly important. MODS usually necessitates highly invasive monitoring and treatments, which provides access for further micro-organisms.

Failure of each vital organ carries significant mortality; mortality from MODS increases with the number of organs involved, failure of all four major organs (lungs, heart, liver, kidneys) being almost invariably fatal.

## Treatments

Human and financial cost of SIRS and MODS remains high, so much research has invested in finding solutions. Survival has improved, but remains poor, and solutions remain evasive. Treatment therefore focuses primarily on treating symptoms and preventing complications.

However caused, shock results in tissue hypoperfusion. Shock creates a syndrome of microcirculatory hypoperfusion, creating an 'oxygen debt'. Reversing oxygen debt improves survival. Despite improvements in monitoring technology, oxygen debt (the difference between oxygen demand and oxygen delivery) cannot directly be measured. Where possible, causes are identified and treated and systems supported. Treatment should focus on early and aggressive resuscitation:

- CVP 8–12 mmHg
- mean arterial pressure ≥65 mmHg
- urine output ≥0.5 ml/kg/hour
- central (or mixed) venous saturation ≥70 per cent (Dellinger *et al.*, 2004).

Aggressive fluid and inotrope therapy is often needed, and may be augmented by vasopressin/terlipressin (Patel *et al.*, 2002) or methylthioninium chloride (methylene blue) (Ghiassi *et al.*, 2004).

Gut mucosa normally receives 70 per cent of *intestinal blood flow* (Tham *et al.*, 2000). Immunoglobulins in the gut wall (IgA, IgM) help prevent pathogen translocation, while hepatic macrophages destroy bacteria that translocate into the hepatic portal vein. However, septic inflammatory response syndrome compromises all of these mechanisms by

- reducing gut perfusion (Tham *et al.*, 2000)
- gut wall atrophy causing hyposecretion of immunoglobulins
- hepatic hypoperfusion impairing kuppfer cell function.

Translocation of gut bacteria is therefore likely to cause or accelerate sepsis.

Gut function can be supported by increasing blood flow and stimulating function. Enteral nutrition should, whenever possible, be given to reduce bacterial translocation (see Chapter 9). Currently, dobutamine appears to be the most effective drug for improving blood flow to the gut (Tham *et al.*, 2000).

*Steroids* should theoretically reduce the inflammatory response that is the underlying problem, but most studies fail to show benefits. In 2002, Annane *et al.* found steroids beneficial, but by 2004 they concluded both that steroids at any dose over any duration failed to reduce mortality and, in apparent contradiction, long courses of low doses reduced 28 day mortality. Wort and Evans (1999) found mortality higher with steroid therapy. Most intensivitists do not prescribe steroids unless there is a specific indication, although the Surviving Sepsis Campaign (Dellinger *et al.*, 2004) recommends steroids for septic shock if adequate fluid has been given and vasopressors (e.g. noradrenaline) are required to maintain blood pressure.

*Plasmapheresis* (see Chapter 40), sometimes called 'high flow haemofiltration' (>35 ml/kg/hr) can remove cytokines and other inflammatory mediators such as TNFα (Busund *et al.*, 2002; Morgera *et al.*, 2003), but benefits are unclear (DeVriese *et al.*, 1999; Cariou *et al.*, 2004), and the Surviving Sepsis Campaign does not support using haemofiltration in the absence of renal failure (Dellinger *et al.*, 2004).

There have been many attempts to mediate abnormal or excessive chemical pathways that accelerate SIRS. Phospholipidase is activated by endotoxin, which then triggers platelet activating factor (Fisher, 2003). Inhibiting phospholipidase can break this cascade.

The endogenous vasodilator nitric oxide (NO) appears to be a major mediator in SIRS, so nitric oxide inhibitors have been developed (Murray *et al.*, 2000), But trials were terminated due to excessive mortality (Brealey & Singer, 2000).

Homeostasis is normally maintained by carefully balancing effects of opposing chemicals. Inflammation normally releases thrombomodulin, which activates protein C, and endogenous anti-inflammatory chemical released by vascular epithelium. SIRS inhibits thrombomodulin, so endogenous protein C levels become abnormally low despite extensive inflammation (Laterre, 2002). Giving exogenous activated protein C (drotrecogin alpha; Xigris®) mimics the missing endogenous homeostatic response. Activated protein C significantly reduces mortality in SIRS (Bernard *et al.*, 2001; Warren *et al.*, 2002; Barie *et al.*, 2004). APC reverses the procoagulant state of SIRS (Levy *et al.*, 2003), but excessive reversal can cause haemorrhage and strokes. Anticoagulants should not be given during APC infusions (Fourrier, 2004). Activated protein C is expensive, and although it appears to improve survival, mortality from SIRS remains high. There are some anecdotal reports that initial improvement is followed by deterioration after a few days.

## Reperfusion injury

Apparent recovery often leads to subsequent reversal. Reperfusion of ischaemic tissues which have survived through anaerobic metabolism flushes toxic oxygen metabolites and radicals into the cardiovascular system. These can trigger a further cascade of vasoactive and other endogenous chemicals (see Chapter 24). Therefore, apparent recovery can be reversed, one or more vital organs failing for a second time. Reperfusion injury is a complication of thrombolysis (from cardio-inhibitory mediators), but cerebral tissue is also particularly susceptible (survivors of MODS frequently suffer neurological damage and impaired function).

## Implications for practice

- SIRS, the most common pathology in most ICUs, is caused by inappropriate, systemic activation of inflammatory responses. This causes excessive vasodilatation, massive capillary leak and coagulopathy.
- CRP is a useful marker of inflammation.
- Vasodilatation usually necessitates vasoconstriction (inotropes/ vasopressures) and often flow monitoring (cardiac output studies).

■ Capillary leak necessitates aggressive fluid therapy, often with colloids, to maintain perfusion and prevent further organ dysfunction.

■ MODS results from pathological processes initiated at cellular level causing systemic inflammatory responses.

■ Many ICU patients develop MODS, so ICU monitoring and care of all patients should detect early signs of progressive organ failure; this is facilitated by holistic, rather than reductionist, careplanning.

■ Mortality rates from MODS remain very high, but early intervention to support failing systems (especially microcirculatory resuscitation) can improve survival.

■ Maintaining high standards of fundamental aspects of care, especially infection control, can reduce incidence and severity.

■ Apparent recovery may be confounded by reperfusion injury, so close monitoring of vital signs should continue after initial recovery.

■ Mortality reflects the number of major organs failing; multidisciplinary teams should consider whether prognosis justifies continued treatment (is death being prolonged); nurses should be actively involved in team decisions.

## Summary

Multiorgan dysfunction complicates many ICU admissions, incurring high human and financial costs. High incidence and paucity of curative (rather than supportive) treatment has encouraged a search for novel solutions. Such is the need that possible solutions are sometimes pursued with little (or even adverse) benefit. This chapter illustrates how progression from single to multiorgan failure remains the greatest challenge facing intensive care.

## Further reading

SIRS remains the most frequent 'ICU pathology'. The *Surviving Sepsis Campaign* has published evidence-based international guidelines (Dellinger *et al.*, 2004), and promises to update them annually. Articles on Sepsis, SIRS and MODS frequently appear – Gordon (1999), Brealey and Singer (2000) and Ruffell (2004) provide useful reviews.

Galley and Webster (2004) provide a useful summary of endothelial function and dysfunction, while Bernard *et al.*'s (2001) favourable study of activated protein C has encouraged its widespread adoption. www.routledge.com/textbooks/0415373239

For clinical scenarios, clinical questions and the answers to them go to the support website at www.routledge.com/textbooks/0415373239

## Clinical scenarios

Mr Reece Owen is a 71-year-old gentleman who was admitted to hospital with an acute exacerbation of COPD. His physical condition deteriorated necessitating admission to the ICU for closer monitoring, flow monitoring, intubation and mechanical ventilation. By the second day, he remains sedated and ventilated (PSIMV, PEEP of 10 cmH$_2$O, FiO$_2$ 0.6). Mr Owen has multiple cannulation sites for haemodynamic monitoring and administration of drugs. He has a urinary catheter in situ draining < 30 ml/hour and a chest drain for an exudative pleural effusion.

Observations on the second day include

| | |
|---|---|
| Temperature | 37.9 °C |
| Heart rate | 108 bpm |
| BP | 110/60 mmHg |
| CVP | 15 mmHg |
| CO | 5.4 litres/minute |
| CI | 2.92 litres/minute/m$^2$ |
| SV | 50 ml |
| SVI | 27 ml/beat/m$^2$ |
| SVR | 750 dynes/second/cm$^5$ |
| SVRI | 1387 dynes/second/cm$^5$/m$^2$ |
| ScvO$_2$ | 73% |
| DO$_2$I | 420 ml/minute/m$^2$ |

Blood results

| Haematology | | Biochemistry | | Arterial blood gas | |
|---|---|---|---|---|---|
| Hb | 8.5 g/dl | CRP | 135 mg/litre | pH | 7.26 |
| WBC | 24.0 × 10$^{-9}$/litre | Na$^+$ | 141 mmol/litre | PaCO$_2$ | 8.08 kPa |
| Neutrophils | 22.8 × 10$^{-9}$/litre | K$^+$ | 4.3 mmol/litre | PaO$_2$ | 12.2 kPa |
| Platelets | 200 × 10$^{-9}$/litre | Cl$^-$ | 109 mmol/litre | HCO$_3$ | 18.4 mmol/litre |
| | | HCO$_3$ | 20 mmol/litre | Base Ex | −7.5 mmol/litre |
| INR | 1.5 | Glucose | 9 mmol/litre | Lactate | 1.5 mmol/litre |
| APTTratio | >5.0 | Urea | 18.5 mmol/litre | | |
| TT | >100 secs | Creatinine | 326 μmol/litre | | |
| | | Albumin | 10 g/litre | | |

Q.1 Using Mr Owen's results identify variables associated with tissue perfusion, organ function and potential survival. Outline the key interventions and optimal goals using perfusion variables which may improve his outcome.

Q.2 Review the inclusion and exclusion criteria for activated protein C (drotrecogin alfa, Xigris®). Consider how Mr Owen would benefit from this therapy and identify possible adverse effects.

Q.3 Justify using renal replacement therapy with Mr Owen. Analyse the evidence supporting this therapy and review potential risks versus benefits for patient with SIRS.

*Same patient is used in scenario for Chapter 30.*

Chapter 34

# Fluid management

 **Contents**

| | |
|---|---|
| Introduction | 363 |
| Crystalloids | 364 |
| Perfusion | 365 |
| Colloids | 366 |
| Blood | 366 |
| Albumin | 367 |
| Other blood products | 368 |
| Gelatins | 368 |
| Dextran | 368 |
| Starches | 368 |
| Oxygen-carrying fluids | 369 |
| Implications for practice | 370 |
| Summary | 370 |
| Further reading | 371 |
| Clinical scenarios | 371 |

Most (60–80%) of the body is water. Body fluid is distributed between:

- extracellular
- intracellular

fluid, with extracellular fluid divided between

- intravascular
- interstitial

compartments. In health, the average adult may have

- 5 litres of blood (3 litres plasma + 2 litres cells)
- 12 litres of interstitial fluid
- 25 litres of intracellular fluid.

Water movement across capillaries is regulated by pressures, while most water movement across cell walls is actively controlled. In health, homeostasis maintains normal fluid balance. With ill-health, gross and problematic fluid imbalance can occur.

When selecting intravenous fluids, choice depends partly on whether the prime target is

- intravascular rehydration
- whole body rehdyration (especially intracellular)

how long the effect is needed for, and whether specific components (e.g. haemoglobin) are needed.

Fluids are usually divided into two main groups: crystalloids and colloids. Crystalloids are mainly water, with small-molecule solutes. Water extravases rapidly, so crystalloids provide extravascular hydration. Colloids have larger molecules, so remain longer within the intravascular compartment. Molecular size is indicated by molecular weight, usually measured in Daltons – Da, or kiloDaltons – kDa ('molecular weight' is slightly different, but approximates to Daltons). Longer intravascular half-life should make colloids preferable for intravascular resuscitation, although comparative benefits of different fluids continue to be debated. Table 34.1 summaries the main fluids. Duration of fluids' effect, like drugs, is measured by *half-life*, although effect in critically ill people is often noticeably shorter.

In good health, each day nearly five times total blood volume moves in and out of the cardiovascular system. Capillaries walls are semipermeable: thin, sqauemous (= scale-like) epithelium, with gaps between cells. Blood from arterioles has sufficient hydrostatic pressure to force water and small solutes

**Table 34.1 Summary of fluids (simplified)**

| Fluid | Half-life (hours) | KDa | COP (mmHg) | Benefits | Disadvantages |
|---|---|---|---|---|---|
| Crystalloids | $<\frac{1}{2}$ | NaCl 58.5 Glucose 180 | | Provide extravascular hydration | Aggravate oedema most are acidic |
| Blood | —— | —— | —— | Carries oxygen | Possible viral contamination |
| Albumin 4.5% | —— | 66.5 | 25 | No evidence of viral infection; hypoallergenic | Limited supply; exogenous albumin effect only transient as 4.5% |
| Albumin 20% | —— | 66.5 | 75–100 | Reduces oedema free radical scavenger | |
| Gelatins | 2–3 | 20–40 | | Cheap, stable during storage | Short half-life (for colloids) |
| Dextrans (almost obsolete) | 4–6 | 40–70 | | Promotes peripheral perfusion prevents thromboembolism | Coagulopathies allergic |
| Starches | 12–24 | 200–450 450 | 280–1088 | Prolonged effect; reduces oedema | Expensive, prolonged clearance |
| Oxygen carrying fluids | 6–48 | | | Can carry oxygen | Novel therapy with multiple problems; vary between products |

through the gaps in capillary walls. As capillary volume reduces, hydrostatic pressure falls, until extravasation ceases. Nearer the venule, large molecules (mainly plasma proteins, especially albumin) exert sufficient *osmotic* pressure to draw extravascular water back into capillaries. Osmotic pressure exerted within the bloodstream is called *colloid osmotic pressure* (COP). Pro-inflammatory mediators released during critical illness can increase capillary leak threefold (Nicholson *et al.*, 2000), while reduced COP draws less fluid back, resulting in both hypovolaemia and interstitial oedema.

## Crystalloids

Crystalloid fluids are water with small-molecule (below 10 kDa) solutes, such as 0.9% sodium chloride and 5% glucose. Small molecules and water readily diffuse across cell membranes, providing interstitial and intracellular hydration, one-fifth to one-tenth remaining in the intravascular compartment after half an hour (Haljamae & Lindgren, 2000), so provide total body hydration ('maintenance'), and are satisfactory for short-term intravascular resuscitation (Choi *et al.*, 1999). Intracellular sodium concentrations being low (about 14 mmol/litre) saline solutions largely remain in interstitial spaces, whereas glucose solutions, including glucose/saline, hydrate both interstitial and intracellular compartments. Crystalloids are less used for the persistent hypovolaemia often seen in ICU, where large volume infusion is three times more likely to cause pulmonary oedema with crystalloids than with colloids (Boldt, 2000a).

Most standard electrolytes are acidic – 0.9% sodium chloride pH 5.0, 5% glucose pH 4.1. This may exacerbate acidosis.

*Normal saline* largely extravases into interstitial spaces. Saline contains 154 mmol/litre of chloride (normal plasma concentration is about 95–105 mmol/litre), so saline infusion can cause hyperchloraemic metabolic acidosis (Durward *et al.*, 2001; Stephens & Mythen, 2003). Some promising studies suggest hypertonic (7.5%) saline may sustain intravascular volume (Järvelä *et al.*, 2003).

*5% glucose* is a little glucose (5 grams per 100 ml) and water. The water therefore moves freely, mainly into intracellular fluid, where most body water should normally be. Glucose solutions are therefore excellent intracellular rehydration solutions, but should be avoided with raised intracranial pressure (Eynon & Menon, 2002). It contains no electrolytes.

*Lactate* solutions (Hartmann's; Ringer's) contain similar electrolytes to plasma, but their main value is the lactate they contain. Lactate is metabolised by the liver into bicarbonate, so provided liver function is reasonable, lactate solutions buffer metabolic acidosis, hence their use during surgery (Wilkes *et al.*, 2001) or following trauma. Lactate solutions should be avoided during diabetic ketoacidosis, as the liver may metabolise lactate into further glucose (the Coricycle). Hartmann's should also be avoided with blood transfusion, as the calcium they contain may cause coagulation (Cooper & Cramp, 2003).

## Perfusion

Tissue perfusion is needed to supply nutrients to cells and remove waste products of metabolism. Tissue perfusion relies on pressure gradients across capillary walls. These gradients are the sum of

- resistance in tissues
- (mean) arterial blood pressure (MAP)
- colloid osmotic pressure.

At the arteriolar end, intracapillary pressure (average: 35 mmHg (Guyton & Hall, 2000)) exceeds combined interstitial and COP, forcing fluid into tissues. As fluid extravases, intracapillary pressure progressively falls, (average: 15 mmHg by venule end (Guyton & Hall, 2000)), so interstitial and COP force most fluid to return into the capillary.

Capillary permeability varies greatly, ranging from the blood–brain barrier (least permeable) to renal glomerular capillaries (most permeable). Glomeruli may filter positively-charged substances up to 70 kDa, although clearance rate reduces as molecular size increases. Plasma half-life of crystalloids (low molecular weight) is brief, and half-life of low molecular weight colloids

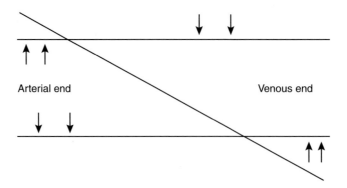

Arterial end

Venous end

**Figure 34.1 Perfusion gradients**

(e.g. gelatine) is limited. Fluids with larger molecular structures remain intravascularly until metabolised into smaller molecules (which can be excreted). So effects of intravascular fluids depends on molecular size and metabolic rate.

## Colloids

Colloids have large molecules. They may be grouped as:

- blood and blood products
- gelatins
- starches.

Each group having advantages and disadvantages, choice (and availability) depend on required effect and the benefit/burden balance. This chapter also describes

- oxygen-carrying artificial fluids

which have little effect on COP, and are not yet commonly used in clinical practice, but may be increasingly used in the near future.

## Blood

Blood for transfusion can be harvested from:

- donors
- recycling (usually perioperative) haemorrhage
- autotransfusion.

Finite resources of blood, together with various hazards, has caused reluctance to transfuse blood unless specific components (e.g. erythrocytes) are needed.

People can survive an 80 per cent loss of erythrocytes, but only a 30 per cent loss of blood volume, and slight anaemia improves perfusion, so blood is normally only given when haemoglobin is below 7 g/dl (Herbert *et al.*, 1999; McLellan *et al.*, 2003).

Donor blood being foreign protein, immunological reactions (both from cellular and plasma components) can occur. Although usually limited to mild fever and slight hypotension, anaphylactic shock can occur.

Cellular metabolism continues during storage. Without access to lungs, kidneys and other organs, progressive cell damage occurs. Hillman and Bishop (2004) suggest that changes to plasma from 35 days storage include

- pH 6.98
- hydrogen ions 106.1 mmol/litre (normal 25.1)
- sodium 155 mmol/litre
- potassium 30.0 mmol/litre
- ATP reduced to 55 per cent of normal quantity
- 2,3 DPG none remaining.

As cells recover following transfusion, intracellular concentrations normalise, potentially causing rebound hypokalaemia within 24 hours (Isbister, 2003).

Recombinant erythropoetin reduces need for blood transfusion, but is expensive, can take four weeks to be fully effective, and its risks and benefits for critical illness are relatively unknown (McLellan *et al.*, 2003). It is not currently widely used in ICU.

## Albumin

Exogenous albumin is normally supplied in two strengths: 4.5% (isotonic, 400 ml) and 20% (hypertonic/salt-poor, 100 ml). For colloid replacement, 4.5 per cent solution is used. Standard bottles contain 17–19 g of albumin in 400 ml. 100 ml of 25% albumin increases intravenous volume by about 450 ml (Boldt, 2000b).

Albumin is heat-treated, so there is no (known) risk of viral transmission (Boldt, 2000a). However, benefits of exogenous albumin are transient; sustained recovery necessitates adequate nutrition for endogenous production of albumin.

Unlike most other colloids, albumin is negatively charged, so is repelled by similarly negatively charged sialoproteins in glomerular capillaries. This normally prevents albumin being filtered by kidneys – glomerular filtrate albumin concentration is only 0.2 per cent of plasma concentration (Ganong, 2003), making protein normally absent on urinalysis. In health, 80 per cent of exogenous albumin remains intravascularly, expanding blood volume for about 24 hours; however, sepsis may limit this effect to little more than an hour.

The Cochrane Injuries Group Albumin Reviewers' (1998) meta-analysis finding that albumin infusion increased mortality has since been disproven (Boldt, 2000b; Wilkes & Navickis, 2001).

## Other blood products

Most blood components are available individually for transfusion, but most blood products (except albumin) carry potential for antigen–antibody reaction and virus infection, so are subject to similar cross-matching safeguards as blood, and are not given unless specifically indicated. Some of the most widely used blood products are Fresh Frozen Plasma (FFP) and platelets, given to reverse haemorrhage. Solvent detergent (SD) plasma, used in the UK, appears free of HIV and HBV, and may also have cytokines (which provoke SIRS) removed (Freeman, 1998). Platelets should be transfused over 30 minutes (British Society for Standards in Haematology, Blood Transfusion Task Force, 2003). Methylthioninium chloride (methylene blue) may be added to FFP to reduce risks of variant CJD (Williamson & Murphy, 2003).

## Gelatins

Gelatins (e.g. Haemaccel®, Gelofusine®), relatively inexpensive and stable plasma substitutes, are useful for resolving simple hypovolaemia, but have the lowest mean molecular weight of colloid fluids – four-fifths of molecules are below 20 kDa (Gutteridge, 2004). Being below renal threshold, this limits their half-life to 2–3 hours (Gutteridge, 2004). Like most fluids, gelatins are iso-osmotic, only expanding blood by the volume infused.

Gelatins are derived from beef extract. Ethical dilemmas of giving them to vegans were compounded by concerns over spread of bovine spongiform encephalopathy (BSE) and Creutzfeld-Jakob Syndrome (CJD). The UK Spongiform Encephalopathy Advisory Committee claim gelatins are safe as they derive from the USA, or UK certified BSE-free herds (Mythen, 2003)

## Dextran

Dextran 40 and Dextran 70 (numbers referring to molecular weight) have largely fallen into disuse. Hypertonic saline dextran (HSD – 7.5 per cent sodium chloride + 6 per cent dextran 70) draws fluid from the extravascular spaces, increasing blood volume by four times the amount infused, and sustains intravascular volume for 3–6 hours. HSD also contains oxygen-free radical scavengers which reduce inflammation (Bradley, 2001a).

## Starches

Starch has a complex chemical structure, giving solutions high molecular weights:

- Pentaspan® 250 kDa
- eloHAES® 200 kDa

- Hemohes (Pentastarch®) 200 kDa
- HAES-steril® 200 kDa
- Voluven 130 kDa.

All starches exceed renal threshold, so remain intravascularly until metabolised (half-lifes of many being about 24 hours). COP of Pentastarch®, the active component of HAES-steril® and Pentaspan®, is 40 mmHg (McDaniel & Prough, 1996), drawing extravascular water back into blood. Because of their prolonged effect, doses are usually limited to 500–1000 ml per day.

Adverse effects of most starches include

- anaphylaxis
- extravasation causing gross oedema from prolonged intravascular osmotic pressure
- coagulopathies (Ekesth *et al.*, 2002)
- hypervolaemia from overinfusion (most units limit to 1 l per patient per day)
- circulatory overload in patients with impaired ventricular function
- long-term pruritis (Morgan & Berridge, 2000; Boldt, 2000a).

Cost, compared to other artificial colloids, also discourages use.

## Oxygen-carrying fluids

Current plasma expanders increase blood volume without increasing oxygen-carrying capacity, resulting in dilutional anaemia. Blood transfusion creates hazards, and supply and shelf-life are limited. Oxygen-carrying fluids attempt to resolve both these problems.

Oxygen-carrying fluids may be grouped as

- haemoglobin derivatives
- chemical (e.g. perfluorocarbon – see Chapter 29).

There are three types of haemoglobin derivatives:

- free haemoglobin (from human blood bank or bovine sources)
- recombinant haemoglobin (genetically engineered *E. coli*)
- modified haemoglobins (e.g. cross-linked haemoglobins).

While haemoglobin derivatives carry oxygen, absence of 2,3 DPG assists oxygen dissociation as tissue level. Haemoglobin being 'free' from erythrocytes, derivatives lack antigenic effects of blood, so cross-matching is unnecessary (Remy *et al.*, 1999). Haemoglobin derivative half-life is 6–8 hours, which although longer than gelatins, limits their usefulness (Vlahakes, 2001). Free deoxyhaemoglobin is highly susceptible to oxidation, so causes oxidative damage, and releases oxygen radicals and other mediators released (Creteur *et al.*, 2000). Free haemoglobin also provides bacteria with a source of iron, so may cause immunocompromise (Creteur *et al.*, 2000).

Oxygen-carrying fluids exert little colloidal osmotic pressure, so are not 'colloids'. Currently, there are many problems and limitations to both groups (e.g. short duration of action, limited oxygen carriage). Limited licences have been granted in the USA; Phase 3 trials show favourable results (Spahn *et al.*, 2002; Sprung *et al.*, 2002), so clinical use may be near.

## Implications for practice

- Prescription of fluid remains a medical decision, but nurses are professionally responsible and accountable for all fluids they administer (so should be aware of efficacy and adverse effects) and their choice of route (e.g. central or peripheral).
- Crystalloid fluid is needed for whole-body hydration.
- Normal saline largely hydrate interstitial spaces; glucose solutions largely hydrate intracellular spaces.
- Colloids have higher molecular weights, so remain for longer in intravascular spaces and may reduce oedema formation (including pulmonary oedema).
- Increasing COP draws extravascular fluid into the intravascular compartment.
- Hypoalbuminaemia reduces COP, hence reducing venous return; giving exogenous albumin only causes transitory increases of serum albumin levels; endogenous production, with adequate nutrition, is the most effective long-term treatment for hypoalbuminaemia.

## Summary

Nurses should recognise advantages and disadvantages of fluids used. Glucose solutes are free water, moving mainly into cells. Saline solutions move mainly into interstitial spaces. Colloids remain largely in intravascular fluid. Extravascular hydration is needed, so most ICU patients receive maintenance crystalloid. But fluid imbalances frequently occur in ICU, with excessive extravascular fluid (oedema) together with hypovolaemia.

Choice of colloids falls into three groups. Blood and blood products usually essential are specific components that are needed, but most carry potential risks of viral transmission. Blood transfusion also creates further complications. Gelatins are useful both for their relative cheapness and stability, but have the shortest half-life of all colloids, so are of limited use for critically ill patients. Starch solutions having the heaviest molecular weight of all colloids are clinically the most useful for volume replacement, but expense and side effects limit their use. Oxygen-carry solutions promise to be a useful development for the not too distant future, but are not yet licensed for UK use.

## Further reading

Most textbooks include chapters of colloids and/or fluid replacement. The British Society for Standards in Haematology, Blood Transfusion Task Force (2003) provide authoritative guidelines on platelet transfusion. Gutteridge's (2004) medical review is comprehensive, while Bradley (2001a) revisits the crystalloid/colloid debate. Farrar and Grocott (2003) and Mackenzie and Bucci (2004) discuss oxygen-carrying fluids. www.routledge.com/textbooks/0415373239

For clinical scenarios, clinical questions and the answers to them go to the support website at www.routledge.com/textbooks/0415373239

## Clinical scenarios

Mr Kenneth McDowall is a 48-year-old known smoker, who had spent an afternoon drinking alcohol and watching sports with friends. While preparing an outdoor barbeque later that day, he collapsed onto the grill, which overturned dropping hot charcoal onto Mr McDowall. He sustained extensive burns down the right side of his head and body.

Mr McDowall was admitted unconscious, vasoconstricted, diaphoretic with full-thickness burns. His ECG on admission revealed large left ventricular infarcted area. Other results included tachycardia (130 bpm), BP 100/78 mmHg, CVP 10 mmHg, tachypnoeic (26 breaths/min) arterial blood gas showed good oxygenation with uncompensated respiratory acidosis, Na+ 148 mmol/litre, K+ 4.5 mmol/litre, blood glucose 12 mmol/litre. He is cannulated with one peripheral cannulae and quad CVC in left jugular vein.

Q.1 Identify the signs which indicate Mr McDowall needs fluid management.

Q.2 Select an appropriate crystalloid & colloid to infuse. Justify this choice, the intravenous route, rate of infusion and list expected effects (include benefits and limitations).

Q.3 Reflect on how fluid challenges are administered in your clinical area (type & volume of fluid, rate and route, use of dynamic indicators or a protocol).

# Chapter 35

# Inotropes and vasopressors

## Contents

Introduction                                     373
Indications                                      373
Receptors                                        374
Safety                                           375
mcg/kg/min                                       376
Adrenaline (epinephrine)                         376
Noradrenaline (norepinephrine)                   377
Dobutamine                                       377
Dopexamine (hydrochloride)                       377
Dopamine                                         378
Phosphodiesterase inhibitors (PDIs)              378
Some other drugs                                 379
Implications for practice                        379
Summary                                          380
Further reading                                  380
Clinical scenarios                               380

## Fundamental knowledge

Sympathetic nervous system
Negative feedback and parasympathetic effect
Renin-angiotensin-aldosterone mechanism

## Introduction

Inotropes are frequently used to maintain adequate blood pressure in critically ill patients. Inotropes (*inos* = 'fibre' in Greek) alter stretch of cardiac and arteriole muscle fibres. Vasopressors (also called 'vasoconstrictors') stimulate vasoconstriction. These effects are mediated through stimulation of the sympathetic nervous system.

Some drugs and other chemicals are described as negative inotropes – for example, digoxin, beta-blockers, tumour necrosis factor, acidosis (especially pH <7.2), but 'inotrope' without any prefix usually presume positive inotropes, drugs which increase muscle fibre stretch, hence increasing cardiac stroke volume or systemic vascular resistance. This chapter discusses only positive inotropes. Blood pressure is the sum volume (cardiac output) multiplied by resistance (systemic vascular resistance, or 'afterload'). Cardiac output is the amount of blood ejected by the left ventricle each minute, so is heart rate multiplied by stroke volume. So

$$BP = HR \times SV \times SVR$$

Provided other factors remain constant, increasing one factor necessarily increases blood pressure. Inotropes increase systemic blood pressure by increasing stroke volume (myocardial stretch) and/or systemic vascular resistance (vasoconstriction).

Positive inotropes may be divided into two main groups:

■  adrenergic agonists (inoconstrictors)
■  phosphodiesterase inhibitors (inodilators).

In ICU adrenergic agonists are used most.

Although the UK has now adopted international names for most drugs, it retains the traditional UK names for adrenaline (elsewhere, 'epinephrine') and noradrenaline (elsewhere, 'norepinephrine').

## Indications

Inotropes and vasopressors are used to increase blood pressure. However, blood volume (CVP) should be optimised before using positive inotropes, as increasing cardiac work, when it has little to work, increases myocardial ischaemia without any benefit. Many patients are hypovolaemic on admission to ICU.

Adrenaline is a first-line drug for cardiac arrest, increasing heart rate, stroke volume and systemic vascular resistance, the three factors that create blood pressure. Other than cardiac arrest, inotropes should only be used where patients can be safely monitored.

## Receptors

The heart and blood vessels contain various types of receptors, many of which have subtypes. Inotropes primarily stimulate either alpha ($\alpha$) or beta ($\beta$) receptors, although none are so pure to solely target only one.

Alpha receptors are located mainly in arterioles and veins, especially in peripheries. Alpha stimulation (e.g. with noradrenaline) causes arteriolar vasoconstriction, hence increasing systemic vascular resistance. Alpha stimulation has little effect on cerebral, coronary and pulmonary bloodflow, hence maintaining perfusion to vital organs.

Alpha stimulation may adversely affect many major organs:

■ heart (dysrhythmias, ischaemia, infarction)
■ pancreas (reduced insulin secretion, causing hyperglycaemia)
■ liver (accentuating immunocompromise and coagulopathies)
■ kidneys (renal failure)
■ gut (translocation of gut bacteria)
■ skin (peripheral blanching or cyanosis; extreme ischaemia may precipitate gangrene, necessitating amputation of digits).

Alpha stimulants are usually given to counter excessive vasodilatation, but excessive vasoconstriction may cause peripheral blanching/cynanosis and cold peripheries. Flow monitoring (cardiac output studies) can estimate systemic vascular resistance.

Beta ($\beta$) receptors are found primarily in the heart and lungs. Beta$_1$ receptors in pacemaker cells, have a *chronotropic* effect; $\beta_1$ receptors on myocardial cells have an inotropic effect. Beta$_1$ stimulation increases cell membrane permeability, hence increasing spontaneous muscle depolarisation. Effects of $\beta_1$ stimulation include

■ increased contractility
■ improved atrioventricular conduction
■ quicker relaxation of myocardium
■ increased stroke volume
■ increased heart rate (with potential dysrhythmias)

and so increased cardiac output.

Beta$_2$ receptors are found mainly in bronchial smooth muscle, but a significant minority are also found in myocardium. Beta$_2$ stimulation is especially chronotropic, increasing myocardial workload and predisposing to dysrhythmias (hence tachycardic/dysrhythmic effects of bronchodilators such as salbutamol). Beta$_2$ receptors are also found in other smooth muscles, such as blood vessels and skeletal muscle. When stimulated, these $\beta_2$ receptors vasodilate arterioles and reduce systemic vascular resistance (afterload).

Beta$_3$ receptors are found in the heart, gall bladder, skeletal muscle and gut. Unlike $\beta_1$ and $\beta_2$ receptors, $\beta_3$ receptors are negatively inotropic when

**Table 35.1 Main target receptors for drugs**

| Effect of stimulation | α vasoconstrict | β₁ (heart) increase cardiac output | β₂ (mainly lungs) bronchodilate | Da (dopamine) renal vasodilation |
|---|---|---|---|---|
| Adrenaline | ✓ | ✓ | ✓ | |
| Noradrenaline | ✓ | | | |
| Dobutamine | | ✓ | | |
| Dopamine | (variable) | ✓ | | ✓ |

stimulated (Moniotte *et al.*, 2001). The number of $\beta_3$ receptors increase with cardiac failure, although decreased contractility is disproportionate to the increase in $\beta_3$ receptors (Moniotte *et al.*, 2001). Beta$_3$ receptors are not significant for inotropic therapy.

Prolonged $\beta_1$ (although not $\beta_2$) stimulation causes '*down regulation*' (Moniotte *et al.*, 2001) or tachyphylaxis – progressive destruction of beta receptors, requiring progressively larger doses of inotropes to achieve the same effect. Destruction starts within minutes of exposure to stimulants, reaching clinically significant levels by 72 hours (Sherry & Barham, 1997). Beta receptors regrow once beta stimulation is removed (Sherry & Barham, 1997).

Main receptor sites targeted are summarised in Table 35.1, although no inotropes purely target only one receptor.

## Safety

Most inotropes have very short half-lives (often 2–5 minutes), and cause profound changes to blood pressure. They should therefore only be used in areas where

- ■ blood pressure and ECG can be monitored continuously (or at least every 5 minutes)
- ■ sufficient staff are available to observe monitors
- ■ staff have sufficient knowledge to understand significance of observations and know how to resolve excessive or insufficient effects.

Appropriate alarm limits should be set on monitors. Effectively, this usually limits inotrope use to ICUs and a few other designated specialist areas, such as CCUs and theatres.

Like most drugs, inotropes are heavier than the fluids they are diluted in, so if given through volumetric pumps may precipitate to the base of bags. When patients are dependent on large doses, interruptions when changing infusions can cause life-threatening hypotension, so many units have a second infusion ready to run ('double pumping'). If changing strength of infusions, deadspace in lines contains a small volume of the previous concentration.

Some inotropes should be dissolved in 5% glucose. Most units dissolve all inotropes in glucose solutions, both reducing risks of error and enabling often limited venous access to be shared by more than one inotrope.

Although some inotropes can be infused peripherally, in practice, they are usually given centrally as poor peripheral circulation and possible alpha vasoconstriction may cause pooling of drugs in peripheries and extravasation into tissues. Lines should be clearly labelled and no bolus or short-term drugs given through lines containing inotropes.

## mcg/kg/min

Traditionally inotropes were measured in micrograms (*mcg* or *μcg*) per kilogram per minute (see later), or variants (e.g. micrograms per minute):

$$\text{mcg/kg/minute} = \frac{\text{mg}}{\text{ml}} \times \frac{1000}{\text{patient's weight}} \times \frac{\text{infusion rate (ml/hour)}}{60}$$

This formula can be expressed in various other ways, for example,

$$\frac{\text{mcg/kg/minute}}{1000} \times \frac{\text{ml}}{\text{mg}} \times \text{patient's weight} \times 60 = \text{infusion rate}$$

So if 500 mg dobutamine is diluted in 250 ml runs at 9 ml/hour for a patient weighing 75 kg:

$$\text{mcg/kg/minute} = \frac{500\,\text{mg}}{250\,\text{ml}} \times \frac{1000}{75} \times \frac{9}{60} = 2 \times \frac{40}{3} \times \frac{3}{20}$$

$$= 2 \times 2 = 4\,\text{mcg/kg/minute}$$

Some units have replaced these potentially cumbersome calculations with simpler measurements (e.g. recording milligrams, as with most other drugs), titrating amounts given to achieve desired effects (e.g. mean arterial pressure). Adequate perfusion pressure being the desired goal, benefits of investing nursing time in complex calculations is questionable, especially with calculations based on estimated weights, which necessitate recalculation when one guess is replaced by another.

## Adrenaline (epinephrine)

The adrenal medulla produces two hormones, both called 'catecholamines'. Adrenaline, the main adrenal medullary hormone, stimulates alpha, $\beta_1$ and $\beta_2$ receptors, triggering the 'fight or flight' stress response via the sympathetic nervous system:

- vasoconstriction (alpha receptors)
- increased cardiac output ($\beta_1$, $\beta_2$).

Acting on both alpha and beta receptors, adrenaline effectively increases all factors contributing to blood pressure, improving bloodflow to coronary and cerebral arteries (Jowett & Thompson, 2003). This makes it valuable for resuscitation from cardiac arrest, where immediate short-term restoration of systemic blood pressure and circulation is essential. Low-dose adrenaline (0.04–0.1 mcg/kg/minute) mainly stimulates (β receptors, while higher dose mainly affects α receptors (Darovic & Simonelli, 2003). Its bronchodilatory qualities (β$_2$) make nebulised adrenaline useful during asthma crises, especially with children. Its use in ICU varies, but it is the cheapest inotrope (Grebenik & Sinclair, 2003) and for many units the catecholamine of choice (Grebenik & Sinclair, 2003).

Adrenaline can cause gross tachycardia, ventricular dysrhythmias, hyperglycaemia, prerenal failure, increased lactate, hypokalaemia, hypophosphataemia and other metabolic complications, so although a first-line drug for resuscitation from myocardial infarction, is not widely used in most ICUs.

## Noradrenaline (norepinephrine)

Noradrenaline primarily stimulates alpha receptors, causing intense arteriolar vasoconstriction, so noradrenaline is useful to normalise systemic vascular resistance (Martin et al., 2000; Kellum & Pinsky, 2003). Normalising afterload significantly improves coronary and renal perfusion (Di Giantomasso et al., 2002). Ideally, doses will be titrated to systemic vascular resistance measurements from flow monitoring; however, low diastolic blood pressure often provides an adequate indication of vascular resistance. Nurses should therefore observe peripheries for perfusion, and delayed capillary refill, pale/mottled skin or cold digits should be reported.

Noradrenaline appears to have fewer metabolic complications (e.g. lactate, glycaemia) than adrenaline. Extravasation of noradrenaline can cause necrosis and peripheral gangrene, so it should be given centrally.

## Dobutamine

Dobutamine, a synthetic analogue of dopamine, is primarily a β$_1$ stimulant. It does have some β$_2$ and α effects, but is less chronotropic and dysrhythmic than most β$_1$ inotropes. It reduces systemic vascular resistance, so together with increased cardiac output, increases oxygen delivery to cells (Eliott, 2003). It is the first-line choice inotrope for ischaemic heart failure (Copper & Cramp, 2003) and septic shock (Beale et al., 2004; Dellinger et al., 2004). Dobutamine also increases diaphragm muscle contractility, so infusion may be useful treatment for diaphragmatic failure (Smith-Blair et al., 2003), although it is not widely used for this at present. Despite these advantages, popularity of dobutamine appears to have waned in practice.

## Dopexamine (hydrochloride)

Dopexamine, a synthetic dopamine derivative, primarily causes arterial vasodilatation (β$_2$ agonist) with weak β$_1$ and dopaminergic effects. Claimed renal and splanchnic benefits appear doubtful (Renton & Snowden, 2005) and it is relatively expensive. It can be given peripherally, but being irritant should be given through a large vein. Its half-life is 5–10 minutes.

## Dopamine

Dopamine is an endogenous catecholamine and noradrenaline precursor. There are specific dopamine receptors ($DA_1$), but dopamine also stimulates alpha and beta receptors. Receptor targeting is partly dose-dependent, but dopamine provides no protection against gut ischaemia (Azar *et al.*, 1996) or renal failure (Australian & New Zealand Intensive Care Society Clinical Trials Group, 2000; Marik, 2002). Exogenous dopamine impairs immunity (Van den Berge & De Zegher, 1996; Grebenik & Sinclair, 2003) and gut motility (Dive *et al.*, 2000). It is therefore rarely used.

Insufficient brain stem production causes neurotransmission failure in Parkinson's disease, but dopamine cannot permeate mature blood–brain barriers (Van den Bergh & De Zehger, 1996), so intravenous dopamine does not affect cerebral receptors.

## Phosphodiesterase inhibitors (PDIs)

Phosphodiesterase is an intracellular enzyme which prolongs cardiac and coronary artery contraction. Inhibiting phosphdiasterase therefore

- increases ventricular filling
- improves myocardial oxygenation
- vasodilates (reduces afterload).

Phosphodiasterase inhibitors combine mild inotropic effects with significant vasodilatation, so are called *inodilators*.

PDIs are protein-bound, giving them half-lifes of about 45 minutes, but also usually necessitating loading doses. Unlike inotropes, they do not rely on receptor site stimulation, so down-regulation does not occur. While useful for cardiology, PDIs have limited value for the ICU, but may be useful for weaning from inotropes. The most widely used PDI is Milrinone/Primacor® (Grebenik & Sinclair, 2003). Calcium sensitizers (e.g. Levosimendan) enhance intracellular contraction.

Adverse effects of PDIs include

- thrombocytopaenia
- gastrointestinal disturbances
- hepatic dysfunction/failure
- dysrhythmias
- hypotension.

## Some other drugs

Some centres use various drugs to 'test' response to, or augment, noradrenaline:

- Methylthioninium chloride (formerly called 'methylene blue' in the UK) (Fielden, 2003; Ghiassi *et al.*, 2004).
- Vasopressin (synthetic anti-diuretic hormone; synacthen) (Holmes *et al.*, 2001; Marik & Zalaga, 2002; Dellinger, 2003).

Steroids enhance inotropes, so current guidelines recommend giving steroid supplements during inotrope therapy (Annane *et al.*, 2002; Dellinger *et al.*, 2004). Vasopressin, with methylprednisolone and thyroxin (T3), is used during transplant retrieval to stabilise organs (Rosendale *et al.*, 2003).

## Implications for practice

- Before commencing drugs to increase blood pressure, blood volume should be optimise, preferably with colloids, to achieve CVP of 10 mmHg (or higher with positive pressure ventilation, PEEP, or chronic heart failure).
- Most inotropes should be diluted in 5% glucose (to prevent oxidation) before preparation.
- Although some (not all) inotropes may be given peripherally, with hypoperfusion (e.g. SIRS) central administration is usually safer, and is generally used in the ICU.
- Within prescribed limits, inotrope doses should be titrated to achieve desired effects, while minimising adverse effects.
- Noradrenaline increases systemic vascular resistance.
- Dobutamine increases cardiac output.
- Adrenaline increases both systemic vascular resistance and cardiac output.
- Methylthioninium chloride and vasopressin increase systemic vascular resistance.
- Inotropes have less effect with acidosis.
- Most inotropes (but not phosphodiesterase inhibitors) have half-lives of only a very few minutes, so should only be used where continuous blood pressure and ECG monitoring is available, where there are sufficient staff to observe monitors, and where staff are familiar with using the drugs.
- With alpha stimulants, monitor peripheral ischaemia. Ideally, measure systemic vascular resistance (flow monitoring), but visual and tactile observation of patients' peripheries is a useful adjunct.
- Many patients become highly dependent on inotropes, becoming hypotensive when infusions are changed; a 'spare' syringe ('double pumping') can reduce changeover time of infusions, so minimising hypotensive effects.
- Traditional practices of measuring inotropes by body weight and calculations, rather than monitored effect, should be reconsidered, especially where units lack facilities to accurately weigh patients on a regular basis.

## Summary

Drugs and chemicals inhibiting myocardial contraction are labelled 'negative inotropes'; drugs increasing muscle contraction should be called 'positive inotropes', but practice usually limits the label 'inotropes' to positive inotropes.

Central blood pressure can be increased by increasing heart rate (chronotrope), increasing stroke volume ($\beta_1$ stimulation or phosphodiesterase inhibition) or increasing systemic vascular resistance (alpha stimulation). Beta$_1$ stimulation, the traditional mainstay on inotrope practice, creates problems of down-regulation, necessitating progressively higher doses.

For $\beta_1$ stimulation, most units rely on dobutamine or adrenaline. Alpha stimulation (from adrenaline or noradrenaline) can usefully raise central blood pressure by increasing systemic vascular resistance, but complications from peripheral (and gut) ischaemia should be considered.

## Further reading

Medical reviews of inotropes include Eliot (2003), Kellum & Pinsky (2002) and Steel and Bihari (2000). Dellinger *et al.* (2004) provide authoritative guidelines. www.routledge.com/textbooks/0415373239

For clinical scenarios, clinical questions and the answers to them go to the support website at www.routledge.com/textbooks/0415373239

## Clinical scenarios

Mrs Caroline Williams, 53 years old, is admitted post laporotomy for faecal peritonitis. During induction she had a cardiac arrest and three cycles of CPR performed. Mrs Williams has no previous cardiac history, is 1.6 m tall and weights 70 kg. She is six days post op, remains sedated and invasively ventilated with signs of septic shock. Arterial blood gas indicates severe metabolic acidosis with pH of 6.9.

Her haemodynamic results include:

| | | |
|---|---|---|
| Temperature | 38.5 °C | |
| BP | 135/72 mmHg (MAP 93 mmHg) | |
| HR | 100 bpm | |
| CVP | 16 mmHg | |
| Stroke Volume | 52 ml | |
| Cardiac Output | 5.4 ml/minute | Cardiac Index *to* |
| SVR | 900 dynes/sec/m$^{-5}$ | *be calculated* |
| SVRi | 1600 dynes/sec/m$^{-5}$/m$^2$ | |
| DO$_2$I | 455 ml/minute/m$^2$ | |

Mrs Williams has continuous infusions of noradrenaline (at 0.19 mcg/kg/minute), hydrocortisone (10 mg/hour) and dopexamine (1.0 mcg/kg/minute) in progress.

Q.1 Describe the therapeutic actions of Mrs Williams' vasoactive drug infusions. Explain their action on specific receptor sites and intended effects. Consider their effect on her haemodynamic values (increase or decrease SV, CO, SVR, $DO_2I$ etc.)

Q.2 Identify other parameters which should be assessed and recorded when evaluating effectiveness (and monitoring for adverse effects) of Mrs Williams'.

Q.3 Over the day, noradrenaline and dopexamine infusion rates are increased. A decision was taken to introduce milnirone and discontinue the dopexamine infusion. Justify the rationale for this change and review approach used when introducing and discontinuing these specific drugs.

Chapter 36

# Vascular surgery

### Contents

Introduction                         383
Aneurysms                            383
Carotid artery disease               384
Nursing care                         385
Implications for practice            387
Summary                              387
Further reading                      387
Clinical scenarios                   388

### Fundamental knowledge

Pathology of atherosclerosis
Thrombolysis (see Chapter 30)
Sternotomy (see Chapter 31)
Anatomy and physiology of large arteries (including aorta,
    femoral, carotid, renal artery)
Pathology of connective tissue disease
How and where to assess pedal pulses

## Introduction

Vascular disease is common, frequently needing medical or surgical intervention, only a few of which usually necessitate ICU admission:

- aneurysm repair
- carotid artery repair.

In addition to needs created by often prolonged and major operations, surgery on major arteries creates risks from

- major bleeds
- organ and tissue damage from perioperative ischaemia distal to the repair
- thrombus/embolus formation (especially strokes)
- patients often having extensive vascular and other diseases that complicate recovery.

Traditionally, surgery involved grafting a synthetic prosthesis (aortic tube graft) into the vessel, but increasingly, major vessels are being repaired through endovascular insertion of fabric or metal stents, inserted through catheters similar to those used for angioplasty. Percutaneous approaches are quicker, create fewer complications, and can be performed with light sedation rather than a general anaesthetic (Latessa, 2002; Prinssen *et al.*, 2004), so seldom need ICU admission. Although endovascular repair mortality is lower (Gravereaux *et al.*, 2002), stenting may not be possible with tortuous, calcified vessels (Carrell & Wolfe, 2005).

Some aspects mentioned in this chapter are covered in other chapters (see Fundamental knowledge), so are not duplicated here.

## Aneurysms

'Aneurysm' means 'widening' (Greek), but traditional concepts of aneurysms simply stretching vessel walls have been replaced by recognition that vessels are remodelled, or grow (Baxter, 2004), usually from atherosclerosis. Progressive deposits eventually separate the wall's layers, causing haemorrhage and rupture. Atherosclerosis being an inflammatory process (Alexander & Franciosa, 2003), C-reactive protein is elevated (Verma *et al.*, 2004). Local inflammation frequently causes pleural effusions. Immediate treatment of aneurysms usually includes antihypertensives, such as beta-blockers, but earlier drug interventions may enable prevention or limitation of atherosclerosis. A minority of aneurysms are caused by trauma, bacterial or fungal infections, and other problems.

Aneurysms can, and do, occur in any vessel, but are usually most life-threatening when they occur in the aorta, carotid arteries or cerebral circulation. Cerebral aneurysms are not described in this chapter. Surgery is usually only indicated if aortic aneurysms exceed 5 cm in diameter (Carrell & Wolfe, 2005).

Aortic aneurysm rupture is a surgical emergency with high mortality, but is almost invariably fatal without intervention (Tambyraja & Chalmers, 2004). Three-quarters of aortic aneurysms are abdominal (AAA or 'triple A'), but thoracic aneurysms may occur in the ascending or descending aorta.

Renal compromise, both from the disease and surgery/repair, stimulates the renin–angiotensin–aldosterone cascade (Adembri et al., 2004), exacerbating problems from hypertension. Open surgery necessitates cross-clamping the aorta. Most abdominal aneurysms occur below the renal artery, so clamps can normally be placed below the renal artery, preserving renal perfusion. But higher aneurysms necessitate clamping above the renal artery which may cause acute tubular necrosis. With endovascular repair, intrarenal damage may be caused by obstruction from the endograft or nephrotoxic dyes, and so damage may accelerate after admission to the ICU. Acute renal failure significantly increases post-operative mortality – possibly tenfold (Jacobs et al., 2004).

Mortality and morbidity from ascending aortic repair is very high, partly because it precedes the carotid arteries, but also because it usually involves aortic vale disease, and so patients need simultaneous aortic valve replacement. For this reason, repair is usually undertaken in specialist centres by cardiothoracic, rather than vascular, surgeons. The ascending aorta stretches from the aortic valve to the carotid arteries, and is especially susceptible to aneurysm in people with Marfan's syndrome (Ranasinghe & Bonser, 2004) and other connective tissue disease. Surgery compromises cerebral perfusion, unless cardiopulmonary bypass is used, so few centres outside cardiothoracic centres undertake this operation. Endovascular approaches may offer a viable alternative provided valve replacement is not needed, but may occlude the brachiocephalic, common carotid and subclavian arteries.

Repair of descending thoracic aortic aneurysms has traditionally involved grafting through left thoracotomy, often a six hour operation (Latessa, 2002) with 5 per cent mortality (Carrell & Wolfe, 2005). Endovascular repair can be completed in one to two hours (Latessa, 2002). 'Endoleak' – blood flowing within the aneursym sac but outside the graft – frequently occurs following surgical or endovascular repair (Veith et al., 2002).

## Carotid artery disease

Atheromatous plaques frequently form in the carotid artery, especially in older people. About one-tenth of people aged over 80 have carotid artery stenosis (Carrell & Wolfe, 2005). Stenosis reduces cerebral bloodflow, so may cause ischaemic strokes. Carotid endarterectomy is an effective way to prevent strokes (Davis et al., 2004). Restenosis, from intimal hyperplasia, frequently occurs, but can be reduced by a small dose of topical Saratin (leech extract) (Davis et al., 2004).

Trauma, such as from sports injuries, may cause carotid artery dissection, one of the most common causes of strokes in people under 50 years of age

(Epley, 2001). Dissection is initially treated with thrombolysis (rt-PA), with endovascular stenting or (rarely) surgical repair if this fails (Epley, 2001). An embolus-protecting device is usually inserted (Yadav *et al.*, 2004). Incidence of post-operative strokes is similar with both endovascular stenting (transluminal angioplasty) and open surgical grafting (Brown *et al.*, 1999) – 3.1 per cent (Halliday *et al.*, 2004), but percutaneous surgery causes less nerve damage and so creates fewer cardiac complications (Brown, 1999).

### Nursing care

In addition to system support, specific individual needs and standard post-operative care (such as observing wound site/dressings), patients with vascular disease are especially susceptible to complications from perfusion failure. Vascular surgery creates the problem of maintaining sufficient perfusion pressure (in patients who usually have extensive vascular disease) while preventing graft damage from excessive pressure. The most common cause of post-operative death is myocardial infarction, often from unidentified coronary artery disease (Carrell & Wolfe, 2005).

To optimise perfusion, mean arterial pressure is usually maintained at 70 mmHg, with perfusion being monitored primarily through urine output (aim >0.5 ml/kg/hour) and observing peripheries distal to the surgical site. Peripheries should be checked for perfusion and possible nerve damage by assessing

- colour
- warmth
- pulses
- movement
- sensation.

Peripheral temperature monitoring can be useful. Aortic surgery (open or endovascular) may occlude the iliac artery, so flow will probably be assessed by Doppler. Doppler assessment may be undertaken by medical or nursing staff, depending on local policies, practice and skills.

Vascular surgery may cause bleeding from surrounding tissue, so drains should be clearly labelled or numbered, volume marked or measured on arrival and drainage initially monitored hourly. If vacuum drains are used, vacuum should be checked hourly.

Endovascular repair, being less invasive, often avoids need for ICU admission unless there are specific concerns. When receiving patients, nurses should handover specific areas of concern. Endovascular surgery uses dye contrast, which may be nephrotoxic, causing allergic reactions or other problems. So despite the less invasive nature of surgery, patients admitted to ICU should be closely monitored, especially for renal function. Once stabilised (especially fluids optimised and clotting normalised) and extubated, recovery is usually quick.

**Table 36.1 Common complications of open surgery to the aorta (after Prinssen et al., 2004)**

System complications
- cardiac – infarction, left ventricular failure, coagulopathies, SIRS
- pulmonary – ventilatory failure, effusions
- acute renal failure
- cerebrovascular (CVA)
- spinal cord (paraplegia)
- bowel ischaemia – paralysis, loss of appetite, nausea

Local – vascular
- haemorrhage (+anaemia)
- graft complication
- graft infection
- endovascular leak
- thromboembolic
- renal artery obstruction
- arterial/graft obstruction

Local – nonvascular
- wound complications – pain
- iatrogenic bowel perforation
- pressure sores

Following abdominal aortic aneurysm repair, many patients develop SIRS (Norwood et al., 2004), necessitating extensive system support. Patients with vascular disease are at high risk of developing pressure sores (Scott et al., 2001) and acute renal failure. Blood pressure should be monitored and regulated to optimise perfusion while protecting grafts from damage. These, and other complications discussed earlier in this chapter, are listed in Table 36.1.

Although the carotid artery is relatively superficial, repair exposes patients to additional specific risks:

- neurological deficit from occlusion, thrombi or emboli
- oedema, compressing the vagus nerve, causing bradycardia, hypotension and possible heart blocks
- displacement of the trachea.

Nurses should therefore observe

- neurological function, report any inappropriate or deteriorating responses
- airway patency. Tracheal shift will probably be detected on X-ray, but any respiratory problems in extubated patients should be reported
- ECG, heart rate and blood pressure, setting appropriate alarms and reporting any signs of excessive vagal stimulation.

Drains used with carotid surgery are usually small, so more likely to occlude and fill more quickly. Arterial flow to, and venous drainage from, the head should not be occluded. With possible oedema on the side of surgery, this necessitates avoiding interventions, such as feeling carotid pulse, on the opposite side of the neck.

Unlike most post-operative patients, anti-thrombotic stockings (TEDs™) are not usually used, as patients are at high risk of bleeding rather than clotting following vascular surgery, and pressure on any femoral incisions may occlude perfusion.

### Implications for practice

- Pulses, colour and warmth should be monitored on limbs distal to surgery.
- Mean arterial pressure should be maintained >70 mmHg.
- Urine output should be maintained >0.5 ml/kg/hour.
- Following carotid artery repair, pressure to the opposite side of the neck should be avoided.
- Anticoagulant therapy is usually omitted post-operatively, and antithrombotic stockings (TEDs™) are usually not used.

### Summary

Most vascular surgery does not necessitate ICU admission, unless patients develop complications or other problems. But following surgery on the aorta or carotid artery, patients usually are admitted to ICU for observation. The main post-operative dangers are

- stroke
- graft/vessel occlusion
- renal failure
- haemorrhage or bleeding from graft leak.

But patients with aortic or carotid artery disease often have extensive cardio-vascular disease, underlying hypertension and often other co-morbidities. Post-operative recovery centres on stabilisation, observation, symptom control and system support.

Endovascular treatments are quicker, less invasive, and so create fewer risks, but are not always possible with tortuous vessels. Developments in endovascular techniques may significantly reduce the numbers of patients admitted to the ICU following vascular surgery.

### Further reading

The *Journal of Vascular Nursing* often includes relevant articles, such as Epley (2001) and Ramage *et al.* (2001). Baxter (2004) provides a useful review of physiology of aneurysms, together with insights into possible medical developments. Carrell and Wolfe (2005) provide a useful medical review of vascular disease, while Morris and Gomez (2004) provide an overview of ICU management. www.routledge.com/textbooks/0415373239

For clinical scenarios, clinical questions and the answers to them go to the support website at www.routledge.com/textbooks/0415373239

## Clinical scenarios

Mr Owen Fowler is an 81-year-old gentleman with hypertension. He has been diagnosed with an abdominal aortic aneurysm (AAA) of 5.2 cm diameter. This was repaired under fluoroscopic guidance using Digital Subtraction Angiography (DSA) to insert an endograft through his femoral arteries. During the endovascular repair, Mr Fowler lost 2 litres of blood and was transfused with 6 units of packed red cells. He was admitted to ICU for further fluid and cardiovascular management, with Hb of 6.2 g/dl, a platelet count of $50 \times 10^{-9}$/litre and a BP of 110/58 mmHg. He has two vacuum drains located in the right and left groin incision wounds.

Q.1 Identify the potential complications for Mr Fowler following his endovascular repair. Why might these occur and consider the effects of contrast dye, position and type of endograft etc.

Q.2 Analyse nursing interventions which monitor and enhance tissue perfusion for Mr Fowler (e.g. fluids, blood products, vasopressors, drain management, limb assessment, use of Doppler, antithrombolytic therapy; drugs versus antiemboli stockings).

Q.3 Compare and contrast patients' selection, recovery and the long-term effects of AAA repair using the endovascular repair and open surgical repair.

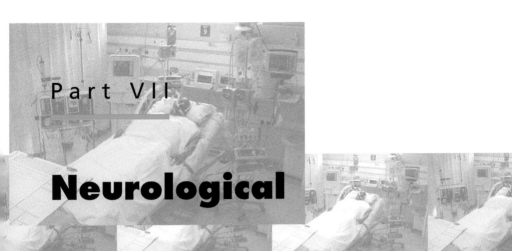

# Part VII

# Neurological

# Chapter 37

# Central nervous system injury

## Contents:

| | |
|---|---|
| Introduction | 392 |
| Airway | 393 |
| Breathing | 393 |
| Circulation | 394 |
| Disability (neurological) | 394 |
| Traumatic brain injury (TBI) | 395 |
| Preventing raised intracranial pressure | 396 |
| Nutrition | 397 |
| Positioning | 397 |
| Pituitary damage | 397 |
| Epilepsy | 398 |
| Spinal cord injury | 399 |
| Autonomic dysreflexia | 400 |
| Haemorrhage | 401 |
| Prognosis | 402 |
| Personality changes | 402 |
| Family care | 403 |
| Legal aspects | 403 |
| Implications for practice | 404 |
| Summary | 404 |
| Further reading | 404 |
| Clinical scenarios | 405 |

## Introduction

Although neurology services are usually focussed in regional centres, patients with acute neurological injuries and complications are admitted to general ICUs. Traumatic brain or spinal injury can cause life-threatening respiratory and cardiovascular failure, necessitating urgent ICU admission. Some patients may later be transferred to regional centres, while others remain due to poor prognosis, their injury being relatively minor, or from lack of beds.

This chapter discusses

■ traumatic brain injury
■ diabetes insipidus
■ spinal cord injury
■ autonomic dysreflexia
■ epilepsy
■ subarachnoid, subdural and extradural haemorrhage.

There are some similarities, but also many differences, about complications from and treatments of this diverse group of pathologies. Intracranial pressure monitoring (see Chapter 23) is often not available in general ICUs, leaving nurses who have less experience of neurological nursing with fewer means to assess problems.

The 'golden hour' of trauma care applies to central nervous system injury. Primary neurological damage is largely irreversible. Secondary damage, mainly from ischaemia (hypotension) or hypoxia causes most in-hospital deaths (Ghajar, 2000). Priorities are therefore early optimisation of

■ ventilation
■ perfusion
■ intracranial pressure.

Immediate priorities are preserving life:

■ airway
■ breathing
■ cardiovascular
■ disability (neurological)

with special emphasis on neuroprotection: hypoxia and hypotension are the most likely causes of death. Traumatic brain injury may have caused death of some brain cells, but the area surrounding the injury will be oedematous, with possible haemorrhage and ischaemic. Ischaemic cells can either recover or die (necrose). Spinal cord injury may cause ischaemia from spinal shock. Management priorities are therefore to optimise perfusion and oxygenation to these at-risk ischaemic brain cells.

## Airway

Airway obstruction may be caused directly by trauma or impaired consciousness. Anyone with a Glasgow Coma Scale score of eight or below may be unable to maintain their own airway, so should be intubated (Eynon & Menon, 2002).

## Breathing

Cerebral oxygen delivery neuroprotects, so severe traumatic brain injury necessitates artificial ventilation. Diaphragmatic nerves normally leave the spinal cord at C3–C5, so spinal injuries involving or above these may cause apnoea, necessitating ventilation. Lower injuries may need initial respiratory support, but problems often resolve later (Ball, 2001). Even if they are able to self-ventilate, hypopnoea and weak cough reflexes expose patients to greater risk of chest infection. Other indications for artificial ventilation may include:

- lung injury from multiple trauma – contusion, pneumothorax, fractured ribs
- hypercapnia – carbon dioxide vasodilates, so controlling levels (target 4.0–4.5 kPa) limits intracranial hypertension.

Former practices of hyperventilation to reduce intracranial pressure have been abandoned, as this reduces cerebral perfusion, and so oxygenation. However, during crises, hyperventilation can rapidly reduce ICP, but should be limited to a few minutes, to buy time for other interventions (Hickey, 2003a).

Sedation is usually needed, for humanitarian reasons, to facilitate effective ventilation, and to reduce brain activity (neuroprotection). Propofol, being short-acting, is usually the sedative of choice.

Paralysing agents may be necessary to facilitate ventilation or reduce metabolism. Nurses should ensure patients are adequately sedated beneath paralysis, both from humanitarian reasons and because stress from being paralysed, but not sedated, will aggravate hypertension (see Chapter 6).

Increased intrathoracic pressure impairs cerebral venous drainage, so unnecessary coughing and straining at stool should be prevented if possible. Antitussive drugs and early tracheostomy may help prevent coughing. Constipation should be prevented through good bowel care which usually necessitates laxatives (see Chapter 9).

## Circulation

Hypovolaemia causes cerebral vasospasm, reducing perfusion. Fluid resuscitation should aim to maintain mean arterial pressure, thus maintaining cerebral perfusion pressure. Glucose solutions should be avoided, as they contain 'free water' which may cause cerebral oedema (Eynon & Menon, 2002; Cree, 2003). Saline is usually used for maintenance and drug infusions, but excessive saline infusions can cause interstitial oedema, so 'filling' is usually with colloids, guided by central venous pressure. Once adequately filled, blood pressure optimisation may necessitate inotropes.

Spinal injury can cause *hypotension*, sympathetic control failing, while unopposed parasympathetic activity causes bradycardia and vasodilation. Hypotension often causes acute renal failure. Dysrhythmias frequently occur within two weeks of injury (Ball, 2001).

## Disability (neurological)

Traumatic brain injury, but not spinal cord injury, exposes patients to secondary dangers from intracranial hypertension. Medical imaging, such as computerised tomography (CT) as magnetic resonance imaging (MRI), may identify specific problems, such as haematoma or excessive cerebral spinal fluid (usually from blockage) which may necessitate urgent drainage or surgery. Secondary brain damage may be prevented by

- sedating (to reduce cerebral oxygen consumption – identified earlier)
- (sometimes) paralysing
- (sometimes) inducing hypothermia
- minimising intracranial pressure

while identifying additional risks, such as

- base of skull fracture
- fitting.

Cerebral oxygen consumption increases about 50 ml each minute for each 1°C (Cooper & Cramp, 2003). Moderate *hypothermia* (32–33°C) reduces metabolism and oxygen demand, so may (Marion *et al.*, 1997; Jalan *et al.*, 1999) or may not (Clifton *et al.*, 2001) be neuroprotective. Profound hypothermia (15–28°C) should be avoided, as it generates toxic metabolites and causes myocardial depression (Werner & Engelhard, 2000).

Cerebral *oedema* is best removed with the osmotic diuretic mannitol. Osmotic diuretics also reduce blood viscosity, thereby improving cerebral perfusion (Werner & Engelhard, 2000). Mannitol is hypertonic, so should be given into a central (or large) vein. Fluid shifts from cells may cause hyperkalaemia.

Cranial venous drainage should be optimised by *positioning* patients at angles of 15–30° (Goh & Gupta, 2002), maintaining good neck alignment

(Sullivan, 2000), ensuring endotracheal tube tapes do not restrict venous drainage (Odell, 1996) and avoiding hip flexion. Rigid neck collars may increase intracranial pressure, so should be removed as soon as injuries allow (Hunt *et al.*, 2001; Goh & Gupta, 2002). If the skull is fractured or has been surgically cut, pressure on any bone flaps should be avoided.

*Base of skull fractures* are not visually obvious and may not have been diagnosed but may still exist. With any cranial trauma, base of skull fracture should be suspected until excluded, and no equipment should be inserted nasally until excluded. Base of skull fractures may cause leakage of cerebrospinal fluid (CSF) from the nose (rhinorrhoea) or ear (otorrhoea). CSF stains on linen look yellow, often as rings around a bloodstain ('halo sign') (Hickey, 2003b). Rhinorrhoea and otorrhea usually seal spontaneously (Watkins, 2000).

Patients should be observed for any signs of *fitting*. If fitting occurs, likely causes (e.g. hypoxia) should be treated. If fitting persists, antiepileptics may be needed.

## Traumatic brain injury (TBI)

Traumatic Brain Injury is the most common cause of death in younger people (Ghajar, 2000), mainly from road traffic accidents (Allen & Ward, 1998). Classification follows Glasgow Coma Scale scoring:

- mild = GCS 13–15
- moderate = GCS 9–13
- severe = GCS 3–8.

Trauma may cause externally visible fracture and bruising, but may also cause internal injuries, such as

- haematoma (extradural, subdural)
- contusion
- contre-coup (the brain hits the opposite side of the skull to the original injury)
- rotation (the brain rotates within the skull, wrenching away nerves and other brain tissue)
- *diffuse axonal injury.*

Victims of TBI often suffer multiple injuries to other parts of the body, so need multisystem support. Some injuries may not be immediately obvious, so nurses should continually assess all body systems and functions.

Following initial stabilisation, main aspects of medical management are listed in Table 37.1. Bayir *et al.* (2003) list the most promising current treatments as

- dexanabinol (currently, only experimental; a synthetic, nonpsychotropic cannabinoid)
- hypertonic saline to reduce cerebral oedema
- mild hypothermia (32–35°C)
- decompressive craniectomy.

**Table 37.1 Possible main aspects of medical management of moderate/severe head injury**

- Diagnostic investigations (computerised tomography – CT, magnetic resonance imaging – MRI, lumbar puncture).
- Surgical (e.g. evacuation if haematoma, ventricular drainage to remove excess/blocked CSF).
- Artificial ventilation, keeping $PaCO_2$ 4.0–4.5 kPa; concurrent sedation + paralysis.
- Osmotic diuretics (mannitol) and/or barbiturates to reduce cerebral oedema and ICP.
- Fluid management.
- Stabilise electrolytes and blood glucose.
- ICP monitoring, maintaining ICP 0–10 and CPP >70 mmHg.
- System support (e.g. vasoactive drugs to normalise blood pressure).
- Induced hypothermia.

## Preventing raised intracranial pressure

In addition to immediate care earlier, nurses have an important role in providing therapeutic care and environments for their patients, primarily by limiting stimuli that may increase intracranial pressure. Ideally, intracranial pressure (ICP) should be maintained at 0–10 mmHg, with cerebral perfusion pressure (CPP) about 60 mmHg (Robertson, 2001). Intracranial pressure exceeding 15 mmHg should be treated, usually by draining cerebrospinal fluid (Ghajar, 2000). However, not all general sections have access to invasive monitoring.

Preventing *pain* has humanitarian and physiological benefits, as stress responses increase intracranial pressure. Codeine phosphate is less likely to mask neurological (diagnostic) signs than other opioids, but once diagnosis is established pain is usually controlled with standard opioids, such as fentanyl. Limbs should be kept in comfortable alignment. Skincare and pressure area care can help prevent pressure sore development, which both cause discomfort and expose patients to potential complications.

Various *activities* have in the past been associated with increasing intracranial pressure, including light and noise (Johnson, 1999), but Rising (1993) found only three interventions significantly affected pressure:

- tracheal suction
- turning
- bed-bathing

and even these only caused transient increases.

Endotracheal *suction*, necessary to remove excessive secretions, is safe provided ICP < 20 mmHg and CPP >50 mmHg (Chudley, 1994). Hypertension can be prevented by bolus analgesia, sedation and 100 per cent oxygen before suction.

*Visits* from friends and family usually bring comfort (Odell, 1996) rather than distress, so should be encouraged. As with all patients, discussing the illness and prognosis may cause distress, so these discussions should be away from the bedside (Hickey, 2003a). Timing of visits may need careful planning to enable sufficient rest between them. As with all patients, supporting the family should help reduce their distress, which benefits both the relatives and patients who sense distress among their loved ones.

## Nutrition

Malnutrition increases risks of infection and delayed rehabilitation in all patients, but head injury significantly increases catabolism (Cree, 2003). Early and aggressive nutrition should be given, which may necessitate drugs (e.g. metoclopramide) to increase gut motility.

Electrolyte imbalances may occur from fluid shifts and loss. Levels should be checked and monitored, with supplements given as necessary.

Blood sugar is often labile following head injury, so should be monitored frequently (e.g. 2–4 hourly). Hyperglycaemia increases intracellular osmotic pressure, causing further cerebral ischaemia, while hypoglycaemia starves neurones of the main fuel used to produce energy. Outcome from severe traumatic brain injury is improved with early tight glycaemic control (Jermitsky *et al.*, 2005). Maintenance fluids should be saline solutions, not glucose (see earlier).

## Positioning

Most ICU patients are at risk of developing pressure sores. Traumatic brain or spinal injury usually cause or necessitate immobility. However, pressure area care interventions should be planned against risks from stimulation. Aggressive manual handling can significantly increase intracranial pressure.

Severe spasticity often occurs following head injury (Collin & Daly, 1998), so assessment and care planning should include active consideration of:

- active/passive exercises
- positioning
- physiotherapy
- any stimuli that reduce muscle tone (e.g. constipation).

Although these aspects will be the focus of later rehabilitation, neglect during the acute phase may prolong or limit rehabilitation.

## Pituitary damage

Although rare, direct trauma from head injury, by central nervous system infection (meningitis) or raised intracranial pressure can cause pituitary damage. The pituitary gland regulates the endocrine system, so damage causes diverse problems, including diabetes insipidus, while damage to the adjacent hypothalamus may cause pryexia.

*Diabetes insipidus* is caused by insufficient antidiuretic hormone (ADH), a hormone produce by the pituitary gland. This only occurs in 1 per cent of patients with head injury (Matta & Menon, 1997). Like diabetes mellitus, it causes polyuria and hypovolaemia, but without glycosuria. Damage might be permanent, but is more often transient, from oedema. Once oedema subsides, diabetes insipidus usually resolves. Until resolution, fluid balance should be carefully monitored and adequate volume replacement prescribed.

*Pyrexia* frequently occurs following head injury and cerebral damage (Collin & Daly, 1998; Rossi *et al.*, 2001). The hypothalamus regulates body temperature, so hypothalamic damage disrupts thermoregulation. Autonomic nervous system dysfunction may cause inappropriate responses. Pyrexia increases cerebral oxygen consumption, potentially causing cerebral hypoxia, fitting and progressive cerebral damage. Temperature should therefore be closely monitored and antipyretic drugs (e.g. paracetamol) prescribed prophylactically or 'as required' for neuroprotection.

## Epilepsy

Epilepsy is the most common serious neurological disease in the UK (Sisodiya & Duncan, 2004), but may occur in ICU patients from cerebral trauma, oedema or hypoxia. Seizures may be

- partial – involving only one hemisphere of the brain
- generalised – involving both hemispheres, and causing loss of consciousness

with sub-classifications of each group. Generalised seizures, usually more problematic, are described in terms of motor (muscle) symptoms:

- tonic – increased muscle tone
- clonic – increased reflex activity
- atonic – sudden loss of tone
- absence – no motor symptoms.

Most generalised seizures are tonic-clonic seizures (formerly called *grand mal*). Absence seizures (formerly *petit mal*), typically causing a blank expression, are usually idiopathic and occur mainly in children. Status epilepticus is prolonged fitting, usually defined as lasting 30 minutes (Chapman *et al.*, 2001; Thomas & Hirsch, 2003; Walker, 2003b).

Patient safety is a priority. If at risk of falling patients may need to be repositioned. Pillows or other padding should be placed between patients and anything on which they may hurt themselves (e.g. cotsides). Tonic-clonic seizures almost invariably cause apnoea, so intubated patients should be fully ventilated and sedated. Facemask ('Ambu-bag'®) ventilation is usually necessary if patients are not intubated. If oxygenation and sedation does not terminate fitting, sedatives (e.g. propofol, midazolam (Marik & Varon, 2004)) are usually given to reduce cerebral irritation. If fitting persists, anti-epileptics drugs may be needed. Fits should be observed, and duration, appearance and effects recorded. Priorities of care are listed in Table 37.2.

**Table 37.2 Priorities of care during fitting**

- Summon help.
- Provide safety and privacy.
- Maintain clear airway (e.g. remove saliva/vomit, insert artificial airway).
- Give 100 per cent oxygen (intubation and artificial ventilation if apnoeic).
- Antiepileptics.
- Reassure family.
- Observing fits: duration, which parts of the body are affected, and record observations.

With traumatic brain injury, fitting more often occurs during recovery. Early post-traumatic seizures appear to have little significance for management or outcome, so prophylactic antiepileptic drugs are not recommended (Ghajar, 2000). Cerebral compression or hypoxia may cause fitting, especially if Glasgow Coma Scale score is below 10 (Menon, 1999).

# Spinal cord injury

Recovery from spinal injury is highest if patients are initially admitted to ICU for 7–14 days (Brain Trauma Foundation, 2001). Even if not admitted with identified spinal injury, multiple trauma may have caused unidentified/unconfirmed injury, so should always be presumed present until excluded. The spinal cord forms the lowest part of the central nervous system, and so damage affects function of all systems and organs regulated by nerves below the injury. Typically, injuries to

- cervical vertebra 1 (C1) to thoracic vertebra 1 (T1) cause tetraplegia
- T2 to lumbar vertebra 1 (L1) cause paraplegia

and injuries above T12 usually cause spasticity and hyperreflexia.

Spinal injury necessitates supine positioning, and may require special ('spinal') beds. Controls for adjusting angles of the head or foot of the bed should be locked if possible. If not possible, control panels should be clearly labelled to identify which controls may and may not be used (with most controls, only the vertical elevation control is safe to use).

Moving can cause further spinal injury, so spinal column alignment should be maintained. Specific instructions about positioning should be clearly visible in the bedarea – for example, multiple trauma may involve the thoracic spine, necessitating maintenance of leg alignment as well. Most ICUs have guidelines for nursing and positioning patients with spinal injury. Sufficient staff should be gathered to safely log-roll patients. Before rolling, a team leader should be identified (normally the person holding the head), readiness of all staff involved should be identified, instructions clarified and the destined angle specified. Additional staff may be required to manage specific injuries or equipment. Cervical and upper thoracic spine injury (C1-T4) necessitates additional stabilisation of the head with a hard collar or head immobiliser, and one additional person holding just to maintain head alignment. Position changes, usually two hourly, should be recorded on observation charts.

Venous stasis causes high risk of thrombus formation. Within three months more than one-third of patients develop deep vein thromboses (Anderson & Spencer, 2003). Prophylaxis (TEDs™, subcutaneous heparin) could be commenced on admission and guidance sought about what passive/active exercises may be performed.

Thermoregulation is impaired and labile due to

- inappropriate cutaneous vasodilatation (hypothermia)
- inability to shiver (hypothermia)
- impaired sweating predisposes (hyperthermia).

Spinal injury care is often prolonged, benefiting from inclusion of various specialists. Neurophysiotherapists should be actively involved in care of spinal injury patients, treating and advising about mobilisation, spasticity (Burchiel & Hsu, 2001), foot drop and other complications caused by loss of peripheral nervous system control. Two-thirds of patients report pain, often severe and disabling (Burchiel & Hsu, 2001), so pain control specialists should be consulted.

## Autonomic dysreflexia ('hyperreflexia')

The autonomic nervous system regulates homeostasis, including vasodilation/constriction and heart rate. Spinal injury blocks normal inhibitory pathways, so parasympathetic compensation occurs only above lesions, with exaggerated sympathetic responses below.

Gradual return of reflex activity after spinal shock causes erratic, uninhibited responses and hypertensive (dysreflexic/hyperreflexic) crises (Glasby & Myles, 2000) – potentially (250/150 mmHg) (Naftchi & Richardson, 1997), with hypertensive symptoms of blurred vision, pounding headaches, nasal congestion, nausea, pupil dilation and profuse sweating and flushing above, with pallor below lesions.

Most spinal injuries above T6 cause autonomic dysreflexia (van Welzen & Carey, 2002) at least 4 weeks, and often 6 months following injury; it can occur with injuries above T10 (Keely, 1998), until resolution (usually after a few years), blood pressure and pulse remain labile. Although usually occurring after transfer to spinal injuries units, ICU nurses may encounter it, especially with patients who have old spinal cord injury (Keely, 1998). Nurses should be able to recognise it should it occur in the ICU and be able to provide appropriate information for patients and their families.

Most crises are caused by distended bladder or bowels (van Welzen & Carey, 2002). Other (rare) stimuli include

- cutaneous – pressure sores, ingrowing toenails, tight/restrictive clothing, seams/creases in clothing and splints
- skeletal – spasm, especially limb contractures, passive movement/exercises

- visceral – internal distension from gastric ulcers or uterine contractures during labour
- miscellaneous – bone fractures, vaginal dilation, ejaculation.

Unable either to feel stimuli or move, spinal reflexes occur without normal protective responses (e.g. changing position).

Treating crises requires urgent intervention – immediately elevating the bedhead to reduce intracranial hypertension and removing possible causes (e.g. straightening creased sheets).

All acute hospitals treating patients with spinal cord injury should have bowel care protocols to prevent dysreflexic crises (National Patient Safety Agency, 2004). Constipation may require manual evacuation (National Patient Safety Agency, 2004) under topical anaesthetic (e.g. lidocaine) cover (Hickey, 2003c). Blood pressure should be recorded very frequently during procedures – continuously or every 2–3 minutes (Wirtz *et al.*, 1996). Antihypertensive (e.g. hydralazine) may be used, but once sympathetic stimuli for hypertension are resolved, circulating drugs and bradycardia may cause excessive rebound hypotension.

Gentle bladder irrigation with 30 ml sterile water may be attempted (van Welzen & Carey, 2002), but blocked urinary catheters are usually replaced urgently (Hickey, 2003c).

For autonomic dysreflexia occurring during rehabilitation from spinal injury, patient and carer education become progressively important. Quadriplegia creates continuing dependency on carers for fundamental aspects of living, including movement. Pressure area care regimes are carefully staged to build skin tolerance until patients can remain in one position for prolonged periods, possibly all night, without developing sores or dysreflexic crises.

Carers should be increasingly involved in aspects of care, which they will have to perform following discharge (e.g. changing urinary catheters, performing manual evacuations). While later stages of rehabilitation are unlikely to be reached before transfer to spinal injury units, ICU nurses may initiate rehabilitation, and should therefore supply appropriate information to patients and carers, as well as being able to recognise and treat complications of autonomic dysreflexia.

## Haemorrhage

Major intracranial haemorrhage is usually caused by severe traumatic brain injury or spontaneous rupture of cerebral blood vessels, usually from aneurysms. Haemorrhage may be

- subdural
- extradural
- subarachnoid.

*Subarachnoid haemorrhage* typically occurs in relatively young people, most often 30–60 years of age (Andrews, 2000).

401

Traumatic brain injury should be managed as mentioned earlier. Spontaneous sub-haemorrhage is ideally treated by either surgical or endovascular obliteration of the aneurysm, but this is not usually available outside neurological centres, the outcome is usually poor (Oliveira-Filho *et al.*, 2001) and transfer may be impractical. Like meningitis, subarachnoid haemorrhage often causes severe photophobia, so patients should be nursed with light levels reduced to the minimum necessary.

## Prognosis

Major intracranial bleeds are often fatal – mortality exceeds 40 per cent, and less than one quarter of patients fully recover (Macmillan, 2003). Recovery from severe traumatic brain injury or spinal cord injury recovery is unpredictable, often prolonged or incomplete. Most (85 per cent) remain disabled one year after traumatic brain injury; even with minor head injury less than half the patients recover fully within one year (Watkins, 2000). Rehabilitation can be a long and often frustrating process for both patients and their relatives, so planning for rehabilitation should begin early. Family will often become carers for these patients, so should be offered support, opportunities to express their feelings and given help to enable them to cope (O'Neill & Carter, 1998).

Many patients experience amnesia, often having no memory of events immediately before the injury (Watkins, 2000). This may be psychologically protective, but can also be psychologically distressing. Once their condition has stabilised, patients may be transferred to specialist rehabilitation centres.

Epilepsy carries a social stigma (Lanfear, 2002) which, although reduced through public education, has been reinforced by restrictions on driving, insurance policies and other restrictions on quality of life. Patients and their families may therefore be fearful of the label, or its potential effects on their lifestyle.

Subarachnoid haemorrhage is frequently fatal – about one-quarter dying immediately (O'Sullivan, 2000; Cairns, 2003), with many subsequent deaths from respiratory failure (Cairns, 2003).

## Personality changes

In addition to general psychological stressors from critical illness and ICU admission, central nervous injury, prolonged recovery and fears about their future can affect psychological function and cause depression (Bénony *et al.*, 2002). Traumatic brain injury can cause temporary or permanent changes in behaviour due to damage; on waking, patients may exhibit

■ lack of inhibition
▓ inflexible thinking

- memory deficits
- irritability.

(O'Neill & Carter, 1998)

Frontal lobe damage is especially likely to cause aggressiveness and loss of inhibition. Damage to other areas of the brain may cause other problems, such as dysphasia. Personality and mood changes are especially distressing for families (Powell, 2004), so family should be warned in advance about possible behavioural change. Victims of road traffic accidents or assault may be anxious about litigation or police involvement. Nurses should therefore assess psychological needs of both patients and families.

## Family care

Prolonged, unpredictable and incomplete recovery expose families to continuing distress. Families need help to enable them to cope (O'Neill & Carter, 1998). ICU staff can offer useful advice and support in the early stages. Social workers, support groups, counsellors or other social supports may be beneficial.

Family and friends often bring comfort, but might cause distress. Where visitors do cause undue distress, nurses may need to intervene to enable patients to rest, but visits that provide therapeutic benefits should be encouraged. Nursing documentation and handover should identify effects of visitors on patients.

While their prime duty is to their patients, care of relatives is an important, albeit secondary, nursing role. Relatives usually appreciate being given appropriate information. They also need adequate rest themselves; they may feel obliged to stay by the bedside, exhausting both themselves and the patient, so planning care with the next-of-kin can prove beneficial to all. Providing somewhere to stay and access to catering facilities can greatly reduce the stress experienced by relatives.

## Legal aspects

Admissions caused by road traffic accidents or other potentially criminal actions may involve the police. There are certain requirements in law for nurses to disclose information, but they are few in number and often require a court order. In the absence of any specific legal requirement, nurses should remember their duty of confidentiality to patients (NMC, 2004). If in doubt about whether the police or other authorities have a right to information or specimens, nurses should seek the advice of their line manager and may need to consult their employer's legal department. Details of legal obligations can be found in Dimond (2005).

DLVA regulations forbid epileptics (with a few specified exceptions) from driving until they have been free from fits for one year (Lanfear, 2002).

## Implications for practice

■ Complications and death from patients admitted with central nervous system injury is usually caused by hypoxia or cerebral ischaemia, so immediate priorities are

  ● airway and breathing – artificial ventilation
  ● cardiovascular – fluid resuscitation, aiming for CPP 60 mmHg
  ● disability – neuroprotection (sedation, possible hypothermia, preventing intracranial hypertension).

■ Following traumatic brain injury, patients should be nursed at 15–30°, with head and neck alignment maintained and nothing (e.g. endotracheal tapes) restricting venous drainage from their head.
■ Spinal injury patients should be nursed supine with their spine in alignment.
■ Spinal injury patients should be turned at least two-hourly. Manual patient handling should always use log-rolls, with sufficient staff to safely turn the patient and manage equipment.
■ Autonomic dysreflexia occurs with most spinal cord injuries above T6, so staff should observe for hypertensive crises, know how to manage them, and appropriate bowel care protocols should be available.
■ Rehabilitation is often .prolonged and may remain incomplete. Patients and families often experience psychological distress, so nurses should assess both patients' and relatives' psychological needs and refer to appropriate support agencies.
■ There are a few instances where police or other authorities have rights to access confidential information; if in doubt, nurses should seek advice before disclosing anything.

## Summary

Neurological admissions may be transferred to regional specialist centres, but early ICU care is more often managed on general units, and when specialist centres consider they cannot offer additional care, patients remain on general units. Head injury can range from mild to severe, and skilled nursing care significantly contributes to survival and recovery following head injury. Prognosis is considerably worse with spinal cord injury and very poor with subarachnoid haemorrhage. But with all central nervous system pathologies, the priorities remain cerebral oxygenation and perfusion. Secondary deaths are often from complications, which should be prevented if possible. Additional aspects of nursing care include supporting fundamental activities of living, co-ordinating care and providing psychological support to patients and families.

## Further reading

The Brain Trauma Foundation (2001) publishes authoritative guidelines. The classic neurological nursing text is Hickey (2003d). Ghajar (2000) reviews traumatic brain injury. Lanfear (2002) reviews epilepsy, while Macmillan

(2003) describes subarachnoid haemorrhage. Powell (2004) is a valuable resource for the families of head injured patients. www.routledge.com/textbooks/0415373239

For clinical scenarios, clinical questions and the answers to them go to the support website at www.routledge.com/textbooks/0415373239

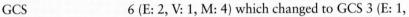

## Clinical scenarios

Claire Healy is 56 years old and sustained a severe head injury after falling 10 feet from an attic. She experienced loss of consciousness for an unknown length of time. Claire was admitted to the ICU via A&E wearing a cervical collar with spinal immobilisation. The results from a neurological examination revealed:

| | |
|---|---|
| GCS | 6 (E: 2, V: 1, M: 4) which changed to GCS 3 (E: 1, V: 1, M: 1) |
| Pupil response | Sluggish, equal response, size 3 mm diameter |

Cough and gag reflex present
Blood discharging from both ears; active bleed in left ear, old dried blood in right ear

Other observations included:

| | |
|---|---|
| Respiratory rate | 29 breaths/minute |
| BP | 150/96 mmHg (mean BP 114 mmHg) |
| HR | 74 bpm |
| CVP | 3 mmHg |
| Central temperature | 36.0°C |
| Blood sugar | 10.5 mmol/litre |

A head CT scan confirmed fractures of basal skull, left occipital, left and right mastoid with a small left subdural haematoma.

Q.1 Interpret the significance of Claire's results in relation to her head injury and explore the physiological implications.

Q.2 The aim of ICU management is to anticipate, prevent and treat secondary physiological insults. Prioritise a plan of care, which incorporates neuroprotection strategies, promotes cerebral perfusion pressure and is likely to improve Claire's outcome after traumatic Brain Injury.

Q.3 Reflect on how head and spinal injured patients are positioned and moved in your clinical area (e.g. equipment, personnel, other resources, specialists, guideline or protocol followed).

Chapter 38

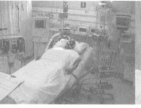

# Peripheral neurological pathologies

## Contents

Introduction                              407
Guillain Barré Syndrome (GBS)             407
Critical illness neuropathy               408
Implications for practice                 409
Summary                                   409
Support groups                            410
Further reading                           410
Clinical scenarios                        410

## Fundamental knowledge

Nerve anatomy and conduction – myelin, nodes of Ranvier

**Introduction**

This chapter discusses two conditions seen with varying frequency in the ICU:

■ Guillain Barré Syndrome
■ Critical illness neuropathy.

Nursing patients with neurological complications can be labour-intensive and stressful. Patients need care and support with many activities of living, while minimising complications significantly improves recovery and survival. Nursing care is therefore especially valuable for patients with these conditions.

Management of both conditions centres on

■ attempts to remove underlying causes
■ prevention of complications
■ system support.

While there is some research evidence, practice varies between units; some approaches described below are anecdotal rather than evidence-based.

**Guillain Barré Syndrome (GBS)**

This syndrome, one of the most common neurological pathologies (Poulter, 1998), may be caused by various pathologies. In Europe and North America the main cause is acute inflammatory demyelinating polyneuropathy (AIDP) (Kuwabara *et al.*, 2002), which often follows minor viral respiratory or gut infections (Seneviratne, 2000; Hudsmith & Menon, 2002).

Progressive destruction of nodes of Ranvier causes ascending demyelination of peripheral motor nerves (Dawson, 2000) resulting in progressive muscle weakness, including respiratory failure. Sensory nerve function is usually altered, causing severe pain.

Steroids are not beneficial (Winer, 2002). Circulating mediators may be removed through plasma exchange (Hudsmith & Menon, 2002; Winer, 2002), or intravenous gamma globulin (Winer, 2002).

If basement membrane remains intact, recovery begins once Schwann cells mitosis remyelinates damaged nerves, often in 2–4 weeks (Skowronski, 2003), but significant weakness can persist after one year (Seneviratne, 2000). ICU mortality from GBS is 5 per cent, usually from myocardial infarction (Seneviratne, 2000).

Muscle weakness and autonomic dysfunction can cause:

■ *Pain,* usually severe (Seneviratne, 2000) and exacerbated by touch and anxiety. Analgesia (often opioids) is needed. Patients should be positioned comfortably; TENS, massage and other interventions may alleviate pain.
■ *Respiratory failure.* Nearly one third of GBS patients develop respiratory failure requiring artificial ventilation (Howard *et al.*, 2003). Being

immunocompromised, noninvasive ventilation is usually used first (Vianello *et al.*, 2000), but invasive ventilation and/or tracheostomy may be needed. Intensive physiotherapy may limit or prevent respiratory failure.

■ *Hypotension* from extensive peripheral vasodilatation (poor sympathetic tone).

■ *Hypertensive* episodes caused by failure of normal negative feedback opposition to sympathetic stimuli.

■ *Dysrhythmias* (sinus tachycardia, bradycardia, asystole) frequently occur.

■ *Thrombosis* from venous stasis (immobility) and hypoperfusion. Like most ICU patients, thromboprophylaxis (subcutaneous heparin) and thromboembolytic stockings (TEDs™) should be given.

■ *Limb weakness,* ascending from distal to proximal muscles, affecting hands, feet or both. Passive exercises may prevent contractures and promote venous return.

■ *Hypersalivation* and loss of swallow from autonomic dysfunction necessitate oral suction for comfort and to prevent aspiration.

■ *Bilateral facial muscle weakness* causing dribbling of saliva and opthalmoplegia, distressing both patients and relatives.

■ *Sweating,* from autonomic dysfunction, is often profuse, so frequent washes and changes of clothing help provide comfort.

■ *Incontinence* from bladder muscle weakness.

■ *Psychological* problems from progressive and prolonged weakness. Mentally fit (often young) adults forced to rely on others to perform fundamental and intimate activities of living causes distress, compounding environmental stressors of ICU (see Chapter 23) and fears about prognosis (many GBS sufferers have extensive knowledge about their disease) often causing psychoses and acute depressive disorders.

■ *Immunocompromise* is multifactoral, aggravated by factors such has hepatic dysfunction, reduced functional residual capacity, sleep disturbance, stress responses and depression, as well as treatments such as intubation. Infection control and preventing opportunistic infection are therefore especially important.

■ *Catabolism,* necessitating aggressive (and early) nutrition to limit muscle wasting.

Depression reduces motivation, needed with protracted debility. Antidepressants are often useful, but should not become a substitute for active human and humane nursing (e.g. making environments as 'normal' as possible). Psychological support should be extended to family and friends.

Patients with critical illness neuropathy suffer similar psychological problems.

## Critical illness neuropathy

One-quarter to one-third of ICU patients develop muscle weakness (Deem *et al.*, 2003). Despite numerous reports and studies, debate persists about what causes critical illness neuropathy, how (or whether) to test for it, how to treat it and even what to call it (Deem *et al.*, 2003) – other names include acute axonal neuropathy. Nates *et al.* (1997) differentiate between

- critical illness neuropathy, which affects nervous tissue
- acute necrotising myopathy, which affects muscles.

Illness and prolonged immobility often result in co-existing muscle flaccidity (Bednarik *et al.*, 2003).

Degeneration of motor nerves (Ghosh *et al.*, 2001) does not delay speed of nerve signals, but does weaken signals. Muscle weakness delays weaning (Druschky *et al.*, 2001) and can cause myocardial fibrillation (Hund *et al.*, 1996).

Various causes have been speculated, including steroids (Jonghe *et al.*, 2002), unidentified serum neurotoxicity (Druschky *et al.*, 2001), and probable cytokine involvement. Most patients with CIP have SIRS/MODS (Druschky *et al.*, 2001).

Muscle necrosis during sepsis increases creatine phosphokinase levels (Bolton, 1999), although diagnosis is usually through electromylogram (EMG) (Ghosh *et al.*, 2001) or clinical picture.

Currently there are no specific treatments for critical illness neuropathy, so diagnosis arguably does not assist management. Aggressive insulin therapy appears to reduce incidence (Deem *et al.*, 2003); physiotherapy and passive exercises also help (Kennedy *et al.*, 2002). Nerves remyelinate by about 3 mm each day, so recovery may take 1–6 months, often necessitating prolonged rehabilitation (Kennedy *et al.*, 2002).

### Implications for practice

- Prolonged admission makes nursing care an especially important factor in recovery for these patients.
- Holistic assessment enables many complications to be avoided.
- Depression and sensory imbalance can easily occur; psychological care should be optimised.
- Neurological deficits impair normal homeostatic mechanisms, so nurses should avoid interventions or lack of interventions that may provoke crises.
- Providing information to patients and families can help them cope and develop any skills they may need following the patient's discharge.

### Summary

This chapter has described three neurological conditions that may be encountered with varying frequency on general ICUs. For nurses with specialist neurological training these conditions can create very real challenges, but more so than many, pathological conditions are largely resolved by nursing rather than medical interventions.

## Support groups

Guillain Barré helpline 0800 374803

## Further reading

Hickey (2003) remains the classic neurology nursing text. Useful medical articles on Guillain Barré Syndrome include Seneviratne (2000) and Winer (2002). Lewis (1999) offers nursing perspectives.

Critical illness neuropathy has generated much debate in the last decade, Druschky *et al.* (2001), Jonghe *et al.* (2002) and Bednarik *et al.* (2003) being recent examples. www.routledge.com/textbooks/0415373239

For clinical scenarios, clinical questions and the answers to them go to the support website at www.routledge.com/textbooks/0415373239

## Clinical scenarios

Donald McLean, 58 years old, presented with a 10 day history of dysphagia, progressive tachypnoea with increasing oxygen requirements, difficulty swallowing, weak cough, slurred speech, general fatigue, deep tendon reflexes absent in all limbs with numbness in both legs and tips of fingers in both hands. When examined the following results were noted:

| | |
|---|---|
| Respiratory rate | 42 breaths/minute |
| $SpO_2$ | 91% on 15 litres of oxygen |
| Vital capacity | 380 ml |
| BP | 150/100 mmHg |
| HR | 80 bpm |
| Temperature | 36.0°C |

Chest X-Ray revealed right middle and lower lobe pneumonia. Arterial blood gas analysis showed uncompensated respiratory acidosis with hypoxia.

In the previous month Donald had flu-like symptoms and was recovering from an upper respiratory tract infection. Acute post-infective polyneuropathy or Guillain Barré Syndrome is suspected and Donald was admitted to the ICU for respiratory support.

Q.1 Review the most suitable type of respiratory support for Donald. Provide a rationale for your suggestion.

Q.2 Identify additional complications associated with polyneuropathy that Donald may experience during his ICU stay. Propose specific nursing interventions to minimise these.

Q.3 Identify and reflect on a range of approaches which may support and strengthen the immune response in Donald and promote an early recovery (e.g. immunonutrition, sleep, administration of IgIV, psychological support, mobilisation, pain management).

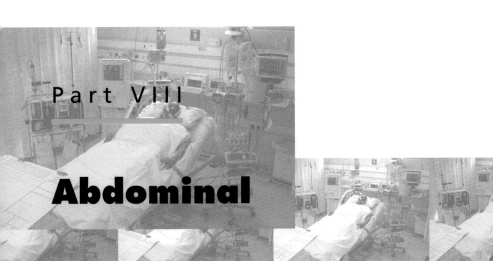

# Part VIII

# Abdominal

Chapter 39

# Acute renal failure

## Contents

Introduction                        414
Prerenal failure                    414
Intrarenal failure                  415
Postrenal failure                   416
Monitoring renal function           416
Effects                             416
Management                          418
Diuretics                           418
Rhabdomyolysis                      418
Implications for practice           419
Summary                             420
Further reading                     420
Clinical scenarios                  420

## Fundamental knowledge

Renal anatomy and physiology
Urea and creatinine (see Chapter 21)

## Introduction

This chapter describes acute renal failure and rhabdomyolysis. Haemofiltration is covered in Chapter 40.

Up to one quarter of ICU patients develop acute renal failure (Bellomo *et al.*, 2001), usually as a complication from poor perfusion during multi-organ dysfunction syndrome (MODS) (Wright *et al.*, 2003). Distinctions between acute and chronic failure are arbitrary, often 100 days, but acute renal failure usually occurs relatively quickly, and is usually reversible (although patients with multisystem failure may die before the kidney recovers). Treatment aims to replace renal function while optimising recovery of renal tissue.

Renal failure is failure of kidneys to perform normal metabolic functions (see Table 39.1). Oliguria (e.g. <0.5 ml/kg/hour) is often a sign of renal failure, but functional failure can occur despite 'normal' or 'polyuric' urine volumes. Oliguria may be caused by

- prerenal
- intrarenal (intrinsic)
- postrenal

problems. Failure of renal function causes many abnormal blood results, including

- raised urea and creatinine
- hyperkalaemia
- metabolic acidosis.

Many of these abnormalities cause further complications.

## Prerenal failure

Prerenal failure is caused by failure to perfuse kidneys; kidney tissue remains undamaged. This is the most common cause of renal failure in the ICU (Rahman & Treacher, 2002), usually from systemic hypotension (e.g. SIRS, cardiac failure) and is immediately reversible by replacing volume. Kidneys are very susceptible to ischaemic damage, especially acute tubular necrosis (ATN), so unreversed prerenal failure almost inevitably progresses to intrarenal failure.

### Table 39.1 Functions of the kidney

- Waste removal
- Fluid balance
- Acid–base balance
- Electrolyte balance
- Hormone production (mainly renin and erythropoetin)
- Part of chain of vitamin D synthesis

Prerenal failure, being caused by hypovolaemia stimulates aldosterone release. Aldosterone increases renal reabsorption of sodium, often reducing urinary sodium <10 mmol/litre, while increasing urine osmolality (specific gravity >0.018) (Rahman & Treacher, 2002).

## Intrarenal failure

In contrast to prerenal failure, intrarenal failure is caused by damage to renal tissue. Damage may be caused by

- ischaemia
- inflammation
- nephrotoxicity.

Many nephrotoxic drugs are used in the ICU, including amphotericin and gentamicin, but the main cause of intrarenal failure in the ICU is acute tubular necrosis from prerenal failure. Whereas prerenal failure is immediately reversible, intrarenal failure persists until cells regrow, which often takes a week or more.

*Acute Tubular Necrosis* used to be attributed to death of renal tubule cells, but pathology is more complex – while the problem is 'acute' and affects tubules, it is caused by ischaemia, rather than (necessarily) necrosis, of tubular cells. Acute tubular necrosis, and most other types of intrarenal failure, can be classified into three stages:

- initiation
- established or maintenance
- recovery or diuretic.

Initially prerenal failure causes ischaemia. Hypoxic damage causes intracellular oedema and, if unreversed, cell death (see Chapter 24). Oliguria (urine production below 0.5 ml/kg/hour) usually occurs within two days of precipitating events and usually lasts up to two weeks, although it can persist far longer. Prognosis worsens with prolonged oliguria. As renal function fails, volume of urine falls, while serum urea and creatinine levels rise.

Cell damage releases vasoactive cytokines provoking further intrarenal vasoconstriction. Preglomerular vasoconstriction reduces glomerular perfusion, and so glomerular filtration. Widespread tubule intracellular oedema physically compresses lumens obstructing flow of what filtrate is produced. Oliguria, and often anuria persists throughout the established phase. Medullary damage from intrarenal failure reduces sodium reabsorption in the Loop of Henle, so urinary sodium is high: >40 mmol/litre. Hypernatraemia in the macula densa activates the renin–angiotensin–aldosterone cascade.

Tubular cells readily regenerate. When they do, the recovery phase begins. This often occurs in 1–2 weeks, but can occasionally take up to one year. As damaged tubules begin to recover function and new (immature) tubule cells

415

grow, filtration improves and obstruction to flow is removed. However recovering and immature tubule cells function inefficiently. Tubular reabsorption and solute exchange being poor, large volumes of poor quality urine are passed (up to 5 l a day), blood urea and creatinine remaining elevated.

When tubular cells mature, normal function is recovered. Urea and creatinine levels fall, urine volumes return to normal, and electrolyte balance is restored.

## Postrenal failure

Postrenal failure, the main cause of renal failure in the community, rarely occurs in ICU. Caused by obstruction between the kidneys and meatus (such as bladder tumours, renal/bladder calculi or an enlarged prostate), resulting back pressure can cause intrarenal damage (glomerulonephritis). Postrenal failure is reversed by removing the obstruction.

## Monitoring renal function

There are many, but no ideal, ways to measure glomerular function, including

- urine volume
- plasma urea
- plasma creatinine
- creatinine clearance (24-hour urine collection).

Like most body systems, healthy kidneys have a large physiological reserve; adequate renal function can usually be maintained with urine outputs of about 450 ml/day. Renal failure occurs when three-quarters of nephrons are non-functional. Endstage renal failure occurs when 90 per cent of nephrons fail, leaving a relatively narrow margin between recoverable and terminal failure.

Urea and creatinine are described in Chapter 21.

Blood creatinine, a waste product of muscle metabolism varies throughout the day – renal clearance is highest during afternoon. Twenty-four-hour urine collections therefore provide a more balanced indication of renal function than isolated blood samples.

## Effects

Renal failure disrupts homeostasis. The main complications to body systems which result from renal failure are:

*Cardiovascular*:

- hyperkalaemia
- acidosis
- dysrhythmias
- anaemia.

*Nervous system*:

■ confusion (from uraemia)
■ twitching
■ coma.

*Respiratory*:

■ compensatory tachypnoea
■ acidosis
■ pulmonary oedema
■ hiccough.

*Gut*:

■ nausea
■ diarrhoea
■ vomiting.

*Metabolic*:

■ electrolyte imbalances
■ acidosis
■ toxicity from active drug metabolites.

*Potassium*: most (90 per cent) potassium loss is in urine, so oliguria usually causes hyperkalaemia, while polyuria causes hypokalaemia.

*Acid–base*: normal renal function maintains acid–base balance by reabsorbing bicarbonate and excreting hydrogen atoms. Many hydrogen ions pass into ultrafiltrate in renal tubules, changing normal blood pH of 7.4 into normal urinary pH of 5–6. Renal failure therefore causes metabolic acidosis.

Acidosis stimulates tachypnoea to compensate metabolic acidosis with respiratory alkalosis. But respiratory failure will limit effectiveness; excessive triggering (e.g. with SIMV or PSV) increases oxygen consumption, aggravating systemic hypoxia.

The main plasma protein creating colloid osmotic pressure, *albumin* weighs 66.5 kDa, so is below renal threshold (68 kDa), but negatively charged sialoproteins in glomerular capillaries normally repel albumin, keeping it in renal capillaries. Nephritis causes

■ loss of glomerular capillary negative charge
■ increased glomerular bed permeability (inflammatory response)

resulting in albumin loss in urine. Hypoalbuminaemia, common in ICU, lowers colloid osmotic pressure, so intravascular fluid is lost into interstitial spaces ('third spacing'), resulting in hypovolaemia and oedema, both of which cause further renal damage.

417

## Management

Too often prerenal failure remains undertreated, and so progresses to intrarenal failure; early intervention can prevent many complications. If renal failure is suspected, cardiovascular status should be optimised by providing adequate *fluids*. With relatively prolonged underlying pathologies (e.g. SIRS, MODS) inappropriate fluid shifts and hypoalbuminaemia will persist, so fluids given to treat hypovolaemia should remain intravascularly. This necessitates using large-molecule fluids, such as hydroxethyl starches (unless patients are receiving renal replacement therapy, these can cause fluid overload, so haemo-dynamic status should be closely monitored) rather than cheaper low molecular weight colloids (see Chapter 34). If cardiac failure is present, hypotension may require inotropic support.

Once blood volume and pressure are optimised, a *fluid challenge* helps identify any failure of renal function. Although much debated, choice between colloid and crystalloid for fluid challenges is probably less important than ensuring that glomerular beds receive sufficient volume to filter. Large volumes should be infused rapidly – at least 500 ml over no more than 30 minutes, preferably with CVP monitoring incase cardiac overload and pulmonary oedema occur.

If kidneys fail to respond to fluid challenges, then medical options are mainly *drugs* and/or *continuous renal replacement therapy* (see Chapter 39). Renal replacement therapy buys time until recovery.

## Diuretics

*Furosemide*, a loop diuretic, blocks sodium reabsorption in the ascending Loop of Henle. Water reabsorption being passive, this increases urine volume. Furosemide is an effective way of treating fluid overload, but can compromise hypovolaemic patients – increasing mortality and development of chronic renal failure of critically ill patients (Mehta *et al.*, 2002). Furosemide is oto-toxic, so intravenous administration should be slow (4 mg/minute), with high doses necessitating continuous infusion. Furosemide can cause hypokalaemia, so with large doses ECG should be monitored and serum potassium levels checked.

*Mannitol*, an osmotic diuretic, is often used for treating cerebral oedema, but seldom used for other problems.

*Dopexamine*, a synthetic analogue of dopamine, has been used for treating renal failure, although benefit is doubtful (see Chapter 35).

## Rhabdomyolysis

Extensive muscle damage, such as from crush injuries, major burns, severe infection/sepsis or prolonged immobilisation, can cause rhabdomyolysis, leading to acute renal failure. Various speculated mechanisms of renal failure

from rhabdomyolysis include

- blockage of tubules with myoglobin precipitate
- myoglobin-induced vasoconstriction of renal arterioles
- oxygen-free radical (mainly from iron-containing haem molecule) damage to renal tubules.

Hydrogen ion excretion by the kidney changes ultrafiltrate from alkali (normal pH 7.4) to acid (often reaching pH 5.0) creating the acid environment in which myoglobin can precipitate. But this traditional explanation is increasingly being replaced by free radical theories (Holt, 1999; Cooper & Cramp, 2003). As myoglobin contains iron, what little urine does filter through is stained a distinctively rusty colour. Rhabdomyolysis is diagnosed by clinical suspicion, but confirmed by elevated serum creatine kinase (CK – see Chapter 30) (Sharp *et al.*, 2004). A few centres can test for myoglobin.

Rhabdomyolysis is treated by rapid intravenous infusion to flush out myoglobin, often 10–12 litres over 24 hours (Holt, 1999; Hunter, 2002). To prevent cardiac overload, CVP monitoring is recommended. Diuretics, usually furosemide (mannitol has also been used), are given to maintain urine at 200–300 ml/hour (Holt, 1999; Meister & Reddy, 2002)

To reduce precipitation and free radical damage, urine may be alkalinised by bicarbonate infusions (Holt, 1999; Hunter, 2002; Meister & Reddy, 2002), although Brown *et al.* (2004) question whether alkalinisation has benefits. Myoglobin may block urinary catheters, so urine flow should be observed closely. Obstructed catheters should be replaced rather than flushed, to prevent returning precipitate into the bladder. Antioxidants may be beneficial (Holt, 1999). Extensive muscle cell damage may cause life-threatening hyperkalaemia (Hunter, 2002), which should be reversed.

Alcoholics appear to be more susceptible to rhabdomyolysis (Hunter, 2002), while incidence of rhabdomyolysis from drug abuse (especially temazepam) appears to be increasing (Deighan *et al.*, 2000).

## Implications for practice

- Renal function should be measured by the ability of the kidneys to achieve maintain homeostasis, not simply by the amount of urine produced.
- The most useful biochemical markers of renal function are urea and creatinine.
- Factors outside the kidneys (e.g. metabolism) may affect glomerular filtration of urea, so blood urea alone is not a reliable marker.
- The most common cause of renal failure in ICU patients is hypovolaemia, causing acute tubular necrosis.
- Prerenal failure can often be prevented if patients receive adequate fluids to maintain perfusion.
- Diuretics can remove excess fluid, but can kill hypovolaemic patients.

■ Renal failure prevents excretion of hydrogen ions from the body, so causes metabolic acidosis.

■ The many other metabolic functions of the kidney mean that renal failure causes complications for all other major systems.

■ Diuretics may restore urine volumes, and are useful for offloading excess fluid, but should be avoided with hypovolaemia.

## Summary

Acute renal failure frequently complicates other pathologies in ICU patients. While mortality from primary renal failure is encouragingly low, mortality from multiorgan dysfunction remains depressingly high. So if the incidence of progression to acute renal failure can be reduced, mortality and morbidity among ICU patients will significantly decrease.

Renal failure is failure of renal function, so causes fluid overload, electrolyte imbalances, acid–base balances and other metabolic disturbances causing further complications. Nurses therefore need knowledge of physiology and effects to optimise prevention and provide holistic care.

## Further reading

Most applied physiology texts include overviews of renal failure, although recent changes in practice limit the value of older texts. Mehta *et al.* (2002) provides convincing evidence against inappropriate use of diuretics. Deighan *et al.* (2000) and Meister and Reddy (2002) discuss rhabdomyolysis. www.routledge.com/textbooks/0415373239

For clinical scenarios, clinical questions and the answers to them go to the support website at www.routledge.com/textbooks/0415373239

## Clinical scenarios

Mr James Roger is 67 years old and has Type II diabetes. He underwent an aortic valve replacement 3 months previously. He was found collapsed at home and was subsequently admitted to the ICU with abnormal clotting and diagnosed with sepsis secondary to endocarditis. Mr Roger had received high dose intravenous antibiotics including Gentamicin, Vancomycin, Rifampicin, Cefotaxime and had been taking oral warfarin. His last recorded weight is 74 kg.

James's blood investigation values include:

| | |
|---|---|
| Urea (mmol/litre) | 28.4 |
| Creatinine (μmol/litre) | 255 |
| Creatine kinase (U/litre) | 294 |
| Sodium (mmol/litre) | 142 |
| Potassium (mmol/litre) | 4.0 |

| | |
|---|---|
| Chloride (mmol/litre) | 119 |
| Bicarbonate (mmol/litre) | 17 |
| Base Deficit (mmol/litre) | 5.8 |
| Lactate (mmol/litre) | 4.7 |

Arterial blood gas results while invasively ventilated on $FiO_2$ of 0.5

| | |
|---|---|
| pH | 7.2 |
| $PaCO_2$ (kPa) | 7.05 |
| $PaO_2$ (kPa) | 9.3 |
| $SaO_2$ (%) | 96.1 |

Vital observations with a noradrenaline infusion at 0.5 mcg/kg/minute were

| | |
|---|---|
| Temperature | 36.2°C |
| Heart rate (bpm) | 107 |
| Rhythm | Atrial fibrillation |
| BP (mmHg) | 76/46 |
| Cardiac Index (litres/minute/m$^2$) | 3.1 |
| CVP (mmHg) | 11 |
| Urine (ml/hour) | 10, 5, 5, 0 trend over 4 hours |

Q.1 Examine Mr Roger's abnormal values and risk factors and give a rationale for developing pre-, intra- or post-renal failure.

Q.2 Compare Mr Roger's results to normal values. Estimate his GFR using the Cockroft–Gault formula (Mallick & Marasi, 1999) (or refer to Chapter 21).

$$\frac{(140 - \text{Age (years)}) \times \text{Weight (kg)}}{\text{Serum creatinine } (\mu mol/l)} \times 1.25 \text{ for males, or } 1.03 \text{ for females}$$

Q.3 Consider the risk factors for developing acute renal failure (ARF) and for each factor explain the physiological processes resulting in ARF. Review the effects of hypoxaemia, hypercapnia, acid–base disturbances and mechanical ventilation on Mr Roger's sympathetic nervous system and ADH release. Formulate a plan of care which may enhance his renal blood flow and renal function.

*Same patient is used in scenario for Chapter 40.*

# Haemofiltration

## Contents

| | |
|---|---|
| Introduction | 423 |
| Haemofiltration | 423 |
| Haemodiafiltration | 425 |
| Factors affecting filtration | 425 |
| Filter membranes | 426 |
| Problems | 427 |
| Plasmapheresis | 429 |
| Implications for practice | 430 |
| Summary | 430 |
| Further reading | 431 |
| Clinical scenarios | 431 |

### Fundamental knowledge

Normal renal anatomy and physiology
Acute renal failure (see Chapter 39)

## Introduction

Renal replacement therapy is used for up to one-third of ICU patients (Rahman & Treacher, 2002). Haemofiltration is the main renal replacement therapy used in ICU (Wright *et al.*, 2003), so nurses should understand principles of haemofiltration, and have a working knowledge of whichever system their section uses. Manufacturers' recommendations differ between systems, so readers should adapt material in this chapter to systems used. Peritoneal dialysis and haemodialysis are rarely used on ICUs, so are not described here. Nurses encountering either therapy should resource specific texts on them. Principles of haemofiltration largely apply to plasmapheresis, sometimes used (usually intermittently rather than continuously) to remove mediators of disease.

Renal replacement therapy for patients in ICU has developed rapidly, 30 years ago being limited to peritoneal dialysis (PD) in most sections, or haemofiltration by renal nurses where hospitals also provided renal sections. Dialysis removes solutes diffusion, passing blood rapidly through a semipermeable membrane. Countercurrent of *dialysate*, fluid with few or no solutes of those to be removed creates a large concentration difference, causing rapid removal of solutes, such as urea and creatinine. Dialysis therefore efficiently removes small molecules, but can aggravate cardiovascular instability, making it unsuitable for ICU.

Haemofiltration, initially *continuous arterial venous haemofiltration* (CAVH), revolutionised renal replacement therapy for the critically ill. CAVH relies on patients having sufficient arterial blood pressure to 'drive' the circuits. Machine-driven *continuous venovenous haemofiltration* (CVVH) proved more successful, most ICU patients being hypotensive. Further developments in renal replacement therapies included combining haemofiltration with CVVH – *continuous venovenous haemodiafiltration* (CVVHD). Table 40.1 lists commonly used terms.

Renal replacement therapies mimic normal renal function by placing semipermeable membranes (filters) between patients' blood and a collection system. *Filtration* occurs when (hydrostatic) pressure forces fluid through this filter, while *dialysis* is movement of solutes by a concentration gradient. In practice, both usually occur together, different options adjusting the ratio, and therefore amount of fluid and solutes removed.

## Haemofiltration

Human glomerular filtration, pressure differences forces plasma through semipermeable capillary tubes (*ultrafiltration*). Haemofiltration mimics this, fluid removed being called *dialysate*. Solutes, especially large to middle-sized molecules, are drawn across the membrane by *convection* ('solvent drag'). Continuous venovenous haemofiltration (CVVH) uses only ultrafiltration and convection. CVVH can effectively remove volume, but solute clearance slows once concentrations on either side of the filter approach similar levels.

**Table 40.1 Renal replacement therapies – commonly used terms**

| | |
|---|---|
| CAPD | chronic ambulatory peritoneal dialysis CAVH continuous arteriovenous haemofiltration; rarely now used in ICU |
| CAVH | continuous arteriovenous haemofiltration (= ultrafiltration, later; rarely now used in ICU |
| CAVHD | continuous arteriovenous haemodialysis; rarely now used in ICU |
| CAVHDF | continuous arteriovenous haemodiafiltration; rarely now used in ICU |
| CRRT | continuous renal replacement therapy blanket term used to describe continuous any mode (e.g. haemofiltration; but not peritoneal dialysis or haemodialysis, which are not continuous) |
| CVVH | continuous venovenous haemofiltration |
| CVVHD | continuous venovenous haemodialysis |
| CVVHDF | continuous venovenous haemodiafiltration |
| dialysis | movement of particles from a highly concentrated to a lower concentration solution, using a semipermeable membrane |
| haemodialysis | renal replacement therapy primarily using extracorporeal dialysis haemofiltration renal replacement therapy primarily using extracorporeal convection of solutes |
| haemodiafiltration | haemofiltration adding a countercurrent, so adding principles of dialysis to haemofiltration |
| HDF | haemodiafiltration |
| HFD | high flux dialysis (also: continuous high flux dialysis – CAVHFD/ CVVHFD) |
| plasmapheresis | haemofiltration, usually with smaller filter pores; sometimes called 'continuous plasma adsorption' |
| SCUF | slow continuous ultrafiltration removal of ultrafiltrate, usually using a small-pore filter, so minimising solute removal; used only for removing/reducing fluid overload (rarely used in ICU) |
| ultrafiltrate | removal of fluid through hydrostatic pressure, solution removed through a small-pore semipermeable membrane |

A large double-lumen cannula is inserted into a large vein, with blood drawn from one side (normally coloured either red or brown) into the circuit and returned to the patient through the other lumen (normally coloured blue). The line from the patient is called 'arterial' or 'afferent' (early haemofilters relied on arterial cannulation). The return line is labelled 'venous' or 'efferent'. Unlike the human kidney, haemofiltration (and haemodialysis) cannot selectively reabsorb, so electrolyte-rich replacement fluid is added to mimic the human kidney's selective reabsorption.

High speed haemofiltration (sometimes called 'high flux dialysis' – HFD or 'continuous high flux dialysis' – CVVHFD) for short periods may achieve better clearance than haemodialysis. Rates of 35 ml/kg/hour have been used mainly to remove mediators of SIRS (Ronco et al., 2000). Circuits are relatively costly, time-consuming to prime and can expose patients to greater risk of cardiovascular instability and error.

## Haemodiafiltration

Solute clearance can be significantly increased by combining the principles of haemofiltration and haemodialysis – adding a countercurrent ('dialysate') to create haemo*dia*filtration (CVVHDF) – ultrafiltration, convection and diffusion. Theoretically, countercurrent clearance is proportional to countercurrent volume, but little benefit is gained by exchanges larger than 1–2 litres each hour.

## Factors affecting filtration

Whatever renal replacement therapy is used, filtration (like human kidneys) relies on *blood flow* through filters and *pressure gradients* across the semipermeable membrane. *Transmembrane pressure* (the pressure across the membrane inside the filter – see Glossary) gradients are created by:

■  driving pressure
■  resistance
■  *oncotic*/osmotic pressure.

*Blood flow* is primarily created by *driving pressure*. In human kidneys driving pressure is afferent arteriole blood pressure; CVVH driving pressure is afferent pump speed. Inadequate flow (e.g. occlusion with changes of patients' position) causes arterial/afferent pressure alarms; readjusting patients' positions usually restores blood flow.

Blood flow through filters is also affected by blood *viscosity* (see Chapter 18), so prediluting blood by adding fluid before the filter reduces viscosity, increasing filtrate volume, urea clearance and filter life (reducing need for anticoagulation) (Kaplan, 1985); but anecdotal reports suggest predilution both hastens coagulation and reduces filter life, perhaps due to activation of clotting factors; further research is needed both to identify mechanisms and to guide practice.

Dialysate flow rate with haemodiafiltration creates counterpressure *resistance* to afferent pump speed. Usually exchanges are 1–2 litres every hour (16.6–33.3 ml/minute), creating a relatively low resistance against afferent flows of 150 ml/minute.

*Oncotic* and osmotic pressure is created by plasma proteins and other large molecules. Predilution reduces oncotic pressure in filters. Some dialysate fluids (e.g. hypertonic glucose) increase osmotic pull.

If circuits are running without achieving aims (removal of volume and/or solutes), they are consuming nursing time and exposing patients to risks needlessly. Effectiveness should therefore be monitored. Means will vary depending on aims, but one way to assess effectiveness is filtration fraction:

$$FF = \frac{\text{ultrafiltrate rate} \times 100}{\text{filter plasma flow rate (QP)}}$$

where QP = blood flow rate (BFR) × (1 − Hct). Filtration fraction should normally be below 20–25 per cent.

## Filter membranes

Filter pore size varies, but many filters used in ICU for haemofiltration have a similar pore size to the glomerulus in the human kidney – 65–70 kiloDaltons (kDa). Although this means they can filter substances of a similar size, filters lacks

- sialoproteins – negatively charged proteins in the glomerular bed which repel other negatively charged ions, such as albumin
- selective renal tubule reabsorbtion.

*Hollow fibres* are usually used. Often containing more than 20,000 fine capillary tubes, creating a large surface area for filtration, using a small volume of blood and, being cylindrical. There are also sturdy. Small capillary tube diameter usually necessitates anticoagulation to prevent thrombosis and obstruction.

*Flat plate* filters contain a series of plates. Although overall surface area is smaller than with hollow fibres, flat plates can clear small molecules more efficiently and are less prone to clotting, so require less anticoagulation.

High *transmembrane pressure* (TMP) can rupture ('blow', 'burst kidney') the filter, necessitating immediate cessation of filtration. No attempt should be made to return blood ('washback') if the membrane is ruptured, as fragments of membrane may be washed back with blood. Maximum transmembrane pressure is usually stated on filters. Transmembrane pressure is created by various factors, but rising pressure usually suggests significantly decreased filtration surface area from thrombus formation. While efferent filters protect patients from emboli, rising transmembrane pressures are usually an indication to discontinue filtration. Maximum transmembrane pressure should not exceed 100 mmHg.

Recommended *priming* volumes normally exceed total circuit volume. While priming removes air emboli, its main purpose is removal of glycerol and ethylene oxide used to protect filters during storage and transportation. These chemicals can cause convulsions, paralysis, renal failure and haemolysis, so priming volumes should follow manufacturer's recommendations and not be abandoned once circuits are filled with fluid.

Similarly, circuits left standing unused should be reprimed before use, and should be used within maximum time allowed by protocols and manufacturer's liability – maximum 72 hours, but sometimes less.

As with human nephrons, *solute clearance* is limited by ultrafiltrate concentrations, ending once equilibrium is reached. Solutes are often referred to as either small or middle (above 500 Da = 0.5 kDa) sized.

## Problems

Initial, usually transient, hypotension can occur when commencing haemofiltration. Likely causes are

- hypovolaemia (bleeding onto circuit; crystalloid bolus replacing blood)
- prostacycline infusion (vasodilates)
- cytokine release (as blood reacts with artificial circuit).

Although filters are biocompatible, to minimise cytokine release, bio-compatibility is relative rather than absolute.

Being continuous, haemofiltration is impractical for prolonged use with mobile patients. Even moving patients onto their side or into chairs often causes problems with filtration.

Extracorporeal circuits are (usually) continuously *anticoagulated* to prevent thrombus (and embolus) formation. Although efferent filters should remove emboli before reaching patients, adsorption of blood proteins onto foreign surfaces (e.g. extracorporeal circuits) occurs within milliseconds of exposure, and platelets adherence to filter membranes triggers thrombus formation. Thrombi rapidly occlud narrow pores of filter membranes, so reducing their efficiency. Thrombus formation is increased by slow blood flow. Signs of thrombus formation include

- dark blood in circuits
- kicking of lines
- high transmembrane pressure.

Anticoagulation may be unnecessary with prolonged clotting. Heparin prime reduces initial platelet aggregation enabling lower dose of subsequent anticoagulants. Anticoagulants are below filter threshold, but some inevitably reaches patients, aggravating coagulopathies; reversal agents (e.g. protamine) can be added after the filter.

Heparin remains the most widely used anticoagulant, but *prostacyclin* (epoprostenol; prostaglandin $I_2$ – $PGI_2$) and citrate are also used (Monchi *et al.*, 2004). Prostacyclin inhibits platelet, and causes vasodilation. Kirby and Davenport (1996) suggest that up to 40 per cent of prostacyclin is removed by filtration, leaving over half remaining. Prostacyclin is more expensive than heparin, and so tends to be used if coagulopathies from heparin become problematic.

Despite extensive monitoring of respiratory and cardiovascular systems on ICU, many units rely on haematology departments and daily blood samples to monitor effects of haemofiltration on clotting.

Poor flow (high afferent pressure), usually from lateral or semi-recumbent position, can sometimes be resolved by swapping connections to the two-way catheter. However, this increases blood recirculation by up to one-fifth, reducing clearance.

*Afferent pump speed* should be commenced slowly (e.g. 100 ml/minute) as some patients develop acute hypotensive crises. If stable, speeds should usually be increased to a minimum 150 ml/minute within 10 minutes, although readers should check manufacturers' recommendations and local protocols. Afferent pump speeds Circuits can safely run at 250–300 ml/minute, which may prolong filter life and/or reduce anticoagulation requirements. Faster speeds, such as would be used with haemodialysis, are unnecessary with continuous haemofiltration and might cause hypotensive crises in critically ill patients.

Lactate-based dialysate reduces metabolic *acidosis* (Cole *et al.*, 2003) but relies on adequate hepatic function to convert lactate to bicarbonate (Hilton *et al.*, 1998). Provided liver function is adequate, the only undesirable effect is hyperglycaemia (Bollman *et al.*, 2004).

Extracoropeal circulation causes convention of heat, so may cause *hypothermia*, especially if circuits hold relatively large volumes of blood. Most manufacturers produce blood warmers for circuits. Body temperature may be reduced by up to 4°C (Keen, 2001), masking pyrexia, so nurses should actively assess for other signs of infection. Foil should not be wrapped around lines, as this prevents nurses from observing bloodflow. Warming blankets should be used with caution, as they may cause peripheral dilatation (Smith, 1999).

Haemofiltraion removes and replaces large volumes of fluid – for example, afferent pump speeds of 150 ml/minute removes 9 litres each hour – nearly double average total blood volume. Despite many safety features on machines, this creates risks of significant fluid imbalance if erroneous figures are charted or therapy is overly aggressive. Risks can be minimised by

- continuous cardiovascular monitoring (with appropriate alarm settings)
- careful monitoring of fluid balance (most units monitor hourly, but some monitor less frequently)
- setting appropriate alarms on haemofiltration machines.

Concern about *drug clearance* by haemofiltration is justified, but factors are complex, requiring advice from unit pharmacists. Some factors are described here to illustrate how problematic this issue is.

All drugs (except some colloidal fluids) used in clinical practice are smaller than filter pore size, weighing at most only a few kiloDaltons, so potentially may be filtered. However, plasma proteins are larger (albumin weighs 66.5 kDa), so protein-bound drugs are retained. All drugs are partly protein bound, but extent of protein binding ranges greatly, from negligible to almost total. Studies of drug clearance may refer to peritoneal dialysis, haemodialysis, haemofiltration or haemodiafiltration. Even within a single technique, different filter pore sizes influence clearance. Clearance may also differ between animal or healthy human volunteers and critically ill patients.

Kaplan (1998) identifies four main factors affecting drug clearance:

- molecular weight – 5–10 kDa substances are readily cleared by haemofiltration

■ degree of protein binding to filter membrane
■ drugs' volume of distribution (water solubility/lipid affinity)
■ drugs' endogenous clearance (hepatic).

Drugs are usually only active if unbound, so binding is normally weak, with volatile shifts between bound and unbound drug molecules. Protein binding alone is affected by

■ acidity (pH) of blood
■ molar drug concentrations
■ bilirubin levels
■ uraemic inhibitors
■ presence of heparin
■ numbers of free fatty acids
■ other (displacing) drugs.

Predilution increases transfer (and so clearance) of protein-bound urea (and other molecules) into plasma (Kaplan, 1998).

Large ultrafiltrate volumes are often smaller than human glomerular filtrate, so drug clearance by filters may be no higher than the Bowmans capsule. But selective reabsorption in the human kidney may restore plasma concentrations. Drug prescriptions may therefore need increasing or decreasing during haemo-filtration. Where drugs are titrated to therapeutic effects such as measured laboratory levels (e.g. Vancomycin) or clinical parameters (e.g. blood pressure with inotropes), dosages can safely be adjusted within prescribed limits to achieve specified aims. With other drugs, advice from unit pharmacists is valuable.

Trace elements may be filtered, calcium and magnesium loss being especially significant, so filtered patients often need additional supplements (Klein *et al.*, 2002).

Gelatins have relatively small molecules (most below 20 kDa), so gelatins are filtered, making their effect relatively transient. Crystalloids are likely to be as beneficial and are cheaper. Alternatively, starch-based colloids are unlikely to be filtered.

Most manufacturers recommend *changing circuits* every 72 hours. Anecdotal reports suggest filters and circuits can function considerably longer, but circuits are highly invasive, so major sources for infection. Not following manufacturer's instructions, or written local protocols, may expose nurses to legal liability for any harm.

## Plasmapheresis

Plasmapheresis resembles haemofiltration, usually with smaller filter pores (30–50 kDa (Meyer, 2000)). Initial enthusiasm for treating SIRS by plasma-pheresis has waned. Plasmapheresis is usually now used to remove mediators in other diseases (e.g. Guillain-Barré Syndrome), drugs (e.g. overdoses) or other small substances without removing large volumes of fluid.

## Implications for practice

- Nurses who have not used haemofiltration equipment should take every opportunity to learn how to manage it before caring for patients being haemofiltered.
- Haemofiltration resembles the human nephron, so although machines can appear daunting, follow through circuits comparing them with nephron function.
- When checking circuits, start from the beginning of the afferent line and work through the circuit until the end of the efferent line.
- Check the circuit and equipment at the start of each shift and whenever necessary.
- Large fluid balance errors can quickly accumulate; fluid balance should be kept as simple as possible avoiding volumes under 1 ml; recheck calculations and running totals.
- Most alarms halt circuits; identify and resolve problems urgently, restarting the system before coagulation blocks the filter.
- Involve unit pharmacists to identify how therapeutic drugs are affected by filtration.
- Hypotension can occur quickly, especially when commencing filtration, so haemodynamic status should be closely monitored.
- Unless instructed otherwise, start afferent pumps at 100 ml/minute; once stable (after 10 minutes) increase pump speed to at least 150 ml/minute.
- Pressures, flow, fluid balance and temperature should be monitored frequently – many units monitor hourly. Precise parameters monitored will vary with machines used, but should ensure patient safety.
- Small substances, including electrolytes and trace elements, are removed through haemofilters, so blood levels should be checked at least daily – especially sodium, potassium magnesium, phosphate, bicarbonate and pH.

## Summary

Renal replacement in most ICUs is provided by haemofiltration (and variants), although hospitals with renal units may use haemodialysis; there is also growing interest in plasmapheresis to treat pathologies such as SIRS/MODS.

Haemofiltration has proved to be a valuable medical adjunct to intensive care. While technology has made circuits and machines safer, haemofiltration is highly invasive exposing patients to various complications and dangers. Renal failure in ICU patients is usually secondary, so caring for patients receiving haemofiltration can create high nursing workloads. Care should be prioritised to ensure a safe environment. Nurses unfamiliar with using haemofiltration are encouraged to find out how to use it in practice before having to care on their own for patients receiving haemofiltration.

## Further reading

Despite widespread use in ICU, few ICU textbooks discuss haemofiltration in sufficient depth. Some useful articles have appeared in specialist journals, although most of these are medical rather than nursing. Wright *et al.* (2003) summarises current use in ICU. Rapid changes in use of haemofiltration limit the value of most older literature. A number of medical studies support bicarbonate filtration, including Bollmann *et al.* (2004). www.routledge.com/textbooks/0415373239

For clinical scenarios, clinical questions and the answers to them go to the support website at www.routledge.com/textbooks/0415373239

## Clinical scenarios

Mr James Roger is a 67-year-old man who developed acute renal failure from sepsis secondary to endocarditis. Mr Roger had received high dose intravenous antibiotics including Gentamicin, Vancomycin, Rifampicin, Cefotaxime and had been taking oral warfarin prior to admission.

He was commenced on continuous venovenous haemofiltration (CVVHF) with 3 litre fluid exchanges. The pump speed was recording 220–50 ml/minute; venous pressure 97 mmHg and transmembrane pressure were 60–70 mmHg. Mr Roger had deranged clotting, and infusions of Heparin at 2500 iu/h and Epoprostenol (Flolan®) at 5 ng/hour are in progress.

Q.1 Reflect on the CVVHF values and anticoagulation regime. Analyse how these drugs may effect Mr Roger's coagulation whilst on CVVHF.

Q.2 The CVVHF venous pressures increase over a 3 hour period to 250 mmHg with trans membrane pressures of 150 mmHg. Analyse this change and review actions you would take.

Q.3 Appraise nursing interventions which help maintain effectiveness and patency of CVVHF.

(a) Explain the nurses' role in monitoring; trouble shooting and maintaining patency of filter and patient safety with circuit (e.g. blood flows, leaks, air, fluid and electrolyte management, patient position).

(b) Justify other nursing approaches aimed at promoting renal recovery (e.g. drugs, temperature management, nutrition, psychological support, infection control, weaning CVVHF, etc.).

(c) Review approaches used for the disposal of ultrafiltrate, manual handling issues, filter changes, workload and resources and nursing skills development.

*Same patient is used in scenario for Chapter 39.*

Chapter 41

# Gastrointestinal bleeds

**Contents**

| | |
|---|---|
| Introduction | 433 |
| Variceal bleeding | 433 |
| Medical treatments | 434 |
| Peptic ulcers | 436 |
| *Helicobacter pylori* colonisation | 437 |
| Stress ulceration | 437 |
| Lower GI bleeds | 438 |
| Implications for practice | 438 |
| Summary | 438 |
| Further reading | 439 |
| Clinical scenarios | 439 |

**Fundamental knowledge**

Gastrointestinal anatomy
Portal pressure

## Introduction

The gastrointestinal (GI) tract is highly vascular, so while bleeding can be a primary pathology necessitating admission, haemorrhage more often complicates other pathologies in ICU patients. Up to one-tenth of ICU patients develop upper GI bleeds (Robertson *et al.*, 1999). Where haemorrhage is the primary problem, mortality is 11 per cent, but one-third of patients with other problems who develop acute bleeds die (British Society of Gastroenterology Endoscopy Committee, 2000). The liver produces most intrinsic clotting factors, so impaired liver function, whether from chronic liver disease or prolonged hypoperfusion during critical illness, impairs haemostasis. Chronic liver disease further increases risks of gastrointestinal bleeding. Lower GI bleeds are less immediately life-threatening, but are briefly mentioned at the end of this chapter.

Risk factors for large and sudden haemorrhage include patients with

■ delayed clotting (e.g. haemofiltration, following cardiac surgery)
■ liver failure (especially chronic)
■ hypertension.

Clotting time should be checked and monitored on admission and then as appropriate. Potentially risk factors that could be modified include

■ removing unneeded invasive equipment
■ avoiding oesophageal equipment if possible, or inserting it under platelet cover
■ adjusting DVT prophylaxis
■ avoiding anti-coagulants
■ controlling blood pressure
■ avoiding traumatic interventions.

Some treatments identified below may also be useful to prevent bleeding, especially beta-blockers.

Severe haemorrhage rapidly causes hypovolaemic *shock*, hypoperfusion predisposing to SIRS and MODS. Urgent fluid resuscitation is usually required, especially with colloids, clotting factors and blood transfusions. Massive blood transfusions further disrupt homeostasis, predisposing to DIC and electrolyte imbalance.

## Variceal bleeding

One-tenth of GI bleeds are from varices (British Society of Gastroenterology Endoscopy Committee, 2000), but half of cirrhotics have varices, and half of these bleed from varices (Fallah *et al.*, 2000; Sharara, 2001). A third of bleeds are fatal (Fallah *et al.*, 2000; Sharara, 2001), two-thirds of survivors will re-bleed (Sharara, 2001) and half of these will die from re-bleeding (Fallah *et al.*, 2000).

The gut is richly supplied with superficial blood vessels flowing to the liver, carrying nutrients from food for processing. These flow eventually into the portal vein, a large vein carrying one litre or more of blood each minute (Smith, 2000). In health, portal pressure is about 5–10 mmHg. Obstructed hepatic bloodflow, typically from cirrhosis, increases pressure in veins before the liver, causing portal hypertension (>12 mmHg, (Smith, 2000)) and varices. Varices form mainly in the oesophagus and stomach. Already distended, and so weak-walled, they rupture easily if pressure increases. Rupture often causes massive, life-threatening haemorrhage.

Urgent treatment should

- stop haemorrhage
- restore blood volume and haematocrit (fluid resuscitation)
- replace clotting factors.

Haemorrhage is usually stopped by

- balloon tamponade
- banding
- sclerosis
- stents.

## Medical treatments

A 'first aid' intervention to stop bleeding is placing direct pressure on bleeding points using *balloon tamponade* (Sengstaken, Sengstaken-Blakemore, Minessota tubes; see Figure 41.1). Tubes usually have three or four ports:

- oesophageal balloon (to stop bleeding)
- oesophageal aspiration port (omitted on 3-port tubes)

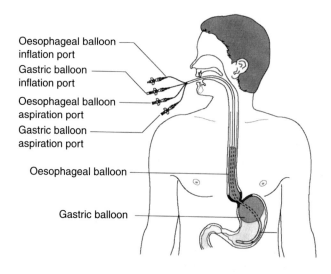

Oesophageal balloon inflation port
Gastric balloon inflation port
Oesophageal balloon aspiration port
Gastric balloon aspiration port
Oesophageal balloon
Gastric balloon

**Figure 41.1 Sengstaken tube**

- gastric balloon (to anchor tubes)
- gastric aspiration port.

Balloon tamponade controls most bleeds, but half rebleed on deflation (Fallah *et al.*, 2000; Therapondos & Hayes, 2002). Balloon tamponade is a temporary (emergency) treatment, use should be limited to 12–24 hours. Rigid tubes are easier to insert (Smith, 2000), so should be stored in a fridge.

Unlike digital pressure on radial arteries, balloon pressure on oesophageal varices creates various problems

- Efficacy is seen only by presence or absence of frank bleeding; extent of subcutaneous bleeding (bruising) remains unseen.
- Surrounding tissue cannot be seen, so ischaemia from arterial/capillary occlusion may remain undetected until damage occurs.
- Staff usually soon tire of digital pressure, but balloon tamponade does not provide staff with sensory feedback.

Oesophageal balloons can hold up to 60 ml of air or water, but should only be inflated if bleeding persists after inflation of the gastric balloon (Stanley & Hayes, 1997). Pressure should be sufficient to control haemorrhage; recommended pressures vary, up to 50–60 mmHg (Sung, 2003). Pressure can be measured by connecting a sphygmomanometer or continuous monitoring system to the oesophageal inflation port.

That external traction can further compress oesophageal varices with the gastric balloon (Steele & Sabol, 2005) is controversial. Gastric varices, already compressed by the gastric balloon, should prevent flow to higher varices. Many centres avoid using traction, but if used, lifting weights should be avoided as tube movement may dislodge clots.

The main complications from prolonged pressure are

- ulceration
- aspiration pneumonia.

To minimise ulceration, if inflated, oesophageal balloons should be deflated for 30 minutes every 4–6 hours (Therapondos & Hayes, 2002). Deflation may traumatise friable healing tissue, causing rebleeding.

*Sclerotherapy* (endoscopic injection of adrenaline or other vasopressors into varices) usually involves progressive obliteration through a series of treatments (usually over 1–4 weeks), so patients may be transferred from ICU before treatment is completed. Endoscopic sclerotherapy stops 90 per cent of bleeds (Vargas *et al.*, 1999; Sharara, 2001).

Endoscopic ligation with bands ('*banding*') is more effective than sclerotherapy (Stiegmann *et al.*, 1992; Gimson *et al.*, 1993). The endoscope suctions the varix, tying it off with an elastic band. The varix sloughs off in 24–72 hours, leaving a shallow ulcer (Vargas *et al.*, 1999). Banding does not usually resolve gastric varices (10–36 per cent of varix bleeds) (Therapondos & Hayes, 2002), so further treatments are often needed later.

*Vasopressin* (antidiuretic hormone) and derivatives (desmopressin, terlipressin) cause splanchnic arterial vasoconstriction, so reducing portal hypertension. It stops 50–70 per cent of bleeds (Fallah *et al.*, 2000). Terlipressin's (triglycyl lysine vasopressin) half-life is longer than vasopressin or desmopressin, is more successful and has fewer side effects, such as vasoconstriction (Vargas *et al.*, 1999; Smith, 2000).

*Beta-blockers* (e.g. propanolol) reduce cardiac output, and constricts mesenteric arteries, so reducing portal pressure. This will not solve acute crises, but reduces risks of rebleeding (Sharara, 2001; Therapondos & Hayes, 2002). However β-blockers may precipitate congestive cardiac failure, asthma and bradycardia (Vargas *et al.*, 1999); nitrates are useful if β-blockers are contra-indicated (Vargas *et al.*, 1999; Sharara, 2001).

The hormone *somatostatin*, and its longer-acting synthetic analogue *octreotide*, constrict splanchnic bloodflow, so control most acute bleeds (Corley *et al.*, 2001) and are useful for preventing further bleeds.

Transjugular intrahepatic portosystemic shunt (*TIPSS*) stops most bleeds, so is the preferred treatment for varices. A percutaneous angioplasty-type catheter creates a fistula between the portal and hepatic veins, which is then kept open with expandable metal stents (usually 8–12 mm diameter) (Therapondos & Hayes, 2002). Because shunted blood bypasses the liver it is not detoxified, so a fifth of patients develop encephalopathy (Smith, 2000).

*Gastric irrigation* to remove blood may also prolong or restart haemorrhage. Cold water may also cause vagal stimulation increasing gastric motility and irritation to ulcers.

*Surgical* oesophageal transection or implantation of portocaval shunts effectively controls bleeding, but without improvement in long-term survival (Sung, 2003). Half develop elcephalopathy, so surgical shunts are rarely performed (Smith, 2000).

## Peptic ulcers

Most upper GI bleeds are from peptic ulcers (British Society of Gastroenterology Endoscopy Committee, 2000; Ghost *et al.*, 2002). A quarter of people with duodenal ulcers develop major bleeds (Shiotani & Graham, 2002).

Gastric mucus maintains wide pH differences between gastric acid (or alkaline bile) and epithelium. Mucosal failure may be caused by

- excess acid production (from gastromas)
- lack of neutralising factors (absence of enteral nutrition)
- bile reflux
- drugs inhibiting cytoprection (e.g. aspirin and non-steroidal anti-inflammatories).

Chronic ulcers often result from non-steroidal anti-inflammatory drugs (NSAIDs) prescribed for chronic conditions such as arthritis. Development of Cox-2 inhibitors to replace NSAIDs has reduced incidence of bleeds.

Treatment may be preventative (protecting against gastric acidity), supportive (replacing blood volume and clotting factors), medical (treating bacteria) or surgical.

## *Helicobacter pylori* colonisation

Most (95 per cent) of duodenal ulcers in people not taking NSAIDs are caused by the bacterium *Helicobacter pylori* (Harris & Misiewicz, 2001), one of the most common and increasing, bacterial human infections (Suerbaum & Michetti, 2002). Colonisation usually begins in childhood (Malaty *et al.*, 2002) and up to half of adults in industrialised countries are colonised (Suerbaum & Michetti, 2002).

To produce the alkaline environment they need to survive, *H. pylori* produce carbon dioxide. Many tests for *H. pylori* measure gastric carbon dioxide.

Ulcers usually heal quickly following eradication of *H. pylori* (Harris & Misiewicz, 2001). However, ulceration only develops in a minority of those colonised by *H. pylori* thus prophylactic eradication is impractical (Calam & Baron, 2001).

## Stress ulceration

Problems of stress ulceration have long been recognised. One-fifth of ICU patients have endoscopic evidence of stress ulceration, although seldom develop significant haemorrhage (Brealey & Singer, 2000). Ventilated patients are at high risk of increased gastric acidity, especially if gut motility is reduced and/or and enteral feeding is not given. Enteral feeding helps protect against gastric ulceration. Enteral feed regimes may, or may not, include rest periods to enable gastric pH to fall (see Chapter 9).

$H_2$-blockers (cimetidine, ranitidine) reduce gastric acid secretion; in ICU ranitidine is widely used to prevent stress ulceration (Williams & Sadler, 2003), although Messori *et al.* (2000) suggest it does not reduce incidence of gastric bleeding.

Sucralfate, an aluminium salt, stimulates mucosal blood flow and mucus secretion, so increasing endogenous defences. Since Cook *et al.*'s (1998) finding that ranitidine prevented more bleeds than Sucralfate, histamine-2 (H2) receptor antagonists have become the most widely used stress ulcer prophylaxis in ICU (Daley *et al.*, 2004). Sucralfate can cause also gastrointestinal obstruction (Bradley, 2001b). Improved management and increased use of enteral feeding has reduced stress ulceration and stress ulcer incidence in ICU decreased, but it still occurs in one-fifth of ICU patients (Williams & Sadler, 2003).

## Lower GI bleeds

A quarter of gastrointestinal bleeds are from the lower tract (Fallah *et al.*, 2000), but these are rarely acutely life-threatening. Most stop spontaneously, seldom necessitating ICU admission. But many ICU patients have coagulopathies, so may bleed from the highly vascular lower GI tract.

Stools should be observed for frank blood; occult bleeding can be confirmed by testing. Observations should be recorded and reported; samples may be required for testing. Bleeding may be fresh (red; usually lower GI bleeds) or old (black, tarry; usually upper GI bleeds).

Most bleeds are small, but if large bleeds do not resolve spontaneously, early surgery (e.g. hemicolectomy) may be needed.

## Implications for practice

- The gut is highly vascular, so upper gastrointestinal haemorrhage is frequently large and life-threatening, requiring urgent fluid resuscitation and close haemodynamic monitoring.
- Risk factors (history, blood pressure, treatment, clotting) should be assessed and risks minimised where possible.
- Balloon tamponade is a quick way to stop bleeding, but is only a temporary measure and removal often restarts bleeding.
- Blood is hazardous, potentially carrying viruses such as hepatitis B and HIV; maintain a safe environment for yourself, other staff and visitors.
- Unless specifically contraindicated, all ventilated patients should receive stress ulcer prophylaxis.
- Seeing blood can make patients and families especially anxious; psychological support/care can help them cope and warn them about possibly seeing/smelling blood; if possible, remove soiled linen.
- Escort visitors to the bedside, encouraging them to sit down (so they do not harm themselves on equipment if they faint).
- Mouthcare helps remove the vile taste of blood and vomit.

## Summary

Stress ulcer prophylaxis and enteral feeding has significantly reduced development of stress ulcers, but patients in ICU can develop major upper gastrointestinal bleeding from ulcers or chronic liver disease. Upper gastrointestinal bleeding is often a life-threatening emergency, and may necessitate ICU admission. ICU nurses necessarily have an important role assisting doctors to control and monitor bleeds, but also have an important role maintaining a safe environment for themselves and others, and meeting the psychological needs of patients and visitors.

## Further reading

The British Society of Gastroenterology Endoscopy Committee (2000) guidelines provide an authoritative resource for all clinical staff. Shiotani and Graham (2002) is a recent medical review of gastric ulceration, while Suerbaum and Michetti (2002) describe *Helicobacter pylori*. Daley *et al.* (2004) review stress ulcer prophylaxis. www.routledge.com/textbooks/0415373239

For clinical scenarios, clinical questions and the answers to them go to the support website at www.routledge.com/textbooks/0415373239

## Clinical scenarios

Victor Newton is a 51-year-old known alcoholic who was admitted to ICU via A&E with a three week history of malaena, recent large volume haematemesis that morning and severe epigastric pain. He had previous episodes of malaena and haematemesis over the Christmas holiday season and was awaiting an out patient endoscopy appointment.

Q.1 List the nursing priorities when preparing for and admitting a patient with an emergency GI bleed. Include resources needed such as equipment, drugs, investigations, specialists.

An emergency endoscopy is performed which confirms three bleeding oesophageal varices that were banded. Victor then re-bled. A balloon tamponade tube was inserted to exert direct pressure on the ruptured and bleeding vessels. His current medications include intravenous infusion of omeprazole at 8 mg/hour and oral sucralfate (antepsin®) suspension of 2 grams every 6 hours.

Q.2 Analyse nursing interventions following balloon tamponade tube insertion which monitor effect and minimise potential complications (e.g. checking tube placement, type of traction methods, free drainage or not, sputum clearance, saliva removal, aspiration pneumonia, tissue pressure necrosis, malaena, metabolic effects of blood in lower GI tract).
Q.3 It is decided to remove the balloon tamponade tube at 24 hours. Consider how this process should be managed to minimise the risk of re-bleeding.

Victor's experience of haematemesis and emergency intervention have made him very anxious. Review possible causes of his ruptured varices and the risk of reoccurrence. Specify the liver function investigations he may undergo.

Design a plan of care for Victor that focuses on reducing his anxiety and the risk of re-bleeding in ICU, following transfer to ward and after discharge from hospital care.

Advice should include the reason for and practical strategies regarding:

- avoiding vigorous coughing and sneezing
- recognition of early signs and symptoms of re-bleeding
- relaxation techniques
- drug action affected by his condition and hepatic impairment (e.g. benzodiazepines, aspirin)
- paracetamol, some antibiotics, alcohol, cigarettes/nicotine
- lifestyle changes
- use of specialist nurses, referral groups.

Chapter 42

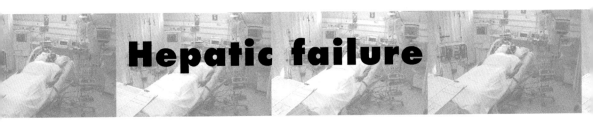

# Hepatic failure

## Contents

Introduction                         442
Acute failure                        442
Chronic failure                      443
Liver function tests                 443
Decompensation                       444
Other complications                  446
Intra-abdominal pressure             447
Artificial livers                    447
Implications for practice            447
Summary                              448
Further reading                      448
Further resources                    448
Clinical scenarios                   449

## Fundamental knowledge

Hepatic anatomy and physiology
Kupffer cell function

## Introduction

The liver has more, and more diverse, functions than any other major organ, including

- nutrition (synthesis of plasma proteins, glucogenesis)
- immunity
- heat production
- synthesis of homeostatic controls (most intrinsic clotting factors, angiotensin 1)
- detoxification (ammonia, drugs)

so hepatic failure affects most other major systems. However, symptoms of liver failure are less immediately apparent than respiratory, cardiac or renal dysfunction, so may be given low priority in ICU patients.

Failure may be acute or chronic. With acute failure, remaining hepatocytes normally regenerate, enabling good recovery. Acute failure is treated mainly by supporting systems and minimise complications to enable hepatocyte recovery. With chronic failure recovery is minimal. Transplantation may be needed, but until available sufficient function may remain for people to normally cope. But demands of acute illness can cause decompensation of chronic failure. Saggs (2000) identifies three main hepatic problems seen in ICU

- fulminant failure
- decompensation of chronic failure
- dysfunction secondary to critical illness.

This chapter describes pathophysiology, major complications and treatments, focussing mainly on acute failure. Main liver function tests are identified, but because liver function is so diverse, no single test exists to identify liver failure. Severe hepatic failure may necessitate referral to specialist centres.

## Acute failure

The term *fulminant hepatic failure* (extensive hepatocyte necrosis together with encephalopathy occurring within eight weeks of onset) is still used, but is increasingly being replaced by

- *hyperacute*: jaundice occurs <7 days before encephalopathy
- *acute*: jaundice occurs 8–28 days before encephalopathy
- *subacute*: jaundice occurs 4–12 weeks before encephalopathy.

This chapter follows terminology of sources cited.

Acute hepatic failure may be caused by

- drugs
- paracetamol

■ chemicals
■ viruses
■ unknown causes.

Although scientifically questionable (paracetamol is a drug, and drugs are chemicals), this apparently arbitrary division is clinically useful. Up to three-quarters of patients die within a few days of onset of acute liver failure (Stockmann *et al.*, 2000), although prognosis varies with the origin of failure. Symptoms of acute failure are similar from all causes.

In the UK, unlike most other countries, paracetamol overdose remains the main cause of liver failure. Many other therapeutic drugs (e.g. isoniazid and other anti-TB drugs, chlorpromazine) can also provoke failure (Rashid *et al.*, 2004). Paracetamol overdose is discussed in Chapter 47.

## Chronic failure

Chronic liver disease is usually caused by

■ alcohol
■ nonalcoholic straetohepatitis (NASH)
■ hepatitis B or C (HBV, HCV)
■ primary hepatocellular carcinoma

but can develop from acute failure, and sometimes causes are unknown.

Alcohol remains the main chemical cause of chronic liver failure. Liver failure can (rarely) be caused by industrial solvents, such as carbon tetrachloride ($CCI_4$, widely used, including for dry cleaning), and by mushroom poisoning (usually Amanita Phalloides – 'death cap').

Hepatic failure may be caused by hepatitis (in the UK, usually B or C) and by many other viruses (e.g. herpes simplex, varicella, CMV, Epstein-Barr). Outside the UK, liver failure is usually viral.

Chronic failure may usually cause

■ hyperdynamic circulation
■ portal hypertension
■ oesophageal varices and bleeding.

End-stage liver disease necessitates transplantation. While some of these problems may necessitate ICU admission, acute failure and hypofunction more often complicate other diseases in ICU, so are the focus of this chapter.

## Liver function tests

The liver metabolises toxins in blood, so with liver failure levels of many solutes increase. The most useful indicators of liver function are usually

■ clotting (especially INR)
■ albumin

**Table 42.1 Main liver function tests**

| Liver function tests | Normal range |
| --- | --- |
| Bilirubin (Bil) | 1–20 µmol/litre |
| Alkaline Phosphatase (Alk Phos) | <100 iu/litre |
| Aspartate Aminotransferase (AST) | <40 iu/litre |
| Alanine Aminotransferase (ALT) | <40 iu/litre |
| Albumin | 30–52 g/litre |
| Total protein (TP) | 60–80 g/litre |
| Gamma glutamyl transpeptidase | 10–48 iu/litre |

- bilirubin
- transaminases (alanine aminotransferase – ALT; aspartate aminotransferase – AST)
- alkaline phosphate (Alk Phos)
- gamma glutamyl transpeptidase (GGT)

(see Table 42.1).

With severe acute failure, INR rises rapidly, potentially exceeding 10 (many laboratories outside transplantation centres cannot measure such high levels). Clotting is discussed in Chapter 21. As the liver detoxifies ammonia into urea, urea levels are also raised.

Bilirubin, a waste product of erythrocyte metabolism, is normally metabolised by the liver into bile, so liver failure causes bilirubinaemia. Serum bilirubin above 50 micromols causes jaundice. Bilirubin is raised with when flow through the liver is obstructed. With chronic liver failure this is typically due to cirrhosis. With most ICU patients obstruction is usually caused by inflammation.

Hepatocyte necrosis releases intracellular enzymes and chemicals – transaminases, Alk Phos, GGT. Although indicating necrosis, levels do not correlate with extent of damage, so cannot be used to predict outcome.

## Decompensation

Failure of liver function causes various symptoms, but the main life-threatening complications of acute failure are usually cerebral oedema and sepsis (Krumberger, 2002). Progressive liver failure causes failure of homeostasis, especially

- encephalopathy
- gross ascites
- hypotension

often occurring together. Major haemorrhage can also occur (see Chapter 41).

Increased permeability of the blood brain barrier, together with failure of liver metabolism, exposes the brain to excessive amounts of ammonia and other toxins. This is proved to be the cause of hepatic *encaphalopathy*. Increased permeability of the blood brain barrier increases cerebrospinal fluid (CSF) protein and sodium concentrations, creating an osmotic pull. Cerebral irritation from oedema may cause fitting, which may be subclinical. Normal sleeping pattern may be reversed, patients remain awake overnight. Increased muscle tone may cause decerebrate postures (Hawker, 2003). Cerebral oedema may be prevented by keeping the head aligned (to facilitate venous drainage), treating underling infections and reduce gut bacterial production of ammonia with lactulose or Neomycin, aiming for 2–4 soft stools each day (Saggs, 2000). It can be reversed with mannitol, an osmotic diuretic. Encephalopathy reduces patients' ability to understand, often making them more agitated and distressing their relatives. Psychological care should include

■   frequent, simple explanations
■   calm, low voice
■   avoiding/minimising conflict
■   supporting relatives.

Some units use intracranial pressure monitoring (see Chapter 23) to guide management, but this is not always available, and this may introduce infection or cause haemorrhage (Saggs, 2000). Jugular venous saturation monitoring may be a useful alternative.

*Ascites* causes mechanical compression of the liver, lungs and other major organs and significantly contributes to hypovolaemia. It may be drained through ascitic tap or paracentesis, but tends to reform, and drainage may introduce infection or cause haemorrhage (Saggs, 2000). Ascites is albumin-rich; hence aggressive fluid replacement, usually including albumin, are needed, both to restore plasma volume and to create an osmotic pull away from remaining ascites into the bloodstream. Intra-abdominal pressure measurement (see later) is useful to prevent liver damage from mechanical compression.

Cardiac output increases, but hypovolaemia causes *hypotension*, mainly due to

■   vasodilatation and increased capillary permeability (inflammatory responses)
■   hypoalbuminaemia (plasma proteins are synthesised in the liver)
■   bleeding (most intrinsic clotting factors are produced in the liver).

Normal compensatory responses fail. Angiotensinogen, the precursor of angiotensin (see Chapter 32), is produced in the liver, so hepatic failure causes failure of the renin-angiotensin-aldosterone mechanism, contributing to vasodilatation.

Prolonged hypotension results in tissue hypoxia, anaerobic metabolism, widespread cell dysfunction, multiorgan dysfunction and eventually death. Hypotension should therefore be treated with aggressive fluid resuscitation. Relatively prolonged effects from liver dysfunction and increased capillary permeability make colloids preferable to crystalloids. Early nutrition provides the protein needed for recovering livers to produce plasma proteins.

## Other complications

Hepatic failure usually causes

- hepatic encephalopathy
- coagulopathy
- jaundice.

The liver synthesises most clotting factors, so bleeding may be an early symptom of acute hepatic failure. Activated clotting factors are not broken down, so disseminated intravascular coagulation (DIC – see Chapter 26) may occur (Krumberger, 2002).

Gastrointestinal and respiratory, although not cerebral, *bleeds* frequently occur (Hawker, 2003). ICU nurses should therefore minimise trauma and observe for bleeding during endotracheal suction or from nasogastric tubes. Oozing around cannulae, or healing of sites after removal, may also cause problems. Cannulae, especially arterial, should remain visible whenever possible.

The liver contributes significantly to immunity through

- producing complements
- Kupffer cells – phagocytotic cells in the liver which destroy bacteria from the gut.

Liver dysfunction therefore causes *immunocompromise*. Most patients with liver failure develop infection, usually within three days of admission to hospital (Caraceni & van Thiel, 1995).

Blood from the liver soon reaches pulmonary vessels, so surviving gut bacteria readily cause *pulmonary* infection; increased capillary permeability enables pulmonary oedema formation, and possible shunting. Endotracheal suction is needed to reduce sputum retention.

Acute *renal failure* is usually caused by hypotension, so should be prevented by optomising perfusion with fluid management.

The liver has over 500 metabolic functions, so hepatic failure causes complex disorders. Many *electrolytes* abnormalities occur, including *hypokalaemia* and *hypocalcaemia* from *hyperaldosteromism* (Saggs, 2000). Magnesium and phosphate deficiencies also frequently occur.

Metabolic *acidosis* occurs in any tissue relying on hypoxic metabolism; but the liver is the main organ that metabolises lactate, so lactate accumulation with hepatic failure inevitably results in metabolic acidosis. Concurrent renal failure aggravates acidosis. Acidosis being negatively inotropic, cardiac output is reduced.

Depleted liver stores of glycogen and elevated circulating insulin levels, which the liver normally metabolises, cause *hypoglycaemia*. Blood sugar levels should therefore be frequently monitored (2–3 hourly), with glucose supplements being given accordingly. Crystalloid fluids should be glucose based, both to avoid sodium (ascites) and provide glucose.

*Jaundice* occurs once serum bilirubin reaches 40 mmol/litre (Saggs, 2000). It is both a symptom and a problem, often causing pruritis. Skincare and dressings should be selected to minimise irritation. If pruritis occurs, drugs such as antihistamines may be useful.

Although severe hepatic failure may necessitate transplantation, aggressive intensive care can valuably stabilise patients' conditions (Shakil *et al.*, 1999). Compared with other body systems, artificial liver support has been slow and problematic, but shortage of donor livers prompted experiments with xenoperfusion (Shakil *et al.*, 1999).

## Intra-abdominal pressure

Increasing recognition that intra-abdominal hypertension causes ischaemic dysfunction of many organs (including lungs, liver, kidneys and gut) has encouraged many sections to monitor intra-abdominal pressure. Various devices are marketed, including intra-abdominal catheters, bladder and urinary collection transducers. Pressures exceeding 20 mmHg significantly increase risk of organ failure (Malbrain *et al.*, 2005), so if intra-abdominal hypertension is identified early

- decompressive laparotomy (possibly with temporary closure)
- paracentesis
- maintaining negative fluid balance
- flatus tube
- intravascular volume resuscitation

(depending on the cause) can preserve organ function.

## Artificial livers

Various 'artificial livers' have been developed, ranging from extracorporeal circulation through cadaver and animal livers to semi and fully synthetic machines. Technological improvements enable people with endstage chronic liver to survive until transplantation. Technology will doubtless further improve, perhaps to permanently implantable devices.

## Implications for practice

- Most ICU patients suffer hepatic dysfunction, usually due to hypoperfusion; nurses should actively assess liver function (e.g. clotting, consciousness), documenting their observations.
- Assess neurological state. Deterioration may indicate encephalopathy.

- Maintain head in alignment and at 15–30°C to facilitate venous drainage.
- Gross ascites should be drained.
- Intravenous volume should be aggressively restored, especially with colloids.
- Whenever possible, keep invasive sites visible.
- If clotting is prolonged, reassess traumatic aspects of nursing care (e.g. shaving, mouthcare); vitamin K and/or folic acid supplements may be needed.
- Blood loss should be assessed (e.g. marking limits of ooze on dressings).
- Hepatic dysfunction impairs immunity, so infection control is essential to maintain a safe environment.
- Monitor blood sugars initially 2–3 hourly and maintain normoglycaemia.
- Electrolytes should be monitored and supplements given – potassium, calcium, magnesium and phosphate imbalances often occur.
- Early nutrition facilitates recovery.
- Intra-abdominal pressure measurement facilitates early identification of, and treatment for, hepatic compromise.
- Patients are often forgetful, confused and agitated, needing simple and frequently repeated explanations. Conflict should be avoided. Relatives should be reassured that altered personality is caused by the disease, and that patience is needed.

## Summary

The liver can be the forgotten vital organ in the ICU; other than transplantation centres, few sections specialise in hepatic failure, but it frequently complicaties most pathologies seen in the ICU. Liver function affects many other organs and systems, so care of patients with liver dysfunction requires a range of knowledge and skills. Extracorporeal liver devices are currently only experimental; for the present, ICU nurses should actively assess liver function and minimise potential complications.

## Further reading

Hawker (2003) is an accessible and useful chapter source in a key text. Saggs (2000) and Ryder and Beckingham (2001) provide useful overviews, while Limdi and Hyde (2003) outline liver function tests. www.routledge.com/textbooks/0415373239

For clinical scenarios, clinical questions and the answers to them go to the support website at www.routledge.com/textbooks/0415373239

## Further resources

Hepatitis C telephone information line: 0800 451451
NHS hepatitis C awareness website: www.hepc.nhs.uk

**Clinical scenarios**

Julia Smith is 60 years old with a past medical history of alcoholic liver disease and remains alcohol dependant. She was admitted to the ICU with respiratory compromise associated with gross ascites, bacterial peritonitis and thrombocytopenia. A peritoneal drain was inserted, 16 l was drained initially with 3 l on second drainage.

An insulin infusion is administered at 10 iu/h and her blood glucose is 8.3 mmol/l.

Blood results include:

| | |
|---|---|
| INR | 2.9 |
| Hb (g/dl) | 9.5 |
| Platelets ($10^{-9}$/litre) | 35 |
| WBC ($10^{-9}$/litre) | 30.6 |
| Neutrophils ($10^{-9}$/litre) | 29.7 |
| Lymphocytes ($10^{-9}$/litre) | 0.5 |
| Monocytes ($10^{-9}$/litre) | 0.5 |
| Urea (mmol/litre) | 22.3 |
| Bilirubin ($\mu$mol/litre) | 223 |
| ALT (iu/litre) | 34 |
| Alkaline Phosphatase (iu/litre) | 89 |
| Gamma GT (iu/litre) | 65 |
| Albumin (g/litre) | 28 |
| Lactate (mmol/litre) | 4.9 |

Arterial Blood Gas results while mechanically ventilated on $FiO_2$ of 0.5

| | |
|---|---|
| pH | 7.25 |
| $PaCO_2$ (kPa) | 5.8 |
| $PaO_2$ (kPa) | 12.2 |
| $SaO_2$ (%) | 94.8 |

Q.1 Examine the results and their significance in terms of Julia's liver function and liver damage.

Q.2 Seven litres of Albumin 4.5% is administered to replace ascetic loss. What are the alternative therapies to the use of albumin with Julie?

Q.3 Consider other treatment strategies she may require. Is she a candidate for transplantation? Justify rationale for transplantation in Julie's case.

Chapter 43

# Obstetric emergencies in ICU

**Content**

Introduction                            451
Normal pregnancy                        451
Pregnancy-induced hypertension          452
Thromboembolism                         453
Amniotic fluid embolus                  453
Haemorrhage                             454
HELLP syndrome                          454
Braindeath incubation                   454
Drugs and pregnancy                     455
Psychology                              455
Implications for practice               455
Summary                                 456
Support groups                          456
Further reading                         456
Clinical scenarios                      456

**Fundamental knowledge**

Normal pregnancy, including normal physiological changes

450

## Introduction

Most deliveries are 'normal', ICU admission rarely being needed, although incidence varies between sections. Obstetric patients can be among the sickest patients in ICU. This, together with limited literature in ICU texts and journals, and few ICU staff being qualified midwives, can provoke special anxieties among staff.

Antenatal emergencies usually necessitate early delivery or termination of pregnancy and are rarely admitted to ICU. Antenatal ICU admissions are more likely to occur for non-obstetric conditions, such as road traffic accidents. Specific obstetric care, if any, depends on foetal age and condition. Antenatal care should optimise conditions for both the mother and the foetus. Foetal mortality may occur in addition to, or independently of, maternal mortality.

ICU obstetric admissions are usually postnatal, necessitated by complications such as respiratory or cardiovascular failure. So, while pregnancy/delivery may trigger crises, medical/nursing care centres on complications–medical treatments supporting failing systems (e.g. ventilation) and the human care familiar to ICU staff. ICU nurses do not need midwifery expertise to care for these admissions, but an understanding of obstetric pathophysiology is useful. Midwives should actively be involved in multidisciplinary teams, to provide both psychological reassurance and practical care, such as expressing breast milk, assessing and monitoring uterine contraction, monitoring vaginal discharge, checking need for anti-rhesus D injections. Midwives also provide valuable links between mother and child while the mother is in ICU.

## Normal pregnancy

Most crises result from physiological changes of pregnancy. Normal physiological changes during pregnancy favour foetal growth but place stress on the mother's body, altering 'normal' biochemical/haematological values from non-pregnant levels.

In the first *trimester* (weeks 1–12) the *cardiovascular* system becomes hyperdynamic:

- Blood volume increases 20–100 per cent (Murray, 1999).
- Stroke volume and heart rate increase, increasing cardiac output by about 40 per cent (McNabb, 2004).
- Systemic vascular resistance halves (Murray, 1999).

If cardiac reserve is limited, increased cardiac work may precipitate cardiac failure. Patients should not be nursed supine, as aortocaval compression may cause hypotension, and hence foetal distress. Increase in erythrocyte numbers does not match increase in blood volume, so causes dilutional anaemia, which improves capillary flow.

Onset of labour accelerates cardiovascular changes. In first stage labour, pain and anxiety increase circulating catecholamines, increasing cardiac output by nearly half. Second stage labour (contractions and delivery) creates a valsalva effect, reducing both venous return and cardiac output. Uterine contraction during the third stage of labour (delivery of placenta) returns 300–400 ml of blood to systemic circulation, potentially precipitating hypertensive crises.

Maternal hearts are usually robust enough to cope with demands of pregnancy, but increased demands may precipitate crises. Increasing survival from congenital heart disease (Thorne, 2004) has significantly increased cardiac complications during pregnancy, with cardiac deaths remaining the single main indirect cause of maternal mortality (RCOG, 2004).

Increased maternal oxygen demand (one-third during pregnancy, a further two-thirds during labour) increases *respiratory* and cardiovascular workload. Minute volume increases by about half, mainly from larger tidal volumes, increasing $PaO_2$ and decreasing $PaCO_2$. Renal function normally compensates for respiratory alkalosis to maintain normal pH. Artificial ventilation should mimic this respiratory alkalosis by maintaining $PaCO_2$ at 4 kPa (Dhond & Dob, 2000). Foetal growth displaces the disphragm up 4 cm (Murray, 1999), reducing functional residual capacity by one-fifth.

Reduced colloid osmotic pressure (dilution), hypertension and vasoconstriction encourage *oedema* formation, including

- pulmonary oedema (impairing gas exchange)
- airway oedema (obstructing airways)
- cerebral oedema (increasing intracranial pressure).

Airway mucosa becomes more vascular and oedematous, increasing risk of haemorrhage (Dhond & Dob, 2000), necessitating smaller endotracheal tubes while increasing airway resistance and pressures.

*Neurological* changes are not normally seen, but cerebral oedema and hypoxia can cause fitting from eclampsia (see later).

*Gastrointestinal* motility is reduced, contributing to nausea/vomiting, malnutrition and potential acid aspiration ('Mendelsohn's syndrome'). Hypertension can cause *liver* dysfunction, resulting in potential hypoglycaemia, immunocompromise, jaundice, coagulopathies, encephalopathy and other neurological complications. However gestational hyperglycaemia is more common due to increased insulin resistance. Hyperglycaemia may facilitate foetal supply, but maternal blood sugar levels should be monitored regularly as insulin supplements may be needed.

*Glomerular filtration* increases by half (McNabb, 2004), so drug clearance may be increased. Increased urine output and antenatal bladder compression from the foetus cause urgency.

Impaired *immunity* during the third trimester prevents foetal rejection, but increases risk of viral infections, especially varicella (chicken pox) and colds.

## Pregnancy-induced hypertension

*Pre-eclampsia* (hypertension and proteinuria, with or without oedema) occurs in 15–25 per cent of hypertensive mothers (Walker, 2000) causing 20–60 per cent of obstetric admissions to ICU (Dhond & Dob, 2000).

Systemic thromboplastin release in severe pre-eclampsia (probably from damaged placental tissue) causes intense arteriolar vasoconstriction and DIC (Bewley, 2004), compounding hypertension and coagulopathies. Pulmonary oedema, often caused by excessive fluid resuscitation (Engelhardt & MacLennan, 1999; Walker, 2000), frequently complicates pre-eclampsia, and is the main cause of pre-eclamptic deaths in the UK (Walker, 2000). Pulmonary oedema typically occurs 48–72 hours after delivery (Engelhardt & MacLennan, 1999), and may occur despite apparently normal CVP, so CVP should not exceed 5 mmHg (Walker, 2000).

*Eclampsia* is a tonic-clonic type fitting, caused by hypertension-induced vasogenic oedema (Zeeman *et al.*, 2004). Eclamptic deaths often occur after only one fit, so convulsions should be controlled (Bewley, 2004). Delivery is essential to resolve eclampsia, usually necessitating caesarian section or termination of pregnancy.

Eclampsia should be controlled with magnesium (Eclampsia Trial Collaborative Group, 1995; Belfort *et al.*, 2003), maintaining plasma levels 2–4 mmol/l (Bewley, 2004). Higher levels may be toxic, causing respiratory and cardiac arrest; hence one gram of the magnesium-antagonist calcium gluconate should be immediately available (Idama & Lindow, 1998). Rapid infusion of magnesium can cause dysrhythmias; Walker (2000) suggests intravenous rates of 1–3 g every hour.

*Acute fatty liver* is a rare variant of pre-eclampsia, causing gross microvascular fatty infiltration without hepatic necrosis or inflammation. Liver disease occurs in less than 1 per cent of pregnancies, but up to 5 per cent may have abnormal liver function tests (Sillender, 2002). Normal hepatic function resumes postnatally.

Analgesia should be given both for humanitarian reasons and to reduce sympathetic stimulation (stress response), which contributes to hypertension.

Plasmapheresis (see Chapter 40) can remove mediators, preventing pre-eclampsia from progressing to eclampsia or other complications (e.g. HELLP).

## Thromboembolism

Pregnancy causes a *procoagulant* state. Thromboembolism remains the single main direct cause of obstetric deaths (RCOG, 2004). Antenatally, oral anticoagulants are contraindicated because they cross the placenta and may cause placental/foetal haemorrhage. For high-risk pregnancy, CLASP (Collaborative Low-dose Aspirin Studies) (1994) recommend low dose aspirin for high-risk pre-eclampsia, although low molecular weight heparin is now often used.

## Amniotic fluid embolus

This rare condition occurs most frequently in older women with higher *parity*, progressing rapidly, and usually being diagnosed postmortem (RCOG, 2004).

Amniotic fluid is derived from plasma, and contains vasoactive mediators (e.g. prostaglandins, leukotrienes and thromboplastins) which can cause severe respiratory failure and DIC (Lindsay, 2004).

453

## Haemorrhage

Bleeding from normal third stage labour is reduced by arterial constriction and with the development of a fibrin mesh over the placental site; placental circulation, about 600 ml/minute at term (Lindsay, 2004), is autotransfused by uterine contraction. Incomplete contraction therefore causes major haemorrhage. Bleeding can also occur from genital tract lacerations and coagulopathies – DIC frequently complicates pregnancy.

Postpartum haemorrhage volume is easily underestimated (e.g. from loss on sheets) (Lindsay, 2004). Specific management of primary postpartum haemorrhage (e.g. oxytocin) is usually supervised by obstetricians or midwives before transfer to ICU for fluid resuscitation and monitoring.

## HELLP syndrome

*Haemolysis*
*Elevated Liver* enzymes and
*Low Platelets*

This syndrome causes severe hypertension, coagulopathies and grossly disordered liver function, although classification and criteria for HELLP are inconsistent (Geary, 1997). Between 4 and 20 per cent of patients with severe pre-eclampsias progress to HELLP (Dhond & Dob, 2000), with maternal mortality potentially reaching 25 per cent (Geary, 1997). HELLP is often the main obstetric emergency requiring ICU admission.

Platelet activation causes thrombi in small blood vessels. Narrowed lumens trigger erythrocyte haemolysis, further reducing haemoglobin levels (aggravating hypoxia) and raising serum bilirubin levels (Turner, 1997).

Early symptoms are often vague and non-specific (e.g. epigastric pain, nausea and vomiting; hypertension and proteinuria may not even be present (Sibai, 1994)), so HELLP may become life-threatening before it is diagnosed. In those diagnosed with HELLP, half suffered cerebral infarctions, and most developed multiple seizures (Zeeman *et al.*, 2004).

Treatments include

- urgent delivery of foetus (induction, caesarian section) (Sibai, 1994)
- seizure prophylaxis (Nutt, 1997)
- antithrombotic agents (heparin, prostacyclin)
- plasmapheresis (removes circulating mediators) (Sibai, 1994; Turner, 1997)
- system support (e.g. ventilation).

## Braindeath incubation

Technology can support body systems following brain death, enabling foetal growth despite maternal death (Diehl *et al.*, 1994). Although rare, admission of braindead mothers creates stress for families and places nurses in a similar (but more prolonged) situation as when caring for organ donors (see Chapter 44).

## Drugs and pregnancy

Additional considerations when giving drugs during pregnancy are:

- Will they cross the placenta?
- Are they expressed in breast milk (if breastfeeding)?
- Is there foetal/newborn drug clearance?

Being professionally accountable for each drug given, nurses should withhold drugs and seek advice from their pharmacist if unsure of likely effects. Pharmacists should actively be involved in multidisciplinary teams.

## Psychology

Most babies are wanted, so obstetric emergencies can be especially devastating. Miscarriages or abortion may create guilt. Other children, usually young, may experience various emotional traumas. Psychological support and care is therefore especially important. Support may be gained from family and friends, chaplains, counselling services or various support groups.

Bereavement is traumatic, but photographs can become treasured mementoes, which parents may not think to ask for, or take, at the time.

Obstetric emergencies can be psychologically traumatic for staff, most nurses being female, of a similar age and possibly planning or raising families of their own.

## Implications for practice

- ICU admission will usually be to provide respiratory and/or cardiovascular support, so care should follow from problems necessitating admission.
- Do not nurse supine; aortocaval compression occludes circulation.
- Pregnancy causes immunocompromise, so minimise infection risks.
- Pregnancy can cause DIC, so clotting should be monitored.
- Significant electrolyte loss/shifts can occur, so levels should be monitored and normalized.
- After the hopes of pregnancy, critical illness can cause devastating stress to patients, partners and family, so psychological needs should be assessed and support provided.
- Midwives are valuable members of the team, providing specialist care and advice.
- Antenatally, the mother's body should provide an optimal environment for foetal development.
- Postnatal obstetric observations should include vaginal examination (amount and type of discharge) and uterine contraction.
- Mothers wishing, but currently unable, to breastfeed should be offered opportunities to express breast milk (breast pump); this also relieves breast pain.
- Bereavement counselling and care may be needed.

## Summary

Pregnancy is a normal physiological function, and most pregnancies occur without serious complications. However lifethreatening complications can and do occur, necessitating ICU admission, usually for cardiovascular or respiratory failure. Antenatal admissions should consider foetal health, but most admissions are postnatal; the precipitating cause (foetus/placenta) being delivered, system support may be all required until homeostasis is restored, although some problems require more aggressive treatments. Interventions used will be familiar to most ICU nurses, but terminology and pathophysiology may differ.

## Support groups

Pre-Eclamptic Toxaemia Society (PETS): 01286 880057
Miscarriage Association: 01924-200799 (Scotland: 0131-354-8883)
Stillbirth and Neonatal Death Society (SANDS): 020-7436-7940; helpline@uk-sands.org

## Further reading

Most ICU textbooks include an overview of obstetric emergencies. Mayes classic midwifery text has been updated by Henderson and Macdonald (2004). The RCOG (2004) triennial report discusses the main causes of maternal mortality, including a specific section on ICU. Critical care journals occasionally print articles on obstetrics, such as Dhond and Dob (2000). Walker (2000) provides a useful medical review. www.routledge.com/textbooks/0415373239

For clinical scenarios, clinical questions and the answers to them go to the support website at www.routledge.com/textbooks/0415373239

## Clinical scenarios

Susan Jackson, a 27-year-old primagravida with recently diagnosed pre-eclampsia, is admitted to the ICU following an emergency caesarean delivery at 34 weeks gestation. Susan was progressively hypertensive, oedematous with proteinuria, experienced visual disturbances and epigastric pain. Susan is mechanically ventilated with intravenous infusions of magnesium and hydralazine. She is cold with tachycardia of 125 bpm, BP of 160/110 mmHg, oliguria and hypoalbuminaemia.

Q.1 Explain the potential causes of Susan's oliguria including the significance of her proteinuria and hypoalbuminaemia. Formulate a plan for her fluid management and renal support.

Q.2 What other investigations should be performed to check for complications associated with pre-eclampsia, e.g. HELLP syndrome, DIC?

Q.3 Appraise the role of others within the interdisciplinary team, including the midwife, in planning collaborative care for Susan while she is mechanically ventilated.

# Chapter 44

# Transplants

## Contents

Introduction     459
Brainstem death     459
Nursing care     461
Donors     462
Ethical issues     463
Living donors     464
Non-heart-beating organ
    donors (NHBOD)     464
Xenografts     465
Postoperative care of recipients     465
Graft versus host disease (GvHD)     466
Immunosuppression     467
Implications for practice     467
Summary     468
Useful contacts     468
Further reading     468
Clinical scenarios     468

## Fundamental knowledge

Brainstem and cranial nerve function

Immune response

Current limitations on what can be donated (an aspect of rapid change and local variation, so check recent local protocols)

## Introduction

In the financial year 2004–5, 2242 organ transplants were performed in the UK (UK Transplant, 2005), enabling people with end-stage disease to survive with significantly improved quality of life. Although viability of donated organs cannot be guaranteed, advanced techniques enable most (up to 90 per cent of kidneys) organs to survive, overall recipient-one-year survival of 85–90 per cent (Bonner & Rudge, 2002). However, 2004–5 ended with 6142 people on the UK register awaiting organ transplantation – more than double the number that received organs during the financial year. There is a continuing shortfall of available organs to meet the needs of those on waiting lists.

Compared with European countries such as France, Austria and Spain, UK donations rates (per million population) are low (Bonner & Rudge, 2002), with a relatively static one quarter of people on waiting lists dying before transplant. Organ and tissue retrieval should be standard practice in ICU and many other clinical areas.

Although historically associated with organs (kidneys, heart, lungs, liver, pancreas, islet cells, small bowel), donation of many body tissues (eyes, skin, bone, ligaments, tendons, heart valves) can help others, and most tissues donated can be retrieved up to 24 hours following death. Brain and spinal cord tissue is not yet transplanted into humans, but is used for research; currently there are hopes that brain tissue may in future provide a cure for Parkinson's Disease.

## Brainstem death

Historically, death was synonymous with cessation of breathing and/or heartbeat. Development of technologies to replace breathing (ventilators) and heartbeat (pacing) coincided with the transfer of organ donation from science fiction to science fact, necessitating revision of concepts of death.

The brainstem, extending between the cerebrum and spinal cord and consisting of the pons, medulla oblongata and midbrain, contains the vital centres (respiratory, cardiac and other), so if the brainstem is dead, higher consciousness and control cannot be regained. Brainstem death, first described in 1959, is established in the UK through the code of practice (Department of Health, 1998).

Diagnosing brainstem death is not required for every death (it is used for ten per cent of ICU deaths (Frid *et al.*, 1998)), but provides protection for vulnerable patients and diagnosing doctors where

- there is any reasonable doubt about whether the patient is dead
- where organs/tissues may be retrieved for transplantation.

Any medical conditions that could prevent brainstem function must be excluded (see Table 44.1) before testing for braindeath. Reflexes and responses of each cranial nerves are then tested (individually or in combination; see

## Table 44.1 Code of practice: preconditions (DOH, 1998)

- There should be no doubt that the patient's condition is due to irremediable brain damage of known aetiology.
- The patient is deeply unconscious.
- There should be no evidence that this state is due to depressant drugs.
- Primary hypothermia as a cause of unconsciousness must be excluded.
- Potentially reversible circulatory, metabolic and endocrine disturbances must be excluded as a cause of the continuation of unconsciousness.
- The patient is being maintained on a ventilator because spontaneous respiration has been inadequate or has ceased altogether.

## Table 44.2 Brainstem death tests

Should establish absence of

- pupil reaction to light
- corneal reflex
- oculo-vestibular reflex
- motor response to central stimulation
- gag reflex
- cough reflex
- respiratory effort.

Table 44.2). If higher centre responses are absent, brainstem death may be diagnosed. Any response from higher centres, however abnormal or limited, prohibits brainstem death diagnosis. Spinal reflex responses ('Lazarus' sign) are not significant, but may be misinterpreted by relatives or other witnesses as signs of life, thereby causing anxiety. One study, reported by Voelker (2000), found 39 per cent of patients diagnosed as brainstem dead exhibited such movements. Spinal reflexes can be removed with muscle relaxants (Booij, 1999), which might reduce distress for relatives. The legal time of death is the first test, although death is not pronounced until confirmed by the second test (DOH, 1998).

Tests should be carried out by two doctors, both of whom have been qualified for more than five years, and at least one of whom is a consultant, usually the patient's own. Neither doctor making the test should be a member of the transplant team. Tests should follow all criteria in the Code. Most centres perform two sets of tests. Timing between the two sets is often relatively brief, partly to facilitate presence of the same team and partly to reduce anxiety for families waiting for confirmation of death, but should be long enough to ensure the second set of tests is meaningful. Bell et al. (2004) found the UK guidelines were interpreted variably, and so needed review.

The *Human Tissues Act* (1961) established that after death the body becomes the property of the next of kin, giving next of kin the right to refuse donation. In 1998 the Department of Health (DOH, 1998) advised that lack of objection, rather than consent, should normally be obtained from relatives. The *Human Tissue Bill* (2004) makes wishes of patients paramount, although how rigorously this law would be invoked, or results from any legal challenges, if relatives' and patients' wishes differed, remain to be seen; it seems unlikely that strongly-held objections by relatives would be disregarded. The *Human Organ Transplants Act* (1989) legislated against making or receiving payment for organs. In the UK, unrelated living donation is managed through the Unrelated Live Transplant Regulatory Authority (ULTRA).

Brainstem death, which was largely defined by Western values, is not always culturally sensitive. Japan has been especially uncomfortable with the concept of brainstem death, although negative attitudes stem partly from a controversial transplant performed in 1968 (Gill, 2000). Kerridge *et al.* (2002) question the validity of the concept of brainstem death, suggesting instead

- death of the 'person' or
- circulatory death.

Circulatory death was arguably the normal definition prior to transplantation creating the concept of brainstem death and is relatively easy to establish. Death of the 'person' is however open to interpretation and potential abuse. Booij (1999) identifies three types of brain death:

- whole brain death
- brainstem death
- neocortical death.

Whole brain death, involving the cerebrum as well as the brainstem, is a criterion for organ donation in most Western countries (Booij, 1999). Neocortical death, the irreversible loss of higher functions, could be applied to people suffering from such conditions as persistent vegetative states, and hence is too problematical to be accepted (Booij, 1999). The legal definition of death determines what tests are required to certify death: for example, whole brain death necessitates evidence of lack of activity throughout the brain (e.g. a flat EEG).

## Nursing care

Caring for donors and their families can be psychologically stressful. Unlike other terminal care, where (hopefully) peaceful death is followed by last offices, diagnosis of brainstem death is followed by optimising organ function for retrieval. Booij (1999) lists the main system problems as

- diabetes inspidus (79 per cent)
- electrolyte shifts (75 per cent)
- autonomic spinal storms (72 per cent)
- cardiac dysrhythmias (62 per cent)
- hypothermia (50 per cent)
- coagulopathy (5 per cent).

461

Some of these are managed with drugs, such as steroids, hormone replacement therapy, hydrocortisone and T4 (Rosendale *et al.*, 2003). Guidelines on this are forthcoming from the Intensive Care Society. Hypovolaemia, largely resulting from the polyuria of diabetes inspidus, necessitates large volumes of fluid replacement (Booij, 1999).

While logical, this focus on supporting body systems in someone who is diagnosed as dead potentially conflicts with nursing values where actions should be in patients' best interests. However, facilitating patients' wishes to donate *is* in their best interests. With death already diagnosed, retrieval of the body is normally transferred to the mortuary; last offices ('letting go') are performed elsewhere. During this dehumanising experience, nurses usually need to support donors' families, yet few nurses find caring for donors to be rewarding (Watkinson, 1995).

In such potentially undignified situations, nurses should optimise their patient's dignity, both before and after diagnosis of death. Privacy can be helped by drawing curtains or transfer into a sideroom. Relatives facing bereavement should be allowed to grieve; they may also gain comfort from knowing that their loved one's organs will help others to live. Relatives' responses vary. Transplant co-ordinators are experienced at comforting relatives and may prove a valuable resource, although some relatives prefer to speak with staff with whom they have already developed rapport and trust.

## Donors

Waiting lists continue to exceed organ/tissue availability. Donation criteria attempt to optimise supply of viable transplantable organs/tissue, without endangering recipients. Viability varies between organs/tissue, but medical progress has generally enabled progressive relaxation of donation criteria. There are very few exclusions for surface tissue (e.g. corneas), but criteria for vital organs usually exclude donors with malignancies or other transferable lifethreatening conditions. The only absolute contraindications to donations are

- history of malignancy
- exclusion by coroner
- (usually) where known or suspected disease may be spread to recipients, such as Creutzfeldt–Jacob disease (CJD).

Organs and tissue from people with HIV may be retrieved, but are mainly used for recipients with HIV. Transplant co-ordinators can clarify whether potential donors meet criteria.

Medical ethics requires that treatment must be for the patient's benefit: intubation and ventilation cannot be initiated in a living person just to preserve organs for retrieval (DOH, 1998). Therefore organ donors are largely limited to patients already being artificially ventilated (i.e. ICU patients), but multiorgan dysfunction and infection, often the cause of death on ICU, leaves few viable organs for retrieval.

In the UK, available donor organs are matched and allocated through UK Transplant. Organs are used for the benefit of UK patients, but where this is not possible, rather than waste precious resources, they are offered to other European organ-sharing organisations.

Inevitably regional variations exist, sometimes from pragmatic considerations (e.g. services available), and sometimes from local criteria of transplant teams. Occasionally, controversial values cause national debate (e.g. should persistent alcoholics be given livers, or smokers be given hearts), but increasing development of multidisciplinary teams including recipient transplant co-ordinators (often from nursing backgrounds) is encouraging greater objectivity and fairness.

## Ethical issues

Transplantation has always maintained a high public profile, ensuring widespread discussion of ethical issues. Organ donation relies on public goodwill, so healthcare staff should encourage public awareness.

Organ donation can literally be life-saving; *moral duty* to facilitate transplantation creates dilemmas between whether the onus of duty falls on society or on individuals. Some nations (e.g. France, Belgium, Austria, Sweden, Norway, Switzerland, Spain) operate systems of presumed consent: people have to actively opt-out if they do not wish to donate. The UK, like most countries, has an opt-in system, donation becoming a gift, although the 1999 British Medical Association conference called for a change to an opt-out system (Beecham, 1999).

Organs and tissues are only considered if the offer in unconditional. So any condition that organs should not be given to recipients with particular diseases or from various social/religious/cultural/ethnic groups will result in transplant services refusing the donation.

*Publicity* significantly influences donor supply: positive publicity (e.g. transplant games) encourages donation, while negative publicity increases refusal rates. The NHS Organ Donor Register enables people to record their willingness to be organ donors and can be accessed by NHS staff to check whether patients are on the register.

Except for Rastafarians, no major *religions* oppose organ donation (Randhawa, 1997), although some ministers (e.g. some Jewish rabbis) (Levine, 1997) may discourage donation, believing the body should remain unmutilated. UK Transplant publishes leaflets about main religious issues related to donation.

Distressed *relatives*, facing inevitable and usually sudden bereavement, may not think to ask about donation, but find consolation/hope through organ donation (Watkinson, 1995). Families usually appreciate the opportunity to donate organs (Hadingham, 1997; Kent, 1997); failing to ask or be asked about donation is often regretted later (Finlay & Dallimore, 1991; Pelletier, 1992). Yet Molzhahn's (1997) Canadian study found that 85 per cent of nurses were reluctant to seek permission for organ donation. Nurses have a professional responsibility to offer choice (Kent, 1997) with sufficient information to make an informed choice. Having often established a close rapport with relatives, nurses can facilitate choice, either by providing information themselves, or contacting appropriate agencies (e.g. transplant co-ordinators). Relatives should be approached openly, without coercion; the best time and method for approaching relatives is necessarily individual, but team collaboration, possibly already involving transplant co-ordinators, is also valuable. Doran (2004) recommends that families should be offered the choice of being present during brainstem death tests. Should tests exclude possible donation, relatives may feel rejected, so nurses should explain why donation is not possible. If criteria prove problematic, donation of some tissue (e.g. corneas) may be possible, providing some compensatory comfort. Donor HIV testing is required; if results are unexpectedly positive, nurses must maintain patient confidentiality.

Transplant co-ordinators *thank* donor families by letter, describing beneficiaries, but without directly identifying them (for mutual safety). The letters are sent at an early stage, in case recipients reject organs.

Macro-economically, transplant surgery can be highly *cost*-effective, replacing years of chronic treatment costs (e.g. renal dialysis). Units providing donors receive financial remuneration through transplant services, but some hidden costs can be difficult to quantify, and demand for ICU beds may discourage facilitating donation (Wright & Cohen, 1997), or cause refusal of other admissions.

## Living donors

Limited supply of cadaver organs has encouraged use of live donors. One-fifth of renal transplants are from living donors, usually related. Sections from the liver, lung and (occasionally) small bowel can also be transplanted from living donors. Combined heart and lung transplants can also be performed from living donors if the recipients heart is sufficiently healthy to transplant into the donor 'domino' transplant. Compared with many countries, the numbers of UK living organ donors have been small (Lumsdaine, 2000), but numbers increased significantly from 33 in the financial year 2003–4 to 482 in 2004–5, probably mainly due to the establishment of ULTRA (see earlier).

## Non-heart-beating organ donors (NHBOD)

In some centres, patients not surviving cardiopulmonary resuscitation may become organ donors. Warm ischaemia (<50 mmHg) adversely affects function of organs retrieved (Talbot & Bonner, 2003), so external compression pumps (mechanical cardiac compression) may perfuse organs until retrieval, while metabolism is reduced through induced hypothermia (Kootstra *et al.*, 1997).

Following (but not preceding) any decision to withdraw treatment, donation should be considered. Because donors will not have been diagnosed brainstem dead, some hospitals delay touching corpses for a stated time, often 5 or 10 minutes.

Currently, numbers of NHBOD donors are small – about 3 per cent of all donors. But as retrieval facilities develop, this will presumably increase. NHBOD donation was initially limited to kidneys, but has already been extended to retrieve hepatocytes and pancreatic islet cells, and is likely to be further extended in the future.

## Xenografts

Using animal organs for transplantation to humans (xenografting) could provide the means to overcome the continuing, and increasing, shortage of human organs. Complications of transplantation between species can be reduced through genetic engineering, which can then be cloned to supply further 'donors'. Currently, only pigs are being seriously considered for transplantation (Goddard *et al.*, 2000).

While genetic engineering currently poses problems for medical scientists, ethical dilemmas, such as whether humans have the right to kill healthy animals for organs, or the loss of altruism (Schlaudraff, 1999), are value-laden issues that nurses, especially those involved with xenografting and transplantation, should consider carefully.

## Postoperative care of recipients

Post-operative care of transplant recipients includes aspects needed for any patient who has undergone major surgery, with the addition of complications created for supporting the grafted organ to function effectively, while preventing infection in patients receiving strong immunosuppressive drugs. Early extubation is therefore a priority (Glaspole & Williams, 1999). Transplant recipients should be monitored closely for signs of

- rejection
- electrolyte imbalance
- infection.

*Nonfunction* transplanted organs may fail to function. Organ-specific function should be monitored; and if *primary nonfunction* occurs urgent further transplantation is usually organised, if possible. Rejection is often classified by time, such as

- hyperacute: within one week
- acute: 1–4 weeks
- chronic.

Various interventions may support the failing organ, but retransplantation is often needed.

465

*Electrolytes* storage and cooling of organs for transportation usually causes electrolyte imbalance and metabolic acidosis, and hence homeostasis should be restored. Imbalances, acidosis and reperfusion injury may all cause dysrhythmias. If biochemistry does not stabilise over the first postoperative day, graft failure should be suspected.

Immunosuppressant drugs and multiple invasive lines make patients particularly susceptible to opportunist *infection*. Patients should be monitored for signs of infection (blood tests to include CRP and WCC; visual signs; temperature).

*Pain* varies both between individuals and the nature of surgery, but epidural analgesia often provides the most effective cover for patient (Glaspole & Williams, 1999).

Additional organ-specific care may also be needed.

## Graft versus host disease (GvHD)

When foreign tissue, such as a tissue transplant, enters the body, the immune system initiates a host reaction. Severe cases may cause organ failure or death. GvHD causes fibrosis, necrosis and necrosis in skin, liver and gut epithelium. Incidence increases with older donors, older recipients or those with human leucocyte antigen (HLA) mismatch.

Symptoms include

- skin rashes (typically: face, palms, soles, ears)
- jaundice
- diarrhoea.

Treatments include corticosteroids and chemotherapy, often with system support.

*Rejection* is classified as hyperacute, acute or chronic:

- Hyperacute rejection occurs within minutes of anastomosis, with pre-existing mediators provoking thrombotic occlusion of graft vasculature and irreversible ischaemia. Hyperacute rejection is mediated by preformed antibodies (Unsworth, 2000) and is relatively rare. Although rare, graft failure necessitates retransplantation; about 10 per cent of hepatic recipients require urgent retransplantation (Heaton & Prachalias, 1999).
- Acute rejection usually occurs (40–70 per cent of transplants) (Heaton & Prachalias, 1999), causing necrosis of individual cells. Acute rejection is mediated mainly by T-lymphoctes, and begins within days to weeks of transplantation (Unsworth, 2000).
- Chronic rejection, which only begins weeks or years after transplantation, is usually caused by inadequate HLA match, immunotherapy or by both (Unsworth, 2000). It causes fibrosis and loss of normal organ structure.

## Immunosuppression

Healthy immunity would reject transplanted tissue (except for corneas), so donor recipients are given immunosuppressants to prevent rejection.

Until the introduction of *ciclosporin* in 1979, transplant surgery was very limited. *Tacrolimus* (Prograf®), a fungal metabolite, is increasingly replacing ciclosporin (Margreiter, 2002; O'Grady *et al.*, 2002). Oral tacrolimusdoses is usually commenced the day after surgery. Binding-to-plasma proteins, tracrolimus often interacts with other binding-to-plasma proteins, such as NSAIDs, oral anticoagulants and oral hypoglycaemics. It has many adverse effects, the main and earliest one usually being fitting; others include nephrotoxicity (Mihatsch *et al.*, 1998) and diabetes mellitus (Knoll, 1999). Tracrolimus levels should be monitored.

Both ciclosporin and tracrolimus can cause hirsuitism, gum hypertrophy, hypertension, renal impairment, hypercholesterolaemia, hypomagnesaemia and central nervous system symptoms (e.g. tremor, headaches, fits) (Glaspole & Williams, 1999). Immunosuppression can cause opportunist infection, so prophylactic antibiotics (often for 48 hours) and antifungal agents (e.g. acyclovir) are usually given to prevent herpes simplex.

### Implications for practice

■ Donation offers families the opportunity to salvage something positive from bereavement.

■ Donor families should be asked whether they have any objection (rather than consent) to organ/tissue retrieval.

■ ICU nurses should facilitate informed choice about organ donation.

■ Donation in the UK remains a gift; coercion (and apparent coercion) should be avoided.

■ Timing and method for approaching families is individual, but teamwork can support both staff and bereaved relatives.

■ Regional transplant co-ordinators can offer useful support and information at all stages of donation.

■ Any medical conditions that may affect brainstem function must be excluded before brainstem death tests.

■ Both sets of brainstem death tests must show absence of all higher responses on both occasions.

■ Spinal reflexes may occur despite absence of brainstem function; staff and relatives should be warned about these – they are not a sign of life.

■ Time of death is the first set of tests, but is only confirmed after the second set of tests.

■ Retrieval and transplantation raise many ethical issues; staff should clarify their thoughts and feelings on these issues; section discussion forums can be useful to share/develop ideas.

■ Immediate postoperative care requires careful planning of roles (e.g. identify staff who will be able to help provide infusion fluids) and equipment (ensure layout is safe and patients will be accessible).

■ Clarify from theatre staff what special infusions and equipment will be needed.

■ In addition to general ICU care, nurses should monitor transplant recipients for signs of

● rejection
● infection (immunosuppression)
● side effects of immunosuppressants and other drugs, especially fitting.

## Summary

Transplantation of organs and tissues can offer possible cures and improved quality of life to people with endstage and life-threatening pathologies, but continuing donor shortage often causes long waiting lists, with many patients dying before suitable organs are found. When most organs are being retrieved from patients already in ICU, ICU nurses should promote (without coercion) awareness about transplantation. The (usually) close rapport with families enables nurses to offer valuable support during crises and discussion.

Nurses are normally present during brainstem death testing, so should be aware of the code of practice (DOH, 1998) and its requirements.

## Useful contacts

UK Transplant: 01179 757575 or www.uktransplant.org

## Further reading

Each ICU should have the current code of practice (DOH, 1998) (also available from transplant coordinators). Collins (2003) gives an overview of both transplantation history and its current state. Howitt (2000) presents arguments for changing to opt-in systems for donation. Transplantation provokes much ethical debate; Kerridge *et al.* (2002) provide useful ethical perspectives. Talbot and Bonner (2003) review non heart-beating donation. www.routledge.com/textbooks/0415373239

For clinical scenarios, clinical questions and the answers to them go to the support website at www.routledge.com/textbooks/0415373239

## Clinical scenarios

Mrs Wallace is 50 years old and suffered an out-of-hospital VF arrest. She was successfully resuscitated at the scene, but on route to hospital required further resuscitation and seven defibrillation shocks. She was admitted to ICU for mechanical ventilation prior to transfer to CT scan the following day. This head scan revealed extensive and diffuse cerebral damage. Her GCS is E1, $V_T$, M1.

Q.1 Identify features from Mrs Wallace's history that would allow her to be considered as a potential organ donor. What other information and actions are required?

Q.2 Review how permission for Mrs Wallace's organ donation might be obtained.

Q.3 Analyse interventions which can optimise Mrs Wallace's organ function. Consider the beneficial and adverse effects of such interventions on Mrs Wallace, her family and the staff on ICU.

Q.4 Following brain stem death confirmation, should Mrs Wallace be resuscitated in the event she has a cardiopulmonary arrest? Discuss this with medical colleagues.

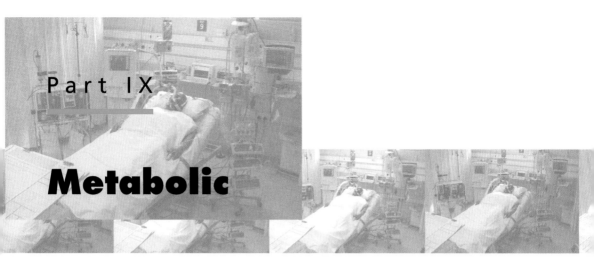

# Part IX

# Metabolic

# Chapter 45

# Pancreatitis

## Contents

| | |
|---|---|
| Introduction | 474 |
| Pathology | 474 |
| Complications | 475 |
| Symptoms | 476 |
| Medical treatments | 477 |
| Implications for practice | 478 |
| Summary | 478 |
| Further reading | 478 |
| Clinical scenarios | 479 |

## Fundamental knowledge

Pancreatic anatomy and physiology – endocrine + exocrine
functions, Sphincter of Oddi

## Introduction

Pancreatitis is a relatively common disease affecting people of all ages, usually caused by

- alcoholism (usually in men under 40)
- biliary obstruction (usually in older women; usually caused by gallstones).

although only a minority of alcoholics or people with gallstones develop pancreatitis.

There are a number of lesser causes, including

- drugs, such as NSAIDs, thiazides, contraceptives (Hughes, 2004)
- animal venoms, rarely seen in the UK
- idiopathic.

Worldwide, gallstones is the main cause (Mitchell *et al.*, 2003), but alcohol is usually the main cause in the UK (Larvin, 1999; Pickworth, 2003). Alcohol causes protein in pancreatic enzymes to precipitate, obstructing pancreatic ductules (Hughes, 2004). UK incidence of pancreatitis, and alcoholism, is increasing (Pickworth, 2003).

Pancreatitis may be acute or chronic. Patients with chronic pancreatitis are seldom admitted to ICUs, so this chapter describes acute pancreatitis. Acute pancreatitis may be

- oedematous/toxic (mild)
- haemorrhagic/necrotising (severe).

*Oedematous* pancreatitis causes congestion and swelling in the pancreas, impairing function, but does not damage cells (Palmer & Penman, 1999), does not affect other organs and resolves after a few days, so should not need ICU admission. *Haemorrhagic* pancreatitis damages cells, releasing proinflammatory mediators, causing progressive ischaemia, oedema and damage, including multiorgan failure. One-fifth of cases of oedematous pancreatitis progress into haemorrhagic, progressing rapidly to multisystem dysfunction and SIRS (Mitchell *et al.*, 2003). Up to a quarter of people developing severe pancreatitis die (Beckingham & Bornman, 2001), usually within one week (Slavin, 2002). Mortality rates have barely changed for three decades (Larvin, 1999). Medical and nursing management focuses on system support to minimise/limit complications. Priorities of nursing care are listed in Table 45.1.

## Pathology

Pancreatic juice, secreted by reflex vagal responses to acidic chyme, enters the duodenum at the Sphincter of Oddi. It is strongly alkaline (pH about 8.0) and contains phospholipidase A, a powerful protein-digesting enzyme.

**Table 45.1 Priorities of nursing care**

- Haemodynamic monitoring (ECG, BP, CVP, flow monitoring) – dysrhythmias + hypovolaemia likely
- Monitor + support ventilation – probable pulmonary oedema/effusions, diaphragmatic splinting
- Pain management – morphine usually needed
- Restore normovolaemia – massive fluid shifts; monitor CVP, give prescribed 'filling' (mainly colloids)
- Monitor + resolve electrolyte imbalances
- Early nutrition, monitor absorption
- Thermoregulation – monitor temperature; blood cultures if infection suspected; antipyretics
- Monitor urine output – CRRT may be needed
- normoglycaemia – frequent blood glucose monitoring, insulin regime.

Phospholipidase A, released as an inactive proenzyme to prevent autodigestion, is normally activated in the duodenum by trypsin. However, with obstruction to flow pancreatic, activated enzymes (trypsin, phospholipidase A, elastase) are released into pancreatic tissue, causing oedema, necrosis and haemorrhage (Hale *et al.*, 2000). If fistulas are formed, pancreatic juices also digest peripancreatic fat.

Obstruction to the Ampulla of Vater leaves acid chyme unneutralised, so stimulus for further pancreatic juice production continues. Congestion eventually ruptures pancreatic ductules, releasing pancreatic juice directly into the gland.

Damage to cell membranes triggers inflammatory responses:

- capillary leak and oedema, including ascites
- vasodilatation and hypotension
- microvascular thromboses
- further release of cytokines and other mediators.

*Serum amylase* (normal 30–100 iu/l) is usually grossly raised, often exceeding 1000 iu/litre within a few hours.

## Complications

*Acute fluid collections* can develop in or near the pancreas (Valencia, 2000). These fluid collections lack a wall of granulation of fibrous tissue (Valencia, 2000).

Acute oedematous pancreatitis may progress to *pancreatic necrosis*, creating an ideal environment for bacterial growth. Infection is usually from colon bacteria (Escherichia coli, Pseudomonas species, Streptococcus faecalis, Enterococcus and Staphylococcus aureus) (Uhl *et al.*, 1998). Mortality from infected severe pancreatitis can exceed 50 per cent (Pickworth, 2003).

*Pancreatic pseudocysts* are collections of pancreatic juice enclosed by a wall of fibrous or granulation tissue (Murphy *et al.*, 2002). Pseudocysts occur in up to half of patients suffering acute pancreatitis (Reece-Smith, 1997). Pseudocysts usually resolve spontaneously, but until resolution, surrounding tissues can be compressed, and fistulae into surrounding tissue can develop, causing haemorrhage (especially hepatic or splenic) or infection (especially with bowel fistulae).

*Pancreatic abscesses* are circumscribed intra-abdominal collections of pus (Murphy *et al.*, 2002). Mortality is 40 per cent (Larvin, 1999). Once confirmed by *CT* scan, abscesses should be drained.

## Symptoms

Oedema and distension of the pancreatic capsule, biliary tree obstruction or chemical peritoneal burning (phospholipidase A) cause severe acute abdominal *pain*, requiring opioid analgesia such as morphine (Mergener & Baillic, 1998; Paulson, 2002). To relieve pain, conscious patients often sit forward, with knees bent (Banks, 1998). Severe pain and opioids, often causes nausea and vomiting, so anti-emetics should also be given.

Thoracic epidural analgesia may also be useful (Johnson, 1998), provided clotting is not impaired. Epidural blockade can cause further vasodilatation (Johnson, 1998), so blood volume should be monitored and replaced as appropriate.

Hypermetabolism is the main cause of *pyrexia*, although infections often occur. Temperature should be monitored. If high, blood cultures should be taken and antipyretics may be needed (see Chapter 8).

*Infection* occurs in one-tenth of patients with acute pancreatitis. About half of patients with acute pancreatitis develop infection within three weeks. Early antibiotic therapy reduces infection rates to one-third (Uhl *et al.*, 1998), so preventing infection is currently the 'most promising...treatment' (Uhl *et al.*, 1999: 103).

Common *electrolyte imbalances* include

- *hyperglycaemia* (from impaired insulin secretion, increased glucagon release, circulating antagonists such as catecholamines, and glucose in parenteral feeds); blood sugars should be closely monitored; sliding scales of insulin may be prescribed
- *hypocalcaemia* is mainly caused by extravasation of albumin (to which calcium is bound) (Hale *et al.*, 2000)
- *hypomagnesaemia* is common, especially with alcohol-related pancreatitis.

*Respiratory* failure, the main cause of death with acute pancreatitis, may be caused by

- pleural effusions, from autodigestion of lung tissue, especially on the left side
- atelectasis and *ARDS* from phospholipidase A impairing surfactant production (Hale *et al.*, 2000)

- pulmonary oedema caused by inflammatory mediators (Pastor *et al.*, 2003) and inappropriate fluid management, especially excessive crystalloid infusion or low molecular weight colloids
- reduced lung volume from diaphragmatic splinting, caused by ascites and the grossly distended pancreas

and often requires artificial ventilation.

*Cardiovascular* instability is caused by SIRS to autodigestion. Gross inflammatory responses cause excessive vasodilatation and capillary leak. Fluid shifts cause electrolyte imbalances. Aggressive fluid resuscitation and inotropes are usually needed, often necessitating flow monitoring (see Chapter 20).

Massive extravasation from inflammation causes severe systemic hypotension pre-renal failure and, if unreversed, *acute tubular necrosis* (Mergener & Baillic, 1998). Aggressive fluid resuscitation should be given (Mergener & Baillic, 1998; Beckingham & Bornman, 2001), especially with large-molecule colloids that will remain in the intravascular space. Renal replacement therapy may be needed. Patients' abdomens should be assessed for bruising or other skin discolouration, indicating haemorrhage ('Grey Turner's sign'; 'Cullen's sign').

Direct damage to the *gastrointestinal* can cause

- peptic ulceration
- gastritis
- translocation of gut bacteria
- bowel infarction
- paralytic ileus.

Hypermetabolism increases energy expenditure, necessitating additional nutritional support.

Enteral nutrition is usually possible with pancreatitis (Wyncoll, 1999; Marik & Zaloga, 2004). If gastric ileus occurs, jejunal feeding should be attempted. Parenteral nutrition (TPN) is a high infection risk, and causes many other complications, so is the least desirable means of nutrition.

## Medical treatments

Treatment, discussed earlier, is largely supporting systems and minimising complications:

- artificial ventilation
- fluids
- (early) antibiotics
- inotropes
- renal replacement therapy
- analgesia
- nutrition
- insulin.

*Gallstones* should be removed with early endoscopic retrograde cholangiopancreatography (ERCP) (Johnson, 1998). Fat necrosis and slough may need surgical removal.

'Magic bullets' for pancreatitis have proved elusive. *Antiproteases* to reduce or neutralise pancreatic enzyme release (e.g. aprotinin, gabexate mesylate) are not beneficial in severe acute pancreatitis (Büchler *et al.*, 1993; Pastor *et al.*, 2003). *Lexipafant*, a platelet-releasing factor antagonist, reduces circulating cytokines (Valencia, 2000), but does not appear to improve outcome (Johnson *et al.*, 2001).

*Surgery* is sometimes necessary, usually to remove infected necrotic tissue.

## Implications for practice

- Pain is severe; analgesia (usually opioid) should be provided and its effectiveness assessed.
- Large fluids shifts can rapidly cause oedema (including ascites and pulmonary oedema) and hypovolaemia; aggressive fluid resuscitation, mainly with colloids, may prevent organ failure. Arterial blood pressure and fluid balance charts give little indication of intravascular volume.
- Respiratory failure is the main cause of death with acute pancreatitis. Respiratory function should be monitored closely, and atelectasis and pleural effusions treated. Severe respiratory failure often progresses to ARDS.
- Fluid shifts/loss can cause various electrolyte imbalances. Biochemistry should be monitored and major imbalances rectified.
- Blood sugars should be monitored regularly and insulin regimes followed.
- Nurses should ensure that nutrition is optimised; if possible use enteral routes, including jejunostomy.

## Summary

Pancreatitis can cause rapid and severe complications in most other major systems. Severe pancreatitis, seen in the ICU, continues to cause high mortality. Current treatment is largely system support to prevent further complications. Pain control being a particularly important nursing role.

## Further reading

Medical reviews of pancreatitis frequently appear. recent examples include Beckingham and Bornman (2001), Mitchell *et al.* (2003) and Pickworth (2003). Nursing reviews occasionally appear, such as Hughes (2004). Much evidence supports enteral nutrition with pancreatitis, including Marik and Zaloga's (2004) meta-analysis.

## Clinical scenarios

Myla Vegas is 56 years old and was admitted to the ICU with sudden acute abdominal pain. The pain radiated towards her back and was accompanied by nausea and vomiting. Two years ago she had an ultrasound which detected gallstones. She is 1.6 metres tall and weighs 74 kg. On admission her abdomen was distended

Other abnormal results from admission assessment include:

| Vital signs | | Blood serum | |
|---|---|---|---|
| Temperature | 38.4°C | Glucose | 12 mmol/litre |
| Respiration | 32 per minute | WBC | $19.3 \times 10^{-9}$/litre |
| SpO$_2$ | 88% on FiO$_2$ of 0.6 | CRP | 151 mg/litre |
| Heart rate | 145 bpm | Amylase | 1 543 iu/litre |
| 3-lead ECG | Sinus rhythm, ST elevation | Alkaline phosphate | 250 iu/litre |
| BP | 110/60 mmHg | Potassium | 3.4 mmol/litre |
| MAP | 77 mmHg | Calcium | 1.8 mmol/litre |
| CVP | 8 mmHg | Magnesium | 0.78 mmol/litre |

Q.1 With reference to physiology, explain Myla's results (e.g. why has her temperature and respiratory rate increased, why does she have low potassium with presenting symptoms and diagnosis?)

A CT scan reveals bilateral pleural effusions, basal consolidation, diffuse pancreatic enlargement with peri-pancreatic fluid and a small amount of fluid around the liver and spleen.

Q.2 Consider the implications of the CT scan results on Myla's condition, and note other complications that may occur. Discuss how these should be managed.

Q.3 Review pain management strategies for Myla's abdominal pain and discomfort caused by nursing, medical and surgical interventions.

# Chapter 46

# Diabetic crises

## Contents

| | |
|---|---|
| Introduction | 481 |
| Diabetes mellitus | 481 |
| Ketones | 482 |
| Complications | 483 |
| Metabolic syndrome | 483 |
| Hyperglycaemia | 484 |
| Severe hypoglycaemia | 484 |
| Diabetic ketoacidosis (DKA) | 484 |
| Hyperosmolar non-ketotic state (HONKS) | 485 |
| Implications for practice | 485 |
| Summary | 485 |
| Useful contacts | 486 |
| Further reading | 486 |
| Clinical scenarios | 486 |

## Fundamental knowledge

Pancreatic anatomy and physiology, especially production of insulin

## Introduction

Diabetes mellitus affects 2–3 per cent of UK adults (DOH, 2002), with many diabetics remaining undiagnosed until a crisis occurs (Audit Commission, 2001). Incidence is higher in people of South Asian, African, African-Caribbean and Middle Eastern descent, increasing with age (5 per cent in over 65s, and 20 per cent in over 85s) (DOH, 2002) and obesity. Incidence will probably double by 2010 due to ageing populations and increasing obesity (Audit Commission, 2001). Human, financial and social costs of diabetes are high, and have prompted the publication of the *National Service Framework for Diabetes* (DOH, 2002).

Insulin transports glucose into cells. Lack therefore deprives cells of their main energy sources, and causes hyperglycaemia. Hyperglycaemia causes acute complications, including

- polyuria (if glucose exceeds the renal reabsorption threshold – blood glucose >10 mmol/litre) and so hypovolaemia
- impaired neutrophil function (immunocompromise can occur if blood glucose exceeds 12 mmol/litre) (Bristow & Hillman, 1999)
- inflammatory responses from vascular endothelium.

Poorly controlled diabetes can cause many diseases, outlined in this chapter. The *metabolic syndrome* is also discussed. Many patients are diabetic, or develop short-term hyperglycaemia in response to stressors of critical illness; even if not the cause of admission, they often complicate recovery, so benefits of glycaemic control in critically ill non-diabetic patients is included. But diabetes can also cause crises which necessitate ICU admission. This chapters discusses

- severe hypoglycaemia
- diabetic ketoacidosis (DKA)
- hyperosmolar non-ketotic state (HONKS; sometimes called 'hyperosmolar hyperglycaemic state'): hyperglycaemia, minimal ketosis, coma; sometimes called Hyperosmolar Hyperglycaemic Syndrome (HHS).

'Diabetes' means 'fountain-like', from the classic symptoms of polyuria and *polydipsia*. Diabetes is popularly used to describe *diabetes mellitus*, a problem with blood sugar control. *Diabetes insipidus* is caused by lack of anti-diuretic hormone (see Chapter 37). Hyperglycaemia from diabetes mellitus causes *glycosuria*. When urinalysis was performed by tasting it, glycosuria gave urine a sweet taste (mellitus is Latin for 'honey').

## Diabetes mellitus

Blood glucose is regulated mainly by the pancreatic hormones insulin and, to a lesser extent, glucagon. This may be caused by deficient production of insulin or excessive resistance of insulin receptors. Diabetes mellitus can be caused by two different pathologies, called diabetes Type1 and diabetes Type 2. With both types, priorities of diabetic care are to control

- glycaemia
- free fatty acids (blood lipids)
- blood pressure.

(Wierzbicki, 2003)

Diabetics with total cholesterol above 5 mmol/litre should receive statins (Winocour & Fisher, 2003).

## Type 1

Previously called 'insulin dependent diabetes mellitus' (IDDM), 'juvenile' and 'Type I', this is an autoimmune disease, which destroys pancreatic beta cells (which produce insulin), but leaves other pancreatic cells unharmed, so glucagons and other pancreatic hormones are produced (Devendra et al., 2004). This disease typically develops in childhood, the almost total destruction of beta cells usually necessitating life-long insulin therapy. Most Type 1 diabetics suffer complications relatively early in life, especially retinopathy, which develops in 90 per cent within 20 years from diagnosis (Walker & Rodgers, 2002). Northern Europe, especially Finland, has the highest incidence of Type 1 diabetes, and incidence is increasing (Lambert & Bingley, 2002).

Transplantation of pancreatic cells is being researched (Markmann et al., 2003), but mortality among recipients is currently higher than from diabetes itself (Venstrom et al., 2003).

## Type 2

Previously called 'non-insulin dependent diabetes mellitus' (NIDDM), 'late-onset', and 'Type II', causes most (90 per cent) (Nolan, 2002) of diabetes. Typically, this develops in later life (65–74 years) (DOH, 2002) partly from age-related pancreatic decline, and often aggravated by obesity – fat causes insulin resistance (Jefrey, 2003). Type 2 is less severe than Type 1, as the pancreas has significant remaining function, but not sufficient to cope with the demands placed upon it. Although usually a disease of later life, incidence of diabetes Type 2 among children is also increasing (Howdle & Wilkin, 2001).

Type 2 diabetics may or may not need insulin. Some can control their diabetes with oral hypoglycaemic tablets or just through diet, especially where they adopt healthier lifestyles.

## Ketones

Glucose is normally the main energy source for mitochondria in cells to produce adenosine triphosphate (ATP). Glucose needs insulin to transport it across cell membrane. Therefore insulin lack deprives cell of their normal main energy source, forcing cells to resort to metabolism of alternative energy sources, mainly free fatty acids (lyposis). Alternative energy source metabolism is relatively inefficient, producing limited energy but much waste, including ketones. Excessive ketones, and other metabolic acids, cause acidosis, which impairs function of many systems (see Chapter 19).

Ketones are filtered by the kidneys, so can be detected on urinalysis. Although less potent than glycosuria, ketonuria causes further osmotic diuresis. Ketones can also cause a distinctive sickly sweet smell to breathe (in unintubated patients).

## Complications

Polyuria (described earlier) causes dehydration, usually provoking thirst (hence polydipsia). Continued, even mild, hyperglycaemia provokes vascular inflammatory responses, resulting in widespread vascular damage. Common complications of vascular damage in diabetes include:

- retinopathy
- strokes – three times more likely with diabetes (Beckman *et al.*, 2002)
- cardiovascular disease – coronary artery disease, atherosclerosis, peripheral vascular disease, renal artery stenosis (Valabhji & Elkeles, 2002; Watkins, 2003)
- chronic renal failure, from intra-renal vascular damage
- neuropathy
- ulcers (Jeffacote & Harding, 2003)
- depression (Grimmer & Mittra, 2001).

In addition to their other needs, caring for critically ill diabetics necessitates holistic assessment, prevention of potential complications treatment of existing complications and health promotion for the future.

## Metabolic syndrome

Chronic hyperglycaemia is often one of various interrelated metabolic problems. As risk factors interact and accumulate, disease progresses. Identifying the metabolic syndrome early enables disease progression to be limited. National Cholesterol Education Program Adult Treatment Panel III (ATP III) criteria for diagnosis (cited Tonkin, 2004) is three or more of

- fasting plasma glucose $\geq$ 6.1 mmol/litre
- abdominal obesity (e.g. waist circumference >102 cm in men, >88 cm in women)
- triglyceride level $\geq$ 1.7 mmol/litre
- high-density lipoprotein cholesterol (HDL-C) <1 mmol/litre in men, 1.3 mmol/litre in women
- BP $\geq$ 130/85 mmHg

483

although other authorities sometimes given slightly different criteria. USA incidence exceeds 20 per cent (Davidson, 2004), while European incidence is very variable (Tonkin, 2004).

Excessive insulin resistance (Wilson & Grundy, 2003; Tonkin, 2004), and so continuing hyperglycaemia, causes widespread inflammatory vascular disease, especially atherosclerosis and myocardial infarction (Reilly & Rader, 2003; Wilson & Grundy, 2003; Malik *et al.*, 2004; Marik & Raghaven, 2004; Sasso *et al.*, 2004).

## Hyperglycaemia

Critical illness usually causes transient hyperglycaemia (Van Den Berghe *et al.*, 2001; Cely *et al.*, 2004) by increasing insulin resistance. Drugs, such as adrenaline or glucocorticosteroids, also increase insulin resistance, while parenteral nutrition infuses large volumes of intravenous glucose. Such transient hyperglycaemia usually resolves with recovery or once treatment is reduced/removed, but maintaining normoglycaemia improves survival and recovery (Van Den Berghe *et al.*, 2001; Jeschke *et al.*, 2003; Cely *et al.*, 2004). Hyperglycaemia (15 mmol/l) triggers release of proinflammatory cytokines (Essposito *et al.*, 2002; Marik & Raghaven, 2004) (see Chapter 24), so aggressive normoglycaemic control reduces systemic inflammatory responses (Jeschke *et al.*, 2003). Tight glycaemic control creates risks for drug errors, necessitating frequent monitoring. Safe management of insulin infusions is helped with continuous nutrition (see Chapter 9). Transient hyperglycaemia may indicate limited pancreatic function, and so possible future development of Type 2 diabetes.

## Severe hypoglycaemia

This may occur if Type 1 diabetics either receive an insulin overdose or have not eaten adequately. Blood glucose below 2 mmol/litre creates a medical emergency (Keays, 2003), as brain cells rely on constant supplies to survive. Severe hypoglycaemia is treated by giving intravenous glucose, stabilising acid–base and electrolyte balances and frequent monitoring. Severe hypoglycaemia is usually managed in Accident and Emergency or acute admission wards, but could occur on ICU, especially if feeds are stopped but insulin infusions continue.

## Diabetic ketoacidosis (DKA)

This is the diabetic crisis, usually occurring when Type 1 diabetics fail to receive insulin, although can occur with Type 2 (Newton & Raskin, 2004) and usually necessitating the ICU admission. DKA causes

■ hyperglycaemia
■ ketosis
■ metabolic acidosis

By the time of admission, blood sugar may be 50–100 mmol/litre which, depending on technology available, may exceed available clinical measurements. Patients may be comatose or acutely confused. Osmotic diuresis from both glyco-suria and ketonuria usually causes hypovolaemic shock. Venous statis and hyperosmolality can cause thromboembolism, epilepsy and strokes.

Priorities are to

- reduce hyperglycaemia with insulin
- rehydrate to reperfuse
- restore electrolytes balance, especially potassium.

This necessitates close monitoring of vital signs, blood sugars, fluid balance, electrolytes and neurological state. Severe acidosis (pH <7.1) may require specific treatment, such as bicarbonate infusion, but mild acidosis usually resolves with recovery.

## Hyperosmolar non-ketotic state (HONKS)

(also called Hyperosmolar Hyperglycaemic Syndrome – HHS)

This rare condition is most likely to occur to Type 2 diabetics, and resembles diabetic ketoacidosis, except that it develops more slowly, and ketosis does not occur, probably because the person has sufficient insulin function to prevent excessive ketogenesis (Charalambous *et al.*, 1999). Hyperglcaemia causes osmotic diuresis and electrolyte imbalance; as HONKS often develops over some days, dehydration is often more severe (Keays, 2003). Dehydration increases serum osmolality, which causes neurological complications, including *tonic-clonic seizures*. Type 2 diabetics are usually more sensitive to insulin (Charalambous *et al.*, 1999), so it should be infused more cautiously and monitored more frequently. Otherwise HONKS is managed as DKA.

### Implications for practice

- Diabetes can cause widespread complications and problems throughout the body, so patients should be assessed and treated holistically.
- In critical illness, insulin protocols should be prescribed to maintain blood sugar 4.4–6.1 mmol/litre. This necessitates frequent (often 2 hourly) monitoring of blood sugar.
- Insulin management should be adjusted with changes in feeding regimes, especially when feeds are stopped.
- Diabetic ketoacidosis and hyperosmolar non-ketotic state should also be treated with aggressive fluid replacement.

### Summary

Diabetes affects an increasing number of people of all ages. Most diabetics have Type 2 diabetes, which becomes increasingly prevalent with age. Poorly controlled diabetes has long been known to cause other problems, especially loss of sight and cardiovascular disease, but progressive deterioration from the metabolic syndrome has only recently been fully recognised. While many diabetics live healthily, diabetes creates an expensive burden on the individual, society and healthcare. This burden is likely to increase as the ageing population and obesity epidemic double the numbers of diabetics in the UK.

Diabetes complicates critical illness, and may cause crises that necessitate ICU admission. Aggressive insulin therapy to maintain normoglycaemia (4.4–6.1 mmol/litre) reduces complications, morbidity and mortality.

## Useful contacts

Diabetes UK, 10 Queen Anne Street, London W1G 9LH:
   020–7323–1531
   fax 020–7637–3644
   info@diabetes.org.uk
   www.diabetes.org.uk

## Further reading

Van Den Berghe *et al.*'s (2001) study significantly changed glycaemic control in most ICUs. The *National Service Framework for Diabetes* (DOH, 2002) has helped focus and develop diabetic care, but provides limited guidance for ICU nurses caring for diabetic patients. General articles on diabetes can frequently be found in both medical and nursing journals, and many textbooks include the topic. Marik and Raghaven (2004) provide a recent medical overview of ICU care. www.routledge.com/textbooks/0415373239

For clinical scenarios, clinical questions and the answers to them go to the support website at www.routledge.com/textbooks/0415373239

## Clinical scenarios

Rosemary Davies, 34-year-old accountant, with no previous medical history was found unconscious and incontinent by her friends. She had been recovering from flu, complaining of fever, thirst, tiredness and feeling confused.

Rosemary was admitted to ICU self-ventilating at 32 breaths/min, HR 120 bpm, BP 80/60 mmHg, CVP 0–1 mmHg, and hypothermic 35.5°C. Blood investigation revealed blood sugar of 40 mmol/litre, $Na^+$ 150 mmol/litre, $K^+$ 4.8 mmol/litre, $HCO_3^-$ 19 mmol/litre with metabolic acidosis. A diagnosis of coma HONK was made.

Q.1 Rosemary is extremely hyperglycaemic. Identify the effects of hyperglycaemia which resulted in Rosemary's admission (hyperglycaemia causes tachycardia, hypothermia, unconsciousness etc. by which physiological process)?

486

Q.2 An intravenous insulin infusion is commenced. Select and give the rationale for infusion rate in units/h to correct Rosemary's hyperglycaemia. What other factors should be considered in correction of hyperglycaemia?

Q.3 Reflect on patient's blood glucose management in your clinical area, consider the benefits and limitations of this strategy (e.g. use of sliding scale insulin prescription versus insulin protocols, equipment required, type of insulin, route and rate of administration, life of infusion, dose adjustments, minimum and maximum dose, methods and frequency of blood glucose assessment, inclusion of 10% glucose and potassium supplementation).

Chapter 47

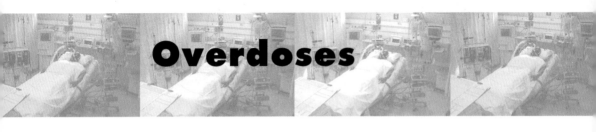

# Overdoses

## Contents

| | |
|---|---|
| Introduction | 489 |
| Deliberate self-harm | 489 |
| Antidepressants | 489 |
| Paracetamol | 490 |
| Illicit drugs | 490 |
| Symptoms | 492 |
| Cardiovascular | 492 |
| Pyrexia | 493 |
| Neurological | 493 |
| Respiratory | 494 |
| Renal | 494 |
| Hepatic | 494 |
| Psychological | 494 |
| Health promotion | 495 |
| Implications for practice | 495 |
| Summary | 496 |
| Support groups | 496 |
| Further reading | 496 |
| Clinical scenarios | 496 |

## Fundamental knowledge

Neurotransmission synapse
Cell metabolism

## Introduction

Many drugs and chemicals have potentially harmful/fatal effects if taken in sufficient quantity. The drugs which cause most ill health are nicotine (and the hundreds of other toxins in cigarettes) and alcohol (Fogarty & Lingford-Hughes, 2004). However, these are relatively socially acceptable drugs, and usually cause insidious rather than sudden changes in health. Deliberate overdoses are usually impulsive, so use easily accessed drugs such as mild analgesics (e.g. aspirin, paracetamol and co-proxamol). This chapter focuses on drugs that more often precipitate crises:

- tricyclic antidepressants
- paracetamol
- cocaine
- 'Ecstasy' (MDMA).

Individual drugs are briefly described, followed by discussion of common physiological effects. Overdoses of drugs not described often cause similar problems, which will be managed similarly. Many wider issues of nursing care discussed in this chapter can be applied to overdose of other drugs, although readers should check applicability before transferring specific aspects.

Overdose may be deliberate or accidental. Further divisions, such as 'calls for help' (sometimes labelled 'parasuicide') are unhelpful labels which can both stigmatise and mislead. Deliberate self-harm is discussed hereafter. Accidental overdose is often due to lack of awareness of the drug.

## Deliberate self-harm

Each year about 140,000 people are treated in UK hospitals for deliberate self-harm (Bennewith *et al.*, 2002), usually from drug overdose (Boyce *et al.*, 2001). Care focuses on

- support for physiological effects
- preventing recurrence of self-harming behaviour (psychiatry)
- dealing with underlying psychopathology.

Although specialist psychological care usually follows ICU discharge, the potential wish to self-harm during ICU stay should be remembered, and so risk factors minimised.

## Antidepressants

Fifteen per cent of depressed people attempt suicide (Finnell & Harris, 2000). People being treated for depression often have access to large numbers of antidepressant tablets (such as amitriptyline), so antidepressants form one of most-frequent overdoses (Finnell & Harris, 2000). In USA antidepressant is the most-frequent type of overdose after analgesics (Mokhlesi *et al.*, 2003).

489

Antidepressants cause

- dysrhythmias, including ventricular tachycardia
- hypotension
- seizures

(Mokhlesi *et al.*, 2003)

and lesser symptoms such as agitation, blurred vision and vomiting. Death usually occurs within 4–6 hours, and all deaths occur within 24 hours (Finnell & Harris, 2000), so Mokhlesi *et al.* (2003) recommend urgent transfer to ICU for 12 hours.

## Paracetamol

The 1998 UK legislation limiting how many paracetamol (= acetaminophen in USA) tablets can be bought at one time has reduced mortality (Hawton *et al.*, 2004). Yet paracetamol remains the most common drug overdose in the UK, causing nearly half of all poison admissions to hospitals, and 100–200 deaths each year (Wallace *et al.*, 2003), prompting calls for paracetamol to be made a prescription only medicine (POM) (Sheen *et al.*, 2002).

Paracetamol is rapidly absorbed, plasma levels peaking within one hour (Mokhlesi *et al.*, 2003). The toxic threshold for liver damage is 150 mg/kg in adults, although as little as 4–6 g can cause injury (Mokhlesi *et al.*, 2003) because metabolism varies greatly between individuals.

Hepatic metabolism of paracetamol forms the potentially toxic metabolite N-acetyl-p-bezoquinone (NAPQI) (Mokhlesi *et al.*, 2003); toxicity rapidly causes hepatocyte necrosis. Plasma levels exceeding 200 mg/litre at 4 hours or 50 mg/litre at 12 hours usually progresses to hepatic damage (Wyncoll, 2003), although severe symptoms may be delayed for 2–3 days, appearing only after significant, possibly fatal, damage. Progressive liver failure often causes:

- metabolic acidosis
- hepatorenal syndrome
- intracranial hypertension
- coagulopathies (prothrombin time exceeds 100 seconds).

Acetylcysteine (Parvolex®) and Methionine can prevent hepatic failure within 10–12 hours of paracetamol overdose, and may still be hepatoprotective up to 24 hours. Overdose may necessitate ICU admission for system support.

Paracetamol overdose is usually impulsive (Turvill *et al.*, 2000; Hawton *et al.*, 2001), so guilt and remorse are likely to be problems for both patients and their families and friends.

## Illicit drugs

Paracetamol and antidepressants are usually obtained legally, but 'recreational' or 'street' drugs are obtained, and often produced, illegally. Purity and strength of recreational drugs is often very variable, whether from deliberate dilution (to reduce cost) or chance contamination during non-aseptic illegal manufacture. Different tablets may have dissimilar strengths, so even users with previous experience of drugs cannot be sure how each dose will affect them. Accidental overdose occurs easily; individual metabolism and tolerance further influence effect.

Drug use among adolescents is declining, although use of 'club drugs' has increased (Koesters *et al.*, 2002). Cannabis is probably the most widely used recreational drug in the UK (Patton *et al.*, 2002; Fogarty & Lingford-Hughes, 2004), but seldom necessitates ICU admission, so is not included here.

Many recreational drugs (such as cocaine and Ecstasy) are taken to achieve desired effects or mood, not with intent to self-harm. Usually, the desired effect will be pleasure, through either

- calming/suppressing/reducing or
- stimulating/increasing

central nervous system function. Drugs which stimulate more often cause acute life-threatening emergencies. Stimulation affects the sympathetic nervous system, so stimulant drugs have many similar effects to inotropes.

Many drugs taken for pleasure become addictive. They replace endogenous neurotransmitters (especially dopamine), causing a 'high' – euphoria, increased libido and energy for all-night dancing. The attractions of many drugs may be seen in raves; the miseries are more often seen in ICU. After a few hours benefits fade, leaving insufficient endogenous neurotransmitters, so causing a 'low' (depression). Drug users often respond by taking further, often larger, dose, becoming progressively addicted or dependent.

Chemical changes in brain tissue cause permanent neurological damage, while effects of other organs often cause acute and sometimes permanent damage. Drugs are also frequently mixed, often with alcohol, tobacco and other recreational drugs. So each patient admitted with an overdose should be individually assessed and treated.

Illicit drugs are often transported in body cavities ('body packing'), using plastic bags or condoms and swallowed or inserted into the rectum. The gut is highly vascular, so if bags break, drugs are efficiently absorbed. Drug traffickers may be admitted with accidental overdoses and, understandably, may be reluctant to admit their continuing rectal drug infusion. Attempts to remove bags may cause further internal spillage (Bulstrode *et al.*, 2002). If drugs have not yet been absorbed, activated charcoal slurry washout may limit absorption within two hours of ingestion (Schofield *et al.*, 1997). Bags may obstruct the gut, causing abdominal pain, distension, vomiting and constipation (Bulstrode *et al.*, 2002). Progress of intact bags can be monitored with abdominal X-rays and CT scans.

Patients may be drug pushers, regular users or novices experimenting with the drug. Whatever their personal views, nurses caring for victims have the same professional duty of care as for other patients (NMC, 2004), so should

- maintain safe environments
- treat with unconditional positive regard
- adopt non-judgmental attitudes.

Patients will usually be in police custody while in hospital, and know they face prison when they recover.

Recreational drugs often have many street names. Some of the more common names are mentioned, but most drugs have many other names.

*Cocaine* ('coke') has long been used as a therapeutic analgesic, but has also a long history as a recreational drug. In 2001 there were an estimated 120,000 regular users and 360,000 occasional users in the UK (Jones & Parsonage, 2002), and increased targeting of the UK market is likely to increase use further.

*Crack* is modified cocaine and causes similar symptoms.

*Amphetamine* sulphate ('speed'). Its effects are similar to cocaine, but usually last far longer. The amphetamine derivative 3–4 methylene-dioxymethamphetamine (MDMA, usually called 'Ecstasy' or 'E') is discussed in the following lines, but other amphetamines have similar effects.

Widespread misuse of *Ecstasy* is a recent phenomenon. In 1990 four deaths were recorded in the USA but none in the UK; between 1997 and 2000 Ecstasy caused 81 deaths in England and Wales (Schifano *et al.*, 2003). Braithwaite (1999) suggests that half a million doses of Ecstasy and related drugs are taken each weekend but cites no source for this figure. Mortality often bears little relation to amounts of Ecstasy taken: single tablet fatalities (serum MDMA levels of 0.424 mg/l) contrast with 42 tablet survival (serum MDMA 7.72 mg/litre) (Wake, 1995).

*Ketamine* ('special K'), used therapeutically as an anaesthetic, is often taken as a cheap alternative to Ecstasy. It induces hallucinations, often nightmare-like (Shehabi & Innes, 2002), can cause nausea, disrupt co-ordination and provoke schizophrenia..

## Symptoms

Life-threatening complications of illicit drugs are usually caused by excessive stimulation of the sympathetic nervous system. Care is often complicated by psychological and social problems.

If the drug remains in the gut, activated charcoal will usually be given. Toxic blood levels may be treated with haemofiltration. If there is an antidote to the drug, it will be started. Otherwise the priorities are system support and psychological care.

## Cardiovascular

Sympathetic nervous system stimulants increase:

- rhythm
- vasoconstriction

Rhythm. Illicit drug overdose victims are usually young, but cardiac health cannot be assumed, and sympathetic stimulation increases myocardial workload while reducing myocardial oxygenation. This may provoke ventricular dysrhythmias and tachycardia (Welsch *et al.*, 2001; Jones & Parsonage, 2002), especially ventricular ectopics (VEs), tachycardia (VT) and fibrillation (VF), and possible myocardial infarction. Prolonged use may cause irreversible cardiomegaly (Ghuran & Nolan, 2000) from prolonged compensatory responses to increased systemic vascular resistance.

Vasoconstriction often causes severe hypertension (Finnell *et al.*, 2000; Jones & Parsonage, 2002). Intravenous drug abuse ('mainlining') and heavy smoking may have caused further previous vascular damage. Vascular damage could cause aortic aneurysms.

Electrolytes and metabolites are often grossly deranged on arrival, including

- hyperkalaemia
- hypercalcaemia
- hyponatraemia
- hypoglycaemia.

Cardiovascular function should be closely monitored. Hypertension often responds to beta-blockers (Lester *et al.*, 2000).

## Pyrexia

Hypermetabolism often induces malignant hyperpyrexia (Crandall *et al.*, 2002), the cause of most Ecstasy-related deaths (Wake, 1995). Malignant hyperthermia should be actively reversed with dantrolene sodium.

## Neurological

Immediate neurological complications are likely to be caused by

- cerebral vasospasm
- intracranial hypertension, causing intracranial bleeding, subarachnoid haemorrhage and CVAs (Welsch *et al.*, 2001)
- hyponatraemic encephalopathy (Hartung *et al.*, 2002)
- seizures.

Cerebral perfusion and oxygenation should be optimised; antiepileptics may be needed (usually benzodiazepines, although these can exacerbate cardiac instability). Major tranquillisers (such as chlorpromazine) should be avoided as they lower seizure threshold, aggravate hypotension and provoke dysrhythmias (MacConnachie, 1997). Treatment for cerebral oedema is discussed in Chapter 37.

Small-scale studies indicate long-term use causes chronic neurological and psychiatric problems (Semple *et al.*, 1999; Reneman *et al.*, 2001), including permanent cognitive impairment (Parrott *et al.*, 1998).

## Respiratory

Many inhaled drugs are smoked, the smoke being far hotter than from cigarettes. Therefore, like burns victims, drug smokers can develop severe larayngeal oedema, necessitating prophylactic intubation. If consciousness is impaired, they may have aspirated, and respiratory failure frequently occurs. Multisystem complications often necessitate intubation and artificial ventilation. Cocaine can cause status asthaticus, upper airway obstruction, pulmonary hypertension, barotrauma and pulmonary oedema (Mokhlesi *et al.*, 2004). Many drugs cause fluid and electrolyte imbalances and trigger inflammatory responses, causing pulmonary oedema (Welsch *et al.*, 2001). Hypercalcaemia may cause trismus (tightening of jaw muscles – 'lockjaw') and bruxism (jaw-clenching) (Koesters *et al.*, 2002), which may make oral intubation difficult.

## Renal

Ischaemia may cause acute renal failure (Schofield *et al.*, 1997), while hypermetabolism often causes rhabdomyolysis (see Chapter 39). Kidneys should be protected with aggressive fluid therapy, but haemofiltration is often needed. Renal failure exacerbates hyperkalaemia.

## Hepatic

Amphetamines are hepatotoxic (Mokhlesi *et al.*, 2004), with further damage caused by ischaemia (Ellis *et al.*, 1996).

## Psychological

The 'low' usually causes generalised fatigue, muscle ache, limited concentration, confusion, anxiety, hypersomnia or insomnia, bizarre and unpleasant dreams, and depression (Chychula & Sciamanna, 2002; Koesters *et al.*, 2002). Survivors often experience frequent and persistent panic attacks ('bad trips'), believing death to be imminent (McGuire *et al.*, 1994).

Patients, relatives and friends often experience guilt about the overdose and fear about prosecution. Parents may have been unaware their children were taking drugs. Drug levels in blood and other specimens will be tested for therapeutic purposes, but there may be legal requirements about saving samples or releasing results to the police or other authorities. Many patients, families and friends are anyway likely to fear what staff will tell other authorities. Warner *et al.* (2003) suggests there should be policies about informed consent for drug testing.

Healthcare professionals have a duty of care to all patients. But negative attitudes to patients considered as 'time-waters', 'bed-blockers', immature or 'mad' or 'sad', may both impair quality of care given, and cause further psychological distress to patients and families. Nurses need to be aware not only of their own attitudes, but also attitudes of others, promoting a team approach of unconditional positive regard.

Many victims of illicit drug overdoses are young; for many nursing staff this can create an uncomfortable reminder of their own mortality.

Psychiatric referral will often be made following recovery.

## Health promotion

With recovery, health promotion for the patient and other significant people, who may be family or friends, can prevent future crises with accidental overdose of prescribed medicines, prescriptions should be reviewed and patients should understand the correct dose and any symptoms of over- or under-dose. Those who have deliberately self-harmed should be referred for psychiatric support. Users of illicit drugs may also benefit from referral to psychiatric or other support services. Health education can raise awareness of dangers and suggest safer ways to take drugs, so users can make their own informed decisions. Friends and families may need support from specialist agencies, such as support groups or counsellors. When providing information to family and friends, nurses should remember their duty of confidentiality to their patient.

Users of illegal drugs, and their friends, are often understandably reluctant to seek medical help until dehydration and collapse occur (Cook, 1995). When help is sought, friends may be reluctant to share information with hospital staff, fearing anything revealed may be passed onto the police. Although many drugs can cause ill-health, ICU admission is usually only needed with immediate life-threatening problems, so drugs unlikely to cause these, such as cannabis, are not discussed here.

Realisation that drugs are not as safe as they previously thought may make patients and friends receptive to health education, so ICU nurses can provide useful information and contacts. However, users often have greater knowledge about recreational drugs than nurses, and may have different values and beliefs; adopting moralistic/righteous attitudes may cause alien-ation. ICU nurses should assess individual needs and offer what support they can. However, they will usually not possess the specialist knowledge of drugs involved, and should therefore work within their limitations, using specialist services that are available locally.

## Implications for practice

- Overdose can affect all major body systems; vital signs should be closely monitored.
- Peak effect often occurs within hours of ingestion, although wide various occur, partly depending on dose and individual tolerance and metabolism.
- Suicide attempts may cause guilt and/or anger among families/friends. Nurses should encourage families to express their needs and emotions, but may need to involve counselling or other services. Listening is often more useful (cathartic) than replying to guilt/anger.

495

- Friends and victims are often reluctant to share information with staff, and often experience guilt and fear.
- Victims are often young, giving friends (and nurses) an uncomfortable reminder of their own mortality.
- Nurses, and other healthcare professionals, have a duty of care to patients, regardless of the cause of illness.
- Nurses should maintain their duty of confidentiality (unless specifically exempted by statute law).
- ICU nurses may be able to offer health information about drugs or support groups.
- Psychiatric support should be offered to those who self-harm.

## Summary

Overdose of various drugs may necessitate ICU admission. Immediate care necessarily focuses on resuscitation and system support. As well as multisystem physiological problems, not usual for younger people, users (and friends) often experience anxiety or guilt. Care therefore needs to integrate urgent multisystem physiological support with skilful psychological care. Caring for such patients is challenging and can cause distress, but holistic nursing care can contribute significantly to every aspect of recovery.

## Support groups

Families Anonymous: 0207-498-4680
Drugline Ltd, Drug Advisory Bureau: 0208-692-4975
Turning Point, Grove Park, Camberwell, London: 0207-274-4883

## Further reading

Social use of drugs can change rapidly. Useful recent medical reviews include Finnell and Harris (2000), Reneman *et al.* (2001), Sheen *et al.* (2002), Mokhlesi *et al.* (2003) and Wallace *et al.* (2003). Since the upsurge in Ecstasy use in the 1990s, there has been little nursing literature, but the devastating effects Ecstasy use can have on both users and their families is poignantly described in Betts *et al.* (1999). www.routledge.com/textbooks/0415373239

For clinical scenarios, clinical questions and the answers to them go to the support website at www.routledge.com/textbooks/0415373239

## Clinical scenarios

Lisa Young is 25 years old and was admitted to ICU 10 hours after ingesting 75 Amitriptyline (50 mg) tablets. A plasma toxicology screen tested positive for heroin and methadone. Lisa's urine also tested positive for opiates, benzodiazepine, cocaine and cannabis. Paracetamol and salicylicate were not detected. Lisa is not receiving any sedation, she is agitated and noncompliant with care. She has a urinary catheter, but has removed her central venous and arterial cannulae.

Other results:

| | |
|---|---|
| Glasgow Coma Scale (GCS) 6 | (E1, V1, M5) |
| All limbs flexing spontaneously without any stimuli | |
| Both pupils' are equal size at 2 mm and increasingly dilated with a brisk response to light | |
| Respiration rate | 34 breaths/minute |
| $SpO_2$ | 97% on $FiO_2$ of 0.6 |
| Temperature | 38.1°C |
| HR | 135 sinus bpm |
| BP | 127/68 mmHg |
| Capillary refill | <1 seconds with warm peripheries |
| Skin feels hot and dry, mouth and tongue are dry | |
| Blood glucose | 6.1 mmol/litre |
| Urine output over previous 4 hours was 1650 ml, 500 ml, 680 ml, 250 ml | |

Q.1 Explain the effects of an amitriptyline overdose on Lisa's cardiovascular system and identify the most common associated arrhythmias. What is the likely cause and significance of her urine output and temperature?

Q.2 Consider interventions to reduce Lisa's risk of seizures and dysrhythmias and justify appropriate fluid management. Discuss other strategies used to monitor and minimise other complications.

Q.3 Review the long-term effects and outcome of this type of overdose. Evaluate the advice and support offered to patients like Lisa in your clinical area, availability of specialist referrals and support groups.

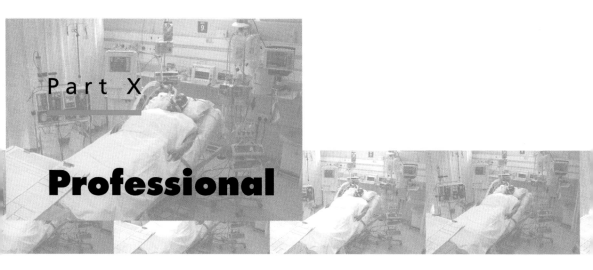

Part X

**Professional**

# Chapter 48

# Professionalism

## Contents

| | |
|---|---|
| Introduction | 502 |
| Accountability | 502 |
| Conflicts of accountability | 504 |
| Accountability in practice | 505 |
| Record keeping | 506 |
| Implications for practice | 506 |
| Summary | 506 |
| Further reading | 506 |
| Clinical questions | 506 |

### Fundamental knowledge

NMC publications:

- Code of Professional Conduct: standards for conduct, performance and ethics
- Guidelines for the Administration of Medicines

Local hospital and unit policies/guidelines/patient group directions

## Introduction

Former subservience of nursing to medicine has been replaced by professional autonomy. Autonomy brings responsibilities and individual accountability. This chapter explores issues of what professional practice means, accountability of nurses, professional standards and civil law of negligence, issues affecting all registered nurses. Every nurse is accountable for their own practice (NMC, 2004), but ICU often heightens problems due to

- critical conditions of patients
- differing roles of ICU nurses (see Chapter 1)
- increased technology.

Enthusiasm to develop skills and knowledge has been rewarded by positive interprofessional relationships of ICU staff; nurses are often trusted to perform specialised tasks. But enthusiasm to develop skills should be tempered by considerations of safety. Tissot *et al.* (1999) found an error rate in ICU drug administration of over 5 per cent; on many shifts, ICU nurses can expect to give 20 drug doses (boluses or changes of infusions), so this finding averages at least one significant drug error per shift per nurse.

Professionalism necessitates accepting

- autonomy
- accountability
- responsibility.

Nursing care should be in patients' best interests. Humans are fallible, so mistakes are inevitable. But risk management seeks to minimise mistakes by altering situations that contribute to error. Nurses should therefore report concerns about actual or potential risks. Where patients are endangered, a clinical incident form should be completed, which will be reviewed by the Trust's clinical risk department.

In law, as in life, we are accountable both for what we do (acts) and for what we do not do (omissions). So conscious or unconscious decisions not to act may be called to account.

Professionals are individually accountable for their own practice (NMC, 2004), so should continue to develop professionally, updating skills and knowledge. Unfortunately many employers under-invest in their nursing staff's development, forcing nurses to invest in themselves (Joshua-Amadi, 2002).

## Accountability

Dimond (2005) identifies four arenas of professional accountability:

- criminal law
- civil law

- employer's contract
- professional body (NMC)

adding that accountability between arenas may conflict.

For civil actions of *negligence* to succeed, three conditions must be met:

- a duty of care must exist
- that duty of care must have been breached
- resulting harm must have been reasonably foreseeable.

Civil cases failing to establish any one condition on the 'balance of probabilities' cannot make a conviction. The word 'negligence' used in different contexts, such as industrial tribunals or the NMC's Professional Conduct Committee, need not carry these same conditions.

While all four of Dimond's arenas can apply to nurses, conflicts with criminal law are rare. Few laws specifically mention nurses or nursing, so legal accountability and rights of nurses are usually the same as for any other citizen. Any individual suffering harm from another may sue that person through civil law; negligence and assault with battery are the charges most frequently brought against healthcare staff. Negligence is briefly outlined later; assault is covered in Chapter 16; nursing accountability through civil law is comprehensively covered in Dimond (2005).

A *duty of care* clearly exists to patients allocated to nurses' care. Breach of that care will usually form the basis of any case. So any case reaching court almost certainly fulfils the first two criteria.

The condition least likely to be established is the third. There are two parts to this third condition:

- breach of care must directly cause harm
- harm suffered must have been reasonably foreseeable.

If the *harm* may reasonably have been caused by other factors (judged by the balance of probabilities), links to breach of duty of care cannot be clearly established. Giving large overdoses of penicillin is reprehensible, but Kay v Ayrshire and Arran Health Board (1987) failed to establish that a child's deafness (harm) was caused by penicillin overdose rather than meningitis (Dimond, 2005), so the case was dismissed. Even where harm can be linked to breach of care, it may not be *reasonably foreseeable*: all drugs and treatments have adverse effects, and nurses should be aware of common effects of whatever they give, and recorded allergies of patients, but cannot reasonably know, or be held accountable for, every possible effect. However, as professional practitioners, nurses are expected to act with reasonable autonomy, so decision-making should have sufficient knowledge to evaluate relative benefits and risks from possible actions and omissions ('reasonable' and 'sufficient' might be evaluated by the '*Bolam*' test – see Glossary). This places an onus on both individual nurses and their employers to maintain relevant knowledge and skills.

The primary, and implicitly primarily important, clause of the *Code of Conduct* (NMC, 2004) emphasises the importance of protecting and supporting the health of individual patients. However, employers pay salaries; nurses failing to satisfy employers' requirements may find themselves unemployed. Pragmatically, resisting instructions of employers, managers or senior staff can prove difficult.

Employment contracts and expectations vary; breach of contract can lead to litigation, or more often dismissal. Although this chapter focuses on professional accountability (through the NMC), readers should remember their concurrent accountability to other arenas.

Accountability raises two main questions:

■ What are the limits of accountability?
■ How can conflicts of accountability be reconciled?

### Limits of accountability

Individual accountability and professional autonomy may seem desirable ideals, but quality healthcare also relies on multidisciplinary teamwork (Mullally, 2001). Responsibility is inevitably partly shared between disciplines and members of the same discipline. Delegation of particular tasks vary between units, and may vary within each unit depending on whoever is best able to perform that task at that time: endotracheal suction may be performed by anaesthetists intubating patients and later by physiotherapists and nurses.

While only individuals on a professional register have professional accountability (i.e. can be removed from the professional register), in law each mentally competent adult remains legally accountable for their actions. Civil law precedent (Nettleship v Weston, 1971) establishes learner/student accountability, despite their inexperience or lack of knowledge (Dimond, 2005). Learners and junior staff may be individually sued if they cause harm, hence the importance of professional indemnity.

Practice should be based on reliable evidence (DOH, 2000d) rather than myth and ritual, but each nurse must individually decide whether (and if so, how) they should perform tasks. Guidelines are widely available, although evidence on which they are based is often poor (Hampton, 2003; Andrews & Redmond, 2004). Individual and local factors may affect applicability and appropriateness of guidelines to individual patient care, but where guidelines are generally reliable, such as those from the National Clinical Institute for Clinical Excellence, failure to follow them could result in legal action (Samanta & Samanta, 2004). However, apparent authoritative guidelines can be legally over-ruled, as shown by, Burke v GMC (2004) which over-ruled the 2002 BMA guidelines on withdrawing treatment.

### Conflicts of accountability

Few tasks are ascribed by law to particular professions, and the DOH (2000d) encourages broadening nursing practice into traditional medical roles.

In civil law, standards of care expected from qualified nurses are those of the ordinary skilled nurse ('Bolam test'). Failure to meet professional standards may also cause removal from the professional register. However, where nursing roles are expanded to work previously performed by other professions (e.g. junior doctors), the standards expected are those of the other professions (Caplin-Davies, 1999). So nurses have a professional duty to ensure they have adequate knowledge and skills to perform tasks they undertake.

## Accountability in practice

*Patient Group Directions* (PGD) are legally recognised prescriptions (DOH, 2000e), but made for patient groups rather than individual patients. They are agreed locally by relevant professions – usually doctors, nurses and pharmacists. Where both patients and nursing staff fulfil agreed criteria for each direction, nurses can give specified drugs. This facilitates prompt administration, and may prevent complications caused by delay. Kingston *et al.* (2002) describe a PGD for haemofiltration.

*Complaints* are a familiar aspect of contemporary healthcare. They highlight deficiencies in services provided, provide a conduit for public accountability, and may diffuse concerns that would otherwise end in litigation, but have unfortunately encouraged defensive nursing. Most complaints result from failures of communication; ironically, those least ill often complain most, so encouraging diversion of time away from those needing it most. Nurses have a professional duty to prioritise care (acts and omissions) so that actions can be justified.

UK NHS *litigation* costs continue to escalate, doubling between 1990 and 1998 (Fenn *et al.*, 2000) to £2.3 billion, nearly doubling again to £4.4 billion in 2001 (National Audit Office, 2002). Litigation diverts substantial funds from patient care to pay compensation. Ironically, fears of litigation foster an ethos of secrecy that conflicts with political rhetoric and professional philosophies of empowerment through providing information. Minimising litigation risks effectively creates substantial income generation, but has the added human values of fostering trust between nurses and patients. Vicarious liability (employers being legally liable for actions of their employees, provided employees follow employers' policies) has been made more robust through the Clinical Negligence Scheme for Trusts (CNST).

Much equipment used in ICUs is disposable. *Disposable equipment* should not be reused (Medical Devices Agency, 1995); recycling disposable equipment may transfer manufacturers' liability to the recycler, such as the nurse. Small savings through recycling disposable equipment may incur greater costs from healthcare litigation. Nurses should therefore follow manufacturer's instructions.

Personal costs of litigation can be substantial: cases may take years to reach court. Protracted (employer, NMC) investigations until, and eventual stress from, the hearing, with possible loss of registration and/or loss of employment can cause significant financial, personal and professional hardship to nurses involved.

## Record keeping

In addition to recording observations, nursing records should be detailed enough both to provide a basis for immediate care, and to provide information in the event of future enquiries. Records should be factual, as under the Freedom of Information Act (2001) individuals have the right to copies of records about them. Any written records, including notes on scraps of paper, may be required as evidence for legal investigations. Poor record keeping is one of the most common causes of professional misconduct hearings (UKCC, 2001).

## Implications for practice

- Concerns should be reported. Where patient safety is compromised, clinical incident forms should be completed.
- Guidelines are useful resources, but are not infallible, and do not replace individual accountability.
- Each nurse remains individually accountable for their actions.
- Nurses should only undertake tasks if competent to do so, refusing any task they do not consider they can safely complete.
- Nursing care should be prioritised by patients' best interests.
- Each nurse is responsible to ensure adequate and current knowledge for their own practice.
- Nurses should be familiar with local policies/procedures/guidelines/standards.

## Summary

Society's demands, and pace of change, are both likely to continue to increase. ICU nurses often respond positively to challenging and changing work, but enthusiasm should be tempered by considerations of safe practice, and how far care meets the holistic needs of each patient. The human and financial costs of professional malpractice can be high for each nurse, employer and patient.

## Further reading

Burnard and Chapman (2003) provide a useful short book about professionalism in nursing. Mullally (2001) offers useful insights into developments of nursing. www.routledge.com/textbooks/0415373239

For clinical scenarios, clinical questions and the answers to them go to the support website at www.routledge.com/textbooks/0415373239

## Clinical questions

Q.1 Identify areas of accountability and responsibility within the ICU. Reflect on the main areas of accountability in your practice while supervising novice ICU nurses.

Q.2 A colleague has failed to attend consecutive mandatory training sessions (resuscitation skills, moving and handling, drug administration, drug calculations, medical devices) for over three years, despite being rostered and given study leave. Identify who is accountable when this nurse makes an error in practice. How should this situation be managed to ensure professional accountability and vicarious liability?

Q.3 You administer a new trial drug which is currently unlicensed in the UK. The patient suffers associated adverse effects and dies. Who is accountable for the patient's death? Examine the extent of nurse accountability in this situation (i.e. nurse's knowledge of drug administration, awareness of adverse effects, appropriateness of drug etc.).

Chapter 49

# Managing the ICU

 **Contents**

Introduction                        509
Time out 1                          509
Starting to manage                  509
Staff morale                        512
Staffing levels                     513
During the shift                    514
Time out 2                          514
Implications for practice           515
Summary                             515
Further reading                     516
Clinical questions                  516

## Introduction

Staff who have gained necessary bedside nursing experience and any required educational developments/qualifications may plan managerial experience as part of their professional development, or find one day they are the most senior person on duty (possibly due to sickness of senior staff) and so expected to manage the unit for that shift. This chapter provides a trouble-shooting introduction for staff not normally in charge of their units (hence the direct address to readers).

Many ICU staff have previous experience of working in, and often managing, other areas; principles of management remain similar, so previous experience should be applied where possible.

Staff may look to the shiftleader (nurse in charge) for direction. The shiftleader therefore needs sufficient knowledge to provide information. Some information may be factual, but much will be sharing experience and ideas to help others make clinical decisions. There are often no right or wrong answers, just different ways of doing things. This chapter therefore raises issues that different readers may differ over. Options, rather than answers, are usually provided; these issues serve their purpose if they help readers clarify their own values.

There is noticeably little literature in ICU nursing journals advising staff how to develop management skills. As many staff are unlikely to resource management journals unless undertaking management courses, this consigns development of management skills to the 'sitting with Nellie' ethos so antithetical to evidence-based nursing. Evidence and theory for nurse management is often, as here, drawn either from management outside healthcare, or about senior healthcare management, such as lead nurse and team leader roles. When specifically discussing the shiftleader of the shift, this chapter uses 'shiftleader', reserving 'managers' either for more senior managers, or from evidence about senior roles which may also be applicable to shiftleaders.

## Time out 1

Compare your own previous experience of being in charge of wards/department with how you have seen others manage the ICU where you work. Note down significant differences. Reflect on why these differences may be necessary.

## Starting to manage

Much has been written about management, mostly from industrial perspectives, although there is a growing body of literature on health service management. Many principles of industrial management or managing other healthcare areas are applicable to the ICU.

Vaughan and Pilmoor (1989) suggest that management is getting the work done through people. A good shiftleader is a good team leader (Firth-Cozens, 2001), enabling other people to do their work. Drucker (1974) identifies five roles for managers:

- setting objectives
- organising
- motivating and communicating
- measuring targets
- developing people, including themselves.

The shiftleader should establish constructive working conditions at the start of each shift, enabling development of staffs' individual strengths and skills, while recognising individual needs and limitations. Managers should individually assess and proactively plan and respond to needs for each shift, rather than seek to impose their own agendas on staff.

You may remember most patients from your previous shift; if not, briefly assess patients before taking handover. You may need to walk through your unit to take handover, but if not a brief look at the unit can suggest both the number and dependency of patients. Many units have data sheets providing brief synopses of patients.

Managers rely on their staff to achieve the work, so staff are the shiftleader's most important resource. Staff numbers are important – are there enough staff for patients already on the unit and expected/potential admissions? Staffing levels were discussed in Chapter 1, although the ratios 1:1 for level 3 patients and 1:2 for level 2 patients reflects medical condition more than nursing care. But abilities and qualities of staff are also important. 'Skill mix' is more than simply counting numbers of staff at each grade. Some staff need more support than others; each has different experience, knowledge and skills to draw on. Most staff will probably be known to you, so scanning the off-duty roster helps your planning; with new or unfamiliar staff (e.g. agency) you may gain insight into their qualities by asking about their experience and what they feel able and not able to do.

Allocating staff may be guided by managerial structures, such as named nursing. Specific allocation should consider:

- maintaining patient safety
- optimising patient treatment
- developing and supporting staff.

Nurses unable to *safely* care for a patient should not be allocated to their care. Each nurse is individually accountable for their actions, and should acknowledge their limitations (NMC, 2004). But staff may be unaware of their limitations, so shiftleaders should actively assess competence of each nurse. The most experienced member of staff may be able to give the *best care* to the sickest patient, but without gaining experience of nursing very sick patients, junior staff will be denied opportunities to develop their skills. If continually *denied developmental* experience, they may become demotivated and leave or be unable to care safely for sicker patients when more experienced staff are not available.

Safety during break cover should also be considered: two junior nurses may safely manage adjacent patients when both are present, but become unsafe if caring for two patients through covering each other's breaks. Nurse managers remain accountable for their actions; unsafe allocation breaches the *Code of Conduct* (NMC, 2004).

The Health and Safety at Work Act (1974) places specific requirements on managers (and employees) to ensure workplaces are safe; the shiftleader also has wider moral responsibilities for health and safety of their staff and patients. Fire exits should remain clear and accessible at all times and safety and emergency equipment should be in complete and in working order. Emergency equipment varies between units, but may include the resuscitation trolley, emergency intubation trolley and (on cardiothoracic units) thoracotomy pack. Any environmental hazards should be minimised, and where possible removed.

The shiftleader is responsible for all patients on their unit, even if some responsibilities are devolved to team/area subleaders. Following handover, the shiftleader should visit each patient to make their own assessment, identify needs of each bedside nurse and pass on any relevant additional information/expectations. Allow sufficient time for bedside nurses to take individual handovers, complete their own safety checks and make their own patient assessment; seeking information before bedside nurses can fully assimilate it creates stress for the nurse without providing information for shiftleaders. Looking through each patient's notes gives bedside nurses time to complete initial assessment and checks, while giving shiftleaders information that may have been missed in handover. Relevant aspects should then be passed on to the bedside nurse.

The shiftleader should ensure imminent shifts are adequately covered: check staff numbers and initiate booking of any additional staff required. Numbers of staff needed for each shift may vary with

- number, location and dependency of patients
- skillmix of other staff
- anticipated specific needs, such as transfer or procedures.

Many agencies provide their main service during office hours, so planning should include all shifts until the next 'office hours'; on-call services may be able to provide emergency cover, but often have few remaining staff to allocate. Other services (e.g. equipment suppliers/repair) may also need to be contacted.

The shiftleader may have to assume direct patient care, but this causes role conflict between responsibility to the whole unit as shiftleader and individual responsibility to your patient, and limits your availability to other members of staff. The experience of many nurses in charge who also assume direct patient care is that their patient tends to get neglected. The RCN recommend that the shiftleader should not provide direct patient care (RCN Critical Care Forum, 2003c). Instead, it may be reasonable to allocate two patients to one member of staff; the appropriateness or otherwise of assuming direct patient care necessarily remains an individual decision, based on resources available, and remembering that you remain accountable for whatever decision you make.

Shiftleaders need to maintain clinical skills and credibility; with career progression and increasing management duties, staff may need to identify shifts when they assume direct patient care without unit management responsibilities. Endacott (1999) identifies four key aspects of shift leadership:

- presence (availability)
- information gathering (from bedside nurses)
- supportive involvement (e.g. fetching equipment, checking drugs, reassuring staff)
- direct involvement (taking over from bedside nurses when they are away or unable to cope).

Shiftleaders may also co-ordinate services, contacting other people/departments or liaising with staff on the unit. Shiftleaders should be present during ward rounds so that they are aware of current plans, can contribute to discussion, support staff and co-ordinate activity.

## Staff morale

Shiftleaders are responsible for enabling others to achieve their work, so should motivate and communicate (Drucker, 1974). Nursing demands high levels of cognitive, affective and psychomotor skills, so the ability of staff to realise their potential is affected by morale. Maintaining staff and unit morale is therefore a management priority (Joshua-Amadi, 2002; Erlen, 2004) – loyal staff are more likely to support shiftleaders during crises.

Management theory often identifies styles of leadership as authoritarian, laissez-faire and democratic. Democratic or authoritarian leaders use their power and authority to achieve goals and objectives (Firth-Cozens & Mowbray, 2001). But healthcare is riddled with an ethos of 'blame' culture, which should be replaced by one of 'safety' (DOH, 2000b). A safety culture recognises that errors will occur, and so an openness about reporting errors allows potential causes to be identified and rectified.

An alternative approach to management is 'Transformational' leadership, which seeks to transform the culture of care through

- staff empowerment
- practice development
- developing other workplace characteristics.

(Manley, 2004)

Shiftleaders therefore need good interpersonal skills and respect for their staff. Shiftleaders seeing unsatisfactory practices should approach staff constructively, identifying why staff are acting that way (rationale, knowledge base), treating incidents as developmental learning opportunities rather than belittling and humiliating experiences for the junior nurse (or possibly shiftleaders). If patient safety is compromised, shiftleaders may need to act before discussion.

Breaks from work provide a psychological coping mechanism. European working time regulations are prescriptive about working time, including the right to breaks every four hours. Delayed, compromised or missed breaks often cause dissatisfaction, so ensuring smooth (and safe) organisation of breaks for staff is an important managerial duty. Organising break relief varies between units and shifts; where units have a system that works and is familiar to staff, this should be followed. Shiftleaders may need to assume some direct patient responsibilities to cover breaks; this can also provide shiftleaders with valuable opportunities to assess patients, and the nurse's skills and needs. Possible conflicts with managerial duties (earlier) should be considered, especially if relieving for breaks in inaccessible areas (e.g. side rooms).

When situations are particularly stressful, shiftleaders may be able to support staff by offering additional 'stress breaks', making themselves (and other experienced staff) available when necessary, and by acknowledging the stress of the situation.

The ICU work is unpredictable; workload will sometimes exceed resources, so shiftleaders and staff should identify priorities, accepting that some lesser priorities are not always achieved. Shiftleaders unable to offer ideal support to staff can still build team rapport and loyalty by acknowledging others' stress. Opinions vary about staff consuming refreshments at bedsides; concerns usually include infection and professionalism. Ideally, staff should take breaks away from their workspace, but busy shifts may sometimes prevent this. If full breaks cannot be taken, providing refreshments at bedsides (this task could be delegated) may help staff function safely, and maintain morale. Anything brought into the bedspace may introduce infection, but stressed nurses are more likely to work inefficiently, skipping more important infection control measures under pressure of time. What is 'unprofessional' is a value judgement, but professional images may be less important than meeting basic physiological needs of staff. Relatives, and patients who are able, may also be offered refreshments, and anecdotal experience suggests that they do not mind, or feel any less confidence in, nurses drinking at bedsides. Staff needing breaks are likely to function inefficiently, give less empathy to others and be more difficult to motivate.

## Staffing levels

Staff levels should be individualised to patient/unit needs (see Chapter 1). If shiftleaders consider unit, patient or staff safety is compromised through inadequate staff (or any other problem they are unable to resolve), they should inform senior managers, who have (higher) responsibility for the unit.

### During the shift

Shiftleader who have established mechanisms for staff to work effectively have achieved their most important role, but throughout the remainder of the shift, shiftleaders should ensure that the unit continues to run smoothly, solving problems as they occur and providing a resource (knowledge, experience) for and support to more junior staff.

Staff need to feel confidence in their shiftleader. While shiftleaders usually have more experience and knowledge than their staff, each member of staff has potential to contribute knowledge, experience or values, and shiftleaders should be prepared to learn from, as well as guide and teach, their staff. Following the Code of Conduct (NMC, 2004), shiftleaders should acknowledge limits of their own knowledge and competence.

Staff need to feel confident that they can approach their shiftleader, so shiftleaders should show positive attitudes and remain accessible, including spending most of their time in the main patient-care area.

The shiftleader is a link between unit nurses and other hospital staff, facilitating active involvement of bedside nurses in ward rounds (Manias & Street, 2001). If medical review of patients does not involve bedside nurses, shiftleaders often become links between medical and nursing staff. Similarly, information to/from other hospital departments, or telephone messages from family members are often ciphered through the nurse-in-charge.

Shiftleaders may be pressurised to accept patients because there is an empty bed, there appear to be enough staff or because patients need the ICU. Rationing is an unfortunate reality of healthcare, and when an 'ultimate' area such as the ICU is involved, the pressure cannot always be relieved by admission to other wards. While medical staff must decide whether patients require ICU admission, shiftleaders must decide whether patients can be safely nursed on the unit. This decision includes

- imminent shifts
- dependency of patients already on the unit
- skills of staff available.

The shiftleader is professionally accountable for decisions about managing nursing on the unit, but faced with coercion or moral blackmail may need considerable skills in assertiveness.

Good shiftleaders may inspire loyalty in their staff, but being in charge can isolate shiftleaders from other support mechanisms. Shiftleaders also need their breaks: a stressed shiftleader is less likely to be able to support their staff.

### Time out 2

Using the cues below, jot down plans for your professional development over the next six months. Aims may be clinical, educational and professional. Be realistic, setting sufficient aims to help you develop, but not too difficult to achieve (six aims is often a reasonable target, but the number and scope vary between individuals). You may wish to share all or part of this with your manager/mentor/colleagues, or retain this as a private document in your professional profile. You may wish to divide aims between short-term (a few weeks), medium-term (up to six months) and long-term (after six months), or cover all aims together. Long-terms aims will not be achieved fully by your six month review, but you may have partially progressed towards them. You will probably find setting target dates for achieving aims helpful.

Over the next six months I would like to achieve (include target times):

I would like to achieve these because:
To achieve these will need (include people and resources):
I will now I have achieved these aims because (i.e. evaluation):
Possible problems I anticipate for myself/others:
Ways to minimise these problems:

## Implications for practice

- Staff who have met minimum criteria to manage their unit should plan a structure to develop their skills before they find themselves unexpectedly in charge.
- Shiftleaders should enable their staff to work safely, efficiently and effectively.
- Shiftleaders rely on their staff, so should encourage morale and meet the needs of their staff (professional development, support, breaks).
- Shiftleaders should co-ordinate unit activity, so participate in decision-making, both during and between ward rounds.
- Shiftleaders should recognise potential role conflicts and priorities.
- Nurse shiftleaders, like all qualified nurses, are professionally accountable for their decisions and actions.

## Summary

This chapter has considered some of the practical issues for ICU nurses who are beginning to develop their management skills. Much has been written elsewhere on wider management issues and theory; nurses developing management careers may need to develop this knowledge further, but should first gain practical management skills through structured experiential programme. The shiftleader is morally and professionally responsible and accountable for their managerial decisions.

## Further reading

Most literature on management is written by non-nurses, and often not specifically about healthcare. How far principles of industrial and commercial management can or should apply to healthcare continue to generate political debate. Drucker (e.g. 1974) is an influential management theorist. Literature on nursing management is rarely ICU specific, but McCormack and Manley (2004) includes many valuable chapters. Endacott (1999) provides a useful study of (paediatric) nursing management.

Management journals include *Nursing Management* (there are both UK and USA journals with this title – both are useful), *Quality in Health Care* and *Journal of Nursing Management*. www.routledge.com/textbooks/0415373239

For clinical scenarios, clinical questions and the answers to them go to the support website at www.routledge.com/textbooks/0415373239

## Clinical questions

Q.1 Describe the responsibilities of the shiftleader within your own clinical practice area (e.g. specify responsibilities toward resource management, people management, monitoring standards and quality)

Q.2 Review the range management style(s) used within your own ICU. Are there differences in styles/behaviours used between different shiftleaders? Analyse any perceived differences in terms of leadership, relationship, personality and change theories.

Q.3 Formulate a training programme to prepare ICU nurses for shift and unit management. Propose and justify the selection criteria, basic nurse competencies required for managing the ICU, resources needed for training and the evaluation and feedback strategy.

# Chapter 50

# Cost of intensive care

## Contents

| | |
|---|---|
| Introduction | 518 |
| Spending on health | 518 |
| Budget | 518 |
| Scoring systems | 519 |
| Mortality | 519 |
| Morbidity | 520 |
| Transfer | 520 |
| Implications for practice | 521 |
| Summary | 521 |
| Further reading | 522 |
| Clinical questions | 522 |

## Introduction

ICU has a high public profile, partly due to its high financial costs. But human-itarian costs of ICU can also be high. Intensive care should be provided where beneficial consequences can be achieved at an acceptable cost (King's Fund, 1989); defining and measuring 'beneficial consequences' and 'acceptable costs' is often problematic. Increasing financial pressures are paralleled by increasingly higher public expectations.

Subjectivity surrounds the human cost, so there are seldom absolute answers, but there are issues which all nurses, and other healthcare profes-sionals, should consider. Having reached the end of this book, nurses devel-oping their ICU careers should be grappling with the following question: what price Intensive Care? Nurses should use their own knowledge and values to decide whether the costs of intensive care are justified.

## Spending on health

The UK spends less of its gross national product (GNP) on health than most developed countries, with a smaller proportion of what it does spend reaching ICUs (Bion, 1995). On average, UK ICUs have 2.6 per cent of hospital beds (Hibbert & Edbrooke, 2002). Although sounding favourable to the 1 per cent of 20–30 years ago, decimation in numbers of hospital beds has resulted in no greater provision of ICU beds, while increasingly sick patients are being managed in fewer beds elsewhere. In Denmark, 4.1 per cent of hospital beds are in ICU (Hibbert & Edbrooke, 2002), while the USA rates are 7 per cent (Rosenberg & Watts, 2000). The NHS is arguably the most cost-effective health service in the world, caring for sicker, so more expensive, ICU patients on a fraction of resources available elsewhere, yet resources (beds) are often insufficient to meet demand (Southgate, 1999).

## Budget

Recent years have seen many changing structures for devolving UK health-care budgets. Historically, ICUs budgets were often hidden in budgets of other departments, such as anaesthetics. Inevitable and increasing high financial costs of ICU patients, and continuing financial pressures, have focussed the economic microscope firmly on intensive care. Currently (2005) budgets devolve through Primary Care Trusts (PCTs), run by profes-sionals who, however empathetic, may have little knowledge or experience of intensive care.

ICU is labour-intensive and expensive. About half ICU costs are from staffing (Intensive Care Society, 2002). Successful cures of simpler pathologies (e.g. single organ failure) have created more complex pathologies (e.g. MODS) which increase both cost per patient day, and length of stay. Increasingly com-plex and expensive technology and drugs (e.g. Xigris®) further strain budgets. But ICU budgets may subsidise other departments by providing support services such as Outreach and programmes for high dependency care. Financially, intensive care has become a victim of its own success (Southgate, 1999).

Treating nonsurvivors inevitably prolongs death, and so from humanitarian perspectives is undesirable; but the cost of treating survivors is only 55–67 per cent that of treating nonsurvivors (Vedio *et al.*, 2000). Predicting survival could reduce both humanitarian and financial burdens of ICU, but raises ethical concerns about reliability and 'playing God'.

## Scoring systems

There are various scoring systems, mostly developed for medical audit, and reviewed in many medical texts. Audit can help staff learn from experience, and inappropriate admission to ICU can cause excessive and unnecessary human suffering, but applying retrospective audit tools to prospective prediction may create dilemmas; Parkinson *et al.* (1996) suggest that most scoring systems have 90 per cent accuracy in predicting survival from ICU, but only 50–70 per cent accuracy in predicting mortality. The Ethics Committee of the Society of Critical Care Medicine (1997) recommend caution when applying such tools to individuals rather than populations, adding that while they measure survival, morbidity is not addressed. This echoes nursing debate around quality against quantity of life. Scoring systems have also been inappropriately used to predict nurse staffing requirements (Chellel *et al.*, 1995).

The Acute Physiology And Chronic Health Evaluation (APACHE) is the most widely used scoring system in ICU; its design is not too dissimilar to the Waterlow pressure scoring system. Most UK units use APACHE II (Knaus *et al.*, 1985), APACHE III (Knaus *et al.*, 1991) requiring purchase of a computerized system from APACHE Medical Systems (Castella *et al.*, 1995). Apache III may (Cho & Wang, 1997) or may not (Beck *et al.*, 1997) be an improvement on APACHE II.

Other scoring systems used include

- SAPS II
- The Riyadh Intensive Care Programme (a computerised adaptation of Apache II)
- Quality Adjusted Life Years system (QALYs).

## Mortality

Mortality rates for general UK ICUs is 15–35 per cent (Audit Commission, 1999), averaging about 21 per cent (Young & Ridley, 2002). However, mortality is usually measured to discharge from units; following discharge mortality is 9–27 per cent (Daly *et al.*, 2001).

Predicting survival is often difficult. Nevertheless 72.6 per cent of ICU deaths follow withdrawal of treatment (Mercer *et al.*, 1998).

## Morbidity

Quality of life is a widely used phrase, but interpreting quality is subjective. Aksoy (2000) argues that QALYs are ageist, sexist, unjust and unfair. Aller and Coeling (1995) identify three major factors affecting quality of life:

- physical environment
- recreational activities
- social environment.

These factors provide a useful guide to assess potential future quality of life for ICU patients.

Most ICU patients suffer significant psychological problems months after discharge. Post traumatic stress disorder appears more widespread than previously suspected (see Chapter 3), and only a minority resume normal work (Garner & Sibthorpe, 2002). While antipsychotic drugs may be useful, nurses should also consider all the nonpharmacological approaches (e.g. reducing sensory imbalance – see Chapter 3) that can reduce/prevent postdischarged psychosis.

Patients discharged during the night fare worse than patients discharged during daytime, presumably because discharge is more likely to be premature (Goldfrad & Rowan, 2000). While this illustrates that the UK has insufficient ICU beds to meet demand, it also implies that staff should consider more carefully whether patients are ready for transfer from ICU. If nurses are to be advocates for their patients, they should voice concerns whenever they consider discharge to be premature.

## Transfer

Premature transfer of patients to lower-cost areas can create false economies, increasing readmission rates, long-term financial costs, and mortality (Goldhill & Sumner, 1998; Rosenberg & Watts, 2000), yet appears to have increased recently (Daly *et al.*, 2001). Australian (Russell, 2000) and USA (Rosenberg & Watts, 2000) studies found that more than 10 per cent of patients were readmitted; UK readmission rates range from 9–16 per cent (Carr, 2002), although development of Critical Care Outreach teams in recent years has probably eased the burden of premature transfer. Daly *et al.* (2001) suggest that ICU bed numbers should be increased by 16 per cent to avoid deaths from inappropriate early transfer.

Leith (1999) found that most patients and families made negative comments about transfer, and recommends that more gradual transfer in level of care is needed. Pressure on beds often encourages premature transfer; however, as patients move towards or reach level 2, nursing staff distancing themselves from patients more may help patients and their families adapt to the lower staffing levels found in wards.

Demand for ICU beds is largely unpredictable, often necessitating interhospital transfer. Since 1996 this has been facilitated in the UK by a National Bed Bureau, but this resources may in part be responsible for increasing numbers of transfers. Between 1994 and 2004 interhospital transfers have doubled, with at least 5 per cent of adult ICU patients being transferred (Smith *et al.*, 2004). Interhospital transfer of critically ill patients creates many risks, so should be managed by experienced and reliable nursing and medical staff.

### Implications for practice

■ Costs involve both financial and human aspects; human costs are subjective, including debateable issues such as quality of life, but are fundamentally central to nursing values.
■ Medical outcome scoring systems are available, but predictive reliability for individuals is debated, so rationing by scoring systems is ethically questionable.
■ Postdischarge followup can reduce psychological costs of intensive care to ex-patients and identify areas of nursing practice needing development. Critical Care Outreach teams can often provide units with valuable insights from former patients.
■ Interhospital transfer requires careful planning, and should be undertaken by experienced, competent and reliable staff.

### Summary

This final chapter has revisited issues raised at the start of this book:

■ What, fundamentally, are we doing for our patients?
■ What should we be doing?
■ How should we be doing it?

There are many possible answers to these questions; discussion in other chapters should have developed readers' awareness of these in everyday practice. As professionals, ICU nurses need to evaluate both financial and humanitarian costs of intensive care to determine its ultimate value. In the United Kingdom's chronically grossly underfunded and bureaucratic NHS, enthusiasm to cut costs can lead to false economies. For example, restricting choice of colours for plastic aprons may achieve price reductions per item, but if colours are used to prevent cross infection (see Chapter 15) could lead to greater financial and humanitarian costs. Cheapest is not always best, and nurse advocacy may include resisting inappropriate and dangerous it decisions at all levels. Attempts to equate financial with humanitarian (morbidity) costs may help nurses justify their value, but also create the danger that (to adapt Oscar Wilde) we know the price of everything but the value of nothing.

### Further reading

Economics of healthcare and intensive care have been much studied and debated, especially when general elections loom. Ridley (2002) provides a detailed resource on economic costs, while Griffiths and Jones (2002) indicate humanitarian costs. National economics can change rapidly, but professional groups such as the Intensive Care Society and the British Association of Critical Care Nurses occasionally publish relevant documents about ICU economics. www.routledge.com/textbooks/0415373239

For clinical scenarios, clinical questions and the answers to them go to the support website at www.routledge.com/textbooks/0415373239

### Clinical questions

Q.1  List the positive benefits of the critical care process and categorise these into

    a)   benefits to patients
    b)   benefits to friends and family
    c)   benefits to health practitioners
    d)   benefits to society and the public.

Q.2  Analyse the cost per day of a typical patient in your own clinical area; break this down into staff costs, treatments, disposables and resources. Include also the recruitment costs incurred over the last 12 months, replacement costs for study leave/mandatory training and temporary staff.

Q.3  Review practical strategies, which can be implemented by ICU nurses, which can have an impact on the long-term survival of ICU patients once discharged home. Consider ICU nurses' role in community health, feasibility of specialist community link nurses, advice booklets and follow-up/discharge clinics.

522

# Glossary

**Allograft** Transplant tissue from the same species (e.g. cadaver heart valves).

**Anabolism** Building up.

**Anacrotic notch** Abnormal notch occurring on arterial blood pressure traces before the main pressure peak.

**Anion** Negatively charged ion.

**Anthropometry** Measurement of body weight using relationships between height, weight and size.

**Anxiolysis** Removing ('breakdown' of) anxiety.

**Arterial tonometry** A noninvasive means of continuously measuring arterial pressure.

**Autologous** From the same individual (e.g. autologous blood = patients' own blood).

**Autologous transfusion** Transfusion of patients' own blood.

**Balloon tamponade** Inflation of balloon-tipped catheters (e.g. Sengstaken tube) places direct pressure on bleeding points, so can stop internal bleeding in the same way nurses use digital pressure to stop bleeding after arterial lines are removed.

**Barotrauma** Damage to alveoli from excessively high (peak) airway pressure.

**Beta ($\beta$) lactam** Class of antibiotics (e.g. ceftazidime, penicillin).

**Blepharitis** Inflammation of eyelash follicles and sebaceous glands.

**Böhr effect** Carbon dioxide and hydrogen reduce affinity of oxygen for haemoglobin, so acidosis increases dissociation.

**Bolam test** Case law precedent establishing that practitioners were not guilty of negligence if their practice conformed to that of a reasonable body of opinion held by practitioners skilled in the area of question.

**Bradycardia** Heart rate below 60 beats per minute.

**Bruxia** Jaw-clenching.

**Calorie (cal, c)** Amount of heat needed to raise one gram of water 1°C at atmospheric pressure (= small calorie).

**Calorie (Cal, C)** Amount of heat needed to raise one kilogram of water 1°C at atmospheric pressure (= large calorie, kilocalorie).

**Capillary occlusion pressure** The pressure at which capillary flow will be prevented, resulting in ischaemia, anaerobic metabolism and (eventually) infarction of tissue (e.g. pressure sore formation).

**Catabolism** Breaking down.

**Cation** Positively charged ion.

**Chemotaxis** Movement of cell/organism to/from chemical substance.

**Chronotrope** Affecting heart rate (*chronos* = time). Positive chronotropes (e.g. atropine) increase heart rate. Negative chronotropes (e.g. beta-blockers) reduce heart rate. Inotropes are usually also chronotropic.

**Circadian rhythm** The 'body clock', an endogenous rhythm around the day. Normal circadian rhythm lasts about 24 hours, but abnormal rhythms can take longer or shorter. Circadian rhythm affects various endogenous hormone levels, so disturbed circadian rhythm results in various abnormal body responses (e.g. wakefulness at night).

**Coagulopathies** Disorders (pathologies) of clotting, such as DIC, sickle cell anaemia.

**Colloid osmotic pressure** The osmotic pressure created by large molecules (e.g. proteins) that retain plasma in the intravascular space. Fluids with high colloid osmotic pressures therefore assist return of extravascular fluid (oedema) into the bloodstream.

**Commensal** Endogenous bacteria helping normal human functions.

**Complements** Plasma proteins (produced in the liver), which facilitate phagocytosis.

**Coning** See tentorial herniation.

**Cori cycle** Glycolysis in contracting muscles produces lactate which the liver converts back into glucose, enabling further glycolysis-induced lactate.

Therefore, lactate solutions are best avoided with uncontrolled hyperglycaemic diabetes mellitus.

**Cullen's sign**   Irregular, bluish-purple discolouration around umbilicus.

**Cytokines**   Secreted by cells of inflammatory and immune processes; interleukins, interferon, coagulation-stimulating factor, TNFα.

**Daltons (Da)**   Molecular weight.

**D-dimer**   Fibrinolysis product used to measure clotting.

**Deadspace**   Space between air/gas mix and alveoli; physiological adult deadspace is about 150 ml; on ventilators deadspace extends from the Y connector to alveoli.

**Depolarisation**   Reduction of membrane potential to a less negative value.

**Dialysis**   Movement of solutes through semipermeable membranes by a concentration gradient, so greater differences in concentrations result in faster movement.

**Dicrotic notch**   The notch normally seen on downstrokes of arterial waveforms, representing closure of the aortic valve, which causes transient slight increases in pressure.

**Diffuse axonal injury**   Widespread injury caused by shearing forces, usually from rotational acceleration (e.g. road traffic accidents).

**Diffusion**   Movement of molecules from an area of higher concentration to an area of lower concentration.

**Eicosanoids**   Fatty acid.

**Ejection fraction**   Stroke volume as a fraction of ventricular blood volume. Normal ejection fraction is 0.6–0.75 (60–70%), but dysfunctional ventricles (e.g. myocardial infarction) eject less. Figures inversely indicate extent of myocardial damage.

**Endogenous**   Inside the person.

**Endoleak**   Continued bloodflow through aneurysm sac around repair/stent.

**Erythropoesis**   Production of erythrocytes (red blood cells).

**Exogenous**   From outside the person.

**Flow monitoring**   Monitoring of cardiovascular flow, previously called 'cardiac output studies'.

**Fowler's position**   Semirecumbent, usually with knees slightly elevated.

**Frank-Starling law**   The force exerted during each heartbeat is directly proportional to the length or degree of myocardial fibre stretch; so increasing fibre length (e.g. with positive inotropes) increases stroke volume.

**Free radicals**   Atoms with one or more unpaired electron in their outer orbit; this makes them inherently unstable, so they react readily with other molecules to pair with the free electron.

**Glucolysis**   Breakdown of glucose.

**Glycosides**   Carbohydrates that, when hydrolysed, produce a sugar and a non-sugar. Digoxin is a cardiac glycoside.

**Glycosuria**   Sugar in urine; blood sugar is filtered by the kidney, but normally is all reabsorbed. When blood sugar exceeds 10 mmol/litre, renal tubules are unable to reabsorb all the sugar. As glucose creates high osmotic pressure, the tubules also reabsorb less water, resulting in polyuria.

**Gravid**   Pregnancy (e.g. primagravida = first pregnancy).

**Grey Turner's sign**   Bluish-purple discolouration of flanks, indicated acute haemorrhagic pancreatitis.

**Haldane effect**   A rise in oxyhaemoglobin shifts the carbon dioxide dissociation curve to the right.

**Half-life**   Time taken for a chemical to lose half of its active effect.

**Heterotopic**   Graft into different site.

**Hypercalcaemia**   High serum concentrations of calcium (normal serum levels are 2.25–2.75 mmol/litre).

**Hyperchloraemia**   High blood chloride (normal = 98–108 mmol/litre).

**Hyperglycaemia**   High serum concentrations of glucose (normal serum levels are 4–8 mmol/litre).

**Hyperkalaemia**   High serum concentrations of potassium (normal serum levels are 3.5–5.0 mmol/litre).

**Hypernatraemia**   High serum concentrations of sodium (normal serum levels are 135–45 mmol/litre).

**Hypertriglyceridaemia**   High serum concentrations of triglycerides; most animal and vegetable fats are triglycerides, so this is the principle lipid found in serum (normal serum levels are 200–300 mg/dl).

**Hypo-**   Low (so hypocalcaemia = serum calcium below 2.25 mmol/litre).

**Hysteresis**   Literally, the difference between two phenomena; medically, usually refers to lung differences between inspiration and expiration (pressure/volume curve), where passive elastic recoil allows greater volume in relation to airway pressure during expiration than during inspiration; so manipulating I:E ratio also manipulates mean airway pressure.

**Iatrogenic**   Problems caused by treatments.

**Idiopathic**   With known causes.

**Interleukin**  See Chapter 24.

**Isothermic saturation boundary**  Where 100 per cent relative humidity is reached at 37°C; normally (in adults) just below the carina.

**Joule**  A unit to measure energy (= $10^7$ ergs or 1 watt second).

**Keratitis**  Inflammation of the cornea.

**Keratopathy**  Non-inflammatory corneal disease.

**Kilocalorie**  Amount of heat needed to raise one kilogram of water 1°C at atmospheric pressure (= Calorie, C).

**KiloDaltons**  1000 Daltons (Da) = 1 kDa; a unit of molecular weight.

**Kilojoule**  1000 joules.

**Krebs' cycle**  A chain of intracellular chemical reactions to metabolise fat for energy(citric acid cycle). Krebs' cycle is efficient at energy (adenosine triphosphate) production, but produces metabolic wastes (acids, ketones, carbon dioxide, water). See Chapter 9.

**Leuckotriene**  Active compound contained in leukocytes; causes allergic and inflammatory response.

**lidocaine**  Formerly called 'lignocaine' in the UK.

**Lipolysis**  Breakdown of fat.

**Marfan's syndrome**  Hereditary connective tissue disorder; symptoms include elongation of limbs and aortic aneurysms.

**Microcirculation**  Capillaries.

**MIDCAB**  Minimally invasive direct coronary artery bypass grafting.

**Millimole**  Unit for measuring chemicals; 1 mole = relative atomic mass in grams of each element.

**Mitochondria**  Organelles within cytoplasm that provide the main source for the cells energy (often called the 'powerhouse' of the cell); Singular: mitochondrion.

**Monoclonal antibodies**  Antibodies (B leucocytes) that have been cloned (in a laboratory) from a single genetic strand, so each monoclonal antibody is identical and specific to a particular antigen.

**Morphology**  Shape.

**Myocytes**  Cardiac muscle cells.

**Nosocomial infection**  Infection acquired in hospital (technically, at least 22 hours following admission).

**Oncotic**  Osmotic pressure of colloids in solution.

**OPCAB**   Off-pump coronary artery bypass.

**Orthotopic**   Tissue graft being placed in its normal anatomical position.

**Osmolarity**   Number of dissolved particles per litre of solution.

**Osmosis**   Movement of solutes through a semipermeable membrane to form a concentration equilibrium on both sides (osmotic = of osmosis).

**Ototoxic**   Toxic to the ear (oto = ear); damage is caused to the eighth cranial nerve or the organs of hearing and balance. Many drugs (e.g. gentamicin, furosemide) can be ototoxic.

**Para**   Birth (e.g. primapara = first birth).

**Parity**   Number of pregnancies (including stillbirths/abortions/miscarriages) reaching 20 weeks gestation.

**Paroxysm**   Sudden.

**Permissive hypercapnia**   Tolerating abnormally high arterial carbon dioxide tensions ($pCO_2$) to enable smaller tidal volumes, and so limit/avoid barotrauma and volutrauma.

**Pleth**   See plethysmograph.

**Plethysmograph**   Instrument for measuring changes in blood volume.

**Polydipsia**   Excessive thirst.

**Prostacyclin ($PGI_2$)**   An active arachidonic acid metabolite; inhibits angiotensin-mediated vasoconstriction, stimulates renin release, inhibits platelet aggregation (so used for anticoagulation).

**Protease inhibitors**   Protease is an essential enzyme for viral replication, so protease inhibitors prevent viral replication.

**Prothrombin time**   A test to measure clotting; normal prothrombin time is 11–12.5 seconds; prolonged prothrombin time indicates deficiency in one or more clotting factors.

**Radicals**   An atom with an unpaired electron (see Free radicals).

**Repolarisation**   Restoration of cell to its resting potential.

**ROS**   Reactive oxygen species ( = oxygen-free radicals).

**Saturated fatty acid**   Fats with univalent bonds joining all atoms; valency determines hydrogen binding capacity of molecules, so saturated fatty acids contribute to hypercholestrolaemia and cardiovascular (especially coronary) disease. Most animal fats are saturated.

**Septal myomectomy**   Open heart surgery to treat severe hypertrophic obstructive cardiomyopathy (HOCM).

**Serotonin**  Tryptophan derivative found in platelets and cells of brain and intestine; vasopressor and neurotransmitter.

**Shunt**  'shunting' describes a conduit between two body compartments. In respiratory medicine this usually describes movement of blood from venous to arterial circulation without effective ventilation, typically from intrapulmonary problems, such as ARDS, but can also be caused by an atrial–septal defect allowing blood to pass between the atria without entering the pulmonary circulation. 'Shunt' can also be used to describe an abnormal conduit directly joining an artery to a vein, such as an arteriovenous shunt used for haemodialysis access, or a drain inserted to remove excess fluid (e.g. an intraventricular shunt to drain CSF from the ventricles of the brain and so relieve intracranial hypertension).

**Shunt (blood)**  Blood 'shunting' from arteries to veins with perfusing tissues.

**Sigh breath**  An occasional, especially large breath. See Chapter 4.

**Solvent drag (convection)**  Movement of fluid by osmotic pressures from solutes moving across a semipermeable membrane.

**Somatotrophin**  Growth hormone.

**Tentorial herniation**  Brainstem forced into spinal column from raised intracranial pressure.

**Thromboxane A$_2$**  (TXA$_2$) unstable derivative of PGG$_2$, stimulates platelet aggregation.

**Tonic-clonic seizures**  Generalised fitting (formerly called 'grand mal').

**Transmembrane pressure**  The pressure across a membrane. Where artificial technologies replicate capillary function, such as the 'artificial kidneys' used for haemofiltration, excessive pressure may rupture the necessarily delicate membrane. Being artificial, damage is permanent and irrepairable. As the surface area of the filter becomes progressively engorged with clots, filtrate is forced through a smaller area, increasing transmembrane pressure. Therefore measuring the transmembrane pressure should identify impending rupture of the artificial kidney. Stopping filters before maximum transmembrane pressure is reached enables blood in the circuit to be safely returned to the patient. See manufacturers' instructions for maximum transmembrane pressures of individual models.

**Trimester**  Pregnancy is divided into 3 trimesters: trimester 1 = up to week 12; trimester 2 = weeks 13–28; trimester 3 = week 29 to delivery.

**Tunica intima**  Inner layer of blood vessel wall.

**Ultrafiltration**  Removal of fluid through a membrane under pressure.

529

**Volutrauma**   High lung volumes (in relation to space available) can cause sheering damage to lung tissue; the concept is similar to barotrauma. Volutrauma is sometimes spelled 'volotrauma'.

**V/Q**   (Alveolar) ventilation to (pulmonary capillary) perfusion ratio; normal V/Q = 0.8.

**Xenograft**   Transplant tissue from another species (e.g. pig heart valves).

**Zymogen**   Granules found in some secretory exocrine cells; contain enzyme precursors.

# References

Abbas, A.K., Lichtman, A.H. and Pober, J.S. (1994) *Cellular and Molecular Immunology*, 2nd edn, Philadelphia, PA: W.B. Saunders Co.

Abbott, R.D., Ando, F., Masaki, K.H., Tung, K.-H., Rodriguez, B.L., Petrovitch, H., Yano, K. and Curb, J.D. (2003) 'Dietary magnesium intake and the future risk of coronary heart disease (The Honolulu Heart Program)', *American Journal of Cardiology*, 92(6): 665–9.

Abraham, E., Gallagher, T.J. and Fink, S. (1996) 'Clinical evaluation of multiparameter intra-arterial blood-gas sensor', *Intensive Care Medicine*, 22(5): 507–13.

Abu-Omar, Y. and Taggart, D.P. (2002) 'Off-pump coronary artery bypass grafting', *Lancet*, 360(9329): 327–9.

ACCP Consensus Conference (1993) 'Mechanical ventilation', *Chest*, 104(6): 1833–59.

ACCP/SCCM (1992) 'Consensus conference: definitions for sepsis and organ failure and guidelines for the use of innovative therapies', *Critical Care Medicine*, 20(6): 864–74.

Ackerman, M.H. (1993) 'The effects of saline lavage prior to suctioning', *American Journal of Critical Care*, 2(4): 326–30.

Ackrill, P. and France, M.W. (2002) 'Common electrolyte problems', *Clinical Medicine*, 2(3): 205–8.

Acute Respiratory Distress Syndrome Network (2000) 'Ventilation with lower tidal volumes as compared with traditional tidal volumes for acute lung injury and the acute respiratory distress syndrome', *New England Journal of Medicine*, 342(18): 1301–8.

Adams, D.C., Heyer, E.J., Simon, A.E., Delphin, E., Rose, E.A., Oz, M.C., McMahon, D.J. and Sun, L.S. (2000) 'Incidence of atrial fibrillation after mild or moderate hypothermic cardiopulmonary bypass', *Critical Care Medicine*, 28(2): 309–11.

Adams, J.P. and Murphy, P.G. (2000) 'Obesity of anaesthesia and intensive care', *British Journal of Anaesthesia*, 85(1): 91–108.

Adams, R. (1996) 'Qualified nurses lack adequate knowledge related to oral health, resulting in adequate oral care of patients on medical wards', *Journal of Advanced Nursing*, 24(3): 552–60.

Adelman, R., Berger, J. and Macina, L. (1994) 'Critical care of the geriatric patient', *Clinics in Geriatric Medicine*, 10(1): 19–30.

Adembri, C., Kastamoniti, E., Bertolozzi, I., Vanni, S., Dorigo, W., Coppo, M., Pratesi, C., De Gaudio, A.R., Gensini, G.F. and Modesti, P.A. (2004) 'Pulmonary injury follows systemic inflammatory reaction in infrarenal aortic surgery', *Critical Care Medicine*, 32(5): 1170–7.

Ahern, J. and Philpot, P. (2002) 'Assessing acutely ill patients on general wards', *Nursing Standard*, 16(47): 47–54.

Akca, O., Kolta, K., Uzel, S., Cakar, N., Pembeci, K., Sayan, M.A., Tutuncu, A.S., Karakas, S.E., Calagnu, S., Ozkan, T., Esen, F., Telci, L., Sessler, D.I. and Akpir, K. (2000) 'Risk factors for early-onset, ventilator-associated pneumonia in critical care patients', *Anesthesiology*, 93(3): 638–45.

Aksoy, S. (2000) 'Can the "quality of life" be used as a criterion in health care services?' *Bulletin of Medical Ethics*, 162: 19–22.

Albarran, J.W. (1998) 'Managing the nursing priorities in the patient with an acute myocardial infarction', in Albarran, J.W. and

Price, T.E. (eds) *Managing the Nursing Priorities in Intensive Care*, Dinton: Quay Books, 134–70.

Alberti, C., Brun-Buisson, C., Burchardi, H., Martin, C., Goodman, S., Artigas, A., Sicignano, A., Palazzo, M., Moreno, R., Boulmé, R., Lepage, E. and Le Gall, J.R. (2002) 'Epidemiology of sepsis and infection in ICU patients from an international multicentre cohort study', *Intensive Care Medicine*, 28(2): 108–21.

Alchaghouri, S. (2004) 'Atrial fibrillation 2: management', *Hospital Medicine*, 65(9): 546–52.

Alexander, R.W. and Franciosa, J.A. (2003) 'Background and overview of a symposium to update the biology of atherosclerosis and its implications for treatment strategies', *American Journal of Cardiology*, 91(3A): 1A–2A.

Allen, C.H. and Ward, J.D. (1998) 'An evidence-based approach to management of increased intracranial pressure', *Critical Care Clinics*, 14(3): 485–95.

Allen, K. (2004) 'Principles and limitations of pulse oximetry in patient monitoring', *Nursing Times*, 100(41): 34–7.

Aller, L.J. and Coeling, H.V.E. (1995) 'Quality of life: its meaning to the long-term care resident', *Journal of Gerontological Nursing*, 21(2): 20–5.

Allison, A. (1994) 'High frequency jet ventilation – where are we now?' *Care of the Critically Ill*, 10(3): 122–4.

Al-Ruzzeh, S., Ambler, G., Asimakopoulos, G., Omar, R.Z., Hasan, R., Fabri, B., El-Gamel, A., DeSouza, A., Zamvar, V., Griffin, S., Keenan, D., Trivedi, U., Pullan, M., Cale, A., Cowen, M., Taylor, K. and Amrani, M. (2003) 'Off-pump coronary artery bypass (OPCAB) surgery reduces risk-stratified morbidity and mortality: a United Kingdom multi-center comparative analysis of early clinical outcome', *Circulation*, 108(supplement II): 1–8.

Amyes, S.G.B. and Thomson, C.J. (1995) 'Antibiotic resistance in the ICU', *British Journal of Intensive Care*, 5(8): 263–71.

Anderson, F.A. and Spencer, F.A. (2003) 'Risk factors for venous thromboembolism', *Circulation*, 23 (supplement): I9–I16.

Andrew, C.M. (1998) 'Optimizing the human experience: nursing the families of people who die in intensive care', *Intensive and Critical Care Nursing*, 14(2): 59–65.

Andrews, E.J. and Redmond, H.P. (2004) 'A review of clinical guidelines', *British Journal of Surgery*, 91(8): 956–64.

Andrews, P.J.D. (2000) 'Medical complications of management following aneurysmal sub-arachnoid haemorrhage', in Galley, H.F. (ed.) *Critical Care Focus 3: Neurological Injury*, London: BMJ Books, 28–38.

Annane, D., Bellisant, E., Bollaert, P.E., Briegel, J., Keh, B.D. and Kupfer, Y. (2004) 'Corticosteroids for severe sepsis and septic shock: a systematic review and meta-analysis', *BMJ*, 329(7464): 480–4.

Annane, D., Sebille, V., Charpentier, C., Bollaert, P.-E., François, B., Korach, J.-M., Capellier, G., Cohen, Y., Azoulay, E., Troché, G., Chaumet-Riffaut, P. and Bellissant, E. (2002) 'Effect of treatment with low doses of hydrocortisone and fludrocortisone on mortality in patients with septic shock', *JAMA*, 288(7): 862–71.

Antman, E.M., Cohen, M., Bernink, P.J.L.M., McCabe C.H., Horacek, T., Papuchis, G., Mautner, B., Corbalan, R., Radley, D. and Braunwald, E. (2000) 'The TIMI risk score for unstable angina/non-ST elevation MI', *JAMA*, 284(7): 835–42.

Arbour, R. (2000) 'Mastering neuromuscular blockade', *Dimensions of Critical Care Nursing*, 19(5): 4–20.

Armstrong, R.F., Bullen, C., Cohen, S.L., Singer, M. and Webb, A.R. (1992) 'Critical care algorithm. Sedation, analgesia and paralysis', *Clinical Intensive Care*, 3(6): 284–7.

Arntz, H.R., Willich, S.N., Schreiber, C., Bruggemann, T., Stern, R. and Schultheiss, H.P. (2000) 'Diurnal, weekly and seasonal variation of sudden death. Population-based analysis of 24,061 consecutive cases', *European Heart Journal*, 21(4): 315–20.

Aronow, H.D., Topol, E.J., Roe, M.T., Houghtaling, P.L., Wolski, K.E., Lincoff, A.M., Harrington, R.A., Califf, R.M., Ohman, E.M., Kleiman, N.S., Keltai, M., Wilcox, R.G., Vahanian, A., Armstrong, P.W. and Lauer, M.S. (2001) 'Effect of lipid-lowering therapy on early mortality after acute coronary syndromes: an observational study', *Lancet*, 357(9262): 1063–8.

Arrowsmith, J.E., Grocott, H.P., Reves, J.G. and Newman, M.F. (2000) 'Central nervous complications of cardiac surgery', *British Journal of Anaesthesia*, 84(3): 378–93.

Artigas, A., Bernard, G.R., Cartlet, B.J., Dreyfuss, D., Gattinoni, L., Hudson, L., Lamy, M., Marini, J.J., Matthay, M.A., Pinsky, M.B., Soragg, R. and Suter, P.M. (1998) 'The American–European consensus conference on ARDS, part 2', *American Journal of Respiratory Critical Care Medicine*, 157(4 part 1): 1332–47.

Ascione, R., Reeves, B.C., Taylor, F.C., Seehra, H.K. and Angelini, G.D. (2004) 'Beating heart against cardio-plegic arrest studies (BHACAS 1 and 2): quality of life at mid-term follow-up in two randomised controlled trials', *European Heart Journal*, 25(9): 765–70.

Ashurst, S. (1997) 'Nursing care of the mechanically ventilated patient in ITU', *British Journal of Nursing*, 6(8): 447–54.

Ashworth, P. (1980) *Care to Communicate*, London: RCN.

Astle, S.M. (2003) 'Beside tracheostomy: a step by step guide', *AJN*, 66(10): 41–5.

Atherton, J.C. (2003) 'Acid-base balance: maintenance of plasma pH', *Anaesthesia and Intensive Care Medicine*, 4(12): 419–22.

Attia, J., Ray, J.G., Cook, D.J., Douketis, J., Ginsberg, J.S. and Geerts, W.H. (2001) 'Deep vein thrombosis and its prevention in critically ill adults', *Archives of Internal Medicine*, 161(10): 1268–79.

Audit Commission (1999) *Critical to Success. The Place of Efficient and Effective Critical Care Services Within the Acute Hospital*, London: Audit Commission.

—— (2001) *Testing Times*, London: Audit Commission.

Ault, M.L. and Stock, M.C. (2004) 'Respiratory monitoring', *International Anaesthesiology Clinics*, 42(1): 97–112.

Australian & New Zealand Intensive Care Society Clinical Trials Group (2000) 'Low-dose dopamine in patients with early renal dysfunction: a placebo-controlled randomised trial', *Lancet*, 356(9248): 2139–43.

Avidan, M.S., Jones, N. and Pozniak, A.L. (2000) 'The implications of HIV for the anaesthetist and the intensivist', *Anaesthesia*, 55(4): 344–54.

Aviles, R.J., Asskari, A.T., Lindahl, B., Wallentin, L., Jia, G., Ohman, E.M., Mahaffey, K.W., Newwby, L.K., Califf, R.M., Simoons, M.L., Topol, E.J. and Lauer, M.S. (2002) 'Troponin T levels in patients with acute coronary syndromes, with or without renal dysfunction', *New England Journal of Medicine*, 346(226): 2047–52.

Ayello, E. and Braden, B. (2002) 'How and why to do pressure ulcer risk assessment', *Advances in Skin & Wound Care*, 15(3): 125–31.

Ayliffe, G.A.J., Babb, J.R. and Taylor, L.J. (2001) *Hospital-Acquired Infection: Principles and Prevention*, 3rd edn, London: Arnold.

Azar, G., Love, R., Choe, E., Flint, L. and Steinberg, S. (1996) 'Neither dopamine nor dobutamine reverses the depression in mesenteric blood flow caused by positive end-expiratory pressure', *Journal of Trauma*, 40(5): 679–85.

Azoulay, E., Chevret, S., Leleu, G., Pochard, F., Barboteu, M., Adrie, C., Canoui, P., Le Gall, J.R. and Schlemmer, B. (2000) 'Half the families of intensive care unit patients experience inadequate communication with physicians', *Critical Care Medicine*, 28(8): 3044–9.

Azoulay, E., Pochard, F., Chevret, S., Arich, C., Brivet, F., Brun, F., Charles, P.-E., Desmettre, T., Dubois, D., Galliot, R., Garrouste-Orgeas, M., Goldgran-Toledano, D., Herbecq, P., Joly, L.-M., Jourdain, M., Kaidomar, M., Lepape, A., Letellier, N., Marie, O., Page, B., Parrot, A., Rodie-Talbere. P.-A., Sermet, A., Tenaillon, A., Thuong, A., Thuong, M., Tulasne, P., Le Gall, J.-R., Schlemner, B. and French Famirea Group (2003) 'Family participation in care to the critically ill: opinions of families and staff', *Intensive Care Medicine*, 29(9): 1498–504.

BACCN (2005) *Position Statement on Nurse–Patient Ratios in Critical Care*, London: British Association of Critical Care Nurses.

Backmän, C.G. and Walther, S.M. (2001) 'Use of a personal diary written on the ICU during critical illness', *Intensive Care Medicine*, 27(2): 426–9.

Bahouth, M.N. and Yarbrough, K.L. (2005) 'Patient management: nervous system', in Morton, P.G., Fontaine, D.K., Hudak, C.M. and Gallo, B.M. (eds) *Critical Care Nursing: A Holistic Approach*, 8th edn, Philadelphia, PA: Lippincott Williams & Wilkins, 775–95.

Bailey, D., Jackson, L. and White, D. (2004) 'HBO therapy: beyond the bends', *RN*, 27(9): 31–5.

Baktoft, B. (2001) 'Nursing care of patients in the prone position', *Connect*, 1(3): 83–6.

Ball, P.A. (2001) 'Critical care of spinal cord injury', *Spine*, 26(24S): S27–S30.

Ballantyne, J.C., McKenna, J.M. and Ryder, E. (2003) Epidural analgesia – experience of 5628 patients in a large teaching hospital derived through audit', *Acute Pain*, 4(3–4): 89–97.

Banks, P.A. (1998) 'Acute and chronic pancreatitis', in Felman, M., Scharschmidt, B.F. and Sleisenger, M.H. (eds) *Sleisenger & Fordtran's Gastrointestinal and Liver Disease*, Philadelphia, PA: WB Saunders Co., 809–62.

Barie, P.S., Williams, M.D., McCollam, J.S., Bates, B.M., Qualy, R.L. and PROWESS Surgical Evaluation Committee (2004) 'Benefit/risk profile of drotrecogin alfa (activated) in surgical patients with severe sepsis', *American Journal of Surgery*, 188(3): 212–20.

Baris, R.R., Israel, A.L., Amory, D.W. and Benni, P. (1995) 'Regional cerebral oxygenation during cardiopulmonary bypass', *Perfusion*, 10(4): 245–8.

Barr, W. (1996) 'Do restraints really protect intubated patients?' *American Journal of Nursing*, 96(6): 51.

Barrett, S.P. (1999) 'Control of the spread of multi-resistant Gram-positive organisms', *Current Anaesthesia and Critical Care*, 10(1): 27–31.

Bartlett, R.H., Roloff, D.W., Custer, J.R., Younger, J.G. and Hirschl, R.B. (2000) 'Extracorporeal life support', *JAMA*, 283(7): 904–8.

Bastacky, S. and Lee, R.E. (2001) 'Disseminated intravascular coagulation,' *New England Journal of Medicine*, 345(10): 1394.

Bateson, S., Adam, S., Hall, G. and Quirke, S. (1993) 'The development of a pressure area scoring system for critically ill patients', *Intensive and Critical Care Nursing*, 9(3): 146–51.

Baxter, B.T. (2004) 'Could medical intervention work for aortic aneurysms?' *American Journal of Surgery*, 188(6): 628–32.

Bayir, H., Clark, R.S.B. and Kochanek, P.M. (2003) 'Promising strategies to minimize secondary brain injury after head trauma', *Critical Care Medicine*, 31(1): S112–S117.

BCSH (1998) 'Guidelines on oral anticoagulation', *British Journal of Haematology*, 3rd edn, 101(2): 374–87.

BCSH Task Force Sickle Cell Working Party (2003) 'Guidelines for the management of the acute painful crisis in sickle cell disease', *British Journal of Haematology*, 120(5): 745–52.

Beale, R.J., Hollenberg, S.M., Vincent, J.-L. and Parrillo, J.E. (2004) 'Vasopressor and inotropic support in septic shock: an evidence-based review', *Critical Care Medicine*, 32(11): S455–S65.

Beauchamp, T.L. and Childress, J.F. (2001) *Principles of Biomedical Ethics*, 5th edn, Oxford: Oxford University Press.

Beck, D.H., Taylor, B.L., Millar, B. and Smith, G.B. (1997) 'Prediction of outcome from intensive care: a prospective cohort study comparing Acute Physiology and Chronic Health Evaluation II and III prognostic systems in a United Kingdom intensive care unit', *Critical Care Medicine*, 25(1): 9–15.

Beckingham, I.J. and Bornman, P.C. (2001) 'Acute pancreatitis', *BMJ*, 322(7286): 595–8.

Beckman, J.A., Creager, M.A. and Libby, P. (2002) 'Diabetes and atherosclerosis: epidemiology, pathophysiology and management', *JAMA*, 287(19): 2570–81.

Bednarik, J., Lukas, Z. and Vondracek, P. (2003) 'Critical illness polyneuropathy: the electrical physiological components of a complex entity', *Intensive Care Medicine*, 29(9): 1505–14.

Beecham, L. (1999) 'BMA wants presumed consent for organ donors', *BMJ*, 319(7203): 141.

Beevers, G., Lip, G.Y.H. and O'Brien, E. (2001) 'Blood pressure measurement', *BMJ*, 322(7292): 981–5.

Behrendt, C.E. (2000) 'Acute respiratory failure in the United States', *Chest*, 118(4): 1100–5.

Bein, T., Reber, A., Ploner, F., Taeger, K. and Jauch, K.-W. (2000) 'Continuous axial rotation and pulmonary fluid balance in acute lung injury', *Clinical Intensive Care*, 11(6): 307–10.

Belfort, M.A., Anthony, J., Saade, G.R., Allen, J.C. and Nimodipine Study Group (2003) 'A comparison of magnesium sulphate and nimodipine for the prevention of eclampsia', *New England Journal of Medicine*, 384(4): 304–11.

Bell, M.D.D., Moss, E. and Murphy, P.G. (2004) 'Brainstem death testing in the UK – time for reappraisal?' *British Journal of Anaesthesia*, 92(5): 633–40.

Belligan, G.J. (2002) 'Resolution of inflammation and repair', in Evans, T.W., Griffiths, M.J.D. and Keogh, B.F. (eds) *ARDS*, Sheffield: European Respiratory Society Journals Ltd., 70–82.

Bellingan, G. (1999) 'Inflammatory cell activation in sepsis', *British Medical Bulletin*, 55(1): 12–29.

Bellingham, G. (1999) 'The early fibrotic response in acute lung injury and the role of steroids in Galley, H.F. (ed.) *Critical Care Focus 2: Respiratory Failure*, London: BMJ Books, 37–51.

Bellomo, R., Kellum, J. and Ronco, C. (2001) 'Acute renal failure: time for consensus', *Intensive Care Medicine*, 27(10): 1685–8.

Bennett, C. and Baker, K. (2001) 'HIV and AIDS: an overview', *Nursing Standard*, 15(24): 45–52.

Bennett, D.H. (2002) *Cardiac Arrhythmias*, 6th edn, London: Arnold.

Bennett, L. (2005) 'Understanding sickle cell disorders', *Nursing Standard*, 19(32): 52–61.

Bennett, N.R. (1999) 'Paediatric intensive care', *British Journal of Anaesthesia*, 83(1): 139–56.

Bennewith, O., Stocks, N., Gunnell, D., Peters, T.J., Evans, M.O. and Sharp, D.J. (2002) 'General practice based intervention to prevent repeat episodes of deliberate self harm: cluster randomised controlled trial', *BMJ*, 324(7348): 1254–557.

Bénony, H., Daloz, L., Bungener, C., Chahraoui, K., Frenay, C. and Auvin, J. (2002) 'Emotional factors and subjective quality of life in subjects with spinal cord injuries', *American Journal of Physical Medicine and Rehabilitation*, 81(6): 437–45.

Bergbom, I. and Askwall, A. (2000) 'The nearest and dearest: a lifeline for ICU patients', *Intensive and Critical Care Nursing*, 16(6): 384–95.

Bergbom, I., Svensson, C., Berggren, E. and Kansula, M. (1999) 'Patients' and relatives' opinions and feeling about diaries kept by nurses in an intensive care unit: pilot study', *Intensive and Critical Care Nursing*, 15(4): 185–91.

Bergeron, B., Dubois, M.-J., Dumont, M., Dial, S. and Skrobik, Y. (2001) 'Intensive care delirium screening checklist: evaluation of a new screening tool', *Intensive Care Medicine*, 27(5): 859–64.

Bergstrom, N., Braden, B.J., Laguzza, A. and Holman, V. (1987) 'The Braden scale for predicting pressure sore risk', *Nursing Research*, 36(4): 205–10.

Bernard, G.R., Artigas, A., Brigham, K.L., Carlet, J., Falke, K., Hudson, L., Lamy, M., LeGall, J.R., Morris, A. and Spragg, R. (1994a) 'Report of the American–European consensus conference on ARDS: definitions, mechanisms, relevant outcomes and clinical trial co-ordination', *Intensive Care Medicine*, 20(3): 225–32.

—— (1994b) American–European consensus conference on ARDS: definitions, mechanisms, relevant outcome and clinical trial co-ordination', *American Journal of Respiratory Critical Care Medicine*, 149(3 part 1): 818–21.

Bernard, G.R., Vincent, J.-L., Laterre, P.-F., LaRosa, S.P., Dhainaut, J.-F., Lopez-Rodriguez, A., Steingrub, J.S., Garber, G.E., Helterbrand, J.D., Ely, E.W. and Fischer, C.J. (2001) 'Efficacy and safety of recombinant human activated protein C for severe sepsis', *New England Journal of Medicine*, 344(10): 699–709.

Berson, A.J., Smith, J.M., Woods, S.E., Hasselfeld, K.A. and Hiratzka, L.F. (2004) 'Off-pump versus on-pump coronary artery bypass surgery: does the pump influence outcome?' *Journal of the American College of Surgeons*, 199(1): 102–8.

Berthelot, P., Grattard, F., Mahul, P., Pain, P., Jospé, R., Venet, C., Carricajo, A., Aubert, G., Ros, A., Dumont, A., Lucht, F., Zéni, F., Auboyer, C.A., Bertrand, J.C. and Pozzetto, B. (2001) 'Prospective study of nosocomial colonization and infection due to *Pseudomonas aeruginosa* in mechanically ventilated patients', *Intensive Care Medicine*, 27(3): 503–12.

Bertrand, M.E., Simoons, M.L., Fox, K.A.A., Wallensttin, L.C., Hamm, C.W., McFadden, E., Feyter, P.J., Specchia, G. and Ruzyllo, W. (2002) 'Task Force on the management of acute coronary syndromes in patients presenting without persistent ST segment elevation', *European Heart Journal*, 23(23): 1809–40.

Bertrand, X., Thouverez, M., Talon, D., Boillot, A., Capellier, G., Floriot, C. and Helias, J.P. (2001) 'Endemecity, molecular diversity and colonisation routes of Pseudomonas aeruginosa in intensive care units', *Intensive Care Medicine*, 27(8): 1263–8.

Bettex, D.A., Hinselmann, V., Hellermann, J.P., Jenni, R. and Schmid, ER. (2004) 'Transosphageal echocardiography is unreliable for cardiac output assessment after cardiac surgery compared with thermodilution', *Anaesthesia*, 29(12): 1184–92.

Betts, J., Betts, P. and Sage, I. (1999) *Leah Betts: The Legacy of Ecstasy*, London: Robson Books.

Bewley, C. (2004) 'Hypertensive disorders of pregnancy', in Henderson, C. and Macdonald, S. (eds) *Mayes' Midwifery: A Textbook for Midwives*, 13th edn, Edinburgh: Baillière Tindall, 780–92.

Bigatello, L.M., Davignon, K.R. and Stelfox, H.T. (2005) 'Respiratory mechanics and ventilator waveforms in the patient with acute lung injury', *Respiratory Care*, 50(2): 235–44.

Bion, J. (1995) 'Rationing intensive care', *BMJ*, 310(6981): 682–3.

Bion, J.F., Elliott, T.S.J. and Glen, L. (2001) 'Infection on the intensive care unit: the scale of the problem', in Galley, H.F. (ed.) *Critical Care Focus 5: Antibiotic Resistance and Infection Control*, London: BMJ Books, 1–11.

Bird, J. (2003) 'Selection of pain measurement tools', *Nursing Standard*, 18(13): 33–9.

Birtwistle, J. (1994) 'Pressure sore formation and risk assessment in intensive care', *Care of the Critically Ill*, 10(4): 154–9.

Blackburn, F. and Bookless, B. (2002) 'Valve disorders', in Hatchett, R. and Thompson, D. (eds) *Cardiac Nursing: A Comprehensive Guide*, Edinburgh: Churchill Livingstone, 260–86.

Blackwood, B. (1999) 'Normal saline instillation with endotracheal suctioning: primum non nocere (first do no harm)', *Journal of Advanced Nursing*, 29(4): 928–34.

Blackwood, B., Wilson-Barnett, J. and Trinder, J. (2004) 'Protocolized weaning from mechanical ventilation: ICU physicians' views', *Journal of Advanced Nursing*, 48(1): 26–34.

Blasi, F. (2004) 'Atypical pathogens and respiratory tract infections', *European Respiratory Journal*, 24(1): 171–81.

Blenkharn, A., Faughnan, S. and Morgan, A. (2002) 'Developing a pain assessment tool for use by nurses in an adult intensive care unit', *Intensive and Critical Care Nursing*, 18(6): 332–41.

Blood Transfusion Task Force (2001) 'Guidelines for the clinical use of red cell transfusions', *British Journal of Haematology*, 113(1): 24–31.

Blumenthal, I. (2001) 'Carbon monoxide poisoning', *Journal of the Royal Society of Medicine*, 94(6): 270–2.

BMA (2002) *Withholding and Withdrawing Life-Prolonging Medical Treatment*, 2nd edn, London: BMJ Books.

Board, M. (1995) 'Comparison of disposable and glass mercury thermometers', *Nursing Times*, 91(33): 36–7.

Boden, D., Hurley, A., Zhang, L., Cao, Y., Guo, Y., Jones, E., Tsay, J., Ip, J., Farthing, C., Limoli, K., Parkin, N. and Markowitx, M. (1999) 'HIV-1 drug resistance in newly infected individuals', *JAMA*, 282(12): 1135–41.

Bodenham, A.R. and Barry, B.N. (2001) 'The role of tracheostomy in ICU', *Anaesthesia and Intensive Care Medicine*, 27(9): 336–9.

Boersma, E., Mercado, N., Poldermans, D., Gardien, M., Vos, J. and Simoons, M.L. (2003) 'Acute myocardial infarction', *Lancet*, 361(9360): 847–58.

Boldt, J. (2000a) 'Volume replacement in the surgical patient – does the type of solution make a difference?' *British Journal of Anaesthesia*, 84(61): 783–9.

—— (2000b) 'The good, the bad, and the ugly: should we completely banish human albumin from our intensive care units?', *Anaesthesia & Analgesia*, 91(4): 887–95.

Bollmann, M.-D., Revelly, J.-P., Tappy, L., Berger, M.M., Schaller, M.-D., Cayeux, M.-C., Martinez, A. and Chioléro, R.-L. (2004) 'Effect of bicarbonate and lactate buffer on glucose and lactate metabolism during hemofiltration in patients with multiple organ failure', *Intensive Care Medicine*, 30(6): 1103–10.

Bolton, C.F. (1999) 'Pathophysiology and causes of neuropathy', in Webb, A.R., Shapiro, M., Singer, M. and Suter, P.M. (eds) *Oxford Textbook of Critical Care*, Oxford: Oxford University Press, 490–4.

Bone, R.C., Balk, R.A., Cerra, F.B., Dellinger, R.P., Fein, A.M., Knaus, W.A., Schein, R.M. and Sibbald, W.J. (1992) 'Definitions for sepsis and organ failure and guidelines for the use of innovative therapies is sepsis', *Chest*, 101(6): 1644–55.

Bonnefoy, E., Godon, P., Kirkorian, G., Fatemi, M., Chevalier, P. and Touboul, P. (2000) 'Serum cardiac troponin I and ST-segment elevation in patients with acute pericarditis', *European Heart Journal*, 21(10): 832–6.

Bonner, S. and Rudge, C. (2002) 'UK Transplant and ITU', *JICS*, 3(2): 47–9.

Booij, L.H.D.J. (1999) 'Brain death and care of the brain death patient', *Current Anaesthesia and Critical Care*, 10(6): 312–18.

Booth, C., Heyland, D.K. and Paterson, W.G. (2002) 'Gastrointestinal promotility drugs in the critical care setting: a systematic review of the evidence', *Critical Care Medicine*, 30(7): 1429–35.

Booth, C.M., Matukas, L.M., Tomlinson, G.A., Rachlis, A.R., Rose, D.B., Dwosh, H.A., Walmsley, S.L., Mazulli, T., Avendano, M., Derkach, P., Ephtimios, I.E., Kitai, I., Mederski, B.D., Shadowitz, S.B., Gold, W.L., Hawryluck, L.A., Rea, E., Chenkin, J.S., Cescon, D.W., Poutanen, S.M. and Detsky, A.S. (2003) 'Clinical features and short-term outcomes of 144 patients with SARS in the greater Toronto area', *JAMA*, 289(21): 2801–9.

Booth, C.M. and Stewart, T.E. (2005) 'Severe acute respiratory syndrome and critical care medicine: the Toronto experience', *Critical Care Medicine*, 33(1 supplement): S53–S60.

Booth, S. (2002) 'A philosophical analysis of informed consent', *Nursing Standard*, 16(39): 43–6.

Boralessa, H., Goldhill, D. and Boralessa, H. (2003) 'Blood and the critically ill', *Care of the Critically Ill*, 19(1): 15–17.

Bouchut, J-C., Godard, J. and Claris, O. (2004) 'High-frequency oscillatory ventilation', *Anesthesiology*, 100(4): 7–12.

Boumendil, A., Maury, E., Reinhard, I., Luquel, L., Offenstadt, G. and Guidet, B. (2004) 'Prognosis of patients aged 80 years and over admitted in medical intensive care unit', *Intensive Care Medicine*, 30(4): 647–54.

Bourne, R.S. and Mills, G.H. (2004) 'Sleep disruption in critically ill patients – pharmacological considerations', *Anaesthesia*, 59(4): 374–84.

Bowling, T.E. (2004) 'Enteral nutrition', *Hospital Medicine*, 65(12): 712–16.

Bowsher, J., Boyle, S. and Griffiths, J. (1999) 'Oral care', *Nursing Standard*, 13(37): 31.

535

Boyce, P., Oakley-Browne, M. and Hatcher, S. (2001) 'The problem of deliberate self-harm', *Current Opinion in Psychiatry*, 14(2): 107–11.

Brackenbury, A.M., Puligandla, P.S., McCaig, L.A., Nikore, V., Yao, L.-J., Veldhuizen, R.A.W. and Lewis, J.F. (2001) 'Evaluation of exogenous surfactant in HCl-induced lung injury', *American Journal of Respiratory and Critical Care Medicine*, 163(5): 1135–45.

Bradley, C. (2001a) 'Crystalloid, colloid or small volume resuscitation?' *Intensive and Critical Care Nursing*, 17(5): 304–6.

—— (2001b) 'Stress ulcer prevention – the controversy continues', *Intensive and Critical Care Nursing*, 17(1): 58–60.

Brady, A.J.B. and Buller, N.P. (1996) 'Coronary angioplasty and myocardial ischaemia', *Care of the Critically Ill*, 12(3): 83–6.

Brain Trauma Foundation (2001) *Guidelines for the Management of Severe Head Injury*, American Association of Neurological Surgeons Joint Section on Neurotrauma and Critical Care, *Journal of Neurotrauma*, guidelines/downloads/btf_guidelines_management.pdf? BrainTrauma_Session=b7dae74 ddb 2d323elf6766c45d344baf (downloaded 4 July 2005).

Braithwaite, R.A. (1999) 'The application of drugs of abuse screening on critically ill patients', *Care of the Critically Ill*, 15(5): 180–4.

Brandstetter, R.D., Sharma, K.C., Dellabadia, M., Cabreros, L.J. and Kabinoff, G.S. (1997) 'Adult respiratory distress syndrome: a disorder in need of improved outcome', *Heart and Lung*, 26(1): 3–14.

Branson, R.D. (2005) 'The role of ventilator graphs when setting dual-control modes', *Respiratory Care*, 50(2): 187–201.

Branson, R.D. and Campbell, R.S. (2001) 'Modes of ventilator operation', in MacIntyre, N.R. and Branson, R.D. (eds) *Mechanical Ventilation*, Philadephia, PA: W.B. Saunders Co.

Bray, K., Hill, K., Robson, W., Leaver, G., Walker, N., O'Leary, M., Delaney, T., Walsh, D., Gager, M. and Waterhouse, C. (2004) 'British Association of Critical Care Nurses position statement on the use of restraint in adult critical care units', *Nursing in Critical Care*, 9(5): 199–211.

Brealey, D. and Singer, M. (2000) 'Multi-organ dysfunction in the critically ill: effects on different organs', *Journal of the Royal College of Physicians of London*, 34(5): 428–31.

Breiburg, A.N., Aitken, L., Reaby, L. Clancy R.L. and Pierce, J.D. (2000) 'Efficacy and safety of prone positioning for patients with acute respiratory distress syndrome', *Journal of Advanced Nursing*, 32(4): 922–9.

Brenner, Z.R. (2002) 'Lessons for the critical care nurse on caring for the dying', *Critical Care Nurse*, 22(1): 11–12.

Bridgewater, B., Grayson, A.D., Hasan, R., Dihmis, W.C., Munsch, C., Waterworth, P. and North West Quality Improvement Programme in Cardiac Interventions (2004) 'Improving mortality of coronary surgery over first four years of independent practice: retrospective examination of prospectively collected data from 15 surgeons, *BMJ*, 329(7463): 421–4.

Brims, F.J.H., Davies, M.G., Elia, A. and Griffiths, M.J.D. (2004) 'The effects of pleural fluid drainage on oxygenation in mechanically ventilated patients after cardiac surgery', *Thorax*, 59: ii40: S129.

Bristow, P. and Hillman, K. (1999) 'Management of hyperglycaemia', in Webb, A.R., Shapiro, M., Singer, M. and Suter, P.M. (eds) *Oxford Textbook of Critical Care*, Oxford: Oxford University Press, 589–91.

British Society for Standards in Haematology, Blood Transfusion Task Force (2003) 'Guidelines for the use of platelet transfusions', *British Journal of Haematology*, 122(1): 10–23.

British Society of Gastroenterology Endoscopy Committee (2000) 'Non-variceal upper gastrointestinal haemorrhage guidelines', *Gut*, 51(supplement IV): iv1–iv6.

British Thoracic Society (2002) 'Non-invasive ventilation in acute respiratory failure', *Thorax*, 57(3): 192–211.

—— (2003) 'British Thoracic Society guidelines for the management of suspected acute pulmonary embolim', *Thorax*, 58(6): 470–84.

Brochard, L. (1999) 'What's new in ventilator weaning?' in Galley, H.F. (ed.) *Critical Care Focus 2: Respiratory Failure*, London: BMJ Books, 26–30.

Brochard, L., Roudot-Thoravel, F., Roupie, E., Delclaux, C., Chastre, J., Fernandez-Mondejar, E., Clementi, E., Mancebo, J., Factor, P., Matamis, D., Ranieri, M., Blanch, L., Rodi, G., Mentec, H., Dreyfuss, D., Ferrer, M., Brun-Buisson, C., Tobin, M. and Lemaire, F. (1998) 'Tidal volume reduction for prevention of ventilator-induced lung injury in acute respiratory distress syndrome', *American Journal of Respiratory and Critical Care Medicine*, 158(6): 1831–8.

Brock, W.A., Nolan, K. and Nolan, T. (1998) 'Pragmatic science: accelerating the improvement of critical care', *New Horizons*, 6(1): 61–8.

Broomhead, R. (2002) 'Percutaneous tracheostomy', *Anaesthesia & Critical Care*, 3(6): 210–12.

Brower, R.G., Ware, L.B., Berthiaume, Y. and Matthay, M.A. (2001) 'Treatment of ARDS', *Chest*, 120(4): 1347–67.

Brown, C.M., Nuorti, P.J., Breiman, R.F., Hathcock, A.L., Fields, B.S., Lipman, H.B., Llewellyn, G.C., Hofmann, J. and Cetron, M. (1999) 'A community outbreak of Legionnaires' disease linked to hospital cooling towers: an epidemiological method to calculate dose of exposure', *International Journal of Epidemiology*, 28(2): 353–9.

Brown, C.V., Rhee, P., Chan, L. Evans, K., Demetriades, D. and Velmahos, G.C. (2004) 'Preventing renal failure in patients with rhabdomyolysis: do bicarbonate and mannitol make a difference?' *The Journal of Trauma*, 56(6): 1191–996.

Brown, M.M. (1999) 'Results of the carotid and vertebral artery transluminal angioplasty study', *British Journal of Surgery*, 86: A710–1.

Brun-Buisson, C. (2001) 'Catheter-related infection', in Galley, H.F. (ed.) *Critical Care Focus 5: Antibiotic Resistance and Infection Control*, London: BMJ Books, 26–33.

Bruton, W.A.T. (1995) 'Infection and hospital laundry', *Lancet*, 345(8964): 1574–5.

Buchan, J. (2002) 'Global nursing shortages', *BMJ*, 324(7340): 751–2.

Büchler, M., Malfertheiner, P., Uhl, W. Schömerich, J., Stöckmann, F., Adler, G., Gaus, W., Rolle, K., Beger, H.G. and German Pancreatitis Study Group (1993) 'Gabexate mesilate in human acute pancreatitis', *Gastroenterology*, 104(4): 1165–70.

Bulstrode, N., Banks, F. and Shrotria, S. (2002) 'The outcome of drug smuggling by "body packers" – the British experience', *Annals of the Royal College of Surgeons of England*, 84(1): 35–8.

Burchiel, K.J. and Hsu, F.P. (2001) 'Pain and spasticity after spinal cord injury: mechanisms and treatment', *Spine*, 26(24S): S146–S160.

Burnard, P. and Chapman, C. (2003) *Professional and Ethical Issues in Nursing*, 3rd edn, London: Baillière Tindall.

Burr, G. (1998) 'Contextualising critical care family needs through triangulation: an Australian study', *Intensive and Critical Care Nursing*, 14(4): 161–9.

Busund, R., Koukline, V., Utrobin, U. and Nedashkovsky, E. (2002) 'Plasmapheresis in severe sepsis and septic shock: a prospective, randomised, controlled trial', *Intensive Care Medicine*, 28(10): 1434–9.

Buswell, C. (1996) 'Beta thalassaemia', *Professional Nurse*, 12(2): 145–7.

Butts, J.B. (2001) 'Outcomes of comfort touch in institutionalized elderly female residents', *Geriatric Nursing*, 22(4): 180–4.

Bytheway, B. (1995) *Ageism*, Buckingham: Open University Press.

Caelli, M., Porteous, J., Carson, C.F., Heller, R. and Riley, T.V. (2000) 'Tea tree oil as an alternative topical decolonisation agent for methicillin-resistant *Staphylococcus aureus*', *Journal of Hospital Infection*, 46(3): 236–7.

Cairns, C.J.S. (2003) 'Cardiac and pulmonary complications of subarachnoid haemorrhage: pathophysiology, diagnosis and management', *International Journal of Intensive Care*, 10(3): 109–18.

Calam, J. and Baron, J.H. (2001) 'Pathophysiology of duodenal and gastric ulcer and gastric cancer', *BMJ*, 323(7319): 980–2.

Callaghan, I. (1998) 'Bacterial contamination of nurses' uniforms: a study', *Nursing Standard*, 13(1): 37–42.

Calne, S. (1994) 'Dehumanisation in intensive care', *Nursing Times*, 90(17): 31–3.

Calzia, E. and Stahl, W. (2004) 'The place of helium in the management of severe acute respiratory failure', *International Journal of Intensive Care*, 11(2): 65–9.

Caplin-Davies, P.J. (1999) 'Doctor–nurse substitution: the workforce equation', *Journal of Nursing Management*, 7(2): 71–9.

Capovilla, J., VanCouwenberghe, C. and Miller, W.A. (2000) 'Noninvasive blood gas monitoring. *Critical Care Nursing Quarterly*, 23(2): 79–86.

Caraceni, P. and Van Thiel, D.H. (1995) 'Acute liver failure', *Lancet*, 345(8943): 163–9.

Cariou, A., Vinsonneau, C. and Dhainaut, J.-F. (2004) 'Adjunctive therapies in sepsis: an evidence-based review', *Critical Care Medicine*, 32(11): S562–70.

Carney, D., DiRocco, J. and Nieman, G. (2005) 'Dynamic alveolar mechanics and ventilator-induced lung injury', *Critical Care Medicine*, 33(3 supplement): S122–8.

Caron, E.A. and Berlandi, J.L.H. (1997) 'Extracorporeal membrane oxygenation', *Nursing Clinics of North America*, 32(1): 125–40.

Carr, K. (2002) 'Ward visits after intensive care discharge: why?' in Griffiths, R.D. and Jones, C. (eds) *Intensive Care Aftercare*, Oxford: Butterworth-Heinemann, 69–82.

Carrell, T.W.G. and Wolfe, J.H.N. (2005) 'Non-cardiac vascular disease', *Heart*, 91(2): 265–70.

Casbolt, S. (2002) 'Communicating with the ventilated patient – a literature review', *Nursing in Critical Care*, 7(4): 198–202.

Casey, A. (1988) 'A partnership with child and family', *Senior Nurse*, 8(4): 8–9.

Casey, G. (2002) 'Physiology of skin', *Nursing Standard*, 16(34): 47–51.

Castella, X., Artigas, A., Bion, J. and Kari, A. (1995) 'A comparison of severity illness scoring systems for intensive care unit patients: results of a multicenter, multinational study', *Critical Care Medicine*, 23(8): 1327–35.

Cavaliere, F., Antonelli, M., Arcangeli, A., Conti, G., Pennisi, M.A. and Proietti, R. (2002) 'Effects of acid-base abnormalities on blood capacity of transporting $CO_2$: adverse effect of metabolic acidosis', *Intensive Care Medicine*, 28(5): 609–15.

Cely, C.M., Arora, P., Quartrin, A.A., Kett, D.H. and Schein, R.M.H. (2004) 'Relationship of baseline glucose homeostasis to hyperglycaemia during medical critical illness', *Chest*, 126(3): 879–87.

Chadda, K., Louis, B., Benaïssa, L., Annane, D., Gajdos, P., Raphaël, J.C. and Lofaso, F. (2002) 'Physiological effects of decannulation in tracheostomized patients', *Intensive Care Medicine*, 28(12): 1761–7.

Chalmers, C.A. (2002) 'Applied anatomy and physiology and the renal disease process', in Thomas, N. (ed.) *Renal Nursing*, 2nd edn, Edinburgh: Baillière Tindall, 27–74.

Chan, J.W.M. and Ng, C.K. (2005) 'Severe acute respiratory distress syndrome (SARS): a brief review with exploration of the outcomes, prognostic factors and sequelae', *Current Respiratory Medicine Reviews*, 1(1): 85–92.

Chaney, J.C. and Derdak, S. (2002) 'Minimally invasive hemodynamic monitoring for the intensivist: current and emerging technology', *Critical Care Medicine*, 30(10): 2338–45.

Chapman, M.G., Smith, M. and Hirsch, N.P. (2001) 'Status epilepticus', *Anaesthesia*, 56(7): 648–59.

Charalambos, C., Schofield, I. and Malik, R. (1999) 'Acute diabetic emergencies and their management', *Care of the Critically Ill*, 15(4): 132–5.

Chassard, D. and Bruguerolle, B. (2004) 'Chronobiology and anesthesia', *Anesthesiology*, 100(2): 413–27.

Chastre, J. (2001) 'Colonisation or infection?' in Galley, H.F. (ed.) *Critical Care Focus 5: Antibiotic Resistance and Infection Control*, London: BMJ Books, 19–25.

Chawala, L.S., Zia, H., Gutierrez, G., Katz, N.M., Seneff, M.G. and Shah, M. (2004) 'Lack of equivalence between central and mixed venous oxygen saturation', *Chest*, 12(6): 1891–6.

Cheever, K.H. (1999) Reducing the effects of acute pain in critically ill patients', *Dimensions of Critical Care Nursing*, 18(3): 14–23.

Chellel, A., Dawson, D., Endacott, R., Andrews, I. and RCN Critical Care Forum (1995) 'Patient scoring systems in critical care', *British Journal of Intensive Care*, 5(8): 250–4.

Chengi, S. and Katz, R. (2000) 'Antioxidant vitamins and coronary artery disease: from CHAOS to HOPE?' *British Journal of Cardiology*, 7(10): 601–12.

Chikwe, J., Walther, A. and Pepper, J. (2004) 'The surgical management of mitral valve disease', *British Journal of Cardiology*, 11(1): 42–7.

Chitnavis, B.P. and Polkey, C.E. (1998) 'Intracranial pressure monitoring', *Care of the Critically Ill*, 14(3): 80–4.

Chlan, L. (1998) 'Effectiveness of a music therapy intervention on relaxation and anxiety for patients receiving ventilatory assistance', *Heart & Lung*, 27(3): 169–76.

Cho, D.Y. and Wang, Y.C. (1997) 'Comparison of the APACHE III, APACHE II and Glasgow Coma Scale in acute head injury for prediction of mortality and functional outcome', *Intensive Care Medicine*, 23(1): 77–84.

Choi, P., Yip, G., Quinonez, L. and Cook, D. (1999) 'Crystalloid vs. colloid in fluid resuscitation: a systematic review', *Critical Care Medicine*, 27(1): 200–10.

Chowdhury, U.K., Airan, B., Mishra, P.K., Kothari, S.S., Subramaniam, K., Ray, R., Singh, R. and Venugopal, P. (2004) 'Hisopathology and morphometry of radial artery conduits: basic study and clinical application', *The Annals of Thoracic Surgery*, 78(5): 1614–23.

Christensen, M. (2002) 'The physiological effects of noise: considerations for intensive care', *Nursing in Critical Care*, 7(6): 300–5.

Chudley, S. (1994) 'The effects of nursing activities on ICP', *British Journal of Nursing*, 3(9): 454–9.

Chychula, N.M. and Sciamanna, C. (2002) 'Help substance abusers attain and sustain abstinence', *The Nurse Practitioner*, 27(11): 30–47.

Clarke, C. and Harrison, D. (2001) 'The needs of children visiting on adult intensive care units: a review of the literature and recommendations for practice', *Journal of Advanced Nursing*, 34(1): 61–8.

Clarke, C.M. (2000) 'Children visiting family and friends on adult intensive care units: the nurse's perspective', *Journal of Advanced Nursing*, 31(2): 330–8.

Clarke, G. (1993) 'Mouthcare and the hospitalised patient', *British Journal of Nursing*, 2(4): 225–7.

CLASP Collaborative Group (1994) 'CLASP: a randomised trial of low-dose aspirin for the prevention and treatment of pre-eclampsia among 9364 pregnant women', *Lancet*, 343(8898): 619–29.

Clay, A.S., Behina, M. and Brown, K.K. (2001) 'Mitochondrial disease', *Chest*, 120(2): 634–48.

Clay, H.D. (2000) 'Validity and reliability of the SjO2 catheter in neurologically impaired patients: a critical review of the literature', *Journal of Neuroscience Nursing*, 32(4): 194–203.

Clay, M. (2002) 'Assessing oral health in older people', *Nursing Older People*, 14(8): 31–2.

Clifton, G.L., Miller, E.R., Choi, S.C., Levin, H.S., McCauley, S., Smith, K.R. Jr, Muizelaar, P., Wagner, F.C., Marion, D.W., Luerssen, T.G., Chesnut, R.M. and Schwartz, M. (2001) 'Lack of effect of induction of hypothermia after acute brain injury', *New England Journal of Medicine*, 344(8): 556–63.

Clopidogrel in Unstable Angina to Prevent Recurrent Events Trial Investigators (2001) 'Effects of Clopidogrel in addition to aspirin in patients with acute coronary syndromes without ST-segment elevation', *New England Journal of Medicinem*, 345(7): 494–502.

Cochrane Injuries Group Albumin Reviewers (1998) 'Human albumin in critically ill patients: systemic review of randomised control trials', *BMJ*, 317(7153): 235–40.

Cohen, A.T. and Kelly, D.R. (1987) 'Assessment of alfentanil by intravenous infusion as a long-term sedation in intensive care', *Anaesthesia*, 45(5): 545–8.

Cohen, J., Brun-Buisson, C., Torres, A. and Jorgensen, J. (2004) 'Diagnosis of infection in sepsis: an evidence-based review', *Critical Care Medicine*, 32(11): S466–94.

Cole, L., Bellomo, R., Baldwin, I., Hayhoe, M. and Ronco, C. (2003) 'The impact of lactate-buffered high-volume hemofiltration on acid-base balance', *Intensive Care Medicine*, 29(7): 1113–20.

Collin, C. and Daly, G. (1998) 'Brain injury', in Stokes, M. (ed.) *Neurological Physiology*, London: Mosby.

Collins, B.H. (2003) 'Organ transplantation', *Annals of Surgery*, 238(6): S72–89.

Combe, D. (2005) 'The use of patient diaries in an intensive care unit', *Nursing in Critical Care*, 10(1): 31–4.

Comfort, A. (1977) *A Good Age*, London: Mitchell Beazey.

Conaway, D.G., House, J., Bandt, K., Hayden, L., Borkon, A.M. and Spertus, J.A. (2003) 'The elderly: heath status benefits and recovery of function one year after coronary artery bypass surgery, *Journal of the American College of Cardiology*, 42(8): 1421–6.

Conrad, S.A., Zwischenberger, J.B., Grier, L.R., Alparo, S.K. and Bidani, A. (2001) 'Total extracorporeal arteriovenous carbon dioxide removal in acute respiratory failure: a phase 1 clinical study', *Intensive Care Medicine*, 27(8): 1340–51.

Conti, G., Antonelli, M., Navalesi, P., Rocco, M., Bufi, M., Spadetta, G. and Meduri, G.U. (2002) 'Noninvasive vs conventional mechanical ventilation in patients with chronic obstructive pulmonary disease after failure of medical treatment in the ward: a randomized trial', *Intensive Care Medicine*, 28(12): 1701–7.

Cook, A. (1995) 'Ecstasy (MDMA): alerting users to the dangers', *Nursing Times*, 91(16): 32–3.

Cook, D., Guyatt, G., Marshall, J., Leasa, D., Fuller, H., Hall, R., Peters, S., Rutledge, F., Griffith, L., McLellan, A., Wood, G. and Kirby, A. (1998) 'A comparison of sucralfate and ranitidine for the prevention of upper gastrointestinal bleeding in patients requiring mechanical ventilation', *New England Journal of Medicine*, 338(12): 791–7.

Cook, M., Hale, C. and Watson, B. (1999) 'Interrater reliability and the assessment of pressure-sore risk using an adapted Waterlow Scale', *Clinical Effectiveness in Nursing*, 3(2): 66–77.

Cook, S. and Palma, O. (1989) 'Diprivan as the sole sedative agent for prolonged infusion in intensive care', *Journal of Drug Development*, 2(supplement 2): 65–7.

Coombs, M. (2001) 'Making sense of arterial blood gases', *Nursing Times*, 97(27): 36–8.

Cooper, A.B., Ferguson, N.D., Hanly, P.J., Meade, M.O., Kachura, J.R., Granton, J.T., Slutsky, A.S. and Stewart, T.E. (1999) 'Long-term follow-up of survivors of acute lung injury: lack of effect of a ventilation strategy to prevent barotrauma', *Critical Care Medicine*, 27(12): 2616–21.

Cooper, D.J. (2003) 'Lactic acidosis', in Bersten, A.D. and Soni, N. (eds) *Intensive Care Manual*, 5th edn, Edinburgh: Butterworth-Heinemann, 107–11.

Cooper, N. and Cramp, P. (2003) *Essential Guide to Acute Care*, London: BMJ Books.

Cooper, S.J. (2004) 'Methods to prevent ventilator-associated lung injury: a summary', *Intensive and Critical Care Nursing*, 20(6): 358–65.

Copson, D. (2003) 'Topical negative pressure and necrotising fasciitis', *Nursing Standard*, 18(6): 71–80.

Corley, D.A., Cello, J.P., Adkisson, W., Ko, W.-F. and Kerlikowske, K. (2001) 'Octreotide for acute esophageal variceal bleeding: a meta-analysis', *Gastroenterology*, 120(4): 946–54.

Corne, J., Carroll, M., Brown, I. and Delany, D. (2002) *Chest X-Ray Made Easy*, 2nd edn, Edinburgh: Churchill Livingstone.

Cotter, G., Kaluski, E., Milo, O., Blatt, A., Salah, A., Hendler, A., Krakover, R., Golick, A. and Vered, Z. (2003) 'LINCS: L-NAME (a NO synthase inhibitor) in the treatment of refractory cardiogenic shock', *European Heart Journal*, 24(14): 1287–95.

Cotter, G., Moshkovitz, Y., Kaluski, E., Cohen, A.J., Miller, H., Goor, D. and Vered, Z. (2004) 'Accurate, noninvasive continuous monitoring of cardiac output by whole-body electrical bioimpedance', *Chest*, 125(4): 1431–40.

Cottle, S. (1997) 'Nurse's under-medication of analgesia in cardiac surgical patients: a personal exploration', *Nursing in Critical Care*, 2(3): 146–9.

Covinsky, K.E., Wu, A.W., Landefeld, C.S., Connors, A.F., Phillips, R.S., Tsevat, J., Dawson, N.V., Lynn, J. and Fortinsky, R.H. (1999) 'Heath status versus quality of life in older patients: does the distinction matter?' *American Journal of Medicine*, 106(4): 435–40.

Cox, W. (2002) 'Cardiac transplantation', in Hatchett, R. and Thompson, D. (eds) *Cardiac Nursing: A Comprehensive Guide*, Edinburgh: Churchill Livingstone, 462–80.

Craid, J.V., Lancaster, G.A., Taylor, S., Williamson, P.R. and Smyth, R. (2002) 'Infrared ear thermometry compared with rectal thermometry in children: a systematic review', *Lancet*, 360(9333): 603–9.

Crandall, C.G., Vongpatanasin, W. and Victor, R.G. (2002) 'Mechanism of cocaine-induced hyperthermia in humans', *Annals of Internal Medicine*, 136(11): 785–91.

Cree, C. (2003) 'Acquired brain injury: acute management', *Nursing Standard*, 18(11): 45–54.

Creteur, J., Sibbald, W. and Vincent, J.-L. (2000) 'Hemoglobin solutions – not just red blood cell substitutes', *Critical Care Medicine*, 28(8): 3025–34.

Cruickshank, J.M. (2000) 'Beta-blockers continue to surprise us', *European Heart Journalm*, 21(5): 354–64.

Cubbin, B. and Jackson, C. (1991) 'Trial of a pressure area risk calculator for intensive care patients', *Intensive Care Nursing*, 7(1): 40–4.

Curry, S. (1995) 'Identifying family needs and stresses in the intensive care unit', *British Journal of Nursing*. 4(1): 15–21.

Curtis, J.R. (1998) 'The "patient-centered" outcomes of critical care: what are they and how should they be used?' *New Horizons*, 6(1): 26–32.

Daffurn, K., Bishop, G.F., Hillman, K.M. and Bauman, A. (1994) 'Problems following discharge after intensive care', *Intensive and Critical Care Nursing*, 10(4): 244–51.

Dakin, J., Kourteli, E. and Winter, R. (2003) *Making Sense of Lung Function Tests*, London: Arnold.

Daley, R.J., Rebuck, J.A., Welage, L.S. and Rogers, F.B. (2004) 'Prevention of stress ulceration: Current trends in critical care', *Critical Care Medicine*, 32(10): 2008–13.

Dallmeyer, R. (2000) 'Pharmacological support in paediatric intensive care', in Williams, C. and Asquith, J. (eds) *Paediatric Intensive Care Nursing*, Edinburgh: Churchill Livingstone, 395–418.

Daly, K., Beale, R. and Chang, R.W.S. (2001) 'Reduction in mortality after inappropriate early discharge from intensive care unit: logistic regression triage model', *BMJ*, 322(7297): 1274–16.

Dang, D., Johantgen, M.E., Pronovost, P.J., Jenckes, M. and Bass, E. (2002) 'Postoperative complications: does intensive care unit staff nursing make a difference?' *Heart & Lung*, 31(3): 219–28.

Daniels, L. (2002) 'Diet and coronary heart disease', *Nursing Standard*, 16(43): 47–52.

Danis, M. (1998) 'Improving end-of-life care in the intensive care unit: what's to be learned from outcomes research?' *New Horizons*, 6(1): 110–18.

Danter, J.H. (2003) 'Geriatric assessment', *Nursing2003*, 33(12): 52–4.

Dardaine, V., Dequin, P.-F., Ripault, H., Constans, T. and Ginies, G. (2001) 'Outcome of older patients requiring ventilatory support in intensive care: impact of nutritional status', *Journal of the American Geriatrics Society*, 49(5): 564–70.

Dark, P.M. and Singer, M. (2004) 'The validity of trans-esophageal doppler ultrasonography as a measure of cardiac output in critically ill adults', *Intensive Care Medicine*, 30(11): 2060–6.

Darovic, G.O. (2002a) 'Physical assessment of the pulmonary system', in Darovic, G.O. (ed.)

*Hemodynamic Monitoring: Invasive and Noninvasive Clinical Application*, 3rd edn, Philadelphia, PA: W.B. Saunders, 43–56.

—— (2002b) 'Arterial pressure monitoring', in Darovic G.O. (ed.) *Hemodynamic Monitoring: Invasive and Noninvasive Clinical Application*, 3rd edn, Philadelphia, PA: W.B. Saunders, 133–60.

Darovic, G.O. and Simonelli, R. (2003) 'Pharmacologic influences on hemodynamic parameters', in Darovic, G.O. (ed.) *Hemodynamic Monitoring: Invasive and Noninvasive Clinical Application*, 3rd edn, Philadelphia, PA: W.B. Saunders Company, 305–45.

Dasgupta, A., Rice, R., Mascha, E., Litaker, D. and Stoller, J.K. (1999) 'Four-year experience with a unit for long-term ventilation (respiratory special care unit) at the Cleveland Clinic Foundation', *Chest*, 116(2): 447–55.

David, M., Weiler, N., Neinrichs, W., Neumann, M., Joost, T., Markstaller, K. and Eberle, B. (2003) 'High-frequency oscillatory ventilation in adult acute respiratory distress syndrome', *Intensive Care Medicine*, 29(10): 1656–65.

Davidhizer, R. and Giger, J.N. (1997) 'When touch is not the best approach', *Journal of Clinical Nursing*, 6(3): 203–6.

Davidhizer, R.E., Poole, V.L. and Giger, J.N. (1995) 'What nurses need to know about sleep', *Journal of Nursing Science*, 1(1/2): 61–7.

Davidson, M.H. (2004) 'Introduction. A Symposium: emerging strategies for the prevention and treatment of atherosclerosis in patients with type 2 diabetes mellitus and the metabolic syndrome', *American Journal of Cardiology*, 93(11): 1C.

Davies, J.H. and Hassell, L.L. (2001) *Children in Intensive Care*, Edinburgh: Churchill Livingstone.

Davis, J.A., Brown, A.T., Alshafie, T., Poirier, L.A., Cruz, C.P., Wang, Y., Eidt, J.F. and Moursi, M.M. (2004) 'Saratin (an inhibitor of platelet-collagen interaction) decreases platelet aggregation and homocysteine-mediated postcarotid endarterectomy intimal hyperplasia in a dose-dependent manner', *American Journal of Surgery*, 188(6): 778–85.

Dawson, D. (2000) 'Neurological care', in Sheppard, M. and Wright, M. (eds) *High Dependency Nursing*, London: Baillière Tindall, 145–82.

—— (2005) 'Development of a new eye care guideline for critically ill patients', *Intensive and Critical Care Nursing*, 21(2): 118–22.

Dawson, M. and Edbrooke, D.L. (2000) 'Troponin assays: are they a useful tool?' *Care of the Critically Ill*, 16(6): 196–7.

De Beauvoir, S. (1970) *Old Age*, London: Penguin.

De Beaux, I., Chapman, M., Fraser, R., Finnis, M., De Keulenaer, B., Liberalli, D. and Satanek, M., (2001) 'Enteral nutrition in the critically ill: a prospective survey in an Australian intensive care unit', *Anaesthesia and Intensive Care*, 29(6): 619–22.

de Castro, F.R. and Torres, A. (2003) 'Optimizing treatment outcomes in severe community-acquired pneumonia', *American Journal of Respiratory Medicine*, 2(1): 39–54.

De Jonghe, B., Cook, D., Appere-De-Vecchi, C., Guyatt, G., Meade, M. and Outin, H. (2000) 'Using and understanding sedation scoring systems: a systematic review', *Intensive Care Medicine*, 26(3): 275–85.

Dean, B. (1997) 'Evidence based suction management in accident and emergency – a vital component of airway care', *Accident and Emergency Nursing*, 5(2): 92–7.

Deby-Dupont, G. and Lamy, M. (1999) 'Pathophysiology of acute respiratory distress syndrome and acute lung injury', in Webb, A.R., Shapiro, M. Singer, M. and Suter, P.M. (eds) *Oxford Textbook of Critical Care*, Oxford: Oxford University Press, 54–9.

Deem, S. Lee, C.M. and Curtis, J.R. (2003) 'Acquired neuromuscular disorders in the intensive care unit', *American Journal of Respiratory & Critical Care Medicine*, 168(7): 735–9.

Deighan, C.J., Wong, K.M., McLaughlin, K.M. and Harden, P. (2000) 'Rhadomyolysis and acute renal failure resulting from alcohol and drug abuse', *QJM*, 93(1): 29–33.

Dellinger, R.P. (2003) 'Cardiovascular management of septic shock', *Critical Care Medicine*, 31(3): 946–55.

Dellinger, R.P., Carlet, J.M., Masur, H., Gerlach, H., Calandra, T., Cohen, J., Gea-Banacloche, J., Keh, D., Marshall, J.C., Parker, M.M., Ramsay, G., Zimmerman, J.L., Vincent, J.-L. and Levy, M.M. (2004) 'Surviving sepsis campaign guidelines for management of severe sepsis and septic shock', *Intensive Care Medicine*, 30(3): 536–55.

Dennesen, P., van der Ven, A., Vlasveld, M., Lokker, L., Ramsay, G., Kessels, A., van den Keijbus, P., van Nieuw Amerongen, A. and Veerman, E. (2003) 'Inadequate salivary flow and poor oral mucosal status in intubated intensive care patients', *Critical Care Medicine*, 31(3): 781–6.

Deogaonkar, A., Gupta, R., DeGeorgia, M., Sabharwal, V., Gopakumaran, B., Schubert, A. and Provencio, J.J. (2004) 'Bispectral index monitoring correlates with sedation scales in brain-injured patients', *Critical Care Medicine*, 32(12): 2403–6.

Depasse, B., Pauwels, D., Somers, Y. and Vincent, J.-L. (1998) 'A profile of European ICU nursing', *Intensive Care Medicine*, 24(9): 939–45.

Derak, S., Mehta, S., Stewart, T.E., Smith, T., Rodgers, M., Buchman, T.G., Carlin, B., Lowson, S., Granton, J. and Multicenter Oscillatory Ventilation for Acute Respiratory Distress Syndrome Trial (MOAT) Study Investigators (2002) 'High-frequency oscillatory ventilation for acute respiratory distress syndrome in adults', *American Journal of Respiratory and Critical Care Medicine*, 166(6): 801–8.

Deroy, R. (2000) 'Crystalloids or colloids for fluid resuscitation – is that the question?' *Current Anaesthesia and Critical Care*, 11(1): 20–6.

Detriche, O., Berre, J., Massaut, J. and Vincent, J.-L. (1999) 'The Brussels sedation scale: use of a simple clinical sedation scale can avoid excessive sedation in patients undergoing mechanical ventilation in the intensive care unit', *British Journal of Anaesthesia*, 83(5): 698–701.

Devendra, D., Liu, E. and Eisenbarth, G.S. (2004) 'Type 1 diabetes: recent developments', *BMJ*, 328(7442): 750–4.

Devlin, M. (2000) 'The nutritional needs of the older person', *Professional Nurse*, 16(3): 951–5.

DeVriese, A.S., Vanholder, R.C., Pascual, M., Lameire, N.H. and Colardyn, F.A. (1999) 'Can inflammatory cytokines be removed efficiently by continuous renal replacement therapies?', *Intensive Care Medicine*, 25(9): 903–10.

DfEE (Department for Education and Employment) (1998) *The Learning Age: A Renaissance for a New Britain*, London: DfEE.

Dhond, G.R. and Dob, D.P. (2000) 'Critical care of the obstetric patient', *Current Anaesthesia and Critical Care*, 11(2): 86–91.

Di Giantomasso, D., May, C.N. and Bellomo, R. (2002) 'Norepinephrine and vital organ blood flow', *Intensive Care Medicine*, 28(12): 1804–9.

Dickens, J.J. (2004) 'Central venous oxygenation saturation monitoring: a role for critical care?' *Current Anaesthesia & Critical Care*, 15(6): 378–82.

Diehl, C., Hass, J. and Schaefer, K.M. (1994) 'The brain-dead pregnant woman: finding meaning to help care', *Dimensions of Critical Care Nursing*, 13(3): 133–41.

Dietrich, W. (2000) 'Cardiac surgery and the coagulation system', *Current Opinion in Anaethesiology*, 13(1): 27–34.

Dimond, B. (2001) 'Legal aspects of consent 2: the different forms of consent', *British Journal of Nursing*, 10(6): 400–1.

—— (2005) *Legal Aspects of Nursing*, 4th edn, Harlow: Pearson.

Dirkes, S. (1996) 'Liquid ventilation: new frontiers in the treatment of ARDS', *Critical Care Nurse*, 16(3): 53–8.

Dive, A., Foret, F., Jamart, J., Bulpa, P. and Installe, E. (2000) 'Effects of dopamine on gastrointestinal motility during critical illness', *Intensive Care Medicine*, 26(7): 901–7.

Djuretic, T., Herbert, J., Drobniewski, F., Yates, M., Smith, E.G., Magee, J.G., Williams, R., Flanagan, P., Watt, B., Rayner, A., Crowe, M., Chadwick, M.V., Middleton, A.M. and Watson, J.M. (2002) 'Antibiotic resistant tuberculosis in the United Kingdom: 1993–1999', *Thorax*, 57(6): 477–82.

Dodds, C. (2002) 'The physiology of sleep', *Current Anaesthesia and Critical Care*, 13(1): 2–5.

DOH (Department of Health) (1997) *A Bridge to the Future – Nursing Standards, Education and Workforce Planning in Paediatric Intensive Care*, London: HMSO.

—— (1998) *Code of Practice for the Diagnosis of Brain Stem Death*, London: HMSO.

—— (1999) *Saving Lives: Our Healthier Nation*, London: HMSO.

—— (2000a) *Comprehensive Critical Care – A Review of Adult Critical Care Services*, London: DOH.

—— (2000b) *An Organisation with a Memory*, London: DOH.

—— (2000c) *National Service Framework for Coronary Heart Disease*, London: DOH.

—— (2000d) *The NHS Plan*, London: DOH.

—— (2000e) *Health Services Circular HSC 2000/26*, London: DOH.

—— (2001a) *Essence of Care*, London: DOH.

—— (2001b) *National Service Framework for Older People*, London: DOH.

—— (2001c) 'Guidelines for preventing infections associated with the insertion and maintenance of central venous catheters', *Journal of Hospital Infections*, 47(Supplement): S47–67.

—— (2001d) 'Standard principles for preventing hospital-acquired infections', *Journal of Hospital Infections*, 47(Supplement): S21–S37.

—— (2001e) *Reference Guide to Consent for Examination or Treatment*, London: DOH.

—— (2002) *National Service Framework for Diabetes*, London: DOH.

Dohgomori, H., Arikawa, K., Gushiken, T. and Kanmuray, Y. (2002) 'Accuracy of portable infusers under hyperbaric oxygenation conditions', *Anesthesia & Intensive Care*, 30(1): 25–8.

Donaldson, I. (1997) 'Acting with restraint', *Elderly Care*, 9(5): 12–14.

Donnelly, C.A., Ghani, A.C., Leung, G.M., Hedley, A.J., Fraser, C., Riley, S., Abu-Raddad, L.J., Ho, L.-M., Thach, T.-Q., Chau, P., Chan, K.-P., Lam, T.-H., Tse, L.-Y., Tsang, T., Liu, S.-H., Kong, J.H.B., Lau, E.M.C., Ferguson, N.M. and Anderson, R.M. (2003) 'Epidemiological determinants of spread of causal agent of severe acute respiratory syndrome in Hong Kong', *Lancet*, 361(9371): 1761–6.

Doran, M. (2004) 'The presence of family during brain stem death testing', *Intensive and Critical Care Nursing*, 20(2): 87–92.

Dougherty, L. and Lister, S. (eds) (2004) *The Royal Marsden Hospital Manual of Clinical Nursing Procedures*, 6th edn, Oxford: Blackwell Science.

Douketis, J.D., Crowther, M.A., Stanton, E.B. and Ginsberg J.S. (2002) 'Elevated cardiac troponin levels in patients with submassive pulmonary embolus', *Archives of Internal Medicine*, 162(1): 79–81.

Dowding, D., Nimmo, S. and Wisiewski, M. (2002) 'An investigation into the accuracy of different types of thermometers', *Professional Nurse*, 18(3): 166–8.

Doyal, L. (2001) 'Why active euthanasia and physician assisted suicide should be legalised', *BMJ*, 323(7321): 1079–80.

Drakulovic, M.B., Torres, A., Bauer, T.T., Nicholas, J.M., Nogue, S. and Ferrer, M. (1999) 'Supine body position as a risk factor for nosocomial pneumonia in mechanically ventilated patients: a randomised trial', *Lancet*, 354(9193): 1851–8.

Draper, H. and Scott, W. (2004) *Ethics in Anaesthesia and Intensive Care*, Edinburgh: Butterworth-Heinemann.

Drucker, P.F. (1974) *Management*, London: Butterworth-Heinemann.

Druschky, A., Herkert, M., Radespiel-Troger, M., Druschky, K., Hund, E., Becker, C.-M., Hilz, M.J., Erbguth, F. and Neundorfer, B. (2001) 'Critical illness neuropathy: clinical features and cell culture assay of neurotoxicity assessed by a prospective study', *Intensive Care Medicine*, 27(4): 686–93.

D'Souza, A.L., Rajkumar, C., Cooke, J. and Bulpitt, C. (2002) 'Probiotics in the prevention of antibiotic associated diarrhea: meta-analysis', *BMJ*, 324(7350): 1361–6.

Dubé, L. and Granry, J.-C. (2003) 'The therapeutic use of magnesium in anesthesiology, intensive care and emergency medicine: a review', *Canadian Journal of Anesthesia*, 50(7): 732–46.

Dubois, M.J., Bergeron, N., Dumont, M., Dial, S. and Skrobik, Y. (2001) 'Delirium in an intensive care unit: A study of risk factors', *Intensive Care Medicine*, 27(8): 1297–304.

Duncan, A.W. (2003) 'Upper respiratory tract obstruction in children', in Bersten, A.D. and Soni, N. (eds) *Intensive Care Manual*, 5th edn, Edinburgh: Butterworth-Heinemann, 1007–14.

Durward, A. (2002) 'Chloride and the anion gap. A clinical guide to establishing the cause of metabolic acidosis', *International Journal of Intensive Care*, 9(1): 26–31.

Durward, A., Skellett, S., Mayer, A., Taylor, D., Tibby, S.M. and Murdoch, I.A. (2001) 'The value of the chloride: sodium ratio in differentiating the aetiology of metabolic acidosis', *Intensive Care Medicine*, 27(5): 828–35.

Dyer, I.D. (1991) 'Meeting the needs of visitors – a practical approach', *Intensive Care Nursing*, 7(3): 135–47.

Dyer, I. (1995) 'Preventing the ITU syndrome, or how not to torture an ITU patient', *Intensive and Critical Care Nursing*, 11(3): 130–9, 11(4): 223–32.

Eastland, J. (2001) 'A framework for nursing the dying patient in ICU', *Nursing Times*, 97(3): 36–9.

Echols, J., Friedman, B., Mullins, R.F. and Still, J.M. Jr (2004) 'Initial experience with a new system for the control and containment of fecal output for the protection of patients in a large burn centre', *Chest*, 126 (4 supplement): 862S.

Eclampsia Trial Collaborative Group (1995) 'Which anticonvulsant for women with eclampsia? Evidence from the Collaborative Eclampsia', *Lancet*, 345(8963): 1455–63.

Edbrooke, D., Hibbert, C. and Corcoran, M. (1999) *Review for the NHS Executive of Adult Critical Care Services: An International Perspective*, Sheffield: Medical Economics and Research Centre.

Eddleston, J., Macdonald, I. and Littler, C. (1997) 'Withdrawal of sedation in critically ill patients', *British Journal of Intensive Care*, 7(6): 216–22.

Edouard, A.R., Vanhille, E., Le Moigno, S., Benhamou, D. and Mazoit, J.-X. (2005) 'Non-invasive assessment of cerebral perfusion pressure in brain injured patients with moderate intracranial hypertension', *British Journal of Anaesthesia*, 94(2): 216–21.

Edvardsson, J.D., Sandman, P.-O. and Rasmussen, B.H. (2003) 'Meanings of giving touch in the care of older patients: becoming a valuable person and professional', *Journal of Clinical Nursing*, 12(4): 601–9.

Edwards, S. (2001) 'Shock: types, classifications and explorations of their physiological effects', *Emergency Nurse*, 9(2): 29–38.

Eggimann, P. and Pittet, D. (2001) 'Infection control in the ICU', *Chest*, 120(6): 2059–93.

Ekesth, K., Abildgaard, L., Vegfors, M., Berg-Johnsen, J. and Engdahl, O. (2002) 'The *in vitro* effects of crystalloids and colloids on coagulation', *Anaesthesia*, 57(11): 1102–33.

El-Ansary, D., Adams, R., Torns, L. and Elkins, M. (2000a) 'Sternal instability following coronary artery bypass grafting', *Physiotherapy Theory and Practice*, 16(1): 27–33.

El-Ansary, D., Adams, R. and Ghandi, A. (2000b) 'Musculoskeletal and neurological complications following coronary artery bypass graft surgery: a comparison between saphenous vein and internal mammary artery grafting', *Australian Journal of Physiotherapy*, 46(1): 19–25.

Eliopoulos, C. (2001) *Gerontological Nursing*, 5th edn, Philadelphia, PA: Lippincott.

Eliott, P. (2003) 'Rational use of inotropes', *Anaesthesia and Intensive Care*, 4(9): 292–6.

Elliott, T.S.J. and Lambert, P.A. (1999) 'Antibacterial resistance in the intensive care unit: mechanisms and management', *British Medical Bulletin*, 55(1): 259–76.

Elliott, T.S.J., Faroqui, M.H., Armstrong, R.F. and Hanson, G.C. (1994) Guidelines for good practice in central venous catheterization'. *Journal of Hospital Infection*, 28(3): 163–76.

Ellis, A.J., Wendon, J.A., Portmann, B. and Williams, R. (1996) 'Acute liver damage and ecstasy ingestion', *Gut*, 38(3): 454–8.

Ellis, R.F. and Halsall, P.J. (2002) 'Malignant hypothermia', *Anaesthesia & Critical Care*, 3(6): 222–4.

Ely, E.W., Evand, G.W. and Haponik, E.F. (1999) 'Mechanical ventilation in a cohort of elderly patients admitted to an intensive care unit', *Annals of Internal Medicine*, 131(2): 96–104.

Ely, E.M., Gautam, S., Margolin, R., Francis, J., May, L., Speroff, T., Truman, B., Dittus, R., Bernard, G.R. and Inouye, S.K. (2001) 'The impact of delirium in the intensive care unit on hospital length of stay', *Intensive Care Medicine*, 27(12): 1892–900.

Ely, E.M., Meade, M.O., Haponik, E.F., Kollef, M.H., Cook, D.J., Guyatt, G.H. and Stoller, J.K. (2001) 'Mechanical ventilator weaning protocols driven by non-physician health-care professionals: evidence-based clinical practice guidelines', *Chest*, 120(6): 454s–463s.

Ely, E.M., Stephens, R.K., Jackson, J., Thomason, J.W.W., Truman, B., Gordon, S., Dittus, R.S. and Bernard, G.R. (2004) 'Current opinions regarding the importance, diagnosis, and management of delirium in the intensive care unit: a survey of 912 healthcare professionals', *Critical Care Medicine*, 32(1): 106–12.

Emmanuel, E.J., Fairclough, D.L. and Emanuel, L.L. (2000) 'Attitudes and desires related to euthanasia and physician-assisted suicide among terminally ill patients and their caregivers', *JAMA*, 284(19): 2460–8.

Emmerson, A.M. (1997) 'Infection control in hospital and community settings', *Research and Clinical Forums*, 19(6): 19–25.

Endacott, R. (1999) 'Role of the allocated nurse and shift leader in the intensive care unit: findings of an ethnographic study', *Intensive and Critical Care Nursing*, 15(1): 10–18.

Engelhardt, T. and MacLennan, F.M. (1999) Fluid management in pre-eclampsia,' *International Journal of Obstetric Anesthesia*, 8 (4): 253–9.

Epley, D. (2001) 'Carotid artery dissection', *Journal of Vascular Nursing*, 19(1): 2–7.

Erlen, J.A. (2004) 'Wanted – Nurses', *Orthopaedic Nursing*, 23(4): 289–92.

Essposito, K., Nappo, F., Marfella, R., Giugliano, G., Guigliano, F., Ciotola, M., Quagliaro, L., Ceriello, A. and Giugliano, D. (2002) 'Inflammatory cytokine concentrations are acutely increased by hyperglycaemia I humans. Role of oxidative stress', *Circulation*, 106(16): 2067–72.

Esteban, A., Alía, A., Gordo, F., de Pable, R., Suarez, J., Gonález, G. and Blanco, J. (2000) 'Prospective randomized trial comparing pressure-controlled ventilation and volume-controlled ventilation in ARDS', *Chest*, 117(6): 1690–6.

Esteban, A., Anzueto, A., Frustos-Vivar, F., Alía, I., Ely, E.W., Brochard, L., Stewart, T.E., Apezteguía, Tobin, M.J., Nightingale, P., Matamis, D., Pimentel, J. and Abrough, F. (2004) 'Outcome of older patients receiving mechanical ventilation', *Intensive Care Medicine*, 30(4): 639–46.

Etchels, M.C., MacAulay, F., Judson, A., Ashraf, S., Ricketts, I.W., Waller, A., Alm, N., Warden, A., Gordon, B., Brodie, J. and Shearer, A.J. (2003) 'ICU-talk: the development of a computerised communication aid for patients in ICU', *Care of the Critically Ill*, 19(1): 4–9.

Ethics Committee of the Society of Critical Care Medicine (1997) 'Consensus statement of the Society of Critical Care Medicine's Ethics Committee regarding futile and other possible inadvisable treatments', *Critical Care Medicine*, 25(5): 887–91.

European Resuscitation Council (2001) 'Guidelines 2000 for adult and paediatric basic life support and advanced life support', *Resuscitation* 48: 199–239.

Evans, B., Duggan, W., Baker, J., Ramsay, M. and Abiteboul, D. (2001) 'Exposure of healthcare workers in England, Wales and Northern Ireland to bloodborne viruses between July 1997 and June 2000: analysis of surveillance data', *BMJ*, 322(7283): 397–8.

Evans, T.W., Griffiths, M.J.D. and Keogh, B.F. (eds) (2002) *ARDS*, Sheffield: European Respiratory Society Journals Ltd.

Ewing, S. and Torres, A. (2002) 'Prevention and management of ventilator-associated pneumonia', *Current Opinion in Critical Care*, 8(1): 58–69.

Eynon, C.A. and Menon, K.D. (2002) 'Critical care management of head injury', *Anaesthesia & Critical Care*, 3(4): 135–9.

Faist, E. and Kim, C. (1998) 'Therapeutic immunomodulatory approaches for the control of systemic inflammatory response syndrome and the prevention of sepsis', *New Horizons*, 6 (Supplement 2): S97–102.

Falk, R.H. (2001) 'Atrial fibrillation', *New England Journal of Medicine*, 344(14): 1067–77.

Fallah, M.A., Prakah, C. and Edmundowica, S. (2000) 'Acute gastrointestinal bleeding', *Medical Clinics of North America*, 84(5): 1183–208.

Farrar, D. and Grocott, M. (2003) 'Intravenous artificial oxygen carriers', *Hospital Medicine*, 64(6): 352–6.

Farrell, M. (1999) 'The challenge of breaking bad news', *Intensive and Critical Care Nursing*, 15(2): 101–5.

Feil, N. (1993) *The Validation Breakthrough*, Baltimore, MD: Health Professionals Press.

Feldkamp, C.S. (2003) 'Immunological reactions', in Kaplan, L.A., Pesce, A.J. and Kazmierczak, S.C. (eds) (2003) *Clinical Chemistry: Theory, Analysis, Correction*, 4th edn, St Louis: Mosby, 216–45.

Feldt, K. (2000) 'The checklist of non-verbal pain indicators', *Pain Management Nursing*, 1(1): 13–21.

Fenn, P., Diacon, S., Gray, A., Hodges, R. and Rickman, N. (2000) 'Current cost of medical negligence in NHS hospitals: analysis of claims database', *BMJ*, 320(7249): 1567–71.

Ferguson, J., Gilroy, D. and Puntillo, K. (1997) 'Dimensions of pain and analgesic administration associated with coronary artery bypass grafting in an Australian intensive care unit', *Journal of Advanced Nursing*, 26(6): 1065–72.

Ferrer, M., Esquinas, A., Arancibia, F., Bauer, T.T., Gonzalez, G., Carillo, A., Rodriguez-Rosin, R. and Torres, A. (2003) 'Noninvasive ventilation during persistent weaning failure', *American Journal of Respiratory and Critical Care Medicine*, 168(1): 70–6.

Fielden, J.M. (2003) 'Sepsis', *Anaesthesia and Intensive Care*, 4(5): 141–3.

File, T.M. Jr and Tsang, K.W.T. (2005) 'Severe acute respiratory syndrome', *Treatments in Respiratory Medicine*, 4(2): 95–106.

Finlay, I. and Dallimore, D. (1991) 'Your child is dead', *BMJ*, 302(6791): 1524–5.

Finnell, J.T. and Harris, C.R. (2000) 'Cardiovascular toxicity of selected drug overdoses', *Topics in Emergency Medicine*, 22(1): 29–41.

Firmin, R.K., and Killer, H.M. (1999) 'Extracorporeal membrane oxygenation,' *Perfusion*, 14(4): 291–7.

Firth, M. and Prather, C.M. (2002) 'Gastrointestinal motility problems in the elderly patient', *Gastroenterology*, 122(6): 1688–1700.

Firth-Cozens, J. (2001) 'Cultures for improving patient safety through learning: the role of teamwork', *Quality in Health Care*, 10(Supplement II): ii26–ii31.

Firth-Cozens, J. and Mowbray, D. (2001) 'Leadership and the quality of care', *Quality in Health Care*, 10(Supplement II): ii3–ii7.

Fisher, S., Walsh, G. and Cross, N. (2002) 'Nursing management of the cardiac surgical patient', in Hatchett, R. and Thompson, D. (eds) *Cardiac Nursing: A Comprehensive Guide*, Edinburgh: Churchill Livingstone, 426–61.

Fitzpatrick, J. (2000) 'Oral health care needs of dependent older people', *Journal of Advanced Nursing*, 32(6): 1325–32.

Fogarty, A. and Lingford-Hughes, A. (2004) 'Addiction and substance misuse', *Medicine*, 32(7): 29–33.

Folwer, R.A., Lapinsky, S.E., Hallett, D., Detsky, A.S., Sibbald, W.J., Slutsky, A.S., Stewart, T.E. and Toronto SARS Critical Care Group (2003) 'Critically ill patients with severe acute respiratory syndrome', *JAMA*, 290(3): 367–73.

Forbes, N. and Rankin, N. (2001) 'Necrotizing fasciitis and non-steroidal anti-inflammatory drugs: a case series and review of the literature', *New Zealand Journal of Medicine*, 114(1124): 3–6.

Forsythe, S.M. and Schmidt, G.A. (2000) 'Sodium bicarbonate for the treatment of lactic acidosis', *Chest*, 117(1): 260–7.

Fort, P., Farmer, C., Westerman, J., Johannigman, J., Beninati, W., Dolan, S. and Derdak, S. (1997) 'High frequency oscillatory ventilation for adult respiratory distress syndrome – a pilot study', *Critical Care Medicine*, 25(6): 937–47.

Foulkes, A. (2001) 'CHD', *Geriatric Medicine*, 31(4): 29–34.

Fourcade, O., Simon, M.-F., Litt, L., Samii, K. and Chap, H. (2004) 'Propofol inhibits human platelet aggregation induced by proinflammatory lipid mediators', *Anesthesia & Analgesia*, 99(2): 393–8.

Fourrier, F., (2004) 'Recombinant human activated protein C in the treatment of severe sepsis: an evidence-based review', *Critical Care Medicine*, 32(11): S534–S541.

Fourrier, F., Cau-Pottier, E., Boutigny, H., Roussel-Delvallez, M., Jourdain, M. and Chopin, C. (2000) 'Effects of dental plaque antiseptic decontamination on bacterial colonization and nosocomial infections in critically ill patients', *Intensive Care Medicine*, 26(9): 1239–47.

Fox, N. (2002) 'Pulse oximetry', *Nursing Times*, 98(40): 65.

Frazier, S.K. (1999) 'Neurohormonal responses during positive pressure mechanical ventilation, *Heart & Lung*, 28(3): 149–65.

Freeman, B.D., Isabellaa, K., Lin, N. and Buchman, T.G. (2000) 'A meta-analysis of prospective trials comparing percutaneous and surgical tracheostomy in critically ill patients', *Chest*, 118(5): 1412–18.

Freeman, J.W. (1998) 'Solvent detergent treated plasma, viral safety and clinical experience', *British Journal of Intensive Care*, 8(5): 172–5.

Frewin, R., Henson, A. and Provan, D. (1998) 'Haematological emergencies', in Provan, D. and Henson, A. (eds) *ABC of Clinical Haematology*, London: BMJ Publishing Group.

Frid, I., Bergbom-Engberg, I. and Haljamae, H. (1998) 'Brain death in ICUs and associated nursing care challenges concerning patients and families', *Intensive and Critical Care Nursing*, 14(1): 21–9.

Friedman, A.L. (1992) 'Acute renal disease', in Fuhrman, B.P. and Zimmerman, J.J. (eds) *Pediatric Critical Care*, St Louis: Mosby, 723–39.

Frisk, U. and Nordström, G. (2003) 'Patients' sleep in an intensive care unit – patients' and nurses' perceptions', *Intensive and Critical Care Nursing*, 19(6): 342–9.

Fujita, M. and Tambara, K. (2004) 'Recent insights into human coronary collateral development', *Heart*, 90(3): 246–54.

Fulbrook, P. (1997) 'Core body temperature measurement: a comparison of axilla, tympanic membrane and pulmonary artery blood temperature', *Intensive and Critical Care Nursing*, 13(5): 266–72.

Funk, G.-C., Doberer, D., Heinze, G., Madl, C., Holzinger, U. and Scchneeweiss, B. (2004) 'Changes of serum chloride and metabolic acid-base state in critical illness', *Anaesthesia*, 59(11): 1111–15.

Furr, L.A., Binkley, C.J., McCurren, C. and Carrico, R. (2004) 'Factors affecting quality of oral care in intensive care units', *Journal of Advanced Nursing*, 48(5): 454–62.

Gacouin, A., Le Tulzo, Y., Lavoue, S., Camus, C., Hoff, J., Bassen, R., Arvieux, C., Heurtin, C. and Thomas, R. (2002) 'Severe pneumonia due to Legionella pneumophila: prognostic factors, impact of delayed appropriate antimicrobial therapy', *Intensive Care Medicine*, 28(6): 686–91.

Gagné, R.M. (1975) *Essentials of Learning for Instruction*, New York: Holt, Reinhart & Winston.

—— (1985) *The Condition of Learning and Theory Instruction*, London: Holt, Reinhart & Winston.

Galley, H.F. and Webster, N.R. (2004) 'Physiology of the endothelium', *British Journal of Anaesthesia*, 93(1): 105–11.

Ganong, W.F. (2003) *Review of Medical Physiology*, 21st edn, New York: Lange Medical Books.

Garner, A. and Sibthorpe, B. (2002) 'Will he get back to normal? Survival and functional status after intensive care therapy', *Intensive and Critical Care Nursing*, 18(33): 138–45.

Garretson, S. (2005) 'Haemodynamic monitoring: arterial catheters', *Nursing Standard*, 19(31): 55–64.

Gattinoni, L., Bombino, M., Pelosi, P. Lissoni A, Pesenti A, Fumagalli R, Tagliabue M. (1994) 'Lung structure and function in different stages of severe adult respiratory distress syndrome', *JAMA*, 271(22): 1772–9.

Gattinoni, L., Presenti, A., Bombino, M., Pelosi, P. and Brazzi, L. (1993) 'Role of extracorporeal circulation in adult respiratory distress syndrome management', *New Horizons*, 1(4): 603–12.

Geary, M. (1997) 'The HELLP syndrome', *British Journal of Obstetrics & Gynaecology*, 104(8): 887–91.

Gelling, L. and Provest, T. (1999) 'The needs of relatives of critically ill patients admitted to a neuroscience critical care unit: a comparison of the perceptions of relatives, nurses and doctors', *Care of the Critically Ill*, 15(2): 53–8.

Germon, T.J., Kane, N.M., Manara, A.R. and Nelson, R.J. (1994) 'Near infrared spectroscopy in adults: effects of extracranial ischaemia and intracranial hypoxia on estimation of cerebral oxygenation', *British Journal of Anaesthesia*, 73(4): 503–6.

Ghajar, J. (2000) 'Traumatic brain injury', *Lancet*, 356(9233): 923–9.

Ghiassi, S., Sun, Y.-S., Kim, V.B., Scott, C.M., Nifong, W., Rotondo, M.F. and Chitwood, R. Jr (2004) 'Methylene blue enhancement of resuscitation after refractory hemorrhagic shock', *The Journal of Trauma, Injury, Infection and Critical Care*, 57(3): 515–21.

Ghosh, I.R., Kennedy, D.D., Fletcher, S.N., Mishra, V.P., Coakley, J.H. and Hinds, C.J. (2001) 'Identical persisting neurophysiological features of chronic denervation found in four cases of resolved critical illness motor syndrome', *Clinical Intensive Care*, 12(5,6): 229–36.

Ghost, S., Watts, D. and Kinnear, M. (2002) 'Management of gastrointestinal haemorrhage', *Postgraduate Medical Journal*, 78(915): 4–14.

Ghuran, A. and Nolan, J. (2000) 'Recreational drug misuse: issues for the cardiologist', *Heart*, 83(6): 627–33.

Gill, J.K., Greene, L., Miller, R., Pozniak, A., Cartledge, J., Misher, M., Nelson, M.R. and Soni, N. (1999) 'ICU admission in patients infected with the human immunodeficiency virus – a multicentre survey', *Anaesthesia*, 54(8): 727–32.

Gill, P. (2000) 'Brain stem death – an anthropological perspective', *Care of the Critically Ill*, 16(6): 217–20.

Gimson, A.E.S., Ramage, J.K., Panos, M.Z., Hayllar, K., Harrison, P., Williams, R. and Westaby, D. (1993) 'Randomised control trial of variceal banding ligation versus injection sclerotherapy for bleeding oesophageal varices', *Lancet*, 342(8868): 391–4.

Girault, C., Breton, L., Richard, J.-C., Tamion, F., Vandelet, P., Aboab, J., Leroy, J. and Bonmarchand, G. (2003) 'Mechanical effects of airway humidification devices is difficult to wean patients', *Critical Care Medicine*, 31: 1306–11.

Girou, E. (2003) 'Prevention of nosocomial infections in acute respiratory failure patients', *European Respiratory Journal*, 22(Supplement 42): 72s–76s.

Girou, E., Loyeau, S., Legrand, P., Oppein, F. and Brun-Buisson, C. (2002) 'Efficacy of handrubbing with alcohol based solution versus standard handwashing with antiseptic soap: randomised clinical trial', *BMJ*, 325(7360): 362–5.

Glasby, M.A. and Myles, L.M. (2000) 'Applied physiology of the CNS', *Surgery*, 18(9): iii–vi.

Glaspole, I.N. and Williams, T.J. (1999) 'Lung transplantation', *Medicine*, 27(11): 146–8.

Goddard, M.J., Foweraker, J.E. and Wallwork, J. (2000) 'Xenotransplantation – 2000', *Journal of Clinical Pathology*, 53(1): 44–8.

Goffman, E. (1963) *Stigma*, London: Penguin.

Goh, J. and Gupta, A.K. (2002) 'The management of head injury and intracranial pressure', *Current Anaesthesia & Critical Care*, 13(3): 129–37.

Goldfrad, C. and Rowan, K. (2000) 'Consequences of discharges from intensive care at night', *Lancet*, 355(9210): 1138–42.

Goldhill, D.R. and Sumner, A. (1998) 'Outcome of intensive care patients in a group of British intensive care units', *Critical Care Medicine*, 26(8): 1337–45.

Goodwin, A.T. and Dunning, J.J. (2000) 'Coronary artery surgery', *Surgery*, 18(11): 273–6.

Gordon, L. (1999) 'The sepsis continuum from systemic inflammatory response syndrome to multiple organ dysfunction syndrome', *Nursing in Critical Care*, 4(5): 238–44.

Gotto, A.M. (2001) 'Statin therapy: where are we? Where do we go next?' *American Journal of Cardiology*, 87(Supplement): 13B–18B.

Gould, D. (2003) 'Legionnaire's disease', *Nursing Standard*, 17(45): 41–4.

Granberg, A., Enberg, I.B. and Lundberg, D. (1996) 'Intensive care syndrome: a literature review', *Intensive and Critical Care Nursing*, 12(3): 173–82.

Gravereaux, E.C., Faries, P.L., Burks, J.A., Latessa, V.R., Spielvogel, D., Hollier, L.H. and Marin, M.L. (2002) 'Risk of spinal cord ischemia after endograft of thoracic aortic aneurysms', *Journal of Vascular Surgery*, 34(6): 997–1003.

Grebenik, C.R. and Sinclair, M.E. (2003) 'Which inotrope?', *Current Paediatrics*, 13(1): 6–11.

Grech, E.D., Jackson, M.J. and Ramsdale, D.R. (1995) 'Reperfusion injury after acute myocardial infarction', *BMJ*, 310(6978): 477–8.

Green, C. (2003) 'DIC and other coagulopathies in the ICU', *Anaesthesia and Intensive Care*, 4(5): 147–9.

Greenough, A. (1996) 'Liquid ventilation', *Care of the Critically Ill*, 12(4): 128–30.

Greenwood, J. (1998) 'Critical care nurse perceptions of family needs', *Heart & Lung*, 20(2): 189–201.

Gries, A., Bode, C., Gross, S., Peter, K., Bohrer, H. and Martin, E. (1999) 'The effect of intravenously administered magnesium on platelet function in patients after cardiac surgery', *Anesthesia & Analgesia*, 88(6): 1213–19.

Griffiths, R.D. and Jones, C. (eds) (2002) *Intensive Care Aftercare*, Oxford: Butterworth-Heinemann.

Grimmer, S. and Mittra, R. (2001) 'An insight into diabetes-associated depression', *Geriatric Medicine*, 31(7): 23–7.

Grubb, B.D. (1998) 'Peripheral and central mechanism of pain', *British Journal of Anaesthesia*, 81(1): 8–11.

Guenter, P.A., Settle, R.G., Perlmutter, S., Marino, P.L., DeSimone, G.A. and Rolandelli, R.H. (1991) 'Tube feeding-related diarrhoea in acutely ill patients', *Journal of Parenteral and Enteral Nutrition*, 15(3): 277–80.

Guerin, C., Gaillard, S., Lemasson, S., Ayzac, L., Girard, R., Beuret, P., Palmier, B., Le, Q.V., Sirodot, M., Rosselli, S., Cadiergue, V., Sainty, J.-M., Barbe, P., Combourieu, E., Debatty, D., Rouffineau, J., Ezineard, E., Millet, O., Guelon, D., Rodriguez, L., Martin, O., Renault, A., Sibille, J.-P. and Kaidomar, M. (2004) 'Effects of systematic prone positioning in hypoemic acute respiratory failure', *JAMA*, 292(19): 2379–87.

Gully, S. (2002) 'Nursing management of necrotising fasciitis', *Nursing Standard*, 16(52): 39–42.

Gunn, J., Grech, E.D., Grossman, D. and Cumberland, D. (2003) 'New developments in percutaneous intervention', *BMJ*, 327(7407): 150–3.

Gunn, T. (1992) *The Man with Night Sweats*, London: Faber.

Gutteridge, G. (2004) 'Crystalloids, colloids, blood products and blood substitutes', *Anaesthesia and Intensive Care Medicine*, 5(2): 42–6.

Guyton, A.C. and Hall, J.E. (2000) *Textbook of Medical Physiology*, 10th edn, Philadelphia, PA: W.B. Saunders.

Guzman, J.A. and Kruse, J.A. (2001) 'Targeting the gut in shock and organ failure', *Clinical Intensive Care*, 12(5,6): 203–9.

Habashi, N.M. (2005) 'Other approaches to open-lung ventilation: airway pressure release ventilation', *Critical Care Medicine*, 33(3): S228–S240.

Haddadin, A.S., Fappiano, S.A. and Lipsett, P.A. (2002) 'Methicillin resistant *Staphylococcus aureus* (MRSA) in

545

the intensive care unit', *Postgraduate Medical Journal*, 78(921): 385–92.

Hadingham, J. (1997) 'Talking about tissue donation', *Professional Nurse*, 12(7): 473.

Hagler, D.A. and Travers, G.A. (1994) 'Endotracheal saline and suction catheters: sources of lower airway contamination', *American Journal of Critical Care*, 3(6): 444–7.

Haider, A.W., Larson, M.G., Franklin, S.S. and Levy, D. (2003) 'Systolic blood pressure, diastolic blood pressure, and pulse pressure as predictors of risk for congestive heart failure in the Framingham study', *Annals of Internal Medicine*, 138(1): 10–16.

Haitsma, J.J. and Lachmann, B. (2002) 'Partial liquid ventilation in acute respiratory distress syndrome', in Evans, T.W., Griffiths, M.J.D. and Keogh, B.F. (eds) *ARDS*, Sheffield: European Respiratory Society Journals Ltd, 208–19.

Haji-Michael, P.G. (2000) 'Antioxidant therapy in the critically ill', *Care of the Critically Ill*, 16(3): 88–92.

Hale, A.S., Moseley, M.J. and Warner, S.C. (2000) 'Treating pancreatitis in the acute care setting', *Dimensions of Critical Care Nursing*, 19(4): 15–21.

Haljamae, H. and Lindgren, S. (2000) 'Fluid therapy: present controversies', in Vincent, J.-L. (ed.) *Yearbook of Intensive Care and Emergency Medicine*, Berlin: Springer, 429–42.

Hall, J.C., Dobb, G., Hall, J., de Sousa, R., Brennan, L. and McCauley, R. (2003) 'A prospective randomized trial of enteral glutamine in critical illness', *Intensive Care Medicine*, 29(10): 1710–16.

Hall, R.L. and Rocker, G.M. (2000) 'End-of-life care in the ICU: treatments provided when life support was or was not withdrawn', *Chest*, 118(5): 1424–30.

Halliday, A., Mansfield, A., Marro, J., Peto, C., Peto, R., Potter, J., Thomas, D. and MRC Asymptomatic Carotid Surgery Trial (ACST) Collaborative Group (2004) 'Prevention of disabling and fatal strokes by successful carotid endarterectomy in patients without recent neurological symptoms: randomised controlled trial', *Lancet*, 363: 1491–502.

Hallworth, D. and McIntyre, A. (2003) 'The transport of critically ill children', *Current Paediatrics*, 13(1): 12–17.

Hambley, H. (1995) 'Coagulation(II) – clinical problems in coagulation disorder', *Care of the Critically Ill*, 11(5): 203–5.

Hammond, F. (1995) 'Involving families in care within the intensive care environment: a descriptive study', *Intensive and Critical Care Nursing*, 11(5): 256–64.

Hampton, J.R. (2003) 'Guidelines – for the obedience of fools and the guidance of wise men?' *Clinical Medicine*, 3(3): 279–84.

—— (2003a) *The ECG made Easy*, 6th edn, Edinburgh: Churchill Livingstone.

—— (2003b) *The ECG in Practice*, 4th edn, Edinburgh: Churchill Livingstone.

—— (2003c) *150 ECG Problems*, 2nd edn, Edinburgh: Churchill Livingstone.

Hanley, M.V., Rudd, T. and Butler, J. (1978) 'What happens to intratracheal saline installations', *American Review of Respiratory Diseases*, 117(Supplement): 124–6.

Harbath, S., Sax, H. and Gastmeier, P. (2003) 'The preventable proportion of nosocomial infections: an overview of published reports', *Journal of Hospital Infection*, 54(4): 258–66.

Harcombe, C. (2004) 'Nursing patients with ARDS in the prone position', *Nursing Standard*, 18(19): 33–9.

Harioka, T., Matsukawa, T., Ozaki, M., Nomura, K., Sone, T., Kakuyama, M. and Toda, H. (2000) ' "Deep-forehead" temperature correlates well with blood temperature', *Canadian Journal of Anaesthesia*, 47(10): 980–3.

Harker, J. (2000) 'Pressure ulcer classification: the Torrence system', *Journal of Wound Care*, 9(6): 275–7.

Harkin, D.W., Barros, A.A.B., McCallion, K., Hoper, M., Halliday, M.I. and Campbell, C.F. (2001) 'Bacterial permeability-increasing protein attenuates systemic inflammation and acute lung injury in porcine lower limb ischaemia reperfusion injury', *Annals of Surgery*, 234(2): 233–44.

Harper, C.R. and Jacobson, T.A. (2001) 'The fats of life. The role of omega-3 fatty acids in the prevention of coronary heart disease', *Archives of Internal Medicine*, 161(18): 2185–92.

Harper, D. (2004) 'Comparing protective measures in Europe', *Health Estate Journal*, 58(7): 55–7.

Harris, A. and Misiewicz, J.J. (2001) 'Management of Helicobacter pylori infection', *BMJ*, 323(7320): 1047–50.

Hart, R.G., Halperin, J.L., Pearce, L.A., Anderson, D.C., Kronmal, R.A., McBride, R., Nasco, E., Sherman, D.G., Talbert, R.L., Marler, J.R. and Stroke Prevention in Atrial Fibrillation Investigators (2003) 'Antithrombotic therapy to prevent stroke in patients with atrial fibrillation: a meta-analysis', *Annals of Internal Medicine*, 138(10): 831–8.

Hartsell, P.A., Frazee, R.C., Harrison, J.B. and Smith, R.W. (1997) 'Early postoperative feeding after elective colorectal surgery', *Archives of Surgery*, 132(5): 518–20.

Hartung, T.K., Schofield, E., Short, A.I., Parr, M.J.A. and Henry, J.A. (2002) 'Hyponatraemic states following 3,4-methylenedioxymethamphetamine (MDMA) "ecstasy") ingestion', *QJM*, 95(7): 431–7.

Harvey, W.R. and Hutton, P. (1999) 'Carbon monoxide: chemistry, role, toxicity and treatment', *Current Anaesthesia and Critical Care*, 10(3): 158–63.

Hatchett, R. and Thompson, D. (eds) (2002) *Cardiac Nursing: A Comprehensive Guide*, Edinburgh: Churchill Livingstone, 3–13.

Hausmann, H., Potapov, E.V., Koster, A., Krabatsch, T., Stein, J., Yeter, R., Kukucka, M., Sodian, R., Kuppe, H. and Hetzer, R. (2004) 'Prognosis after the implantation of an intra-aortic balloon pump in cardiac surgery calculated with a new score', *Circulation*, 106(12): I203–6.

Hawker, F. (2003) 'Hepatic failure', in Bersten, A.D. and Soni, N. (eds) *Intensive Care Manual*, 5th edn, Edinburgh: Butterworth-Heinemann, 431–41.

Hawthorne, J. and Redmond, K. (1998) *Pain: Causes and Management*, Oxford: Blackwell.

Hawton, K., Simkin, S., Deeks, J. Cooper, J., Johnston, A., Waters, K., Arundel, M., Bernal, W., Gunson, B., Hudson, M., Suri, D. and Simpson, K. (2004) 'UK legislation on analgesic packs: before and after study of long term effects on poisonings', *BMJ*, 329(7474): 1076–9.

Hawton, K., Townsend, E., Deeks, J., Appleby, L., Gunnell, D., Bennewith, O. and Cooper, J. (2001) 'Effects of legislation restricting pack size of paracetamol and salicylate on self-poisoning in the United Kingdom: before and after study', *BMJ*, 322(7296): 1203–7.

Hayes, J. and Jones, C. (1995) 'A collaborative approach to oral care during critical illness', *Dental Health*, 34(3): 6–10.

Hayward, J. (1975) *Information – A Prescription Against Pain*, London: Scutari.

Hazinski, M.F. (1998) 'Children in the adult ICU: preparation and practice', *Critical Care Nurse*, 18(6): 82–7.

Hazzard, A. (2002) 'Audit of a psychology service for intensive care', *Nursing in Critical Care*, 7(1): 15–18.

Heals, D. (1993) 'A key to well-being', *Professional Nurse*, 8(6): 391–8.

Heames, R.M., Gill, R.S., Ohri, S.K. and Hett, D.A. (2002) 'Off-pump coronary artery surgery', *Anaesthesia*, 57(7): 676–85.

Heart Protection Study Collaborative Group (2002a) 'MRC/BHF Heart protection. Study of cholesterol lowering with simvastatin in 20 536 high-risk individuals: a randomised placebo-controlled trial', *Lancet*, 360(9326): 7–22.

—— (2002b) 'MRC/BHF Heart protection. Study of antioxidant vitamin supplementation in 20 536 high-risk individuals: a randomised placebo-controlled trial', *Lancet*, 360(9326): 23–33.

Heath, H. and Schofield, I. (eds) (1999) *Healthy Ageing*, London: Mosby.

Heath, H. and Watson, R. (2005) *Older People: Assessment for Health and Social Care*, London: Age Concern.

Heaton, K. (2004) *Understanding Your Bowels*, London: Family Doctor Publications Ltd.

Heaton, K.W., Radvan, J., Cripps, H., Mountford, R.A., Braddon, F.E.M. and Hughes, AO. (1992) 'Defecation frequency and timing, and stool form in the general population: a prospective study', *Gut*, 33(6): 818–24.

Heaton, N.D. and Prachalias, A.A. (1999) 'Principles and current status of liver transplantation', *Surgery*, 17(19th September): 216–19.

Hemmila, M.R., Rowe, S.A., Boules, T.N., Miskulin, J., McGillicuddy, J.W., Schuerer, D.J., Haft, J.W., Swaniker, F., Arbabi, S., Hirschl, R.B. and Bartlett, R.H. (2004) 'Extracorporeal life support for severe acute respiratory distress syndrome in adults', *Annals of Surgery*, 240(4): 595–607.

Henderson, C. and Macdonald, S. (eds) (2004) *Mayes' Midwifery: A Textbook for Midwives*, 13th edn, Edinburgh: Baillière Tindall.

Hendricks-Thomas, J. and Patterson, E. (1995) 'A sharing in critical thought by nursing faculty', *Journal of Advanced Nursing*, 22(3): 594–9.

Henker, R., Rogers, S., Kramer, D.J., Kelso, L., Kerr, M. and Sereika, S. (2001) 'Comparison of fever treatments in the critically ill', *American Journal of Critical Care*, 10(4): 276–80.

Herbert, P.C., Wells, G., Blajchman, M.A., Marshall, J., Martin, C., Pagliarello, G., Tweeddale, M., Schweitzer, I., Yetisir, E. and Transfusion Requirements Investigators for the Canadian Critical Care Trials Group (1999) 'A multicenter random, controlled clinical trial of transfusion requirements in critical care', *New England Journal of Medicine*, 340(6): 409–17.

Herridge, M.S., Cheung, A.M., Tansey, C.M., Matte-Martyn, A., Diaz-Granados, N., Al-Saidi, F., Cooper, A.B., Guest, C.B., Mazer, C.D., Meehta, S., Stewart, T.E., Barr, A., Cook, D., Slutsky, A.S. and Canadian Critical Care Trials Group (2003) 'One-year outcomes in survivors of the Acute Respiratory Distress Syndrome', *NEJM*, 348(8): 683–93.

Hess, D.R. (2002) 'Mechanical ventilation strategies: what's new and what's worth keeping?' *Respiratory Care*, 47(9): 1007–17.

Hett, D.A and Jonas, M.M. (2004) 'Non-invasive cardiac output monitoring', *Intensive and Critical Care Nursing*, 20(2): 103–8.

Hewitt, J. and Jordan, S. (2004) 'Prescription drugs: uses and effects Opioids', *Nursing Standard*, 19(6): insert.

Heyland, D.K. (1998) 'Nutritional support in the critically ill patient', *Critical Care Clinics*, 14(3): 423–40.

Hibbert, C. and Edbrooke, D. (2002) 'Economic outcomes', in Ridley, S. (ed.) *Outcomes in Critical Care*, Oxford: Butterworth-Heinemann, 202–22.

Hickey, J.V. (2003a) 'Intracranial hypertension: theory and management of increased intracranial pressure', in Hickey, J.V. (ed.) *The Clinical Practice of Neurological and Neurosurgical Nursing*, 5th edn, Philadelphia, PA: Lippincott, 285–318.

—— (2003b) 'Craniocerebral trauma', in Hickey, J.V. (ed.) *The Clinical Practice of Neurological and Neurosurgical Nursing*, 5th edn, Philadelphia, PA: Lippincott, 373–406.

—— (2003c) 'Vertebral and spinal cord injuries', in Hickey, J.V. (ed.) *The Clinical Practice of Neurological and Neurosurgical Nursing*, 5th edn, Philadelphia, PA: Lipincott, 407–50.

Hickey, J.V. (ed.) (2003d) *The Clinical Practice of Neurological and Neurosurgical Nursing*, 5th edn, Philadelphia, PA: Lippincott.

Higgins, C. (2000) *Understanding Laboratory Investigations*, London: Blackwell Science.

Higgins, J., Estetter, B., Holland, D., Smith, B. and Derdak, S. (2005) 'High-frequency oscillatory ventilation in adults: respiratory therapy issues', *Critical Care Medicine*, 33(3 supplement): S196–203.

Higgins, P.A. (1998) 'Patient perceptions of fatigue while undergoing long-term mechanical ventilation: incidence and associated factors', *Heart & Lung*, 27(3): 177–83.

Higgs, D. (2004) 'Outreach', in Moore, T. and Woodrow, P. (eds) *High Dependency Nursing Care*, London: Routledge, 368–75.

Hilbert, G. (2003) 'Difficult to wean chronic obstructive pulmonary disease patients: avoid heat and moisture exchangers?', *Critical Care Medicine*, 31(5): 1580–1.

Hillman, K. and Bishop, G. (2004) *Clinical Intensive Care*, 2nd edn, Cambridge: Cambridge University Press.

Hilton, P.J., Taylor, J., Forni, L.G. and Treacher, D.F. (1998) 'Bicarbonate-based haemofiltration in the management of acute renal failure with lactic acidosis', *QJM*, 91(4): 279–83.

Hindiyeh, M. and Carroll, K.C. (2000) 'Laboratory diagnosis of atypical pneumonia', *Seminars in Respiratory Infections*, 15(2): 101–13.

Hinds, C.J. and Watson, D. (1996) *Intensive Care: A Concise Textbook*, 2nd edn, London: W.B. Saunders.

Hingley, M. (2000) 'Gastric tonometry: a useful tool or just another piece of equipment?' *Nursing in Critical Care*, 5(6): 300–3.

Hlatky, M.A., Boothroyd, D.B., Melsop, K.A., Brooks, M.M., Mark, D.B., Pitt, B., Reeder, G.S., Rogers, W.J., Ryan, T.J., Whitlow, P.L. and Wiens, R.D. (2004) 'Medical costs and quality of life 10 to 12 years after randomization to angioplasty or bypass surgery for multivessel coronary artery disease', *Circulation*, 110(14): 1960–6.

Ho, A.M.-H., Lee, A., Karmakar, M.K., Dion, P.W., Chung, D.C. and Contardi, L.H. (2003) 'Heliox vs air–oxygen mixtures for the treatment of patients with acute asthma', *Chest*, 123(3): 882–90.

Hodis, H.N., Mack, W.J., LaBree, L., Mahrer, P.R. and Sevanian, A. (2002) 'Alpha-Tocopherol supplementation in healthy individuals reduces low-density lipoprotein oxidation but not atherosclerosis', *Circulation*, 106(12): 1453–9.

Holden, J., Harrison, L. and Johnson, M. (2002) 'Families, nurses and intensive care patients', *Journal of Clinical Nursing*, 11(2): 140–8.

Hollenberg, S.M., Kavinsky, C.J. and Parrillo, J.E. (1999) 'Cardiogenic shock', *Annals of Internal Medicine*, 131(1): 45–59.

Holloway, T. and Penson, J. (1987) 'Nursing education as social control', *Nurse Education Today*, 7(5): 235–41.

Holm, C., Melcer, B., Horbrand, F., Wörl, H., von Donnersmarck, G.H. and Mühlbauer, W. (2000) 'Intrathoracic blood volume as an endpoint in resuscitation of the severely burned: an observational study of 24 patients', *Journal of Trauma*, 48(4): 728–34.

Holme, I. (2000) 'Lipid lowering in the patient at risk – the next decade of discovery', *British Journal of Cardiology*, 7(4): 223–30.

Holmes, C.L., Walley, K.R., Chittock, D.R., Lehman, T. and Russell, J.A. (2001) 'The effects of vasopressin on haemodynamics and renal function in severe septic shock: a case series', *Intensive Care Medicine*, 27(8): 1416–21.

Holmes, S. (2004) 'Enteral feeding and percutaneous endoscopic gastrostomy', *Nursing Standard*, 18 (20): 41–3.

Holt, S.G. (1999) 'Rhabdomyolysis', in Galley, H.F. (ed.) *Critical Care Focus 1: Renal Failure*, London: BMJ Books, 15–20.

Hon, K.L.E., Leung, C.W., Cheng, W.T.F., Chan, P.K.S., Chu, W.C.W., Kwan, Y.W., Li, A.M., Fong, N.C., Hg, P.C., Chiu, M.C., Li, C.K., Tam, J.S. and Fok, T.F. (2003) 'Clinical presentations and outcome of severe acute respiratory syndrome in children', *Lancet*, 361(9370): 1701–3.

Hopkins, R.O., Weaver, L.K., Pope, D., Collingridge, D., Parkinson, R.B., Chan, K.J. and Prme, J.F. Jr (1999) 'Neuropsychological sequelae and impaired health status in survivors of severe acute respiratory distress syndrome', *American Journal of Respiratory and Critical Care Medicine*, 160(1): 50–6.

Horvath, K.D., Gray, D., Benton, L., Hill, J. and Swanstrom, L.L. (1998) 'Operative outcomes of minimally invasive saphenous vein harvest', *American Journal of Surgery*, 175(5): 391–5.

Hotchkiss, R.S., Tinsley, K.W., Swanson, P.E. and Karl, I.E. (2002) 'Endothelial cell apoptosis in sepsis', *Critical Care Medicine*, 30(5) Supplement: S225–8.

Houghton, A.R. and Gray, D. (2003) *Making Sense of the ECG*, 2nd edn, London: Edward Arnold.

House of Lords Judgement (1993) *Airedaile NHS Trust v Bland(HL)*, 2WLR 317.

Houwing, R., Overgoor, M., Kon, M., Jansen, G., van Asbeck, B.S. and Haalboom, J.R.E. (2000) 'Pressure-induced skin lesions in pigs: reperfusion injury and the effects of vitamin E', *Journal of Wound Care*, 9(1): 36–40.

Howard, A., Zaccagnini, D., Ellis, M., Williams, A., Davies, A.H. and Greenhalgh, R.M. (2004) 'Randomized clinical trial of low molecular weight heparin with thigh-length or knee-length antiembolism stockings for patients undergoing surgery', *British Journal of Surgery*, 91(7): 842–7.

Howard, R.S., Kullmann, D.M. and Hirsch, N.P. (2003) 'Admission to neurological intensive care: who, when and why?' *Neurology in Practice*, 74(Supplement iii): 2–9.

Howdle, S. and Wilkin, T. (2001) 'Type 2 diabetes in children', *Nursing Standard*, 15(18): 38–42.

Howitt, R. (2000) 'Organ donation: is there a need for new legislation', *Professional Nurse*, 15(4): 236–9.

Hu, F.B., Bronner, L., Willett, W.C., Stampfer, M.J., Rexrode, K.M., Albert, C.M., Hunter, D. and Manson, J.E. (2002) 'Fish and Omega-3 fatty acid intake and risk of coronary heart disease in women', *JAMA*, 287(14): 1815–21.

Hubbard, R.E., O'Mahony, M.S., Cross, E., Morgan, A., Hortop, H., Morse, R.E. and Topham, L. (2004) 'The ageing of the population: implications for multidisciplinary care in hospital', *Age & Ageing*, 33(5): 479–82.

Hudsmith, J.G. and Menon, K.D. (2002) 'Neuromuscular disorders: relevance to anaesthesia and intensive care', *Anaesthesia & Critical Care*, 3(5): 169–73.

Hughes, E. (2004) 'Understanding the care of patients with acute pancreatitis', *Nursing Standard*, 18(18): 45–52.

Hughes, M., MacKirdy, F.N., Norrie, J., Grant, I.S. and Scottish Intensive Care Society (2003) 'Acute respiratory distress syndrome: an audit of incidence and outcome in Scottish intensive care units', *Anaesthesia*, 58(9): 838–45.

Humphreys, H. (2001) 'Infection control on the intensive care unit', in Galley, H.F. (ed.) *Critical Care Focus 5: Antibiotic Resistance and Infection Control*, London: BMJ Books, 12–18.

Humphreys, M. (2002) 'Hyperkalaemia: a dangerous electrolyte disturbance', *Connect*, 2(1): 28–30.

Hund, E.F., Fogel, W., Krieger, D., DeGeorgia, M. and Hacke, W. (1996) 'Critical illness polyneuropathy: clinical findings and outcomes of a frequent cause of neuromuscular weaning failure', *Critical Care Medicine*, 24(8): 1328–33.

Hunt, J.O., Hendrata, M.V. and Myles, P.S. (2000) 'Quality of life 12 months after coronary artery bypass graft surgery', *Heart & Lung*, 29(6): 401–11.

Hunt, K., Hallworth, S. and Smith, M. (2001) 'The effect of a rigid collar on intercranial and cerebral perfusion pressures', *Anaesthesia*, 56(6): 511–13.

Hunter, J.J. and Chien, K.R. (1999) 'Signalling pathways for cardiac hypertrophy and failure', *New England Journal of Medicine*, 341(17): 1276–83.

Hunter, J.P. (2002) 'Rhabdomyolysis', *Care of the Critically Ill*, 18(2): 52–5.

Hynes-Gay, P. and MacDonald, R. (2001) 'Using high-frequency oscillatory ventilation to treat adults with acute respiratory distress syndrome', *Critical Care Nurse*, 21(5): 38–47.

ICN (2000) 'Code of ethics for nurses', *International Nursing Review*, 47(1): 138–41.

Idama, T.O. and Lindow, S.W. (1998) 'Magnesium sulphate: a review of clinical pharmacology applied to obstetrics', *British Journal of Obstetrics and Gynaecology*, 105(3): 260–8.

Idell, S. (2003) 'Coagulation, fibrinolysis, and fibrin deposition in acute lung injury', *Critical Care Medicine*, 31(4): S213–20.

Intensive Care Society (2002) *Framework for Financial Management in Intensive Care*, London: Intensive Care Society.

International Council of Nurses (1991) (revision) *Position Statement: Nursing Care of the Elderly*, Geneva: International Council of Nurses.

Isaac, R. and Taylor, B.L. (2003) 'Fever in ICU patients', *Anaesthesia and Intensive Care*, 4(5): 153–5.

Isbister, J.P. (2003) 'Blood transfusion', in Bersten, A.D. and Soni, N. (eds) *Intensive Care Manual*, 5th edn, Edinburgh: Butterworth-Heinemann, 915–26.

Jaber, S., Fodil, R., Carlucci, A., Boussarsar, M., Pigeot, J., Lemair, F., Harf, A., Lofaso, F., Isabey, D. and Brochard, L. (2000) 'Noninvasive ventilation with helium-oxygen in acute exacerbations of chronic obstructive pulmonary disease', *American Journal of Respiratory and Critical Care Medicine*, 161(4): 1191–200.

Jackson, C. (1999) 'The revised Jackson/Cubbin pressure area risk calculator', *Intensive and Critical Care Nursing*, 15(3): 169–75.

Jacobs, L.G. (2003) 'Prophylactic anticoagulation for venous thromboembolic disease in geriatric patients', *Journal of the American Geriatrics Society*, 51(10): 1472–8.

Jacobs, M.J., van Eps, R.G.S., de Jong, D.S., Schurink, G.W.H. and Mochtar, B. (2004) 'Prevention of renal failure in patients undergoing thoracoabdominal aortic aneurysm repair', *Journal of Vascular Surgery*, 40(6): 1067–73.

Jalan, R., Damink, S.W., Deutz, N.E., Lee and A., Hayes, P.C. (1999) 'Moderate hypothermia for uncontrolled intracranial hypertension in acute liver failure', *Lancet*, 354(9185): 1164–8.

Jallali, N. (2003) 'Necrotising fasciitis: its aetiology, diagnosis and management', *Journal of Wound Care*, 12(8): 297–300.

Jansen, M.J., Hendriks, T., Knapen, M.F.C.M., van Kempen, L.C., van der Meer, J.W. and Goris, R.J. (1998) 'Chlorpromazine down-regulates tumor necrosis factor-alpha and attenuates experimental multiple organ dysfunction syndrome in mice', *Critical Care Medicine*, 26(7): 1244–50.

Järvelä, K., Koskinen, M. and Kööbi, T. (2003) 'Effects of hypertonic saline (7.5%) on extracellular fluid volumes in healthy volunteers', *Anaesthesia*, 58(9): 878–81.

Jastremski, C.A. (2000) 'ICU bedside environment', *Critical Care Clinics*, 16(4): 723–34.

Jastremski, C.A. and Harvey, M. (1998) 'Making changes to improve the intensive care unit experience for patients and their families', *New Horizons*, 6(1): 99–109.

Jeffacote, W.J. and Harding, K.G. (2003) 'Diabetic foot ulcers', *Lancet*, 361(9368): 1545–51.

Jefrey, A. (2003) 'Insulin resistance', *Nursing Standard*, 17(32): 47–53.

Jenkins, D.A. (1989) 'Oral care in the ICU: an important nursing role', *Nursing Standard*, 4(7): 24–8.

Jenkins, P.F. (2005) *Making Sense of the Chest X-Ray*, London: Hodder Arnold.

Jensen, L.A., Onyskiw, J.E. and Prasad, N.G.N. (1998) 'Meta-analysis of arterial oxygen saturation monitoring by pulse oximetry in adults', *Heart & Lung*, 27(6): 387–408.

Jensen, L.O., Thayssen, P., Pedersen, K.E., Stender, S. and Torben, H. (2004) 'Regression of coronary atherosclerosis by Simvastatin', *Circulation*, 110(3): 265–70.

Jermitsky, E., Omert, L.A., Dunham, M., Wilberger, J. and Rodriguez, A. (2005) 'The impact of hyperglycemia on patients with severe brain injury', *The Journal of Trauma, Injury, Infection and Critical Care*, 58(1): 47–50.

Jeschke, M.G., Klein, D. and Herndon, D.N. (2003) 'Insulin treatment improves the systemic inflammatory reaction to severe trauma', *Annals of Surgery*, 239(4): 553–60.

Jevon, P. (2003) *ECGs for Nurses*, Oxford: Blackwell.

Jewitt, J. (2002) 'Psycho-affective disorder in intensive care units', *Journal of Clinical Nursing*, 11(5): 575–84.

Jiggins, M. and Talbot, J. (1999) 'Mouth care in PICU', *Paediatric Nursing*, 11(10): 23–6.

Joanna Briggs Institute (2002) 'Eye care for intensive care patients', *Best Practice*, 6(1): 1–6.

John, J.H., Ziebland, S., Yudkin, P., Rose, L.S. and Neil, H.A.W. (2002) 'Effect of fruit and vegetable consumption on plasma antioxidant concentrations and blood pressure: a randomised controlled trial', *Lancet*, 359(9322): 1969–74.

Johns, C. (2005) 'Reflection on the relationship between technology and caring', *Nursing in Critical Care*, 10(3): 150–5.

Johnson, C.D. (1998) 'Severe acute pancreatitis: a continuing challenge for the intensive care team', *British Journal of Intensive Care*, 8(4): 130–7.

Johnson, C.D., Kingsnorth, A.N., Imrie, C.W., McMahon, M.J., Neoptolemos, J.P., McKay, C., Toh, S.K.C., Skaife, P., Leeder, P.C., Wilson, P., Larvin, M., Curtis, L.D. and UK Acute Pancreatitis Study Group (2001) 'Double blind, randomised, placebo controlled study of a platelet activating factor antagonist, lexipafant, in the treatment and prevention of organ failure in predicted severe acute pancreatitis', *Gut*, 48(1): 62–9.

Johnson, L. (1999) 'Factors known to raise intracranial pressure and the associated implications for nursing management', *Nursing in Critical Care*, 4(3): 117–27.

Johnson, L.G. and McMahan, M.J. (1997) 'Postoperative factors contributing to prolonged length of stay in cardiac surgery patients', *Dimensions in Critical Care Nursing*, 16(5): 243–50.

Joint European Society of Cardiology/American College of Cardiology Committee (2000) 'Myocardial infarction redefined – a consensus document of the Joint European Society of Cardiology/American College of Cardiology Committee for the redefinition of myocardial infarction', *European Heart Journal*, 21(18): 1502–13.

Jones, C. and Griffiths, R.D. (2002) 'Physical and psychological recovery', in Griffiths, R.D. and Jones, C. (eds) *Intensive Care Aftercare*, Oxford: Butterworth-Heinemann, 53–65.

Jones, C. and Parsonage, M. (2002) 'Cocaine related chest pain: are we seeing the tip of an iceberg?' *Accident and Emergency Nursing*, 10(3): 121–6.

Jones, C., Skirrow, P., Griffiths, R.D., Humphris, G., Ingleby, S., Eddleston, J., Waldmann, C. and Gager, M. (2004) 'Post traumatic stress disorder-related symptoms in relatives of patients following intensive care, *Intensive Care Medicine*, 30(3): 456–60.

Jones, C.V. (2004) 'The importance of oral hygiene in nutritional support', in White, R. (ed.) *Trends in Oral Health Care*, Dinton: Quay Books, 72–83.

Jones, I. (2003) 'Acute coronary syndromes', *Professional Nurse*, 18(5): 289–92.

Jonghe, B. de, Sharshar, T., Lefaucheur, J.-P., Authier, F.J., Durand-Zaleski, I., Boussarsar, M., Cerf, C., Renaud, E., Mesrati, F., Cartlet J., Raphael, J.C., Outin, H. and Bastuji-Garin, S. (2002) 'Paresis acquired in the intensive care unit', *JAMA*, 288(22): 2859–67.

Joshipura, K.J., Hu, F.B., Manson, J.E., Stampfer, M.J., Rimm, E.B., Speizer, F.E., Colditz, G., Ascherio, A., Rosner, B., Spiegelman, D. and Willett, W.C. (2001) 'The effects of fruit and vegetable intake on risk for coronary heart disease', *Annals of Internal Medicine*, 134(12): 1106–14.

Joshua-Amadi, M. (2002) 'Recruitment and retention', *Journal of Nursing Management*, 9(8): 17–21.

Jowett, N.I. and Thompson, D.R. (2003) 'Comprehensive coronary care', 3rd edn, London: Baillière Tindall.

Kallas, H.J. (1998) 'Non-conventional respiratory support modalities applicable in the older child', *Critical Care Clinics*, 14(4): 655–83.

Kam, P.C.A. and Ferch, N.I. (2000) 'Apoptosis: mechanisms and clinical implications', *Anaesthesia*, 55(11): 1081–93.

Kaplan, A.A. (1985) 'Predilution versus post-dilution for CAVH', *Transactions of the American Society of Artificial Internal Organs*, 31: 28–32.

—— (1998) 'Continuous renal replacement therapy (CRRT) in the intensive care unit', *Journal of Intensive Care Medicine*, 13(2): 85–105.

Kass, J.E. (2003) 'Heliox redux', *Chest*, 123(3): 673–6.

Kass, J.E. and Terregino, C.A. (1999) 'The effect of Heliox in acute severe asthma', *Chest*, 116(2): 296–300.

Kaye, P. and O'Sullivan, I. (2002) 'The role of magnesium in the emergency department', *Emergency Medical Journal*, 19(4): 288–91.

Keays, R. (2003) 'Diabetic emergencies', in Bersten, A.D. and Soni, N. (eds) *Intensive Care Manual*, 5th edn, Edinburgh: Butterworth-Heinemann, 551–8.

Keely, B.R. (1998) 'Preventing complications. Recognition and treatment of autonomic dysreflexia', *Dimensions in Critical Care Nursing*, 17(4): 170–6.

Keen, A. (2001) 'Issues related to the nursing management of haemofiltration', *Nursing in Critical Care*, 6(6): 273–8.

Kellum, J. and Pinsky, M. (2002) 'Use of vasopressor agents in critically ill patients', *Current Opinion in Critical Care*, 8(3): 236–41.

Kelly, J., Rudd, A., Lewis, R.R. and Hunt, B.J. (2002) 'Plasma D-dimers in the diagnosis of venous thromboembolism', *Archives of Internal Medicine*, 162(7): 747–56.

Kemp, M., Donovan, J., Higham, H. and Hooper, J. (2004) 'Biochemical markers of myocardial injury', *British Journal of Anaesthesia*, 93(1): 63–73.

Kemper, M.J., Harps, E. and Muller-Wiefel, D.E. (1996) 'Hyperkalaemia: therapeutic options in acute and chronic renal failure', *Clinical Nephrology*, 46(1): 67–9.

Kennedy, A. (2003) 'Meningitis and encephalomyelitis', in Bersten, A.D. and Soni, N. (eds) *Intensive Care Manual*, 5th edn, Edinburgh: Butterworth-Heinemann, 521–9.

Kennedy, D.D., Coakley, J. and Griffiths, R.D. (2002) 'Neuromuscular problems and physical weakness', in Griffiths, R.D. and Jones, C. (eds) *Intensive Care Aftercare*, Oxford: Butterworth-Heinemann, 7–18.

Kennedy, J.F. (1997) 'Enteral feeding for the critically ill patient', *Nursing Standard*, 11(33): 39–43.

Kennedy, M.S. (2004) 'Kinetic therapy: in search of the evidence: it may prevent some pulmonary complications', *AJN*, 104(12): 22.

Kent, B. (1997) 'Understanding attitudes towards tissue donation', *Professional Nurse*, 12(7): 482–4.

Keogh, B.F. and Cordingley, J.J. (2002) 'Current invasive ventilatory strategies in acute respiratory distress syndrome', in Evans, T.W., Griffiths, M.J.D. and Keogh, B.F. (eds) *ARDS*, Sheffield: European Respiratory Society Journals Ltd., 161–80.

Kern, L.S. (2004) 'Postoperative atrial fibrillation: new directions in prevention and treatment', *The Journal of Cardiovascular Nursing*, 19(2): 103–15.

Kerridge, I.H., Saul, P., Lowe, M., McPhee, J. and Williams, D. (2002) 'Death, dying and donation: organ transplantation and the diagnosis of death', *Journal of Medical Ethics*, 28(2): 89–94.

Kessler, P., Neidhart, G., Bremerich, D.H., Aybek, T., Dogan, S., Lischke, V. and Byhahn, C. (2002) 'High thoracic epidural anesthesia for coronary artery bypass grafting using two different surgical approaches in conscious patients', *Anesthesia & Analgesia*, 95(4): 791–7.

Khan, N.E., de Sousa, A., Mister, R., Flather, M., Clague, J., Davies, S., Collins, P., Wang, D., Sigwart, U. and Pepper, M. (2004) 'A randomized comparison of off-pump and on-pump multivessel coronary-artery bypass-surgery', *NEJM*, 351(1): 21–8.

Khan, N.E., de Sousza, A.C. and Pepper, J.R. (2001) 'Off-pump coronary artery surgery – a review', *British Journal of Cardiology*, 8(8): 459–65.

Kiening, K.L., Unterberg, A.W., Bardt, T.F., Schneider, G.H. and Lanksch, W.R. (1996) 'Monitoring of cerebral oxygenation in patients with severe head injuries. Brain tissue $pO_2$ versus jugular vein oxygen saturation', *Journal of Neurosurgery*, 85(5): 751–7.

King's Fund (1989) 'ICU in the United Kingdom: report from the King's Fund Panel', *Intensive Care Nursing*, 5(2): 76–81.

Kingston, D., Sykes, S. and Raper, S. (2002) 'Protocol for the administration of haemofiltration fluids and electrolytes using a patient group direction', *Nursing in Critical Care*, 7(4): 193–7.

Kirby, S.A. and Davenport, A. (1996) 'Haemofiltration/dialysis treatment in patients with acute renal failure', *Care of the Critically Ill*, 12(2): 54–8.

Kite, K. and Pearson, L. (1995) 'A rationale for mouth care: the integration of theory with practice', *Intensive and Critical Care Nursing*, 11(2): 71–6.

Klein, C.J., Moser-Veillon, P.B., Schweitzer, A., Douglass, L.W., Reynolds, H.N., Patterson, K.Y. and Veillon, C. (2002) 'Magnesium, calcium, zinc, and nitrogen loss in trauma patients during continuous renal replacement therapy', *JPEN*, 26(2): 77–93.

Klodgie, F.D., Gold, H.K., Burke, A.P., Fowler, D.R., Kruth, H.S., Weber, D.K., Farb, A., Guerrero, B.S., Motoya-Haayase, Kutys, R., Narula, J., Finn, A.V. and Virmani, R. (2003) 'Intraplaque hemorrhage and progression of coronary atheroma', *NEJM*, 349(24): 2316–25.

Knaus, W.A., Draper, E.A., Wagner, D.P. and Zimmerman, J.E. (1985) 'APACHE II: a severity of disease classification system', *Critical Care Medicine*, 13(10): 818–29.

Knaus, W.A., Wagner, D.P, Draper, E.A., Zimmerman, J.E., Bergner, M., Bastos, P.G., Sirio, C.A., Murphy, D.J., Lotring, T., Damiano, A. and Harrell, F.E. Jr (1991) 'The APACHE III prognostic system. Risk prediction of hospital mortality for critically ill hospitalised adults', *Chest*, 100(6): 1619–36.

Knoll, G.A. (1999) 'Tacrolimus versus cyclosporin for immunosuppression in renal transplantation: meta-analysis of randomised trials', *BMJ*, 318(7191): 1104–7.

Koesters, S.C., Rogers, P.D. and Rajasingham, C.R. (2002) 'MDMA ("ecstasy") and other "club drugs". The new epidemic', *The Pediatric Clinics of North America*, 49(2): 415–33.

Koksal, G.M., Sayilgan, C., Sen, O. and Oz, H. (2004) 'The effects of different weaning modes on the endocrine stress response', *Critical Care*, 8: R31–4.

Kootstra, G., Kievit, J.K. and Heineman, E. (1997) 'The non heart-beating donor', *British Medical Bulletin*, 53(4): 844–53.

Kress, J.P., Pohlman, A.S. and O'Connor, M.F. (2000) 'Daily interruptions of sedative infusions in critically ill patients undergoing mechanical ventilation', *New England Journal of Medicine*, 342(20): 1471–7.

Krishnan, J.A. and Brower, R.G. (2000) 'High-frequency ventilation for acute lung injury and ARDS', *Chest*, 118(3): 795–807.

Krishnan, J.A., Moore, D., Robeson, C., Rand, C.S. and Fessler, H.E. (2004) 'A prospective, controlled trial of a protocol-based strategy to discontinue mechanical ventilation', *American Journal of Respiratory and Critical Care Medicine*, 169(6): 673–8.

Krumberger, J. (2002) 'When the liver fails', *RN*, 65(2): 26–9.

Krumholz, W., Endrass, J. and Hempelmann, G. (1995) 'Inhibition of phagocytosis and killing of bacteria by anaesthetic agents in vitro', *British Journal of Anaesthesia*, 75(1): 66–70.

Kucher, N. and Goldhaber, S.Z. (2003) 'Cardiac biomarkers for risk stratification of patients with acute pulmonary embolism', *Circulation*, 108(18): 2191–4.

Kudst, K.A. (2003) 'Effect of route and type of nutrition on intestine-derived inflammatory responses', *American Journal of Surgery*, 185(1): 16–21.

Kuo, J. and Butchart, E.G. (1995) 'Sternal wound dehiscence', *Care of the Critically Ill*, 11(6): 244–8.

Kuperberg, K.G. and Grubbs, L. (1997) 'Coronary artery bypass patients' perceptions of acute postoperative pain', *Clinical Nurse Specialist*, 11(3): 116–22.

Kuwabara, S., Ogawara, K., Sing, J.-Y., Mori, M., Kanai, K., Hattori, T., Yuki, N., Lin, C.S., Burke, D. and Bostock, H. (2002) 'Differences in membrane properties of axonal and demyelinating Guillain-Barré Syndromes', *Annals of Neurology*, 52(2): 180–7.

Laing, A.S.M. (1992) 'The applicability of a new sedation scale for intensive care', *Intensive and Critical Care Nursing*, 8(3): 149–52.

Lambert, P. and Bingley, P.J. (2002) 'What is type 1 diabetes?', *Medicine*, 30(1): 1–5.

Lamerton, M. and Albarran, J.W. (1997) 'Percutaneous balloon mitral valvuloplasty: advancing the nursing perspective', *Nursing in Critical Care*, 2(2): 88–92.

Lanfear, J. (2002) 'The individual with epilepsy', *Nursing Standard*, 16(4): 43–53.

Lange, N.R., Kozlowski, J.K., Gust, R., Shapiro, S.D. and Schuster, D.P. (2000) 'Effect of partial liquid ventilation on pulmonary vascular permeability and edema after experimental acute lung injury', *American Journal of Respiratory and Critical Care Medicine*, 162(1): 271–7.

Lapinsky, S.E. and Granton, J.I. (2004) 'Critical care lessons from severe acute respiratory syndrome', *Current Opinion in Critical Care*, 10(1): 53–8.

Lapinsky, S.E. and Hawryluck, L. (2003) 'ICU management of severe acute respiratory syndrome', *Intensive Care Medicine*, 29(6): 870–5.

Larvin, M. (1999) 'Acute pancreatitis', *Surgery*, 17(11): 261–5.

Laterre, P.-F. (2002) 'Activated protein C and severe sepsis', in Galley, H.F. (ed.) *Critical Care Focus 8: Blood and Blood Transfusion*, London: BMJ Books, 38–48.

Latessa, V. (2002) 'Endovascular sent-graft repair of descending thoracic aortic aneurysms: the nursing implications for care', *Journal of Vascular Nursing*, 20(3): 86–93.

Latman, N. (2003) 'Clinical thermometry: possible causes and potential solutions to electronic, digital thermometer inaccuracies', *Biomedical Instrumentation & Technology*, 37(3): 190–6.

Laupland, K.B., Zygun, D.A., Davies, H.D., Church, D.L., Louie, T.J. and Doig, C.J. (2002) 'Population-based assessment of intensive care unit-acquired bloodstream infections in adults: Incidence, risk factors, and associated mortality rate', *Critical Care Medicine*, 30(11): 2462–7.

Law, C. (2000) 'A guide to assessing sputum', *Nursing Times*, 96(24): 7–10.

Lawes, E.G. (2003) 'Hidden hazards and dangers associated with the use of HME/filters in breathing circuits. Their effect on toxic metabolite production, pulse oximetry and airway resistance', *BJA*, 91(2): 249–64.

Lee, M.S. and Makkar, R.R. (2004) 'Stem-cell transplantation in myocardial infarction: a status report', *Annals of Internal Medicine*, 140(9): 729–37.

Lee, N., Hui, D., Wu, A., Chan, P., Cameron, P., Joynt, G.M., Ahuja, A., Yung, M.Y., Leung, C.B., To, K.F., Lui, S.F., Szeto, C.C., Chung, S. and Sung, J.J.Y. (2003) 'A major outbreak of severe acute respiratory syndrome in Hong Kong', *New England Journal of Medicine*, 348(20): 1986–94.

Leigh Brown, A.J. (1999) 'Viral evolution and variation in the HIV pandemic', in Dalgleish, A.G. and Weiss, R.A. (eds) (1999) *HIV and the New Viruses*, 2nd edn, San Diego, CA: Academic Press, 29–42.

Leith, B.A. (1999) 'Patients' and family members' perceptions of transfer from intensive care', *Heart & Lung*, 28(3): 210–18.

Leliopoulou, C., Waterman, H. and Chakrabarty, S. (1999) 'Nurses failure to appreciate the risks of infection due to needlestick stick accidents: a hospital based survey', *Journal of Hospital Infection*, 42(1): 53–9.

Lester, S.J., Baggott, M., Welm, S., Schiller, N.B., Jones, R.T., Fostrer, E. and Mendelson, J. (2000) 'Cardiovascular effects of 3,4-methylenedioymethamphetamine', *Annals of Internal Medicine*, 133(12): 969–73.

Lever, A. (2001) 'HIV: the virus', *Medicine*, 29(4): 1–3.

Levi, M. and ten Cate, H. (1999) 'Current concepts: disseminated intravascular coagulation', *New England Journal of Medicine*, 341(8): 586–92.

Levine, E. (1997) 'Jewish views and customs on death', in Parkes, C.M. (ed.) *Death and Bereavement Across Cultures*, London: Routledge, 98–130.

Levy, M.M., Fink, M.P., Marshall, J.C., Abraham, E., Angus, D., Cook, D., Cohen, J., Opal, S.M., Vincent, J.-L., Ramsay, G. and International Sepsis Definition

Conference (2003) '2001 SCCM/ESICM/ACCP/ATS/ SIS International Sepsis Definition Conference', *Intensive Care Medicine*, 29(4): 530–8.

Lew, T.W.K., Kwek, T.-K., Tai, D., Earnest, A., Loo, S., Singh, K., Kwan, K.M., Chan, Y., Yim, C.F., Bek, S.L., Kor, A.C., Yap, W.S., Chelliah, Y.C. and Goh, S.-K. (2003) 'Acute respiratory distress syndrome in critically ill patients with severe acute respiratory syndrome', *JAMA*, 290(3): 374–80.

Lewis, A.M. (1999) 'Neurologic emergency!', *Nursing 99*, 29(10): 54–6.

Lewis, S.J., Egger, M., Sylvester, P.A. and Thomas, S. (2001) 'Early enteral feeding versus "nil by mouth" after gastro-intestinal surgery: systematic review and meta-analysis of controlled trials', *BMJ*, 323(7316): 773–6.

Lewis, S.J. and Heaton, K.W. (1997) 'Stool form scale as a useful guide to intestinal transit time', *Gut*, 41(4S supplement): 122A–123A.

L'Her, E., Renault, A., Robaux, M-A. and Boles, J.-M. (2002) 'A prospective survey of early 12-h prone positioning effects in patients with the acute respiratory distress syndrome', *Intensive Care Medicine*, 28(5): 570–5.

Li, T., Buckley, T.A., Yap, F.H.Y., Sung, J.J.Y. and Joynt, G.M. (2003) 'Severe acute respiratory syndrome (SARS): infection control', *Lancet*, 361(9366): 1386.

Light, R.W., Rogers, J.T., Moyers, J.P., Lee, Y.C.G., Rodriguez, R.M., Alford, W.C. Jr, Ball, S.K., Burrus, G.R., Coltharp, W.H., Glassford, D.M. Jr, Hoff, S.J., Lea, J.W. IV, Nesbitt, J.C., Petracek, M.R., Starkey, T.D., Stoney, W.S. and Tedder, M. (2002) 'Prevalence and clinical course of pleural effusions at 30 days after coronary artery and cardiac surgery', *American Journal of Respiratory and Critical Care Medicine*, 166(12): 1567–71.

Lim, W.S., Macfarlane, J.T., Boswell, T.C., Harrison, T.G., Rose, D., Leinonen, M. and Saikku, P. (2001) 'Study of community acquired pneumonia aetiology (SCAPA) in adults admitted to hospital: implications for management guidelines', *Thorax*, 56(4): 296–301.

Limdi, J.K. and Hyde, G.M. (2003) 'Evaluation of abnormal liver function tests', *Postgraduate Medical Journal*, 79(932): 307–12.

Lin, S.-M., Liu, C.-Y., Wang, C.-H., Lin, H.-C., Huang, C.-D., Huang, P.-Y., Fang, Y.-F., Shieh, M.-H. and Kuo, H.-P. (2004) 'The impact of delirium on the survival of mechanically ventilated patients', *Critical Care Medicine*, 32(11): 2254–59.

Lindholm, M.G., Kober, L., Boesgaard, S., Torp-Pedersen, C., Aldershvile, J. and TRACE study group (2003) 'Cardiogenic shock complicating acute myocardial infarction', *European Heart Journal*, 24(3): 258–65.

Lindsay, P. (2004) 'Complications of the third stage of labour', in Henderson, C. and Macdonald, S. (eds) *Mayes' Midwifery: A Textbook for Midwives*, 13th edn, Edinburgh: Baillière Tindall, 987–1002.

Livesey, S. (2002) 'Coronary artery bypass', *Medicine*, 30(4); 85–8.

Liwu, A. (1990) 'Oral hygiene in intubated patients', *Australian Journal of Advanced Nursing*, 7(2): 4–7.

Lloyd, C. and Lewis, V.M. (1999) 'Common medical disorders associated with pregnancy', in Bennett, V.R. and Brown, L.K. (eds) *Myles Textbook for Midwives*, 13th edn, Edinburgh: Churchill Livingstone, 279–314.

Lobo, S.M.A., Lobo, F.R.M., Bota, D.P., Lopes-Ferreira, F., Soliman, H.M., Mélot, C. and Vinent, J.L. (2003) 'C-reactive protein levels correlate with mortality and organ failure in critically ill patients', *Chest*, 123(6): 2043–9.

Locke, G.R., Pemberton, J.H. and Phillips, S.P. (2000) 'AGA technical review on constipation', *Gastroenterology*, 119(6): 1766–78.

Lorenz, B.T. and Coyte, K.M. (2002) 'Coronary artery bypass graft surgery without cardiopulmonary bypass: a review and nursing implications', *Critical Care Nurse*, 22(1): 51–60.

Lorgeril, M. de, Salen, P., Marin, J.-L., Boucher, F., Paillard, F. and Leiris, J. de (2002) 'Wine drinking and risks of cardiovascular complications after recent acute myocardial infarction', *Circulation*, 106(12): 1465–69.

Loussert-Ajaka, T.D.L., Chaix, M.L., Ingrand, D., Saragosti, S., Courouce, A.M., Brun-Vezinet, F. and Simon, F. (1994) 'HIV-1/HIV-2 seronegativity in HIV-1 subtype O infected patients', *Lancet*, 343(8910): 1393–4.

Lower, J. (2003) 'Using pain to assess neurologic response', *Nursing2003*, 33(6): 56–7.

Lowery, M.T. (1995) 'A pressure sore risk calculator for intensive care patients: the Sunderland experience', *Intensive and Critical Care Nursing*, 11(6): 344–53.

Lowthian, P. (1997) 'Notes on the pathogenesis of serious pressure sores', *British Journal of Nursing*, 6(16): 907–12.

Lueckenotte, A.G. (2000) *Gerontologic Nursing*, 2nd edn, St Louis: Mosby.

Lumb, A. (2000) *Nunn's Applied Respiratory Physiology*, 5th edn, Oxford: Butterworth-Heinemann.

Lumsdaine, J.A. (2000) 'Care of the living kidney donor and recipient', *Professional Nurse*, 16(2): 885–7.

Lynn-McHale, D.J., Corsetti, A., Brady-Avis, E., Shaffer, R., McGregory, J. and Rothenberger, C. (1997) 'Preoperative ICU tours: are they helpful?' *American Journal of Critical Care*, 6(2): 106–15.

Lytle, B.W. and Sabik, J.F. (2004) 'On-pump and off-pump bypass surgery. Tools for revasularisation', *Circulation*, 109(7): 810–12.

McAuley, D.F., Giles, S., Fichter, H., Perkins, G.D. and Gao, F. (2002) 'What is the optimal duration of ventilation in the prone position in acute lung injury and acute respiratory distress syndrome?', *Intensive Care Medicine*, 28(4): 414–18.

McCaffery, M. and Pasero, C. (1999) *Pain Clinical Manual*, 2nd edn, St Louis: Mosby.

McClave, S.A., Sexton, L.K., Spain, D.A., Adams, J.L., Owens, N.A., Sullins, M.B., Blandford, B.S. and Snider, H.L. (1999) 'Enteral tube feeding in the intensive care unit: factors impeding adequate delivery', *Critical Care Medicine*, 27(7): 1252–6.

McClave, S.A., Marsano, L.S. and Lukan, J.K. (2002a) 'Enteral access for nutritional support: rationale for utilization', *Journal of Clinical Gastroenterology*, 35(3): 209–13.

McClave, S.A., DeMeo, M.T., DeLegge, M.H., DiSario, J.A., Heyland, D.K., Maloney, J.P., Metheny, N.A., Moore, F.A., Scolapio, J.S., Spain, D.A. and Zaloga, G.P. (2002b) 'North American summit on aspiration in the critically ill patient: consensus statement', *Journal of Parenteral & Enteral Nutrition*, 26(6 Supplement): S80–S85.

McClave, S.A., Lukan, J.K., Stefater, J.A., Lowen, C.C., Looney, S.W., Matheson, P.J., Gleeson, K. and Spain, D.A. (2005) 'Poor validity of residual volumes as a marker for risk of aspiration in critically ill patients', *Critical Care Medicine*, 33(2): 324–30.

McClelland, A.J.J., Owens, C.G., Walsh, S.J., McCarty, D., Matthew, T., Stevenson, M., Gracey, H., Khan, M.M. and Adgey, A.A.J. (2005) 'Percutaneous coronary intervention and 1 year survival in patients treated with fibrionolytic therapy for acute ST-elevation myocardial infarction', *European Heart Journal*, 26(6): 544–8.

McClune, B. and Franklin, M. (1987) 'The Mead model for nursing – adapted from the Roper/Logan/Tierney model for nursing', *Intensive Care Nursing*, 3(3): 97–103.

MacConnachie, A.M. (1997) 'Ecstasy poisoning', *Intensive and Critical Care Nursing*, 13(6): 365–6.

McCormack, B. and Manley, K. (eds) (2004) *Practice Development in Nursing*, Oxford: Blackwell Publishing.

McCormick, J. Blackwood, B. (2001) 'Nursing the ARDS patient in the prone position', *Intensive and Critical Care Nursing*, 17(6): 331–40.

McCulloch, J. (1998) 'Infection control: principles for practice', *Nursing Standard*, 13(1): 49–53.

McCusker, J., Cole, M., Abrahamowicz, M., Primeau, F. and Belzile, E. (2002) 'Delirium predicts 12 month mortality', *Archives of Internal Medicine*, 162(4): 457–63.

McDaniel, L.B. and Prough, D.S. (1996) 'Fluid therapy during and after anaesthesia', in Prys-Roberts, C. and Brown, B.R. Jr (eds) *International Practice of Anaesthesia*, Oxford: Butterworth-Heinemann; 1/47/1–17.

MacDonald, C. and Armstrong, D. (2000) 'The prone position – a nursing perspective', *Nursing in Critical Care*, 5(5): 215–19.

McFadzean, J. and Dexter, T. (1999) 'Consent in the intensive care unit', *Care of the Critically Ill*, 15(4): 129–31.

MacFie, J. (2004) 'Current status of bacterial translocation as a cause of surgical sepsis', *British Medical Bulletin*, 71: 1–12.

McGuire, P.K., Cope, H. and Fahy, T.A. (1994) 'Diversity of psychopathy associated with use of 3,4-methylenedioxymethamphetamine ("Ecstasy")', *British Journal of Psychiatry*, 165(3): 391–5.

Maciel, A.T., Creteur, J. and Vincent, J.-L. (2004) 'Tissue capnotmetry: does the answer lie under the tongue', *Intensive Care Medicine*, 30(12): 2157–65.

McInroy, A. and Edwards, S. (2002) 'Preventing sensory alteration: a practical approach', *Nursing in Critical Care*, 7(5): 247–54.

MacIntosh, I. and Britto, J. (2000) 'How to guide: high frequency oscillatory ventilation', *Care of the Critically Ill*, 16(4): centre insert.

MacIntyre, P. and Ready, L. (2001) *Acute Pain Management: A Practical Guide*, London: W.B. Saunders.

MacKenzie, C.F. and Bucci, C. (2004) 'Artificial oxygen carriers for trauma: myth or reality?', *Hospital Medicine*, 65(10): 582–8.

McKinley, S., Coote, K. and Stein-Parbury, J. (2003) 'Development and testing of a Faces Scale for the assessment of anxiety in critically ill patients', *Journal of Advanced Nursing*, 41(1): 73–9.

McLaughlin, A., McLaughlin, B., Elliott, J. and Campalini, G. (1996) 'Noise levels in a cardiac surgical intensive care unit: a preliminary study conducted in secret', *Intensive and Critical Care Nursing*, 12(4): 226–31.

McLean, B. (2001) 'Rotational kinetic therapy for ventilation/perfusion mismatch', *Connect*, 1(4): 113–18.

McLean-Tooke, A.P.C., Bethune, A., Far, A.C. and Spickett, G.P. (2003) 'Adrenaline in the treatment of anaphylaxis: what is the evidence?', *BMJ*, 327(7427): 1333–5.

McLellan, S.A., McClelland, D.B.L. and Walsh, T.S. (2003) 'Anaemia and red blood cell transfusion in the critically ill patient', *Blood Reviews*, 17(4): 195–208.

MacLennan, J. (2001) 'Meningococcal group C conjugate vaccines', *Archives of Diseases in Childhood*, 84(5): 383–6.

McLeod, G.A., Davies, H.T.O., Munnoch, N., Bannister, J. and Macrae, W. (2001) 'Postoperative pain relief using thoracic epidural analgesia: outstanding success and disappointing failures', *Anaesthesia*, 56(1): 75–81.

McLoughlin, C. (2004) 'Statins', *Professional Nurse*, 19(11): 51–2.

MacMillan, C.S.A. (2003) 'Cardiorespiratory compromise after SAH: a life-threatening syndrome', *British Journal of Intensive Care*, 13(2): 62–7.

McMurry, S.A. and Hogue, C.W. (2004) 'Atrial fibrillation and cardiac surgery', *Current Opinion in Anaesthesiology*, 17(1): 63–70.

McNabb, M. (2004) 'Maternal and fetal physiological responses to pregnancy', in Henderson, C. and Macdonald, S. (eds) *Mayes' Midwifery: A Textbook for Midwives*, 13th edn, Edinburgh: Baillière Tindall, 288–311.

McQuay, H. and Moore, A. (1998) *An Evidence-Based Resource for Pain Relief*, Oxford: Oxford Medical.

Maddox, M., Dunn, S.V. and Pretty, L.E. (2001) 'Psychological recovery following ICU: experiences and influences upon discharge to the community', *Intensive and Critical Care Nursing*, 17(1): 6–15.

Maggiore, S.M., Lelloche, F., Pigeot, J., Taille, S., Deye, N., Durrmeyer, X., Richard, J.-C., Mancebo, J., Lemaire, F. and Brochard, L. (2003) 'Prevention of endotracheal suctioning-induced alveolar derecruitment in acute lung injury', *American Journal of Respiratory and Critical Care Medicine*, 167(9): 1215–24.

Mahon, A. and Hattersley, J. (2002) 'Investigations in renal failure', in Thomas, N. (ed.) *Renal Nursing*, 2nd edn, Edinburgh: Baillière Tindall, 143–70.

Mak, S. and Newton, G.E. (2001) 'The oxidative stress hypothesis of congestive heart failure', *Chest*, 120(6): 2035–46.

Malaty, H.M., El-Kasabany, A., Graham, D.Y., Miller, C.C., Reddy, S.G., Srinivasan, S.R., Yamaoka, Y. and Berenson, G.S. (2002) 'Age at acquisition of *Helicobactor pylori* infection: a follow-up study from infancy to adulthood', *Lancet*, 359(9310): 931–5.

Malbrain, M.L.N.G., Chiumello, D., Pelosi, P., Bihari, D., Innes, R., Ranieri, V.M., del Turco, M., Wilmer, A., Brienza, N., Malcangi, V., Cohen, J., Japiassu, A., de Keulenaer, B.L., Daelemans, R., Jacquet, L., Laterre, P.-F., Frank, G., de Souza, P., Cesana, B. and Gattinoni, L. (2005) 'Incidence and prognosis of intraabdominal hypertension in a mixed population of critically ill patients: a multiple-center epidemiological study', *Critical Care Medicine*, 33(2): 315–32.

Malik, S., Wong, N.D., Franklin, S.S., Kamath, T.V., L'Italien, G.J., Pio, J.R. and Williams, R. (2004) 'Impact of the metabolic syndrome on mortality from coronary heart disease, cardiovascular disease, and all causes in United States adults', *Circulation*, 110(10): 1245–50.

Maloney, D.G., Appadurai, R. and Vaughan, R.S. (2002) 'Anions and the anaesthetist', *Anaesthesia*, 57(2): 140–54.

Manias, E. and Street, A. (2000) 'The handover: uncovering the hidden practices of nurses', *Intensive and Critical Care Nursing*, 16(6): 373–84.

—— (2001) 'Nurse-Doctor interactions during critical care ward rounds', *Journal of Clinical Nursing*, 10(4): 442–50.

Manley, K. (2004) 'Transformational culture', in McCormack, B. and Manley, K. (eds) *Practice Development in Nursing*, Oxford: Blackwell Publishing.

Mann, D.L. (1999) 'HLA and HIV-1 infection', in Dalgleish, A.G. and Weiss, R.A. (eds) *HIV and the New Viruses*, 2nd edn, San Diego, CA: Academic Press, 155–72.

Manns, B.J., Lee, H., Doig, C.J., Johnson, D. and Donaldson, C. (2002) 'An economic evaluation of activated protein C treatment for severe sepsis', *New England Journal of Medicine*, 347(13): 993–1000.

Manocha, S., Walley, K.R. and Russell, J.A. (2003) 'Severe acute respiratory distress syndrome (SARS): a critical care perspective', *Critical Care Medicine*, 31(11): 2684–92.

Manson, J.E., Greenland, P., LaCroix, A.Z., Stefanik, M.L., Mouton, C.P., Oberman, A., Perri, M.G., Sheps, D.S., Pettinger, M.B. and Siscovick, D.S. (2002) 'Walking compared with vigorous exercise for the prevention of cardiovascular events in women', *New England Journal of Medicine*, 347(10): 716–25.

Margreiter, R., (2002) 'European Tacrolimus vs Ciclosporin microemulsion tranel transplantation study group', *Lancet*, 359(9308): 741–6.

Marieb, E.N. (2004) *Human Anatomy and Physiology*, 6th edn, San Fransisco, CA: Pearson/Benjamin Cummings.

Marik, P.E. (2000) 'Fever in the ICU', *Chest*, 117(3): 855–69.

—— (2002) 'Low-dose dopamine: a systematic review', *Intensive Care Medicine*, 28(7): 877–83.

Marik, P.E. and Raghaven, M. (2004) 'Stress-hyperglycaemia, insulin and immunodulation in sepsis', *Intensive Care Medicine*, 30(5): 748–56.

Marik, P.E. and Varon, J. (2004) 'The management of status epilepticus', *Chest*, 126(2): 582–91.

Marik, P.E. and Zaloga, G.P. (2002) 'Adrenal insufficiency in the critically patients', *Chest*, 122(5): 1784–96.

—— (2004) 'Meta-analysis of parenteral nutrition versus enteral nutrition in patients with acute pancreatitis', *BMJ*, 328(7453): 1407–10.

Marion, D.W., Penrod, L.E., Kelsey, S.F., Obrist, W.D., Kochanek, P.M., Palmer, A.M., Wisniewski, S.R. and DeKosky, S.T. (1997) 'Treatment of traumatic brain injury with moderate hypothermia', *New England Journal of Medicine*, 336(8): 540–6.

Markmann, J.F., Deng, S., Huang, X., Velidedeoglu, E.H., Lui, C., Frank, A., Markmann, E., Palanjian, M., Brayman, K., Wolf, B., Bell, E., Vitamaniul, M., Dolba, N., Matschinsky, F., Barker, C.F. and Naji, A. (2003) 'Insulin independence following isolated islet transplantation and single islet infusions', *Annals of Surgery*, 237(6): 741–50.

Marsh, M. (2000) 'Respiratory anatomy and physiology in infants and children', in Williams, C. and Asquith, J. (eds) *Paediatric Intensive Care Nursing*, Edinburgh: Churchill Livingstone, 61–79.

Marshall, A.P. and West, S.H. (2003) 'Gastric tonometry and enteral nutrition: a possible conflict in critical care nursing practice', *American Journal of Critical Care*, 12(4): 349–56.

Marshall, W.J. (2000) *Clinical Chemistry*, 4th edn, Edinburgh: Mosby.

Marthaler, M., Keresztes, P. and Tazbir, J. (2003) 'SARS: what have we learned?' *RN*, 66(8): 58–64.

Martin, L. (1999) *All You Really Need to Know to Interpret Arterial Blood Gases*, 2nd edn, Philadelphia, PA: Lippincott, Williams & Wilkins.

Martin, C., Viviand, X., Leone, M. and Thirion, X. (2000) 'Effects of norephinephrine on the outcome of septic shock', *Critical Care Medicine*, 28(8): 2758–65.

Maslow, A.H. (1954/1987) *Motivation and Personality*, 3rd edn, New York: Harper & Row.

—— (1971) *The Farthest Reaches of Human Nature*, London: Penguin.

Matta, B.F. and Menon, D.K. (1997) 'Management of acute head injury', in Kaufman, L. and Ginsburg, R. (eds) *Anaesthesia Review 13*, New York: Churchill Livingstone, 163–200.

Matthews, P.J. and Matthews, L.M. (2000) 'Reducing the risks of ventilator-associated pneumonia', *Dimensions of Critical Care Nursing*, 17(1): 17–21.

Maunder, T. (1997) 'Principles and practice of managing difficult behaviour situations in intensive care', *Intensive and Critical Care Nursing*, 13(2): 108–10.

Mavrommatis, A.C., Theodoridis, T., Orfanidou, A., Roussos, C., Christopoulou-Kokkinou, V. and Zakynthinos, S. (2000) 'Coagulation system and platelets are fully activated in uncomplicated sepsis', *Critical Care Medicine*, 28(2): 451–7.

Medical Devices Agency (1995) *The Reuse of Medical Devices Supplied for Single-Use Only*, London: Medical Devices Agency.

—— (2001) 'Tissue necrosis caused by pulse oximeter probes', *Medical Devices Agency Safety Notice, MDA SN 2001 (08)*, March 2001, London: Medical Devices Agency.

Meduri, G.U., Headley, A.S. and Golden, E. (1998) 'Effect of prolonged methylprednisolone therapy in unresolving acute respiratory distress syndrome: a randomized controlled trial', *JAMA*, 280(2): 159–65.

Meek, S. and Morris, F. (2002) 'ABC of clinical electrocardiography: introduction II – basic terminology', *BMJ*, 324(7335): 470–3.

Mehta, R.L., Paascual, M.T., Soroko, S., Chertow, G.M., PICARD Study Group (2002) 'Diuretics, mortality, and nonrecovery of renal function in acute renal failure', *JAMA*, 188(19): 2547–53.

Meister, J. and Reddy, K. (2002) 'Rhabdomyolysis: an overview', *AJN*, 102(2): 75–9.

Melzack, R. and Wall, P. (1988) *The Challenge of Pain*, 2nd edn, London: Penguin.

Menon, D.K. (1999) 'Cerebral protection in severe brain injury: physiological determinants of outcome and their optimisation', *British Medical Bulletin*, 55(1): 226–58.

Mercer, M., Winter, R., Dennis, S. and Smith, C. (1998) 'An audit of treatment withdrawal in one hundred patients on a general ICU', *Nursing in Critical Care*, 3(2): 63–6.

Mergener, K. and Baillic, J. (1998) 'Acute pancreatitis', *BMJ*, 316(7124): 44–8.

Messori, A., Trippoli, S., Vaiani, M., Gorini, M. and Corrado, A. (2000) 'Bleeding and pneumonia in intensive care patients given ranitidine and sucralfate for prevention of stress ulcer: meta-analysis of randomised controlled trials', *BMJ*, 321(7269): 1103–6.

Metheny, N. (1993) 'Minimising respiratory complications of nasogastric tube feedings. State of the science', *Heart & Lung*, 22(3): 213–22.

Metheny, N., Reed, L., Worseck, M. and Clark, J. (1993) 'How to aspirate fluid from small-bore feeding tubes', *American Journal of Nursing*, 93(5): 86–8.

Metheny, N.A. and Titler, M.G. (2001) 'Assessing placement of feeding tubes', *AJN*, 101(5): 36–44.

Meyer, M.M. (2000) 'Renal replacement therapies', *Critical Care Clinics*, 16(1): 29–58.

Michel, M. and Gutmann, L. (1997) 'Methacillin-resistant *Staphylococcus aureus* and vancomycin-resistant Enterococci: therapeutic realities and possibilities', *Lancet*, 349(9069): 1901–2006.

Michie, C.A. and Shah, V. (2003) 'Managing toxic shock syndrome', *Nursing Times*, 99(5): 26–7.

Mick, D.J. and Ackerman, M.H. (2004) 'Critical care nursing for older adults: pathophysiological and functional considerations', *Nursing Clinics of North America*, 39(3): 473–93.

Mihaljevic, T., Cohn, L.H., Unic, D., Aranki, S.F., Couper, G.S. and Byrne, J.G. (2004) 'One thousand minimally invasive valve operations', *Annals of Surgery*, 240(3): 529–34.

Mihatsch, M.J., Kyo, M., Morozumi, K., Yamaguchi, Y., Nickeleit, V. and Ryffel, B. (1998) 'The side-effects of cyclosporin-A and tacrolimus', *Clinical Nephrology*, 49(6): 356–63.

Minnaganti, V.R., Patel, P.J., Iancu, D., Schoch, P.E. and Cunha, B.A. (2000) 'Necrotising fasciitis caused by *Aeromonas hydrophila*', *Heart & Lung*, 29(4): 306–8.

555

Minors, D.S. (2004) 'Physiology of red and white blood cells', *Anaesthesia and Intensive Care Medicine*, 5(5): 174–8.

Mitchell, R.M.S., Byrne, M.F. and Baillie, J. (2003) 'Pancreatitis', *Lancet*, 361(9367): 1447–55.

Mocroft, A., Katlama, C., Johnson, A.M., Pradier, C., Antunes, F., Mulcahy, F., Chiesi, A., Phillips, A.N., Kirk, O., Lundgren, J.D. and EuroSIDA Study Group (2000) 'AIDS across Europe, 1994–98: the EuroSIDA study', *Lancet*, 356(9226): 291–6.

Mokhlesi, B., Garimella, P.S., Joffe, A. and Velho, V. (2004) 'Street drug abuse leading to critical illness', *Intensive Care Medicine*, 30(8): 1526–36.

Mokhlesi, B., Leikin, J.B., Murray, P. and Corbridge, T.C. (2003) 'Adult toxicity in critical care. Part II: specific poisonings', *Chest*, 123(3): 897–922.

Molnar, Z., Shearer, E. and Lowe, D. (1999) 'N-acetylcysteine treatment to prevent the progression of multisystem organ failure: a prospective, randomised, placebo-controlled study', *Critical Care Medicine*, 27(6): 1100–4.

Molzhahn, A.E. (1997) 'Knowledge and attitudes of critical care nurses regarding organ donation', *Canadian Journal of Cardiovascular Nursing*, 8(2): 13–18.

Monchi, M., Berghmans, D., Ledoux, D. Canivet J-L, Dubois B, Damas P. (2004) 'Citrate vs heparin for anticoagulation in continuous venovenous hemofiltration: a prospective randomized study', *Intensive Care Medicine*, 30(2): 260–5.

Moniotte, S., Kobzik, L., Feron, O. Trochu JN, Gauthier C, Balligand JL. (2001) 'Upregulation of $\beta_3$-adonoreceptors and altered contractile response to inotropic amines in human failing myocardium', *Circulation*, 103(12): 1649–55.

Montaye, M., De Bacquer, D., De Backer, G. Amouyel P. (2000) 'Overweight and obesity: a major challenge for coronary heart disease secondary prevention in clinical practice in Europe', *European Heart Journal*, 21(10): 808–13.

Montejo, J.C. (1999) 'Enteral nutrition-related gastrointestinal complications in critically ill patients: a multicenter study', *Critical Care Medicine*, 27(8): 1447–53.

Moore, T. (2004) 'Suctioning', in Moore, T. and Woodrow, P. (eds) *High Dependency Nursing Care*, London: Routledge, 290–300.

Moore, T. and Woodrow, P. (eds) (2004) *High Dependency Nursing Care*, London: Routledge.

Morgan, I. and Campanella, C. (1998) 'Transmyocardial laser revascularisation in Edinburgh', *British Journal of Theatre Nursing*, 7(12): 4–9.

Morgan, M., Evans-Williams, D., Salmon, R., Hosein, I., Looker, D.N. and Howard, A. (2000) 'The population impact of MRSA in a country: the national survey of MRSA in Wales, 1997', *Journal of Hospital Infection*, 44(3): 227–39.

Morgan, P.W. and Berridge, J.C. (2000) 'Giving long-persistent starch as volume replacement can cause pruritis after cardiac surgery', *British Journal of Anaesthesia*, 85(11): 696–9.

Morgan, W.M. 3rd and O'Neill, J.A. Jr (1998) 'Hemorrhagic and obstructive shock in pediatric patients', *New Horizons*, 6(2): 150–4.

Morgera, S., Rocktäschel, J., Hasse, M., Lehmann, C., von Heeymann, C., Ziemer, S., Priem, F., Hocher, B., Göhl, Kox, W.J., Buder, H.-W. and Neumayer, H.-H. (2003) 'Intermittent high permeability hemofiltration in septic patients with acute renal failure', *Intensive Care Medicine*, 29(11): 1989–95.

Morris, A., Creasman, J., Turner, J. Luce JM, Wachter RM, Huang L. (2002) 'Intensive care of Human Immunodeficiency Virus-infected patients during the era of highly active antiretroviral therapy', *American Journal of Respiratory and Critical Care Medicine*, 166(3): 262–7.

Morris, H. and Gomez, C.M.H. (2004) 'Critical care management of the vascular patient', *Surgery*, 22(11): 303–7.

Morris, R.J. and Woodcock, J.P. (2004) 'Evidence-based compression: prevention of stasis and deep vein thrombosis', *Annals of Surgery*, 239(2): 162–71.

Moser, D., Chung, M., McKinley, S., Riegel, B., An, K., Cherrington, C.C., Blakely, W., Biddle, M., Frazier, S.K. and Garvin, B.J. (2003) 'Critical care nursing practice regarding patient anxiety assessment and management', *Intensive and Critical Care Nursing*, 19(5): 276–88.

Mostafa, S.M., Bhandari, S., Ritchie, G. Gratton N, Wenstone R. (2003) 'Constipation and its implications in the critically ill patient', *British Journal of Anaesthesia*, 91(6): 815–19.

Muecke, S.N. (2005) 'Effects of rotating night shifts', *Journal of Advanced Nursing*, 50(4): 433–9.

Mullally, S. (2001) 'Future clinical role of nurses in the United Kingdom', *Postgraduate Medical Journal*, 77(907): 337–9.

Munro, N. (2003) 'Cardiac bypass without the pump', *RN*, 66(10): 29–32.

Murdoch, J. and Larsen, D. (2004) 'Assessing pain in cognitively impaired older adults', *Nursing Standard*, 18(38): 33–9.

Murdoch, S. and Cohen, A. (2000) 'Intensive care sedation: a review of current British practice', *Intensive Care Medicine*, 26(6): 922–8.

Murphy, J., Mehigan, B.J. and Keane, F.B.V. (2002) 'Acute pancreatitis', *Hospital Medicine*, 6(8): 487–92.

Murray, I. (1999) 'Change and adaptation in pregnancy', in Bennett, V.R. and Brown, L.K. (eds) *Myles Textbook for Midwives*, 13th edn, Edinburgh: Churchill Livingstone, 167–89.

Murray, P.R., Kobayashi, G.S., Pfaller, M.A. and Rosenthal, K.S. (1994) *Medical Microbiology*, 2nd edn, St Louis: Mosby.

Murray, P.T., Wylam, M.E. and Umans, J.G. (2000) 'Nitric oxide and septic vascular dysfunction', *Anesthesia and Analgesia*, 90(1): 89–101.

Mythen, M. (2003) 'Colloids and blood products', in Bersten, A.D. and Soni, N. (eds) *Intensive Care Manual*, 5th edn, Edinburgh: Butterworth-Heinemann, 927–32.

Naftchi, N.E. and Richardson, J.S. (1997) 'Autonomic dysreflexia: pharmacological management of hypertensive crises in spinal cord injured patients', *Journal of Spinal Cord Medicine*, 20(3): 355–60.

Nakagawa, N., Macchione, M., Petrolino, M.S., Guimaraes, E.T., King, M., Saldiva, P.H.N. and Lorenzo-Filho, G. (2000) 'Effects of a heat and moisture exchanger and a heated humidifier on respiratory mucus in patients undergoing mechanical ventilation', *Critical Care Medicine*, 28(2): 312–17.

Nakos, G., Tsangaris, I., Kostanti, E., Nathanail, C., Lachana, A., Koulouras, V. and Kastani, D. (2000) 'Effect of the prone position on patients with hydrostatic pulmonary edema compared with patients with acute respiratory distress syndrome and pulmonary fibrosis', *American Journal of Respiratory and Critical Care Medicine*, 161(2 part 1): 360–8.

Narasinghan, M., Posner, A.J., De Palo, V.A., Mayo, P.H. and Rosen, M.J. (2004) 'Intensive care in patients with HIV infection in the era of highly active antiretroviral therapy', *Chest*, 125(5): 1800–4.

Nates, J.L., Cooper, D.J., Day, B. and Tuxen, D.V. (1997) 'Acute weakness syndromes in critically ill patients – a reappraisal', *Anaesthesia and Intensive Care*, 25(5): 502–13.

Nathan, A.T. and Singer, M. (1999) 'The oxygen trail: tissue oxygenation', *British Medical Bulletin*, 55(1): 96–108.

National Audit Office (2002) *Summarised Accounts 2000–2001*, London: National Audit Office.

National Institute for Clinical excellence (2003) *Head Injury, Triage Assessment, Investigation and Early Management of Head Injury in Infants, Children and Adults – Clinical Guideline 4*, London: NICE.

National Patient Safety Agency (2004) *Bowel Care for Patients with Established Spinal Cord Lesions*, 15th September, London: National Patient Safety Agency.

Neal, M. (1994) 'Necrotising fasciitis', *Nursing Times*, 90(41): 53–4.

Newcombe, P. (2002) 'Pathology of sickle cell disease crisis', *Emergency Nurse*, 9(9): 19–22.

Newton, C.A. and Raskin, P. (2004) 'Diabetic ketoacidosis in type 1 and type 2 diabetes mellitus', *Archives of Internal Medicine*, 164(17): 1925–31.

Nicholls, J.M., Poon, L.L.M. and Lee, K.C. (2003) 'Lung pathology of fatal severe acute respiratory syndrome', *Lancet*, 361(9371): 1773–8.

Nicholson, J.P., Wolmarans, M.R. and Park, G.R. (2000) 'The role of albumin in critical illness', *British Journal of Anaesthesia*, 85(4): 599–610.

Nierman, D.M., Schechter, C.B. and Cannon, L.M. (2001) 'Outcome prediction model for very elderly critically ill patients', *Critical Care Medicine*, 29(10): 1853–9.

Nightingale, F. (1859/1980) *Notes on Nursing: What It Is, and What It Is Not*, Edinburgh: Churchill Livingstone.

Nissen, S.E. (2002) 'Who is at risk for atherosclerotic disease? Lessons from intravascular ultrasound', *American Journal of Medicine*, 112(Supplement 8A): 27S–33S.

NMC (2002) *Guidelines for the Administration of Medicines*, London: NMC.

—— (2004) *The NMC Code of Professional Conduct: Standards for Conduct, Performance and Ethics*, London: NMC.

Nolan, J.J. (2002) 'What is type 2 diabetes?', *Medicine*, 30(1): 6–10.

Norman, I.J. and Redfern, S.J. (eds) (1997) *Mental Health Care for Elderly People*, Edinburgh: Churchill Livingstone.

Norwood, M.G.A., Bown, M.J., Lloyd, G., Bell, P.R.F. and Sayers, R.D. (2004) 'The clinical value of the systemic inflammatory response syndrome in abdominal aortic aneurysm repair', *British Journal of Surgery*, 91(Supplement 1): 112.

NPSA (2002) *Patient Safety Alert. Ref PSA 01*, London: National Patient Safety Agency.

—— (2005) *Safety Alert 0180Jan05. Reducing the harm caused by misplaced nasogastric feeding tubes*, London: National Patient Safety Agency.

Ntoumenopoulos, G., Presneill, J.J., McElholum, M. and Cade, J.F. (2002) 'Chest physiotherapy for the prevention of ventilator-associated pneumonia', *Intensive Care Medicine*, 28(7): 850–6.

Nunn, J.F. (1996) 'Oxygen consumption and delivery', in Prys-Roberts, C. and Brown, B.R. Jr (eds) *International Practice of Anaesthesia*, Oxford: Butterworth-Heinemann, 1/61/1–10.

Nutt, J. (1997) 'HELLP syndrome', *British Journal of Midwifery*, 5(1): 8–11.

Nye, K.J., Leggett, V.A. and Watterson, L. (2005) 'Provision and decontamination of uniforms in the NHS', *Nursing Standard*, 19(33): 41–45.

O'Connor, T.M., O'Halloran, D.J. and Shanahan, F. (2002) 'The stress response and the hypothalamic-pituitary-adrenal axis: from moleule to melancholia', *QJM*, 93(6): 323–33.

Odell, A., Allder, R., Bayne, R., Everett, C., Scott, S., Still, B. and West, S. (1993) 'Endotracheal suction for adult, non-head-injured, patients', *Intensive and Critical Care Nursing*, 9(4): 274–8.

Odell, M. (1996) 'Intracranial pressure monitoring, nursing in a district general hospital', *Nursing in Critical Care*, 1(5): 245–7.

Oesterie, S.N., Sanborn, T.A., Ali, N., Resar, J., Ramee, S.R., Heuser, R., Dean, L., Knopf, W., Schofield, P., Schaer, G.L., Masden, R., Yeung, A.C. and Burkhoff, D. (2000) 'Percutaneous transmyocardial laser revascularisation for severe angina: the PACIFIC randomised trial', *Lancet*, 356(9243): 1705–10.

O'Grady, J.G., Burroughs, A., Hardy, P., Elbourne, D., Truesdale, A. and UK and Republic of Ireland Liver Transplant Study group (2002) 'Tacrolimus versus micromulsified ciclosporin in liver transplantations: the TMC randomised controlled trial', *Lancet*, 360(9340): 1119–25.

O'Grady, N.P., Barie, P.S., Bartlett, J., Bleck, T., Garvey, G., Jacobi, J., Linden, P., Maki, D.G., Nam, M., Pasculle, W., Pasquale, M.D., Tribett, D.L. and Masur, H. (1998) 'Practice parameters for evaluating new fever in critically ill patients', *Critical Care Medicine*, 26(2): 392–408.

Oh, T.E. (2003) 'Oxygen therapy', in Bersten, A.D. and Soni, N. (eds) *Intensive Care Manual*, 5th edn, Edinburgh: Butterworth-Heinemann, 275–82.

Oliveira–Filho, J., Ezzeddine, M.A., Segal, A.Z., Buonanno, F.S., Chang, Y., Ogilvy, C.S., Rordorf, G.,

Schwamm, L.H., Koroshetz, W.J. and McDonald, C.T. (2001) 'Fever in subarachnoid hemorrhage: relationship to vasospasm and outcome', *Neurology*, 56(10): 1299–304.

Olleveant, N., Humphris, G. and Roe, B. (1998) 'A reliability study of the modified New Sheffield sedation scale', *Nursing in Critical Care*, 3(2): 83–8.

O'Neill, L.J. and Carter, D.E. (1998) 'Adult/elderly care nursing. The implications of head injury for family relationships', *British Journal of Nursing*, 7(14): 842–6.

Opal, S., Kessler, C., Roemisch, J. and Knaub, S. (2002) 'Antithrombin, heparin and heparin sulphate', *Critical Care Medicine*, 30(5 Supplement): S325–31.

O'Reilly, M. (2003) 'Oral care of the critically ill: a review of the literature and guidelines for practice', *Australian Critical Care*, 16(3): 101–9.

Orme, J., Romney, J.S., Hopkins, R.O., Pope, D., Chan, K.J., Thomsen, G., Crapo, R.O. and Weaver, L.K. (2003) 'Pulmonary function and health-related quality of life in survivors of acute respiratory distress syndrome', *American Journal of Respiratory and Critical Care Medicine*, 167(5): 690–4.

O'Shea, P. (1997) 'Altered consciousness and stroke', in Goldhill, D.R. and Withington, P.S. (eds) *Textbook of Intensive Care*, London: Chapman & Hall, 495–502.

O'Sullivan, G.F. and Park, G.R. (1990) 'The assessment of sedation in critically ill patients', *Clinical Intensive Care*, 1(3): 116–22.

O'Toole, S. (1997) 'Alternatives to mercury thermometers', *Professional Nurse*, 12(11): 783–6.

Packer, M., Coats, A.J., Fowler, M.B., Katus, H.A., Krum, H., Monacsi, P., Roulen, J.L., Tendera, M., Castaigne, A., Roecker, E.B., Schultz, M.K., DeMets, D.L. and Carvedilol Prospective Randomized Cumulative Survival Study Group (2001) 'Effect of carvedilol on survival in severe chronic heart failure', *New England Journal of Medicine*, 344(22): 1651–8.

Padwal, R., Straus, S.E. and McAlister, F.A. (2001) 'Cardiovascular risk factors and their effects on the decision to treat hypertension: evidence based review, *BMJ*, 322(7292): 977–80.

Palmer, K.R. and Penman, I.D. (1999) 'Diseases of the alimentary tract and pancreas,' in Haslett, C., Chilvers, E.R., Hunter, J.A.A. and Boon, N.A. (eds) *Davidson's Principles and Practice of Medicine,'* 18th edn, Edinburgh: Churchill Livingstone, 599–681.

Pamba, A. and Maitland, K. (2004) 'Capillary refill: prognostic value in Kenyan children', *Archives of Diseases in Childhood*, 89(10): 950–5.

Pandharipande, P.P., Shintani, A., Peterson, J. and Ely, W. (2004) 'Sedative and analgesic medications are independent risk factors for ICU patients for transitioning into delirium', *Critical Care Medicine*, 32(12 Supplement): A19.

Paparella, D., Brister, S.J. and Buchanan, M.R. (2004) 'Coagulation disorders of cardiopulmonary bypass: a review', *Intensive Care Medicine*, 30(10): 1873–81.

Parker, L.J. (1999) 'Managing and maintaining a safe environment in the hospital setting', *British Journal of Nursing*, 8(16): 1053–66.

—— (2002) 'Infection and diseases', in Walsh, M. (ed.) *Watson's Clinical Nursing and Related Sciences*, 6th edn, Edinburgh: Baillière Tindall, 125–49.

Parker, R.I. (1997) 'Etiology of acquired coagulopathies in the critically ill adult and child', *Critical Care Clinics*, 13(3): 591–609.

Parker, T.J., Stevens, J.E., Rice, A.S.C., Greenaway, C.L., Bray, R.J., Smith, P.J., Waldman, C.S. and Verghese, C. (1992) 'Metabolic acidosis and fatal myocardial failure after propofol infusion in children: five case reports', *BMJ*, 305(6854): 613–16.

Parkinson, E., Beale, R. and Bihari, D. (1996) 'Prediction of outcome in the ICU', *British Journal of Intensive Care*, 6(2): 55–9.

Parnaby, C. (2004) 'A new anti-embolism stocking', *British Journal of Perioperative Nursing*, 14(7): 302–7.

Parrillo, J.E. (2001) 'The heart and vasculature in sepsis and septic shock', in Galley, H.F. (ed.) *Critical Care Focus 6: Cardiology in Critical Illness*, London: BMJ Books, 46–56.

Parrott, A.C., Lees, A., Garnham, N.J., Jones, M. and Wesnes, K. (1998) 'Cognitive performance in recreational users of MDMA of "ecstasy": evidence for memory deficits', *Journal of Psychopharmacology*, 12(1): 79–83.

Parthasarathy, S. and Tobin, M.J. (2004) 'Sleep in the intensive care unit', *Intensive Care Medicine*, 30(2): 197–206.

Pastor, C.M., Maatthay, M.A. and Frossard, J.-L. (2003) 'Pancreatitis-associated acute lung injury', *Chest*, 124(6): 2341–51.

Patel, B.M., Chittock, D.R., Russell, J.A. and Walley, K.R. (2002) 'Beneficial effects of short-term vasopressin infusion during severe septic shock', *Anaesthesia*, 96(3): 576–82.

Patel, D. and Meakin, G.H. (2000) 'Paediatric airway management', *Current Anaesthesia & Critical Care*, 11(5): 262–8.

Patil, B.B. and Dowd, T.C. (2000) 'Physiological functions of the eye', *Current Anaesthesia & Critical Care*, 11(6): 291–8.

Patton, G.C., Coffey, C., Carlin, J.B., Degenhardt, L., Lynskey, M. and Hall, W. (2002) 'Cannabis use and mental health in young people: cohort study', *BMJ*, 325(7374): 1195–8.

Paulson, C. (2002) 'Meperidine or morphine for the treatment of pancreatic pain', *RN*, 65(5): 10.

Pearce, C.B. and Duncan, H.D. (2002) 'Enteral feeding: nasogastric, nasojejunal, percutaneous endoscopic gastrostomy, or jejunostomy: it's indications and limitations', *Postgraduate Medical Journal*, 78(918): 198–204.

Pearson, L.S. (1996) 'A comparison of the ability of foam swabs and toothbrushes to remove dental plaque: implications for nursing practice', *Journal of Advanced Nursing*, 23(1): 62–9.

Peate, I. (2004) 'An overview of meningitis: signs, symptoms, treatment and support, *British Journal of Nursing*, 13(3): 796–801.

Peiris, J.S., Chu, C.M., Cheng, V.C., Guan, Y., Yam, L.Y.C., Lim, W., Nicholls, J., Yee, W.K.S., Yan, W.W.,

Cheung, M.T., Cheng, V.C.C., Chan, K.H., Tsang, D.N.C., Yung, R.W.H., Ng, T.K., Yuen, K.Y. and Sars Study Group (2003) 'Clinical progression and viral load in a community outbreak of coronavirus-associated SARS pneumonia: a prospective study', *Lancet*, 361(9371): 1767–72.

Pelletier, M.L. (1992) 'The organ donor family members perception of stressful situations during the organ donation experience', *Journal of Advanced Nursing*, 17(1): 90–7.

Pelosi, P., Brazzi, L. and Gattinoni, L. (2002) 'Prone position in acute respiratory distress syndrome', in Evans, T.W. Griffiths, M.J.D. and Keogh, B.F. (eds) *ARDS*, Sheffield: European Respiratory Society Journals Ltd, 143–60.

Pelosi, P., Chiumello, B.D., Caironi, P., Panigada, M., Gamberoni, C., Colombo, G., Bigatello, L.M. and Gattinoni, L. (2003) 'Sigh in supine and prone position during acute respiratory distress syndrome', *American Journal of Respiratory and Critical Care Medicine*, 167(4): 521–7.

Pender, L.R. and Frazier, S.K. (2005) 'The relationship between dermal pressure ulcers, oxygenation and perfusion in mechanically ventilated patients', *Intensive and Critical Care Nursing*, 21(1): 29–38.

Penzer, R. and Finch, M. (2001) 'Promoting healthy skin in older people', *Nursing Older People*, 13(8): 22–8.

Perlino, C.A. (2001) 'Postoperative fever', *Medical Clinics of North America*, 85(5): 1141–9.

Perrins, J., King, N. and Collings, J. (1998) 'Assessment of long-term psychological well-being following intensive care', *Intensive and Critical Care Nursing*, 14(3): 108–16.

Petter, A.H., Chiolero, R.L., Cassina, T., Chassot, P.-G., Muller, X.M. and Revelly, J.-P. (2003) 'Automatic "respirator/weaning" with adaptive support ventilation, the effect on duration of endotracheal intubation and patient management', *Anesthesia & Analgesia*, 97(6): 1743–50.

Pickworth, T. (2003) 'Acute pancreatitis', *Anaesthesia and Intensive Care*, 4(4): 106–7.

Pierce, J.D., Cackler, A.B. and Arnett, M.G. (2004) 'Why should you care about free radicals?', *AJN*, 67(1): 38–42.

Pierce, L.N.B. (1995) *Guide to Mechanical Ventilation and Intensive Respiratory Care*, Philadelphia, PA: W.B. Saunders.

Pilcher, T. and Odell, M. (2000) 'Position statement on nurse–patient ratios in critical care', *Nursing Standard*, 15(1): 38–41.

Pinhu, L., Whitehead, T., Evans, T. and Griffiths, M. (2003) 'Ventilator-associated lung injury', *Lancet*, 361(9354): 332–40.

Pinosky, M.L., Kennedy, D.J., Fishman, R.L., Reeves, S.T., Alpert, C.C., Ecklund, J., Kribbs, S., Spinale, F.G., Kratz, J.M., Crawford, R., Gravalee, G.P. and Dorman, B.H. (1997) 'Tranexamic acid reduces bleeding after cardiopulmonary bypass when compared to epsilon aminocaproic acid and placebo', *Journal of Cardiac Surgery*, 12(5): 330–8.

Pitkin, A., Scott, R. and Salmon, J. (1997) 'Hyperbaric oxygen therapy in intensive care', *British Journal of Intensive Care*, 7(3): 107–13.

Pittet, D. and Boyce, J.M. (2001) 'Hand hygiene and patient care: pursing the Semmelweis legacy', *Lancet, Infection diseases* (April): 9–20.

Plant, P.K., Owen, J.L. and Elliott, M.W. (2001) 'Non-invasive ventilation in acute exacerbation of chronic obstructive pulmonary disease: long term survival and predictors of in-hospital outcome', *Thorax*, 56(9): 708–12.

Platt, A.T. (2001) 'MRSA in intensive care', *Nursing Standard*, 15(31): 27–32.

Plowright, C.I. (1995) 'Needs of visitors in the intensive care unit', *British Journal of Nursing*, 4(18): 1081–3.

Pochard, F., Azoulay, E., Chevret, S., Lemaire, F., Hubert, P., Canoui, P., Grassin, M., Zittoun, R., le Gall, J.-R., Dhainaut, J.F. and Schlemmer, B. (2001) 'Symptoms of anxiety and depression in family members of intensive care patients: ethical hypothesis regarding decision-making capacity', *Critical Care Medicine*, 29(10): 1893–7.

Polderman, K.H. and Girbes, A.R.J. (2002) 'Central venous catheter use. Part 1: mechanical complications', *Intensive Care Medicine*, 28(1): 1–17.

Poulter, A. (1998) 'The patient with Guillain Barré syndrome: implications for critical care nursing practice', *Nursing in Critical Care*, 3(4): 182–9.

Póvoa, P. (2002) 'C-reactive protein: a valuable marker of sepsis', *Intensive Care Medicine*, 28(3): 235–43.

Powell, T. (2004) *Head Injury: A Practical Guide*, 2nd edn, Bicester: Speechmark.

Prandoni, P., Lensing, A.W.A., Prins, M.H., Frulla, M., Marchiori, A., Bernardi, E., Tormene, D., Mosena, L., Pagnan, A. and Girolami, A. (2004) 'Below-knee elastic compression stockings to prevent the post-thrombotic syndrome', *Annals of Internal Medicine*, 141(4): 249–56.

Pratt, R. (2003) *HIV & AIDS*, 5th edn, London: Arnold.

Pratt, R.J., Pellowe, C., Loveday, H.P., Robinson, N., Smith, G.W. and *epic* guidelines team (2001) 'Guidelines for preventing infections associated with the insertion and maintenance of central venous catheters', *Journal of Hospital Infection*, 47 (supplement): S47–S67.

Price, T.E. (1998) 'Managing the nursing priorities in the patient with a cerebral insult', in Albarran, J.W. and Price, T.E. (eds) *Managing the Nursing Priorities in Intensive Care*, Dinton: Quay Books, 86–116.

Priestly, M. (1999) 'How nurses identify and meet the needs of visitors to intensive care units', *Nursing In Critical Care*, 4(1): 27–30.

Prinssen, M., Verhoeven, E.L.G., Buth, J., Cuypers, P.W.M., van Sambeek, M.R.H.M., Balm, R., Buskens, E., Grobbee, D.E. and Blankensteijn, J.D. (2004) 'A randomised trial comparing conventional and endovascular repair of abdominal aortic aneurysms', *New England Journal of Medicine*, 351(16): 1607–18.

Pugin, J., Auckenthaler, R., Lew, P.D. and Suter, P.M. (1991) 'Oropharyngeal decontamination decreases incidence of ventilator associated pneumonia', *JAMA*, 265(20): 2704–10.

Quinlan, G.J. and Evans, T.W. (2000) 'Acute respiratory distress syndrome in adults', *Hospital Medicine*, 61(8): 561–3.

Raaijmakers, E., Faes, J.C., Scholten, R.J., Goovaerts, H.G. and Heethaar, R. (1999) 'A meta-analysis of three decades of validating thoracic impedance cardiography', *Critical Care Medicine*, 27(6): 1203–13.

Rachels, J. (1986) *The End of Life*, Oxford: Oxford University Press.

Raeburn, C.D., Sheppard, F., Barsness, K.A., Ayra, J. and Harken, A.H. (2002) 'Cytokines for surgeons', *American Journal of Surgery*, 183(3): 268–73.

Rahman, T.M. and Treacher, D. (2002) 'Management of acute renal failure on the intensive care unit', *Clinical Medicine*, 2(2): 108–13.

Rajaratnam, S.M.W. and Arendt, J. (2001) 'Health in a 24 hour society', *Lancet*, 3581(9286): 999–1005.

Rakel, B. and Herr, K. (2004) 'Assessment and treatment of postoperative pain in older adults', *Journal of Peri-Anesthesia Nursing*, 19(3): 194–208.

Ramage, D., Lovell, M., DeRose, G., Harris, K.A. and Kribs, S. (2001) 'Establishing an endovascular abdominal aortic program – decisions, decisions, decisions: the London Health Sciences Centre experience', *Journal of Vascular Nursing*, 19(1): 10–13.

Ramnarayan, P., Thomas, D., Tanna, A. Britto J, Alexander S. (2002) 'The impact of specialised paediatric retrieval services on the management of sick children at the referring hospital', *Archives of Disease in Childhood*, 86(supplement 1): A27.

Ramsay, M.A., Savege, T.M., Simpson, B.R. and Goodwin, R. (1974) 'Controlled sedation with alphaxolone-alphadolone', *BMJ*, 1974–2(920): 656–9.

Ramsay, S.J. and Gomersall, C.D. (2003) 'Severe acute respiratory syndrome', *JICS*, 4(2): 42–3.

Ranasinghe, A.M. and Bonser, R.S. (2004) 'Interventions for thoracic aortic disease', in Treasure, T., Hunt, I. and Keogh, B. and Pagan, D. (eds) *The Evidence for Cardiothoracic Surgery*, Harley, Shrewsbury: tfm Publishing Limited, 253–72.

Rance, M. (2005) 'Kinetic therapy positively influences oxygenation in patients', *Nursing in Critical Care*, 10(1): 35–41.

Randhawa, G. (1997) 'Enhancing the health professional's role in requesting transplant organs', *British Journal of Nursing*, 6(8): 429–34.

Randolph, A.G. (1998) 'An evidence-based approach to central venous catheter management to prevent catheter-related infections in critically ill patients', *Critical Care Clinics*, 14(3): 411–21.

Rang, H.P., Dale, M.M. and Ritter, J.M. (1999) *Pharmacology*, 4th edn, Edinburgh: Churchill Livingstone.

Ranieri, V.M., Suter, P.M., Tortorella, C., Tullio, R., De, Dayer, J.M., Brienza, A., Bruno, F. and Slutsky, A.S. (1999) 'Effect of mechanical ventilation on inflammatory mediators in patients with acute respiratory distress syndrome, *JAMA*, 282(1): 54–61.

Ranieri, V.M., Vitale, N., Grraso, S., Puntillo, F., Mascia, L., Paparella, D., Tunzi, P., Giuliani, R., deLuca Tupputi, L. and Fiore, T. (1999) 'Time-course of impairment of respiratory mechanics after cardiac surgery and cardiopulmonary bypass', *Critical Care Medicine*, 27(8): 1454–60.

Rashid, M., Goldin, R. and Wright, M. (2004) 'Drugs and the liver', *Hospital Medicine*, 65(8): 456–61.

Rathbun, S.W., Whitsett, T.L., Vesely, S.K. and Raskob, G.E. (2004) 'Clinical utility of D-dimer in patients with suspected pulmonary embolism and nondiagnostic lung scans or negative CT findings, *Chest*, 125(3): 851–5.

Rathore, S.S., Epstein, A.J., Volpp, K.G.M. and Krumholz, H.M. (2004) 'Hospital coronary artery bypass graft surgery volume and patient mortality 1998–2000', *Annals of Surgery*, 239(1): 110–11.

Rattenbury, N., Mooney, G. and Bowen, J. (1999) 'Oral assessment and care for inpatients', *Nursing Times*, 95(49): 52–3.

Ravenscroft, A.J. and Bell, M.D.D. (2000) ' "End-of-life" decision making within intensive care – objective, consistent, defensible?' *Journal of Medical Ethics*, 26(6): 435–40.

Ravi, R. and Morgan, R.J. (2003) 'Intracranial pressure monitoring', *Current Anaesthesia and Critical Care*, 14(5–6): 229–35.

Rayner, D. (2004) 'Tuberculosis and HIV infection: minimising transmission', *Nursing Standard*, 19(4): 47–53.

RCN (Royal College of Nursing) Critical Care Forum (1999) *Restraint Revisited – Rights, Risks and Responsibility*, London: RCN.

—— (2000) *Digital Rectal Examination and Manual Removal of Faeces. Guidelines for Nurses*, London: RCN.

—— (2003a) *Guidance for Nurse Staffing in Critical Care*, London: RCN.

—— (2003b) *Standards for Infusion Therapy*, London: RCN.

—— (2003c) 'Guidance for nurse staffing in critical care', *Nursing in Critical Care*, 19(5): 257–66.

—— (2005) *Methicillin-resistant Staphylococcus aureas* (MRSA), London: RCN.

RCOG (2004) *Why Mothers Die*, London: Royal College of Obstetricians and Gynaecologists.

Redfern, S.J. and Ross, F.M. (eds) (1999) *Nursing Older People*, 3rd edn, Edinburgh: Churchill Livingstone.

Redmond, M.C. (2001) 'Malignant hyperpyrexia: perianesthesia recognition, treatment, and care', *Journal of Peri Anesthesia Nursing*, 16(4): 259–69.

Reece-Smith, H. (1997) 'Pancreatitis', *Care of the Critically Ill*, 13(4): 135–8.

Reid, C.L. and Campbell, I.T. (2004) 'Metabolic physiology', *Current Anaesthesia & Critical Care*, 15(3): 209–17.

Reid, J. and Morison, M.J. (1994) 'Classification of pressure sore severity', *Nursing Times*, 90(20): 46–50.

Reilly, D.E. (1980) *Behavioural Objectives – Evaluation in Nursing*, New York: Appleton Century Crofts.

Reilly, M.P. and Rader, D.J. (2003) 'The metabolic syndrome: more than the sum of its parts', *Circulation*, 108: 1546–51.

Remy, B., Deby-Dupont, G. and Lamy, M. (1999) 'Red blood cell substitutes: fluorocarbon emulsions and haemoglobin solutions', *British Medical Bulletin*, 55(1): 277–98.

Renehan, A.G., Booth, C. and Potten, C.S. (2001) 'What is apoptosis, and why is it important?' *BMJ*, 322(7301): 1536–8.

Reneman, L., Booij, J., de Bruin, K., Reitsma, J.B., de Wolff, F.A., Gunning, W.B., den Heeten, G.J. and van den Brink, W. (2001) 'Effects of dose, sex and long-term abstention from use on toxic effects of MDMA (ecstasy) on brain serotonin levels', *Lancet*, 358(9296): 1864–9.

Renton, M.C. and Snowden, C.P. (2005) 'Dopexamine and its role in the protection of hepatospanchnic and renal perfusion in high-risk surgical and critically ill patients', *British Journal of Anaesthesia*, 94(4): 459–67.

Reuben, A.D. and Harris, A.R. (2004) 'Heliox for asthma in the emergency department: a review of the literature', *Emergency Medicine Journal*, 21(2): 131–5.

Revelley, J.P., Tappy, L., Berger, M.M., Gerbach, P., Cayeux, C. and Chiolero, R. (2001) 'Early metabolic and splanchnic responses to enteral nutrition in post-operative cardiac surgery patients with circulatory compromise', *Intensive Care Medicine*, 27(3): 540–7.

Ricard, J.-D., Dreyfus, D. and Saumon, G. (2003) 'Ventilator-induced lung injury', *European Respiratory Journal*, 22(Supplement 42): 2s–9s.

Ridker, P.M., Rifai, N., Clearfield, M., Downs, J.R., Weiss, S.E., Miles, J.S., Gotto, A.M. and Airforce/Texas Coronary Atherosclerosis prevention study investigators (2001) 'Measurement of C-reactive protein for the targeting of statin therapy in the primary prevention of acute coronary events', *New England Journal of Medicine*, 344(26): 1959–65.

Ridley, S (ed.) (2002) *Outcomes in Critical Care*, Oxford: Butterworth-Heinemann.

Ridwan, B., Mascini, E., van der Reijden, N., Verhoef, J. and Bonte, M. (2002) 'What action should be taken to prevent spread of vancomycin resistant Enterococci in European hospitals', *BMJ*, 324(7338): 666–8.

Riker, R.R., Fraser, G.L., Simmons, L.E. and Wilkins, M.L. (2001) 'Validation the sedation-agitation scale with the bispectral index and visual analog scale in adult ICU patients after cardiac surgery', *Intensive Care Medicine*, 27(5): 853–8.

Riley, J. (2002) 'Raise a drink to good health', *Professional Nurse*, 17(3): 299.

Rising, C.J. (1993) 'The relationship of selected nursing activities to ICP', *Journal of Neuroscience Nursing*, 25(5): 302–8.

Rivers, E., Ander, D. and Powell, D. (2001) 'Central venous oxygen saturation monitoring in the critically ill patient', *Current Opinion in Critical Care*, 7(3): 204–11.

Roberts, B. and Chaboyer, W. (2004) 'Patients' dreams and unreal experiences following intensive care unit admission', *Nursing in Critical Care*, 9(4): 173–80.

Roberts, B.L. (2001) 'Managing delirium in adult intensive care patients', *Critical Care Nurse*, 21(1): 48–55.

Robertson, C.S. (2001) 'Management of cerebral perfusion pressure after traumatic brain injury', *Anesthesiology*, 95(6): 1513–17.

Robertson, M.S., Cade, J.F. and Clancy, R.L. (1999) '*Helicobacter pylori* infection in intensive care: increased prevalence and a new nosocomial infection', *Critical Care Medicine*, 27(7): 1276–80.

Rogers, C.R. (1951) *Client-Centred Therapy*, London: Constable.

—— (1967) *On Becoming a Person*, London: Constable.

—— (1983) *Freedom to Learn for the 80s*, New York: Merrill.

Romyn, D.M. (2001) 'Disavowal of the behaviorist paradigm in nursing education: what makes it so difficult to unseat?', *Advances in Nursing Science*, 23(3): 1–10.

Ronco, C., Bellomo, R., Homel, P. Brendolan, A., Dan, M., Piccinni, P. and Le Graca, G. (2000) 'Effects at different doses in continuous venovenous haemofiltration on outcomes of acute renal failure: a prospective randomised trial', *Lancet*, 356(9223): 26–30.

Roper, N., Logan, W. and Tierney, A. (1996) *The Elements of Nursing*, 4th edn, Edinburgh: Churchill Livingstone.

Ros, I., Depasse, B., Schroeder, M. Dumont J. and Vincent, J.-L. (2000) 'Information needs of the ICU patient: a Belgium experience, *Clinical Intensive Care*, 11(1): 13–18.

Rosenberg, A.L. and Watts, C. (2000) 'Patients readmitted to ICUs', *Chest*, 118(2): 492–502.

Rosendale, J.D., Kauffman, H.M., McBride, M.A., Chabalewski, F.L., Zaroff, J.G., Garrity, E.R., Delmonico, F.L. and Rosengard, B.R. (2003) 'Aggressive pharmacologic donor management results in more transplanted organs', *Transplantation*, 75(4): 482–7.

Rossi, S., Zanier, E.R., Mauri, I., Columbo, A. and Stocchetti, N. (2001) 'Brain temperature, body core temperature, and intracranial pressure in acute cerebral damage', *Journal of Neurology, Neurosurgery and Psychiatry*, 71(4): 448–54.

Rouby, J.J., Lu, Q. and Goldstein, I. (2002) 'Selecting the right level of positive end-expiratory pressure in patients with acute respiratory distress syndrome', *American Journal of Respiratory and Critical Care Medicine*, 165(8): 1182–6.

Rowlee, S.C. (1999) 'Monitoring neuromuscular blockade in the intensive care unit: the peripheral nerve stimulator', *Heart & Lung*, 28(5): 352–62.

Rubinovitch, B. and Pittet, D. (2001) 'Screening for methicillin-resistant *Staphylococcus aureus* in the endemic hospital: what have we learned?', *Journal of Hospital Infection*, 47(1): 9–18.

Ruffell, A.J. (2004) 'Sepsis strategies: an ICU package', *Nursing in Critical Care*, 9(6): 257–63.

Russell, S. (2000) 'Continuity of care after discharge from ICU', *Professional Nurse*, 15(6): 497–500.

Ryan, D. (1997) 'Euricus-1', *Care of the Critically Ill*, 13(1): 4.

Ryan, J. (2004) 'Aesthetic physical caring – valuing the visible', *Nursing in Critical Care*, 9(4): 181–7.

Ryder, S.D. and Beckingham, I.J. (2001) 'Acute hepatitis', *BMJ*, 322(7279): 151–3.

Safar, M.E., Levy, B.I. and Struijker-Boudier, H. (2003) 'Current perspectives on arterial stiffness and pulse pressure in hypertension and cardiovascular diseases', *Circulation*, 107(22): 2864–9.

561

Safdar, N. and Maki, D.G. (2004) 'The pathogenesis of catheter-related bloodstream infection with noncuffed short-term central venous catheters', *Intensive Care Medicine*, 30(1): 62–7.

Saggs, P. (2000) 'Liver failure in the critically ill', *Nursing in Critical Care*, 5(1): 40–8.

Sakka, S.G., Klein, M., Reinhart, K. and Meier-Hellmann, A. (2002) 'Prognostic value of extravascular lung water in critically ill patients', *Chest*, 122(6): 2080–6.

Salmon, J.B. and Garrard, C. (1999) 'Acute lung injury and acute respiratory distress syndrome', *Medicine*, 27(11): 142–5.

Salukhe, T.V. and Wyncoll, D.L.A. (2002) 'Volumetric haemodynamic monitoring and continuous pulse contour analysis – an untapped resource for coronary and high dependency care units?' *British Journal of Cardiology*, 9(1 AIC): 20–5.

Samanta, A. and Samanta, J. (2004) 'NICE guideline and law: clinical governance implications for trusts', *Clinical Governance*, 9(4): 212–15.

Sandin, R.H., Enlund, G., Samuelsson, P. and Lenmarken, C. (2000) 'Awareness during anaesthesia: a prospective study', *Lancet*, 355(9205): 707–11.

Sanmuganathan, P. (2001) 'Cholesterol reduction: how low should cholesterol go?', *British Journal of Cardiology*, 8(4): 219–29.

Sarvimaki, A. and Sanderlin Benko, S. (2001) 'Values and evaluation in health care', *Journal of Nursing Management*, 9(3): 129–37.

Sasso, F.C., Carbonara, O., Nasti, R., Campana, B., Marfalla, R., Torella, M., Nappi, G., Torella, R. and Cozzolino, D. (2004) 'Glucose metabolism and coronary heart disease in patients with normal glucose tolerance', *JAMA*, 291(15): 1857–63.

Sawyer, N. (1997) 'Back from the twilight zone', *Nursing Times*, 93(7): 28–9.

Say, J. (1997) 'Nutritional assessment in clinical practice: a review', *Nursing in Critical Care*, 2(1): 29–33.

Scannapieco, F.A., Stewart, E.M. and Mylotte, J.M. (1992) 'Colonization of dental plaque by respiratory pathogens in medical intensive care patients', *Critical Care Medicine*, 20(6): 740–5.

Scheibmeir, H.D., Christensen, K., Whitaker, S.H., Jegaethesan, J., Clancy, R. and Pierce, J.D. (2005) 'A review of free radicals and antioxidants for critical care nurses', *Intensive and Critical Care Nursing*, 21(1): 24–8.

Scheinkestel, C.D., Bailey, M., Myles, P.S., Jones, K., Cooper, D.J., Millar, I.L. and Tuxen, D.V. (1999) 'Hyperbaric or nomobaric oxygen for acute carbon monoxide poisoning: a randomised controlled clinical trial', *Medical Journal of Australia*, 170(5): 203–10.

Schifano, F., Oyefeso, A., Webb, L., Pollard, M., Corkery, J. and Ghodse, A.H. (2003) 'Review of deaths related to taking ecstasy, England and Wales, 1997–2000', *BMJ*, 326(7380): 80–1.

Schlaudraff, U. (1999) 'Xenotransplantation: benefits and risks to society', *Bulletin of Medical Ethics*, 146: 13–15.

Schlicher, M.L. (2001) 'Using liquid ventilation to treat patients with acute respiratory distress syndrome: a guide to a breath of fresh liquid', *Critical Care Nurse*, 21(5): 55–65.

Schoenhofer, S.O. (1989) 'Affectional touch in critical care nursing: a descriptive study', *Heart and Lung*, 18(2): 146–54.

Schofield, E., Lawman, S., Volans, G. and Henry, J. (1997) 'Drugs of abuse: clinical features and management', *Emergency Nurse*, 5(6): 17–22.

Schreuder, F.M. and Jones, U.F. (2004) 'The effect of saline instillation on sputum yield and oxygen saturation measurement in adult intubated patients: single subject design', *Physiotherapy*, 90(2): 109.

Schwacha, M.G. and Chaudry, I.H. (2000) 'Sex hormone-mediated modulation of the immune response after trauma, haemorrhage or sepsis', in Galley, H.F. (ed.) *Critical Care Focus 4: Endocrine Disturbance*, London: BMJ Books, 36–56.

Schweickert, W.D., Gehlbach, B.K., Pohlman, A.S., Hall, J.B. and Kress, J.P. (2004) 'Daily interruption of sedative infusions and complications of critical illness in mechanically ventilated patients', *Critical Care Medicine*, 32(6): 1272–6.

Scott, E.M., Leaper, D.J. and Clark, M. (2001) 'Effects of warming therapy on pressure ulcers – a randomised trial', *AORN*, 73(5): 921–38.

Seaton-Mills, D. (2000) 'Prone positioning in ARDS: a nursing perspective', *Clinical Intensive Care*, 11(4): 203–8.

Sedrakyan, A., Treasure, T. and Elefteriades, J.A. (2004) 'Effect of aprotinin on clinical outcomes in coronary artery bypass graft surgery: a systematic review and meta-analysis of randomized clinical trials', *Journal of Thoracic & Cardiovascular Surgery*, 128(3): 442–8.

Selby, I.R. and James, M.R. (1995) 'Severe metabolic and respiratory acidosis', *British Journal of Intensive Care*, 5(7): 222–5.

Seligman, M.E.P. (1975) *Helplessness: On Depression, Development and Death*, New York: W.H. Freeman.

Semple, D.N., Ebmeier, K.P., Glabus, M.F., O'Carroll, R.E. and Johnstone, E.C. (1999) 'Reducing *in vivo* binding to the serotonin transporter in the cerebral cortex of MDMA ("ecstasy") users', *British Journal of Psychiatry*, 175: 63–9.

Seneviratne, U. (2000) 'Guillain-Barré syndrome', *Postgraduate Medical Journal*, 76(902): 774–82.

Sessler, D.I. (2002) 'Temperature measurements', *Anesthesia & Analgesia*, 96(4): 1236–7.

Shakil, A.O., Mazariegos, G.V. and Kramer, D.J. (1999) 'Fulminant hepatic failure', *Surgical Clinics of North America*, 79(1): 77–107.

Shangraw, R.E. (2000) 'Acid-base balance', in Miller, R.D. (ed.) *Anesthesia*, 5th edn, Philadelphia, PA: Churchill Livingstone, 1383–401.

Shannon, S.A., Mitchell, P.H. and Cain, K.C. (2002) 'Patients, nurses, and physicians have differing views of quality of critical care', *Journal of Nursing Scholarship*, 34(2): 173–9.

Sharara, A.I. (2001) 'Gastroesophageal variceal hemorrhage', *New England Journal of Medicine*, 345(9): 669–81.

Sharp, L.S., Rozycki, G.S. and Feliciano, D.V. (2004) 'Rhabdomyolysis and secondary renal failure in critically ill surgical patients', *American Journal of Surgery*, 188(6): 801–6.

Sheen, C.L., Dillon, J.F., Bateman, D.N., Simpson, K.J. and Macdonald, T.M. (2002) 'Paracetamol toxicity: epidemiology, prevention and costs to the health-care system', *QJM*, 95(9): 609–19.

Shehabi, Y. and Innes, R. (2002) 'Sedation and analgesia in the 21st century', *Egyptian Journal of Anaesthesia*, 18: 143–55.

Sherry, K.M. and Barham, N.J. (1997) 'Cardiovascular pharmacology', in Goldhill, D.R. and Withington, P.S. (eds) *Textbook of Intensive Care*, London: Chapman & Hall, 245–53.

Shiotani, A. and Graham, D.Y. (2002) 'Pathogenesis and therapy of gastric and duodenal ulcer disease', *Medical Clinics of North America*, 86(6): 1447–66.

Shirai, K., Lansky, A.J., Mehran, R., Dangas, G.D., Costantini, C.O., Fahy, M., Slack, S., Mintz, G.S., Stone, G.W. and Leon, M.B. (2004) 'Minimally invasive coronary artery bypass grafting versus stenting for patients with proximal left anterior descending coronary artery disease', *American Journal of Cardiology*, 93(8): 953–8.

Shishehbor, M.H., Brennan, M.-L., Aviles, R.J., Fu, X., Penn, M.S., Specher, D.L. and Hazen, S.L. (2003) 'Statins promote potent systemic antioxidant effects through specific inflammatory pathways', *Circulation*, 108(4): 426–31.

Short, A.F., McVeigh, S.K., Flynn, J.M. Moores LK. (2001) 'Intensive care unit outcomes for patients with thrombotic thrombocytopenic purpura', *Clinical Intensive Care*, 12(2): 73–9.

Sibai, B.M. (1994) 'Pre eclampsia – eclampsia', in Queenan, J.T. (ed.) *Management of High Risk Pregnancy*, Boston, MA: Blackwell Scientific Publications, 377–85.

Sillender, M. (2002) 'The liver and pregnancy', *Care of the Critically Ill*, 18(6): 181–6.

Silvestri, L., Lenhart, F.P. and Fox, M.A. (2001) 'Prevention of intensive care unit infections', *Current Anaesthesia & Critical Care*, 12(1): 34–40.

Simini, B. (1999) 'Patients' perceptions of intensive care', *Lancet*, 354(9178): 571–2.

Simpson, H. (2004) 'Interpretation of arterial blood gases: a clinical guide for nurses', *British Journal of Nursing*, 13(9): 522–8.

Singer, M. and Webb, A.R. (1997) *Oxford Handbook of Critical Care*, Oxford: Oxford University Press.

Sisodiya, S.M. and Duncan J. (2004) 'Epilepsy, epidemiology, clinical assessment and natural history', *Medicine*, 32(10): 47–51.

Sivasothy, P., Brown, L., Smith, I.E. and Shneerson, J.M. (2001) 'Effect of manually assisted cough and mechanical insufflation on cough flow of normal subjects, patients with chronic obstructive pulmonary disease (COPD), and patients with respiratory muscle weakness', *Thorax*, 56(6): 438–44.

Skinner, B.F. (1971) *Beyond Freedom and Dignity*, London: Penguin.

Skinner, R. and Watson, D. (1997) 'Renal failure', in Goldhill, D.R. and Withington, P.S. (eds) *Textbook of Intensive Care*, London: Chapman & Hall, 435–40.

Skowronski, G. (2003) 'Neuromuscular disease in intensive care', in Bersten, A.D. and Soni, N. (eds) *Intensive Care Manual*, 5th edn, Edinburgh: Butterworth-Heinemann, 537–47.

Slavin, J. (2002) 'Acute pancreatitis', *Surgery*, 20(10): 227–30.

Slovis, C. and Jenkins, R. (2002) 'ABC of clinical electrocardiography: conditions not primarily affecting the heart', *BMJ*, 324(7349): 1320–3.

Smith, P.K. and Shah, A.S. (2004) 'The role of aprotinin in a blood-conservation programe', *Journal of Cardiothoracic and Vascular Anesthesia*, 18(4, supplement): 24S–28S.

Smith, P.M. (2000) 'Portal hypertension', *Surgery*, 18(7): 153–6.

Smith, R. (1999) 'Temperature regulation in intensive care patients receiving continuous renal replacement therapies', *Nursing in Critical Care*, 4(6): 298–300.

Smith, R., Hay, A., Hilditch, G. and Wallace, P. (2004) 'Transfer of adults between intensive care units in the United Kingdom: demographics', *Journal of the Intensive Care Society*, 5(3): 125–8.

Smith-Blair, N., Pierce, J.D. and Clancy, R.L. (2003) 'The effect of dobutamine infusion on fractional diaphragm thickening and diaphragm blood flow during fatigue', *Heart & Lung*, 32(2): 111–20.

Snell, C.C. Fothergill-Bourbonnais, F. and Durocher-Henriks, S. (1997) 'Patient controlled analgesia and intramuscular injections: a comparison of patient pain experiences and postoperative outcomes', *Journal of Advanced Nursing*, 25(4): 681–90.

Somme, D., Maillet, J.-M., Gisselbrecht, M., Novara, A., Ract, C. and Fagon, J.-Y. (2003) 'Critically ill old and the oldest-old patients in intensive care: short- and long-term outcomes', *Intensive Care Medicine*, 29(12): 2137–43.

Sontag, S. (1989) *AIDS and its Metaphors*, London: Penguin.

Soo, L.H., Gray, D., Young, T. and Hampton, J.R. (2000) 'Circadian variation in witnessed out of hospital cardiac arrest', *Heart*, 84(4): 370–6.

Southgate, H.M.L. (1999) 'Critical analysis of access to and availability of intensive care', *Intensive and Critical Care Nursing*, 15(4): 204–9.

Spahn, D.R., Waschke, K.F., Standl, T., Motsch, J., Van Huynegem, L., Welte, M., Gombotz, H., Coriat, P., Verkh, L., Faithfull, S., Keipert, P. and the European Perflubron Emulsion in Non-Cardiac Surgery Study Group (2002) 'Use of Perflubron emulsion to decrease allogeneic blood transfusion in high-blood-loss non-cardiac surgery: results of a European Phase 3 Study', *Anesthesiology*, 97(6): 1338–49.

Spapen, H., Diltoer, M., van Malderen, C., Opdenacker, G., Suys, E. and Huygens, L. (2001) 'Soluble fibre reduces the incidence of diarrhoea in septic patients receiving total enteral nutrition', *Clinical Nutrition*, 20(4): 301–5.

Spencer, L. and Willats, S. (1997) 'Sedation', in Goldhill, D.R. and Withington, P.S. (eds) *Textbook of Intensive Care*, London: Chapman & Hall, 95–101.

Spodick, D.H. (2003) 'Acute cardiac tamponade', *NEJM*, 349(7): 684–90.

Spragg, R.G., Lewis, J.F., Wurst, W., Häfner, D., Baughman, R.P., Wewers, M.D. and Marsh, J.J. (2003) 'Treatment of acute respiratory distress syndrome with recombinant surfactant protein C surfactant', *American Journal of Respiratory and Critical Care Medicine*, 167(11): 1562–6.

Sprung, J., Kindscher, J.D., Wahr, J.A., Levy, J.H., Monk, T.G., Moritz, M.W. and O'Hara, P.J. (2002) 'The use of bovine hemoglobin glutamer-250(Hemopure®) in surgical patients: results of a multicenter, randomized, single-blinded trial', *Anesthesia & Analgesia*, 94(4): 799–808.

Stack, C. and Dobbs, P. (2004) *Essentials of Paediatric Intensive Care*, London: Greenwich Medical Media Ltd.

Stanley, A.J. and Hayes, P.C. (1997) 'Portal hypertension and variceal haemorrhage', *Lancet*, 350(9036): 1235–9.

Stansfeld, S.A. and Matheson, M.P. (2003) 'Noise pollution: non-auditory effects on health', *British Medical Bulletin*, 68: 243–57.

Steel, A. and Bihari, D. (2000) 'Choice of catecholamine: does it matter?', *Current Opinion in Critical Care*, 6(5): 347–53.

Steele, A.G. and Sabol, V. (2005) 'Common gastrointestinal disorders', in Morton, P.G., Fontaine, D.K., Hudak, C.M. et al. (eds) *Critical Care Nursing: A Holistic Approach*, 8th edn, Philadelphia, PA: Lippincott Williams & Wilkins, 953–92.

Stephens, R. and Mythen, M. (2003) 'Optimizing intraoperative fluid therapy', *Current Opinion in Anaesthesiology*, 16(4): 385–92.

Stewart, D. (2001) 'The percussion technique for restoring patency to central venous catheters', *Care of the Critically Ill*, 17(3): 106–7.

Stiegmann, G.V., Goff, J.S., Michaletz-Onody, P.A. Korula, J., Lieberman, D., Saeed, Z.A., Reveilee, R.M., Sun, J.H., Lowenstein, S.R. (1992) 'Endoscopic sclerotherapy as compared with endoscopic ligation for bleeding esophageal varices', *New England Journal of Medicine*, 326(23): 1527–32.

Stockmann, H.B.A.C., Hiemstra, C.A., Marquet, R.L. and Jzermans, J.N.M. (2000) 'Extracorporeal perfusion for the treatment of acute liver failure', *Annals of Surgery*, 231(4): 460–70.

Stout, J.E. and Yu, V.L. (1997) 'Legionellosis', *New England Journal of Medicine*, 337(10): 682–7.

—— (2003) 'Hospital-acquired Legionnaires' disease: new developments', *Current Opinion in Infectious Diseases*, 16(4): 337–41.

Strahan, E.H.E. and Brown, R.J. (2005) 'A qualitative study of the experience of patients following transfer from intensive care', *Intensive and Critical Care Nursing*, 21(3): 160–71.

Stuart, J. (1996) 'Legal restraint', *Nursing Management*, 2(10): 26–7.

Suerbaum, S. and Michetti, P. (2002) 'Helicobacter pylori infection', *New England Journal of Medicine*, 347(15): 1175–86.

Sullivan, J. (2000) 'Positioning of patients with severe traumatic brain injury: research-based practice', *Journal of Neuroscience Nursing*, 32(4): 204–9.

Sung, J.J.Y. (2003) 'Acute gastrointestinal bleeding', in Bersten, A.D. and Soni, N. (eds) *Intensive Care Manual*, 5th edn, Edinburgh: Butterworth-Heinemann, 413–21.

Suresh, P., Mercieca, F., Morton, A. and Tullo, A.B. (2000) 'Eye care for the critically ill', *Intensive Care Medicine*, 26(2): 162–6.

Szaflarski, N.L. (1996) 'Preanalytic error associated with blood gas/pH measurement', *Critical Care Nurse*, 16(3): 89–100.

Talbot, D. and Bonner, S. (2003) 'Non heart beating donation and the intensive care unit', *Care of the Critically Ill*, 19(3): 77–82.

Tambyraja, A.L. and Chalmers, R.T.A. (2004) 'Aortic aneurysms', *Surgery*, 22(11): 294–6.

Tanaka, A., Kawarabayashi, T., Fukuda, D., Nishibori, Y., Sakamoto, T., Nishida, Y., Shimada, K. and Yashikawa, J. (2004) 'Circadian variation of plaque rupture in acute myocardial infarction', *American Journal of Cardiology*, 93(1): 1–5.

Tarnow-Mordi, W.O., Hau , C., Warden, A. and Shearer, A.J. (2000) 'Hospital mortality in relation to staff workload: a 4 year study in an adult intensive care unit', *Lancet*, 356(9225): 185–9.

Taylor, M.D., Tracy, J.K., Meyer, W., Pasquale M. and Napolitano LM. (2002) 'Trauma in the elderly: intensive care unit resource use and outcome', *Journal of Trauma*, 53(3): 407–14.

Teare, J. and Smith, J. (2004) 'Using focus groups to explore the views of parents whose children are in hospital', *Paediatric Nursing*, 16(5): 30–4.

Teoh, L.S.G., Gowardman, J.R., Larsen, P.D., Green, R. and Galletly, D.C. (2000) 'Glasgow Coma Scale: variation in mortality among permutations of specific total scores', *Intensive Care Medicine*, 26(2): 157–61.

Tham, L.C.H., Martin, C.M. and Sibbald, W.J. (2000) 'Intestinal microcirculation: changes in sepsis and effect of vasoactive manipulation', in Vincent, J.-L. (ed.) *Yearbook of Intensive Care and Emergency Medicine*, Berlin: Springer, 72–9.

Theaker, C., Mannan, M., Ives, N. and Soni, N. (2000) 'Risk factors for pressure sores in the critically ill', *Anaesthesia*, 55(1): 221–4.

Theaker, C., Ormond-Walshe, S., Azadian, B. and Soni, N. (2001) 'MRSA in the critically ill', *Journal of Hospital Infection*, 48(2): 98–102.

Therapondos, G. and Hayes, O.C. (2002) 'Management of gastro-oesophageal varices', *Clinical Medicine*, 2(4): 297–302.

Thomas, C.F. Jr and Limper, A.H. (2004) 'Pneumocystis pneumonia', *NEJM*, 351(24): 2487–98.

Thomas, G. and Hirsch, N. (2003) 'Generalized convulsive status epilepticus', *Anaesthesia and Intensive Care*, 4(4): 120–2.

Thomas, N.J. and Carcillo, J.A. (1998) 'Hypovolemic shock in pediatric patients', *New Horizons*, 6(2): 120–9.

Thompson, D.S. (2004) 'Methicillin-resistant *Staphylococcus aureus* in a general intensive care unit', *JRSM*, 97(11): 521–6.

Thorne, S.A. (2004) 'Pregnancy in heart disease', *Heart*, 90(4): 450–6.

Thorpe, D. and Harrison, L. (2002) 'Bowel management: development of guidelines', *Connect*, 2(2): 61–6.

Thuong, M., Arvaniti, K., Ruimy, R., de la Salmonière, P., Scanvic-Hameg, A., Lucet, J.C. and Régnier, B. (2003) 'Epidemiology of *Pseudomonas aeruginosa* and risk factors for carriage acquisition in an intensive care unit', *Journal of Hospital Infection*, 53(4): 274–82.

Tibballs, J. (2003) 'Equipment for paediatric intensive care', in Bersten, A.D. and Soni, N. (eds) *Intensive Care Manual*, 5th edn, Edinburgh: Butterworth-Heinemann, 1075–86.

Tidswell, M. (2001) 'Prone ventilation', *Clinical Intensive Care*, 12(5,6): 193–201.

Tissot, E., Cornette, L., Demoly, P., Jacquet, M., Barale, F. and Capellier, G. (1999) 'Medication errors at the administration stage in an intensive care unit', *Intensive Care Medicine*, 25(4): 353–9.

Todaro, J.F., Shen, B.J., Niaura, R., Spiro, A. III and Ward, K.D. (2003) 'Effect of negative emotions on frequency of coronary heart disease(The Normative Aging Study)', *American Journal of Cardiology*, 92(8): 901–6.

Todres, L., Fulbrook, P. and Albarran, J. (2000) 'On the receiving end: a hermeneutic-phenomenological analysis of a patient's struggle to cope while going through intensive care', *Nursing in Critical Care*, 5(6): 277–87.

Toh, C.H. and Dennis, M. (2003) 'Disseminated intravascular coagulation: old disease, new hope', *BMJ*, 327(7421): 974–7.

Tolomiczenko, G.S., Kahan, M., Ricci, M., Strathern, L., Jeney, C., Patterson, K. and Wilson, L. (2005) 'SARS: coping with the impact at a community hospital', *Journal of Advanced Nursing*, 50(1): 101–10.

Tonkin, A. (2004) 'The metabolic syndrome – a growing problem', *European Heart Journal*, 6(Supplement A): A37–A42.

Torpy, D.J. and Chrousos, G.P. (1997) 'Stress and critical illness: the integrated immune/hypothalamic-pituitary-adrenal axis response', *Journal of Intensive Care Medicine*, 12(5): 225–38.

Tough, J. (2004) 'Assessment and treatment of chest pain', *Nursing Standard*, 18(37): 45–53.

—— (2005) 'Thrombolytic therapy in acute myocardial infarction', *Nursing Standard*, 19(37): 55–64.

Tousoulis, D., Davies, G., Stefanadis, C., Toutouzas, P. and Ambrose, J.A. (2003) 'Inflammatory and thrombotic mechanisms in coronary atherosclerosis', *Heart*, 89(9): 993–7.

Trehan, N., Mishra, Y. and Mehta, Y. (1998) 'Transmyocardial laser as an adjunct to minimally invasive CABG for complete myocardial revascularization', *Annals of Thoracic Surgery*, 66(3): 1113–18.

Treloar, D.M. (1995) 'Use of a clinical assessment tool for orally intubated patients', *American Journal of Critical Care*, 4(5): 355–60.

Tsang, K.W. and Lam, W.K. (2003) 'Management of severe acute respiratory syndrome', *American Journal of Respiratory & Critical Care Medicine*, 168(4): 417–24.

Tschudin, V. (2003) *Ethics in Nursing*, 3rd edn, Edinburgh: Butterworth-Heinemann.

Tsui, S.S.L. and Large, S.R. (1998) 'The current state of heart transplantation', *Care of the Critically Ill*, 14(1): 20–4.

Turner, A. (1997) 'The holistic management of the patient with pre-eclampsia', *Nursing in Critical Care*, 2(4): 169–73.

Turvill, J.L., Burroughs, A.K. and Moore, K.P. (2000) 'Change in occurrence of paracetamol overdose in UK after introduction of blister packs', *Lancet*, 355(9220): 2048–9.

Uhl, W., Buchler, M.W., Malfertheiner, P., Beger, H.G., Adler, G., Gaus, W. and German Pancreatitis Study Group (1999) 'A randomised, double-blind, multicentre trial of octreotide in moderate to severe acute pancreatitis', *Gut*, 45(1): 97–104.

Uhl, W., Isenmann, R. and Buchler, M.W. (1998) 'Infections complicating pancreatitis: diagnosing, treating, preventing', *New Horizons*, 6(supplement 2): S72–9.

UK Transplant (2005), website. Available online at: www.uktransplant.org.uk/ukt/statistics/latest_statistics/latest_statistics.jsp (accessed 10th May 2005).

UKCC (2001) *Professional Conduct Annual Report 2000–2001*, London: UKCC.

Unsworth, D.J. (2000) 'Immune response to transplantation', *Surgery*, 18(5): iii–vi.

Vacca, A.F. (1999) 'Nursing staff workload as a determinant of methicillin-resistant *Staphylococcus aureus* spread in an adult intensive therapy unit', *Journal of Hospital Infection*, 43(2): 109–13.

Vahanian, A. and Palacios, I.F. (2004) 'Percutaneous approaches to valvular disease', *Circulation*, 109(13): 1572–9.

Valabhji, J. and Elkeles, R.S. (2002) 'Macrovascular disease in diabetes', *Medicine*, 30(2): 47–50.

Valdix, S.W. and Puntillo, K.A. (1995) 'Pain, pain relief and accuracy of their recall after cardiac surgery', *Progress in Cardiovascular Nursing*, 10(3): 3–11.

Valencia, E. (2000) 'Pancreatitis: slowly improving the approach', *Care of the Critically Ill*, 16(3): 98–102.

Valta, P., Usaro, A., Nunes, S. Ruokonen, E. and Takala, J. (1999) 'Acute respiratory distress syndrome: frequency, clinical course and cost of care', *Critical Care Medicine*, 27(11): 2367–74.

Van Den Berghe, G. and De Zegher, F. (1996) 'Anterior pituitary function during critical illness and dopamine treatment', *Critical Care Medicine*, 24(9): 1580–90.

Van Den Berghe, G., Wouters, P., Weekers, F., Verwaest, C., Bruyninckx, F., Schetz, M., Vlasselaers, D., Ferdinande, P., Lauwers, P. and Bouillon, R. (2001) 'Intensive insulin therapy in critically ill patients', *New England Journal of Medicine*, 345(19): 1359–67.

van Dijk, D., Jansen, E.W.L., Hijman, R., Nierich, A.P., Diephuis, J.C., Moons, K.G.M., Lahpor, J.R., Borst, C., Keizer, A.M.A., Nathoe, H.M., Grobbee, D.E., De Jaegere, P.P.T., Kalkman, C.J. and Octopus Study Group (2002) 'Cognitive outcome after off-pump and on-pump coronary artery bypass graft surgery', *JAMA*, 287(11): 1405–12.

Van Horn, E. and Tesh, A. (2000) 'The effect of critical care hospitalization on family members: stress and responses', *Dimensions of Critical Care Nursing*, 19(4): 40–9.

Van Nieuwenhoven, C.A., Buskens, E., van Thiel, F.H. and Bonten, M.J.M. (2001) 'Relation between methodological trial quality and the effects of selective digestive decontamination on pneumonia and mortality in critically ill patients', *JAMA*, 286(3): 335–40.

van Welzen, M. and Carey, T. (2002) 'Autonomic dysreflexia: guidelines for practice', *Connect*, 2(1): 13–21.

Vanhoutte, P.M. (2002) 'Ageing and endothelial dysfunction', *European Heart Journal*, 4(Supplement A): A8–A17.

Vargas, H.E., Gerber, D. and Abu-Elmagd, K. (1999) 'Management of portal hypertension-related bleeding', *Surgical Clinics of North America*, 79(1): 1–22.

Vaughan, B. and Pillmoor, M. (1989) *Managing Nursing Work*, London: Scutari.

Vedio, A.B., Chinn, S., Warburton, F.G., Griffiths, M.P., Leach, R.M. and Treacher, D.F. (2000) 'Assessment of survival and quality of life after discharge from a teaching hospital general intensive care unit', *Clinical Intensive Care*, 11(1): 39–46.

Veith, F.J., Baum, R.A., Ohki, T., Amor, M., Adiseshiah, M., Blankensteijn, J.D., Buth, J., Chuter, T.A.M., Fairman, R.M., Gilling-Smith, G., Harris, P.L., Hodgson, K.J., Hopkinson, B.R., Ivancev, K., Katzen, B.T., Lawrence-Brown, M., Meier, G.H., Malina, M., Makaroun, M.S., Parori, J.C., Richter, G.M., Rubin, G.D., Stelter, W.J., White, G.H., White, R.A., Wisselink, W. and Zarins, C.K. (2002) 'Nature and significance of endoleaks and endotension: summary of opinions expressed at an international conference', *Journal of Vascular Surgery*, 35(5): 1029–35.

Velmahos, G.C., Chan, L.S., Tatevossian, R., Cornwell, E.E. III, Dougherty, W.R., Escudero, J. and Demetriades, D. (1999) 'High-frequency percussive ventilation improves oxygenation in patients with ARDS', *Chest*, 116(2): 440–6.

Venet, L., Guyomarch, S., Migeot, C., Bertrand, M., Gery, P., Page, D., Vermesch, R., Bertrand, J.C. and Zeni, F. (2001) 'The oxygenation variations related to prone positioning during mechanical ventilation: a clinical comparison between ARDS and non-ARDS hypoxemic patients', *Intensive Care Medicine*, 27(8): 1352–9.

Venstrom, J.M., McBride, M.A., Rother, K.I. Hirshberg, B., Orchard, T.J. and Harlain, D.M. (2003) 'Survival after pancreas transplantation in patients with diabetes and preserved kidney function', *JAMA*, 290(21): 2817–23.

Venugopal, S.K., Devaraj, S., Yuhanna, I., Shaul, P. and Jialal, I. (2002) 'Demonstration that C-reactive protein decreases eNOS expression and bioactivity in human aortic endothelial cells', *Circulation*, 106(12): 1439–41.

Verma, S., Szmitko, P.E. and Yeh, E.T.H. (2004) 'C-Reactive protein: structure affects function', *Circulation*, 109(16): 1914–17.

Verstraete, M. (2000) 'Third-generation thrombolytic drugs', *American Journal of Medicine*, 109(1): 52–8.

Vianello, A., Bevilacqua, M., Arcaro, G., Gallan, F. and Serra, E. (2000) 'Non-invasive ventilatory approach to treatment of acute respiratory failure in neuromuscular disorders. A comparison with endotracheal intubation', *Intensive Care Medicine*, 26(4): 384–90.

Vilar, F.J. and Wilkins, E.G.L. (1998) 'Management of pneumocysystis carinii pneumonia in intensive care', *British Journal of Intensive Care*, 8(2): 53–62.

Vincent, J.-L. (2003) 'Nosocomial infections in adult intensive-care units', *Lancet*, 361(9374): 2068–77.

Vincent, J.L., Bihari, D.J., Suter, P.M., Bruining, H.A., White, J., Nicholas-Chanoin, M.H., Wolff, M., Spencer, R.C. and Hemmer, M. (1995) 'The prevalence of nosocomial infection in intensive care units in Europe. Results of the European prevalence of infection in intensive care', *JAMA*, 274(8): 639–44.

Vint, P.E. (2005) 'An exploration of the support available to children who may wish to visit a critically adult in ITU', *Intensive and Critical Care Nursing*, 21(3): 131–4.

Vlahakes, G.J. (2001) 'Haemoglobin solutions in surgery', *British Journal of Surgery*, 88(12): 1553–5.

Voelker R. (2000) 'Movement after brain death', *JAMA*, 283(6): 734.

Vollman, K.M. (1997) 'Critical care nursing technique. Prone position for the ARDS patient', *Dimensions in Critical Care Nursing*, 16(4): 184–93.

Wahr, J.A. and Tremper, K.K. (1996) 'Oxygen measurement and monitoring techniques', in Prys-Roberts, C. and Brown, B.R. Jr (eds) *International Practice of Anaesthesia*, Oxford: Butterworth-Heinemann, 2/159/1–19.

Wainberg, M.A. (1999) 'HIV resistance to antagonists of viral reverse transcriptase', in Dalgleish, A.G. and Weiss, R.A. (eds) (1999) *HIV and the New Viruses*, 2nd edn, San Diego, CA: Academic Press, 223–50.

Wakai, A. and O'Neill, J.O. (2003) 'Emergency management of atrial fibrillation', *Postgraduate Medical Journal*, 79(932): 313–19.

Wake, D. (1995) 'Ecstasy overdose: a case study', *Intensive and Critical Care Nursing*, 11(1): 6–9.

Waldmann, C. and Barnes, R. (2004) 'Cannulation of central veins', *Anaesthesia and Intensive Care Medicine*, 5(1): 6–9.

Walker, C. (2003a) 'Cardiac arrest and resuscitation', *Surgery*, 21(8): 202–8.

Walker, C. (2003b) 'How should serial seizures and status epilepticus be treated?' *Journal of the Royal College of Physicians of Edinburgh*, 33(Supplement 11): 31–8.

Walker, J.J. (2000) 'Pre-eclampsia', *Lancet*, 356(9237): 1260–5.

Walker, R. and Rodgers, J. (2002) 'Diabetic retinopathy', *Nursing Standard*, 16(45): 46–52.

Wall, P.D. and Melzack, R.W. (eds) (1999) *Textbook of Pain*, 4th edn, Edinburgh: Churchill Livingstone.

Wallace, C.I., Dargan, P.I. and Jones, A.L. (2003) 'Paracetamol overdose: an evidence based flowchart to guide management', *Emergency Medicine Journal*, 19(3): 202–5.

Walter, T. (1997) 'Secularization', in Parkes, C.M., Laungani, P. and Young, B. (eds) *Death and Bereavement Across Cultures*, London: Routledge, 166–87.

Walz, M.K., Peitgen, K., Thürauf, N., Trost, H.A., Wolfhard, U., Sander, A., Ahmadi, C. and Eigler, F.W. (1998) 'Percutaneous dilational tracheostomy – early results and long-term outcome of 326 critically ill patients', *Intensive Care Medicine*, 24(7): 685–90.

Wang, K., Asinger, R.W. and Marriott, H.L. (2003)
'ST-segment elevation in conditions other than acute
myocardial infarction', *NEJM*, 349(22): 2128–35.

Wang, S.-M., Kulkarni, L., Dolev, J. and Kain, Z.N.
(2002) 'Music and preoperative anxiety: a randomized
controlled study', *Anesthesia & Analgesia*, 94(6):
1489–94.

Ward, B. and Park, G.R. (2000) 'Humidification of
inspired gases in the critically ill', *Clinical Intensive
Care*, 11(4): 169–76.

Warkentin, T.E. (2003) 'Heparin-induced thrombocytopenia: pathogenesis and management', *British
Journal of Haematology*, 121(4): 535–55.

Warner, E.A., Walker, R.M. and Friedman, P.D. (2003)
'Should informed consent be required for laboratory
testing for drugs of abuse in medical settings?'
*American Journal of Medicine*, 115(1): 54–8.

Warren, B.L., Eid, A., Singer, P., Pillay, S.S., Carl, P.,
Novak, I., Chalupa, P., Atherstone, I., Penzes, I.,
Kubler, A., Knaub, S., Keinecke, H.-O., Heinrichs, H.,
Schindel, F., Juers, M., Bone, R.C., Opal, S.M. and
KyberSept Trial Study Group (2001) 'High dose
antithrombin III in severe sepsis: a randomized
controlled trial', *JAMA*, 286(15): 1869–78.

Warren, H.S., Suffredini, A.F., Eichacker, P.Q. and
Munford, R.S. (2002) 'Risks and benefits of activated
protein C treatment for severe sepsis', *New England
Journal of Medicine*, 347(13): 1027–30.

Waterhouse, C. (2005) 'The Glasgow Coma Scale and
other neurological observations', *Nursing Standard*,
19(33): 56–64.

Waterlow, J. (2005) *Pressure Sore Prevention Manual*,
Taunton: Waterlow.

Waterlow, J.A. (1985) 'A risk assessment card', *Nursing
Times*, 81(48): 49–55.

—— (1995) 'Pressure sores and their management', *Care
of the Critically Ill*, 11(3): 121–5.

Watkins, L.D. (2000) 'Head injuries: general principles
and management', *Surgery*, 18(9): 219–24.

Watkins, P.J. (2003) 'Cardiovascular disease, hypertension,
and lipids', *BMJ*, 326(7394): 874–6.

Watkinson, G.E. (1995) 'A study of the perception and
experiences of critical care nurses in caring for potential
and actual organ donors: implications for nurse
education', *Journal of Advanced Nursing*, 22(5):
929–40.

Watremez, C., Liistro, G., deKock, M., Roesseler, J.,
Clerbaux, T., Detry, B., Reynaert, M., Gianello, P. and
Jolliet, P. (2003) 'Effects of helium-oxygen on respiratory mechanics, gas exchange, and ventilation-perfusion
relationships in a porcine model of stable methachlo-
line-induced brochospasm', *Intensive Care Medicine*,
29(9): 1560–6.

Watson, J.B. (1924/1998) *Behaviourism*, New Brunswick,
NJ: Transaction Publishers.

Watson, R. (2000a) 'Altered presentation in old age',
*Nursing Older People*, 12(3): 19–21.

—— (2000b) 'Assessing pulmonary function in older
people', *Nursing Older People*, 12(8): 27–8.

—— (2001) 'Assessing gastrointestinal(GI) tract functioning
in older people', *Nursing Older People*, 12(10): 27–8.

—— (2002) 'Assessing the need for restraint in older
people', *Nursing Older People*, 14(4): 31–2.

Weaver, W.D., Reisman, M.A., Griffin, J.J., Buller, C.E.,
Leimgruber, P.P., Henry, T., D'Heam, C., Clark, V.L.,
Martin, J.S., Cohen, D.J., Neil, N., Every, N.R. and OPUS-
1 Investigators (2000) 'Optimum percutaneous transluminal coronary angioplasty compared with routine stent
strategy trial (OPUS 1)', *Lancet*, 355(9222): 2199–203.

Weinert, C. and McFarland, L. (2004) 'The state of intubated patients', *Chest*, 126(6): 1883–90.

Welch, J. (2002) 'Kinetic therapy', *Care of the Critically
Ill*, 18(6): centre insert.

Weller, A.S. (2001) 'Body temperature and its regulation',
*Anaesthesia and Intensive Care Medicine*, 2(5): 195–8.

Wells, P.S., Anderson, D.R., Rodger, M., Forgie, M.,
Kearon, C., Dreyer, J., Kovacs, G., Mitchell, M.,
Lewandowski, B. and Kovacs, M.J. (2003) 'Evaluation
of D-dimer in the diagnosis of suspected deep-vein
thrombosis', *NEJM*, 349(13): 1227–35.

Welsch, D., Tilley, R. and Rhodes, A. (2001)
'Cardiovascular complications of cocaine', *Clinical
Intensive Care*, 12(5,6): 241–4.

Werner, C. and Engelhard, K. (2000) 'Cerebral resuscitation:
current concepts and perspectives', in Adams, A.P. and
Cashman, J.N. (eds) *Recent Advances in Anaesthesia and
Analgesia 21*, Edinburgh: Churchill Livingstone, 77–90.

West, E., Raffery, A.M and Lankshear, A. (2004) *The
Future Nurse: Evidence of the Impact of Registered
Nurses*, London: RCN.

Westaby, S. (2001) 'Artificial hearts', in Galley, H.F. (ed.)
*Critical Care Focus 6: Cardiology in Critical Illness*,
London: BMJ Books, 15–22.

Wheeler, A.P. and Bernard, G.R. (1999) 'Treating patients
with severe sepsis', *New England Journal of Medicine*,
340(3): 207–14.

White, R. (ed.) (2004) *Trends in Oral Health Care*,
Dinton: Quay Books.

White, R.J. (2000) 'Nurse assessment of oral health',
*British Journal of Nursing*, 9(5): 260–6.

Whitman, G.R., Kim, Y., Davidson, L.J. Wolf GA, Wang S.
(2002) 'The impact of staffing on patient outcomes
across speciality units', *Journal of Nursing
Administration*, 32(12): 633–9.

Whyte, D. and Robb, Y. (1999) 'Families under stress:
how nurses can help', *Nursing Times*, 95(30): 50–2.

Wierzbicki, A.S. (2003) 'Statin therapy in people with
diabetes and high-risk patients', *Hospital Medicine*,
64(1): 16–19.

Wilkes, M.M. and Navickis, R.J. (2001) 'Patient survival
after human albumin administration. A meta-analysis
of randomized, controlled trials', *Annals of Internal
Medicine*, 135(3): 205–8

Wilkes, N.J., Woolf, R., Mutch, M., Mallett, S.V.,
Peachey, T., Stephens, R. and Mythen, M.G. (2001)
'The effects of balanced versus saline-based Hetastarch
and crystalloid solutions on acid-base and electrolyte
status and gastric mucosal perfusion in elderly surgical
patients', *Anesthesia & Analgesia*, 93(4): 811–16.

Wilkin, K. (2003) 'The meaning of caring in the practice
of intensive care nursing', *British Journal of Nursing*,
12(20): 1178–85.

Wilkins, R.L., Hodgekin, J.E. and Lopez, B. (2004) *Fundamentals of Lung and Heart Sounds*, 3rd edn, St Louis: Mosby.

Wilkinson, K. (1997) 'Paediatric physiology and general considerations', in Goldhill, D.R. and Withington, P.S. (eds) *Textbook of Intensive Care*, London: Chapman & Hall, 345–53.

Wilkinson, P. (1992) 'The influence of high technology care on patients, their relatives and nurses', *Intensive and Critical Care Nursing*, 8(4): 194–8.

Williams, A.M. and Irurita, V.F. (2004) 'Therapeutic and non-therapeutic interpersonal interactions: the patient's perspective', *Journal of Clinical Nursing*, 13(7): 806–15.

Willams, C. and Asquith, J. (eds) (2000) *Paediatric Intensive Care Nursing*, Edinburgh: Churchill Livingstone.

Williams, J., Oenning, V. and Tuomaia, B. (2005) 'Cardiovascular alterations', in Sole, M.L., Klein, D.G. and Moseley, M.J. (eds) *Critical Care Nursing*, 4th edn, St Louis: Elsevier Saunders, 291–350.

Williams, M. and Sadler, P.J. (2003) 'Gastrointestinal tract haemorrhage and ulcer prophylaxis in ICU', *Anaesthesia and Intensive Care*, 4(4): 117–22.

Williams, T.A. and Leslie, G.D. (2004) 'A review of the nursing care of enteral feeding tubes in critically ill adults: part I', *Intensive and Critical Care Nursing*, 20(6): 330–43.

Williamson, L. and Murphy, M. (2003) 'Update on project to provide imported methylene blue treated fresh frozen plasma', *Blood Matters*, 12: 2–4.

Willis, J. (1997) 'Shock absorbers', *Nursing Times*, 93(24): 36–7.

Wilson, J., Woods, I., Fawcettt, J., Whall, R., Dibb, W., Morris, C. and McManus, E. (1999) 'Reducing the risk of major elective surgery: randomised controlled trial of preoperative optimisation of oxygen delivery', *BMJ*, 318(7191): 1099–103.

Wilson, J.N., Pierce, J.D. and Clancy, R.L. (2001) 'Reactive oxygen species in acute respiratory distress syndrome', *Heart & Lung*, 30(5): 370–5.

Wilson, P.W.F. and Grundy, S.M. (2003) 'The metabolic syndrome: practical guide to origins and treatment: part 1', *Circulation*, 108(12): 1422–5.

Windecker, S. and Meier, B. (2000) 'Intervention in coronary artery disease', *Heart*, 83(4): 481–90.

Winer, J.B. (2002) 'Treatment of Guillain-Barré syndrome', *QJM*, 95(11): 717–21.

Winocour, P.H. and Fisher, M. (2003) 'Prediction of cardiovascular risk in people with diabetes', *Diabetic Medicine*, 20(7): 515–27.

Winser, H. (2001) 'An evidence base for adult resuscitation', *Professional Nurse*, 16(7): 1210–13.

Winslow, E.H. and Jacobson, A.F. (1998) 'Dispelling the petroleum jelly myth', *American Journal of Nursing*, 98(11): 16.

Winter, G. (2005) 'A bug's life', *Nursing Standard*, 19(33): 16–18.

Wirtz, K.M., La Favor, K.M. and Ang, R. (1996) 'Managing, chronic spinal cord injury: issues in critical care', *Critical Care Nurse*, 16(4): 24–37.

Woeltje, K.F. and Fraser, V.J. (1998) 'Preventing nosocomial infections in the intensive care unit – lessons learned from outcomes research', *New Horizons*, 6(1): 84–90.

Wolff, A.J. and O'Donnell, A.E. (2001) 'Pulmonary manifestations of HIV infection in the era of highly active antiretroviral therapy', *Chest*, 120(6): 1888–93.

Wong, H.L.C., Lopez-Nahas, V. and Molassiotis, A. (2001) 'Effects of music therapy on anxiety in ventilator-dependent patients', *Heart & Lung*, 30(5): 376–87.

Wong, H.R. (1998) 'Potential protective role of the heat shock response in sepsis', *New Horizons*, 6(2): 194–200.

Wood, A.M. (1993) 'A review of literature relating to sleep in hospital with emphasis on the sleep of the ICU patient', *Intensive and Critical Care Nursing*, 9(2): 129–36.

Wood, C.J. (1998) 'Endotracheal suctioning: a literature review', *Intensive and Critical Care Nursing*, 14(3): 124–36.

Woodman, R. (1999) 'UN warns that AIDS deaths are set to reach record level', *BMJ*, 319(7222): 1387.

Woodrow, P. (2004a) 'Death and dying', in Moore, T. and Woodrow, P. (eds) *High Dependency Nursing: Observation, Intervention and Support*, London: Routledge, 70–9.

—— (2004b) 'Bilevel non-invasive ventilation', in Moore, T. and Woodrow, P. (eds) *High Dependency Nursing Care*, London: Routledge, 161–70.

—— (2004c) 'Temporary tracheostomies', in Moore, T. and Woodrow, P. (eds) *High Dependency Nursing Care*, London: Routledge, 151–60.

Woolf, N. (2000) *Cell, Tissue and Disease,* 3rd edn, Edinburgh: W.B. Saunders Company Ltd.

Working Party Report (1999) 'Revised guidelines for the control of methicillin-resistant *Staphylococcus aureus* infection in hospitals', *Journal of Hospital Infection*, 49(4): 253–90.

World Medical Association (2000) 'Declaration of Helsinki(2000)', *Bulletin of Medical Ethics*, 162: 8–11.

Wort, S.J. and Evans, T.W. (1999) 'The role of the endothelium in modulating vascular control in sepsis and related conditions', *British Medical Bulletin*, 55(1): 30–48.

Wright, C. and Cohen, B. (1997) 'Organ shortages: maximising the donor potential', *British Medical Bulletin*, 53(4): 817–28.

Wright, F., Heyland, D.K., Drover, J.W., McDonald, S. and Zoutman, D. (2001) 'Antibiotic coated central lines: do they work in the critical care setting?', *Clinical Intensive Care*, 12(2): 21–8.

Wright, S.E., Bodenham, A., Short, A.I.K. and Turney, J.H. (2003) 'The provision and practice of renal replacement therapy on adult intensive care units in the United Kingdom', *Anaesthesia*, 58(11): 1063–9.

Wyncoll, D.L. (1999) 'The management of severe acute necrotizing pancreatitis: an evidence-based review of the literature', *Intensive Care Medicine*, 25(2): 146–56.

Wyncoll, D.L.A. (2003) 'Management of acute poisoning', in Bersten, A.D. and Soni, N. (eds) *Intensive Care Manual*, 5th edn, Edinburgh: Butterworth-Heinemann, 823–32.

Xavier, G. (2000) 'The importance of mouth care in preventing infection', *Nursing Standard*, 14(18): 47–51.

Yadav, J.S., Wholey, M.H., Kuntz, R.E., Fayad, P., Katzen, B.T., Mishkel, G.J., Bajwa, T.K., Whitlow, P., Strickman, N.E., Jaff, M.R., Popma, J.J., Snead, D.B., Cutlip, D.E., Firth, B.G., Ouriel, K. and Stenting and Angioplasty with Protection in Patients at High Risk for Endarterectomy Investigators (2004) 'Protected carotid-artery stenting versus endarterectomy in high-risk patients', *New England Journal of Medicine*, 351(15): 1493–1501.

Yassin, J. and Wyncoll, D. (2005) 'Management of intractable diarrhoea in the critically ill', *Care of the Critically Ill*, 21(1): 20–4.

Yates, S.L. and Alston, R.P. (2000) 'Neurological, psychological and cognitive sequelae of cardiac surgery', *Current Anaesthesia & Critical Care*, 11(4): 187–93.

Young, D. and Ridley, S. (2002) 'Mortality as an outcome measure for intensive care', in Ridley, S. (ed.) *Outcomes in Critical Care*, Oxford: Butterworth-Heinemann, 25–46.

Young, J.D. (1999) 'Non-ventilatory treatment of acute respiratory distress syndrome', *British Medical Bulletin*, 55(1): 165–80.

Young, P.J. and Ridley, S.A. (1999) 'Ventilator-associated pneumonia', *Anaesthesia*, 54(12): 1183–97.

Yu, M., Nardella, A. and Pechet, L. (2000) 'Screen tests of disseminated intravascular coagulation: guidelines for rapid and specific laboratory diagnosis', *Critical Care Medicine*, 28(6): 1777–80.

Zacharias, A., Habib, R.H., Schwann, T.A., Riordan, C.J., Durham, S.J. and Shah, A. (2004) 'Improved survival with radial artery versus vein conduits in coronary bypass surgery with left internal thoracic artery to left anterior descending artery grafting', *Circulation*, 109(12): 1489–96.

Zamvar, V., Williams, D., Hall, J., Payne, N., Cann, C., Young, K., Karthikeyan, S. and Dunne, J. (2002) 'Assessment of neuroprotective impairment after off-pump and on-pump techniques for coronary artery bypass graft surgery: prospective randomised controlled trial', *BMJ*, 325(7375): 1268–71.

Zaritsky, A.L. (1998) 'Recent advances in pediatric cardiopulmonary resuscitation and advanced life support', *New Horizons*, 6(2): 201–11.

Zarzaur, B.L., Fukatsu, K. and Kudsk, K.A. (2000) 'The influence of nutrition on mucosal immunology and endothelial cell adhesion molecules', in Vincent, J.-L. (ed.) *Yearbook of Intensive Care and Emergency Medicine*, Berlin: Springer, 63–71.

Zeeman, G.G., Fleckenstein, J.L., Twicker, D.M. and Cunningham, F.G. (2004) 'Cerebral infarction in eclampsia', *American Journal of Obstetrics & Gynecology*, 190(3): 714–20.

Zhong, N.S. and Zeng, G.Q. (2003) 'Our strategies for fighting severe acute respiratory distress syndrome', *American Journal of Respiratory and Critical Care Medicine*, 168(1): 7–9.

# Index

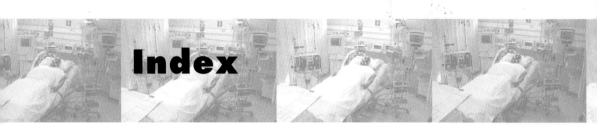

accountability *see* professionalism
ACE inhibitors *see* angiotensin converting
  enzyme inhibitors
acid-base balance 183–8
  base excess 191
  cardiac postoperative care 336
  chemical buffers 186–7
  renal function 186
acid, *definition* 183
acidosis 187–8
  metabolic 185–6, 446
  respiratory 184–5
action potential
  ECG 229–30
  sodium-potassium pump 263
acute axonal neuropathy *see* critical illness
  neuropathy
acute fatty liver 453
acute hepatic failure 442–3
acute myocardial infarction 316–26
  angiogenesis 323
  health promotion 324
  markers 319
  NSTEMI 322
  percutaneous intervention 323
  postoperative cardiac care 337
  thrombolysis 321
  treatment 319–21
acute phase proteins 265
acute renal failure 413–22
  effects 416–17
  intrarenal failure 415–16
  management 418
  monitoring 416
  postrenal failure 416
  prerenal failure 414–15
acute respiratory distress syndrome (ARDS)
  288–96
  cardiac management 294

fluid management 293
high frequency oscillatory ventilation
  (HFOV) 308
inflammatory response 293
pathology 288–9
psychological support 293–4
pulmonary hypertension reduction 293
treatment 289
ventilation 289–90
  prone positioning 290–2
adaptive support ventilation (ASV) 41
Addenbrookes/Cambridge sedation scale 63
adenosine triphosphate (ATP) molecules 263
adrenaline (epinephrine) 376–7
advance directives (living wills) 151–2
AF *see* atrial fibrillation
ageing *see* older patients
agranulocytes 214
AIDS *see* HIV infection
air composition 171
air emboli, haemodynamic monitoring 202
airway, biphasic/biphasic positive airway
  pressure (BIPAP) 44
airway management 48–58
  children 124
  extubation stridor 56
  hyperinflation 56
  intubation 48–9
  problems 50–1
  saline instillation 55
airway obstruction, head injury 393
airway pressure release ventilation
  (APRV) 40–1
albumin 215, 367–8
  hypoalbuminaemia 92
alcohol, acute myocardial infarction
  (AMI) 318
alfentanil, pain management 76
alpha 2 agonists 61

alpha receptors 374
alteplase® 321
alveolar collapse 309
  atelectasis 307
alveoli
  A-a gradient, blood analysis 190
  deadspace 171–2
  partial pressure 171–2
amiodarone, dysrhythmias 233, 236, 237, 243, 337
amnesia 25
amniotic fluid embolus 453
amphetamine (speed) 492
AMV see assisted mandatory ventilation
amylase, serum 475
anaemia 212
  and oximetry 166
anaesthetic agents 61
analgesia see pain management
anaphylactic shock 350–1
aneurysms 383–4
angina 316
angiography, acute myocardial infarction (AMI) 323
angiotensin converting enzyme (ACE) inhibitors, acute
    myocardial infarction (AMI) 322
anion gap 191
anthropometric chart, nutritional assessment 92
antibiotics, cautions 142
anticoagulants 321
antidepressants 489–90
antiemetics 78
antioxidants, acute myocardial infarction (AMI) 322
antipsychotics 62
antipyretics 84
APACHE scoring system 519
  APACHE II scores 118, 135
apoptosis see cell death
aprons 144
APRV see airway pressure release ventilation
ARDS see acute respiratory distress syndrome
arrhythmias see dyrhythmias
arterial blood gas analysis 188–94
  compensation 192
  reading samples 189–92
arterial pressure
  children 126
  intra-aortic balloon pumps (IABPs) 331–2
  mean (MAP) 197, 249–50
  monitoring 196–7
artificial liver 447
artificial tears 111
artificial ventilation see ventilation
ascites, and hepatic failure 445
aspiration 51
aspirin, cardiac dosage 320–1
assisted mandatory ventilation (AMV) 40
ASV see adaptive support ventilation
asystole 244
atelectasis 307
  alveolar collapse 309
atherosclerosis 317–21
  pathology 318

ATP molecules see adenosine triphosphate molecules
atrial ectopics 234–5
atrial fibrillation (AF) 235–6
  cardiac postoperative care 337
atrial flutter 236–7
atrial/junctional dysrhythmias 231–8
atrial tachycardia 233
atrioventricular conduction pathways, blocks 238–40
atrioventricular dyssynchrony 227
auscultation 161–3
autonomic dysfunction 407
autonomic dysreflexia (hyperreflexia) 400–1
autonomy, ethical principle 150–2
axonal neuropathy see critical illness neuropathy

bacteria 140–2
bacterial infection, oral 101
balloon tamponade, gastrointestinal bleeds 434–5
base, definition 183
base excess (BE) 191
BE see base excess
behaviourism 12–14
beneficence 152–3
benzodiazepine 60–1
  antidote 61
beta blockers
  acute myocardial infarction (AMI) 322
  dysrhythmias 230
  gastrointestinal bleeds 436
beta receptors 374–5
bicarbonate 176
  infusions 187–8
  standardised (SBC) 190
bicarbonate ion $HCO_3^-$ 187
  arterial blood analysis 190
bigeminy, ventricular
  ectopics 241–2
bilevel/biphasic positive airway pressure (BIPAP) 44
bilirubin, hepatic failure 444
BIPAP see biphasic/biphasic positive airway pressure
Birty's assessment tool, skincare 117
Bispectral index (BIS) 65
blood 210–22
  biochemistry 216–20
  clotting studies 215–16
  D-dimers 216
  pH 183–4
  platelets 215
  RBCs 210–11
  warming 428
  WCCs 212–13
  see also haemodynamic monitoring
blood flow, haemofiltration 425–6
blood gases 171–81
  analysers 183–94
  carbon dioxide transport 175–6
  oxygen transport 172
  partial pressure 171–2
  samples 188–9
  support groups 180
  see also arterial blood analysis; haemoglobin

blood pressure
  noninvasive measurement 197
  see also arterial pressure
blood transfusion 366–7
  autologus 329
Bloomsbury sedation scale 63
B-lymphocytes 214
bowel management 92–5
Braden assessment tool, skincare 116
brain
  cross-section of cranium 255
  intracranial haemorrhage 401–2
  intracranial hypertension and tissue injury 250
  intracranial physiology, pressure/volume curve 248–9
  see also head injury; intracranial pressure; neurological monitoring
brain death
  incubation, obstetric emergencies 454
  types 461
brainstem death 459–62
  code of practice 460
breathing
  assisted see ventilation
  children 124
  sounds 161–3
  waveform 163–5
Bristol stool form chart 93
bronchus, intubation 48
buccal activity, and salivary glands 99–100
buffering 183, 187, 204
burns, and oximetry 166–7
bypass grafts 330–1

cachectin see tumour necrosis factor alpha (TNFα)
calcium channel blockers 230
  acute myocardial infarction (AMI) 322
calcium, hypocalcaemia 219–20
capillaries
  occlusion pressure 115
  perfusion gradients 365–6
  refill 196
capnography 167
carbon dioxide
  dissociation curve 176
  extracorporeal removal (ECCO₂R) 306
  PaCO₂, blood analysis 190
  partial rebreathing 204
  transport 175–6
  and ventilation 32–4
  see also capnography
carbon monoxide 177–8
  hyperbaric oxygen 309–10
  and oximetry 166
cardiac arrest
  adrenaline 373
  children 126
cardiac failure 331–2
cardiac index (CI) 204
cardiac markers 319

cardiac output 202–7
cardiac surgery 328–42
  bypass grafts 330–1
  intra-aortic balloon pumps (IABPs) 331–2
  minimally invasive surgery 329–30
  neurological complications 339
  normalisation 340
  open heart surgery 328–9
  pain control 338–9
  percutaneous cardiac interventions (PCI) 323
  postoperative care 333–41
  psychological considerations 339–40
  valve surgery 330
  ventricular assist devices (VAD) 331–2
cardiac transplantation 332–3
  issues 340–1
cardiogenic shock 348
  adrenaline 376–7
cardioplegia 329
cardiopulmonary bypass see cardiac surgery, open heart surgery
cardiovascular failure
  shock 347
  ventilation 36–7
care, duty of 8–9
carotid artery disease 384–5
catecholamines 376–8
  circadian rhythm 23
catheters
  airway management 55
  pulmonary artery 203
cell death 264
cell membrane 262–3
cell structure
  cellular pathology 262–8
  chemical mediation 265
  inflammatory response 264–5
cellular respiration 174–5
central nervous system injury see head injury
central venous cannulae 199
central venous pressure (CVP) 199–200
  measurement 200–2
cerebral oedema 251, 445
  treatment 394
cerebral perfusion pressure (CPP) 249–50
children see paediatrics
chloral hydrate, children 127
chlorhexidine 141
chloride, hyperchloraemia 218
chronic hepatic failure 443
chronic obstructive pulmonary disease (COPD)
  breath waveform 164
chronotropes 230
  beta receptors 374
CI see cardiac index
ciclosporin 467
circadian rhythms 23
  acute myocardial infarction 318
  sleep 24

circulation
  children 124
  collateral 323
  microcirculation 196
citric acid cycle 88–90
closed circuit suction, airway management 55
clothing 144
coagulation see disseminated intravascular
  coagulation (DIC)
coagulopathies 306, 335–6
  consumptive see disseminated intravascular
  coagulation (DIC)
cocaine (coke) 492
Cohen and Kelly sedation scale 63
coliforms 142
collateral circulation 323
colloids 366–9
  osmotic pressure (COP) 215, 364
colostomy 95
confusion 18–19
  older patients 133
consent
  for children 151
  relatives to organ donation 460–1, 463
  validity 151
constipation 94–5
continuous positive airway pressure (CPAP) 44
continuous renal replacement therapies (CRRT) 424
Cooley's anaemia see thalassaemia
COPD see chronic obstructive pulmonary disease
coronary angioplasty, percutaneous (PTCA) 323
coronary artery disease 317
  bypass grafts 330–1
  collateral circulation 323
  inferior myocardial infarction 317
  see also myocardial infarction
cost of intensive care 518–22
co-trimoxazole, HIV infection 274
cough reflex 50
  respiratory monitoring 160
CPAP see continuous positive airway pressure
CPP see cerebral perfusion pressure
cranium, cross-section 255
C-reactive protein (CRP) 216–17
creatine kinase, acute myocardial infarction
  (AMI) 319
creatinine and urea, acute renal failure 220
cricoid pressure 48
critical illness neuropathy 408–9
CRP see C-reactive protein
CRRT see continuous renal replacement therapies
crystalloids 364–5
CVP see central venous pressure
cytokines 265

dantrolene, malignant hyperpyrexia 85
D-dimers 216
deadspace, alveoli 171–2
death, ethical issues 153
deep vein thromboses (DVT) 282–3
defence mechanisms, non-specific/specific immunity 270

dentures 105–6
deontology (duty-based theory) 154
dextran 368
diabetes insipidus 397–8
diabetes mellitus 481–7
  complications 483
  ketones 482–3
  metabolic syndrome 483–4
  types 482
diabetic ketoacidosis (DKA) 484–5
dialysis 423–4
diamorphine (heroin), pain management 76
diarrhoea 93–4
DIC see disseminated intravascular coagulation
disseminated intravascular coagulation
  (DIC) 278–84
  pathophysiology 278–9
  progression 279
  related pathologies 281
  symptoms 279–80
  treatment and care 280–1, 282
distributive shock 350
diuretics 418
  osmotic 394
DKA see diabetic ketoacidosis
dobutamine 377
dopamine 378
  synthetic analogues 377–8
dopexamine (hydrochloride) 377–8, 418
double effect doctrine 153
drug administration, central venous cannulae 199
drug clearance, haemofiltration 428–9
DVT see deep vein thromboses
dysrhythmias 201, 224–46
  asystole 244
  atrial fibrillation (AF) 235–6
  atrial flutter 236–7
  atrial/junctional 231–8
  atrial tachycardia 233
  blocks 238–40
    bundle branch 240
    first degree 238
    second degree 239
    third degree 239–40
  ectopics 234
    atrial 234–5
    ventricular 241–2
  junctional (nodal) rhythm 237–8
  postoperative cardiac care 337
  pulseless electrical activity (PEA) 245
  sick sinus syndrome 233–4
  sinus arrhythmia 231–2
  sinus bradycardia 232
  sinus tachycardia 232–3
  torsades de pointes 243–4
  treatments 230–1
  vagal stimulation 231
  ventricular 240–1
  ventricular fibrillation (VF) 244
  ventricular tachycardia 242–3
  Wolff-Parkinson-White syndrome 237

ECG *see* electrocardiography
eclampsia 453
ECMO *see* extracorporeal membrane oxygenation
Ecstasy overdose 490–5
  complications 492–5
  symptoms 492
ectopics 234
  atrial 234–5
  ventricular 241–2
education, humanism 14–15
Einthoven's triangle 225
electrocardiography (ECG) 224–46
  action potential 229–30
  atrial kick 227
  basic principles 225–7
  framework for interpretation 228
  lead changes 227
  ST abnormalities 227–9
  U waves 229
  vagal stimulation 231
electrolyte imbalance, cardiac surgery 337–8
emphysema *see* chronic obstructive pulmonary
    disease (COPD)
encephalopathy, and hepatic failure 445
endotracheal suction 53–5
endotracheal tube (ETT)
  children 49, 124
  high and low pressure cuffs 51
  placement 48–9
enteral nutrition 90–1
*Enterococci* (VRE) 142
epidural analgesia 76–7
epilepsy 398–9
epinephrine *see* adrenaline
erythrocytes (RBCs) 210–11
erythrocyte sedimentation 188
escape ectopics 234
ethics 149–56
  death 153
  dilemmas 150
  HIV infection 274–5
  principles 150–4
  rights 155
  theories 154–5
  transplantation 463–4
ETT *see* endotracheal tube
euthanasia 153
  ethical issues 153
extracorporeal membrane oxygenation
    (ECMO) 305–6
  children 305
  variants 306
extracorporeal ventilation
  carbon dioxide removal
      (ECCO$_2$R) 306
  membrane oxygenation (ECMO) 305–6
extubation stridor, airway management 56
eyecare 109–13
  assessment 110–11
  interventions 111–12
  ocular damage 109–10

fatty liver 453
fentanyl, pain management 76
filter membranes 426
fluid balance
  cardiac postoperative care 336
  children 126
fluid management 363–71
  albumin 367–8
  blood 366–7
  colloids 366
  crystalloids 364–5
  dextran 368
  gelatins 368
  other blood products 368
  oxygen-carrying fluids 369–70
  perfusion 365–6
  starches 368–9
flumazenil 61
foam sticks 104
foramen of Monro 254–5
free radicals 266
fungal infections 142
furosemide 418

GABA *see* gamma-aminobutyric acid
gallstones 474, 478
gamma-aminobutyric acid (GABA) 60
gas carriage *see* blood gases
gastric infection, enteral nutrition 90
gastric pH 91
gastrointestinal bleeds 433–40
  lower 438
  peptic ulcers 436–7
  stress ulceration 437
  variceal bleeding 433–6
gastrointestinal dysfunction, HIV infection 273
gastrointestinal tract
  older patients 134
  selective digestive decontamination
      (SDD) 145
GBS *see* Guillain Barré syndrome
GCS *see* Glasgow Coma Scale
gelatins 368
Geliperm® 112
Glasgow Coma Scale (GCS) 251–2
glomerulonephritis 416
*glossary* 523–30
glucose, hyperglycaemia 218
glycerine 111
goal-based (utilitarian) theory 154–5
graft versus host disease (GvHD) 466
gram negative bacteria 140–1
gram positive bacteria 140
granulocytes 213
Guillain Barré syndrome (GBS) 407–8
GvHD *see* graft versus host
    disease

haemodiafiltration 425
  factors affecting filtration 425–6
haemodialysis 423–4

haemodynamic monitoring 196–208
  arterial pressure 196–7
  ultrasound 207
  see also blood
haemofiltration 423–31
  filter membranes 426
  problems 427–9
haemoglobin 211–12
  arterial blood gas analysis 172–3
  carbon dioxide carriage 176
  foetal (HbF) 173
  oxygen carriage 172
  oxygen dissociation curve 173–4
haemoglobinopathies 177–9
  and oximetry 166
haemolysis, elevated liver enzymes and low platelets
  (HELLP) syndrome 454
haemolytic uraemic syndrome (HUS) 281
haemorrhage
  cardiac surgery 335–6
  head injury 401–2
  obstetric emergencies454
  tamponade 335, 348–9
  see also gastrointestinal bleeds
haemorrhagic shock see hypovolaemic shock
haemostasis, stages 278
handwashing, control of infections 143–4
HbS disease see sickle cell disease
head injury 391–405
  airway 393
  breathing 393
  disability 394–5
  family care 403
  haemorrhage 401–2
  intracranial pressure, preventing raised 396
  legal aspects 403
  nutritional aspects 397
  personality changes 402–3
  pituitary damage 397–8
  positioning 397
  see also brain; neurological monitoring
Health and Safety at Work Act (1974) 511
hearing, sensory imbalance 20
heatstroke 83
Helicobacter pylori 437
heliox 176–7
HELLP syndrome see haemolysis, elevated liver
  enzymes, and low platelets, syndrome
heparin
  anticoagulation 427
  disseminated intravascular coagulation (DIC) 281
heparin-induced thrombocytopenia and thrombosis
  syndrome (HITTS) 198, 281
hepatic failure 442–9
  acute 442–3
  chronic 443
  decompensation 444–6
  liver function tests 443–4
  older patients 134
  other complications 446–7
  ventilation 37

HFJV see high frequency jet ventilation
HFOV see high frequency oscillatory ventilation
HFV see high frequency ventilation
HHS see hyperosmolar non-ketotic state
high frequency jet ventilation (HFJV) 308
high frequency oscillatory ventilation
  (HFOV) 307–8
high frequency percussive ventilation 308
high frequency ventilation (HFV) 306–8
histidine 187
HITTS see heparin-induced thrombocytopenia and
  thrombosis syndrome
HIV infection 271–5
  ethical and health issues 274–5
HONKS see hyperosmolar non-ketotic state
humanism 12, 14
Human Organ Transplants Act (1989) 461
Human Tissues Act (1964) 460
Human Tissues Bill (2004)
  460–1
humidification, airway management 52–3, 307
HUS see haemolytic uraemic syndrome
hyperbaric oxygen 309–10
hypercapnia
  oximetry 166
  permissive 289–90
  respiratory acidosis 185
hyperchloraemia 218
hyperglycaemia 218, 484
hyperinflation, airway
  management 56
hyperkalaemia 218, 347
hyperosmolar hyperglycaemic syndrome
  (HHS) see hyperosmolar non-ketotic state
  (HONKS)
hyperosmolar non-ketotic state (HONKS) 485
hyperphophosphaemia 219
hyperpyrexia 83
  malignant 85
hyperreflexia see autonomic dysreflexia
hypersalivation 51
hypertension
  cardiac postoperative care 335
  intracranial pressure, tissue injury 249, 250
  intraocular 110
  pregnancy-induced 452–3
hypocalcaemia 219–20
hypoglycaemia, hepatic failure 446–7
hypokalaemia 217–18
hypomagnesiumaemia 219
hyponatraemia 217
hypoperfusion, metabolism 89
hypotension
  cardiac surgery 335
  hepatic failure 445
hypothermia
  cardiac surgery 329
  haemofiltration 428
hypovolaemic (haemorrhagic) shock 349
hypoxia, bronchoconstriction 54
hysteresis 42, 164

IABPs *see* intra-aortic balloon pumps
ICP *see* intracranial pressure
immunity 270–6
  nonspecific 270–1
  specific 271
  support groups 276
immunocompromise 51
  mouth care 104
immunodeficiency 271
  and HIV infection 271–5
immunoglobulins, B-lymphocytes 214
immunosuppression,
    transplantation 467
independent lung ventilation 42
infections 139–47
  bacteria 101, 140–2
  control 142–5
  mouth care 101
inotropes and vasopressors 373–81
  indications 373
  receptors 374–5
  safety 375–6
  units of measurement 376
interleukins 265
intermittent positive pressure breathing (IPPB) 39
intra-abdominal pressure 447
intra-aortic balloon pumps (IABPs) 331–2
intra-arterial measurement 197–9
intracellular ions 263–4
intracranial haemorrhage 401–2
intracranial pressure (ICP) 248–9
  measurement 254–5
  preventing raised 396–7
intraocular hypertension 110
intrathoracic pressure 309
intravenous dyes, and oximetry 166
intravenous fluids 363
intravenous oxygenators (IVOX) 306
intubation 22, 48–9
invasive procedures 142
inverse ratio ventilation (IRV) 42, 290
IPPB *see* intermittent positive pressure breathing
IRV *see* inverse ratio ventilation
isolation 21
  SARS 300
IVOX *see* intravenous oxygenators

jaundice 447
Jenkins oral assessment tool 102
Jiggins & Talbot's oral assessment 103–4
jugular venous bulb saturation 254
junctional (nodal) rhythm 237–8
justice 154

ketamine (special K) 492
Krebs (citric acid) cycle 88–90

lactic acid, anaerobic metabolism 191–2
left cardiac work/index (LCW/I) 205
left ventricular stroke work/index (LVSW/I) 205
legionella 301–2

leucocytes 213–14
lexipafant 478
limbs, neurological monitoring 253–4
lipcare 105
liquid ventilation 308–9
litigation, accountability and professionalism 505
liver
  artificial 447
  function tests 443–4
  *see also* hepatic failure
living wills *see* advance directives
lung
  damage, ventilation 37–8
  rest 290
  sounds *see* auscultation

magnesium, hypomagnesiumaemia 219
malignant hyperpyrexia 85
malnutrition
  HIV infection 273
  older patients 134
management of ICUs 509–16
  shift 514
  staff morale 512–13
mannitol, cerebral oedema 418
MAP *see* mean arterial pressure
mattresses, skincare 118
MDMA *see* Ecstasy
mean arterial pressure (MAP) 197, 249–50
meningitis, children 128
metabolic acidosis 185–6
  hepatic failure 446
metabolic analysers 92
metabolic failure, shock 347
metabolism, acid-base balance 185–6
methaemoglobin 173
microcirculation 196
midazolam 60
mitochondria 263
mitral valve surgery 330
MODS *see* multi-organ dysfunction
    syndrome
monitoring
  acid-base balance 183–8
  airway management 48–58
  arterial blood gas analysis 188–94
  artificial ventilation 32–46
  ECGs and dysrhythmias 224–46
  gas carriage 171–81
  haemodynamics 196–208
  neurological 248–57
  respiratory 160–9
monocytes 214
Monro-Kellie hypothesis 248
morbidity, cost of intensive care 520
morphine, pain management 320
mortality, cost of intensive care 519
mouth care 99–107
  anatomy 99–100
  infection 101
  oral assessment 101–4

MRSA *see* staphylococcus aureus
multi-organ dysfunction syndrome (MODS) 357
muscle atrophy, older patients 134
music 25
myocardial infarction *see* acute myocardial infarction
myocardial oxygen supply 317
myocardial stunning 321
myoglobin, cardiac markers 319

nasal cavity, anatomy 52
necrosis 264
  acute tubular necrosis (ATN) 414, 415
  hepatocyte 444
  muscle 409
  pancreatic 475
necrotising fasciitis 119
neurogenic shock 350
neurological monitoring 248–57
  cerebral blood flow 249–50
  cerebral oedema 251
  intracranial pressure (ICP) 248–9
  limb assessment 253–4
  pupil size and response 252–3
  *see also* head injury
neuromuscular blockade, sedation 65–7
Newcastle sedation scale 63–4
New Sheffield sedation scale 64
nitrates, acute myocardial infarction (AMI) 320
nitric oxide
  cellular pathology 266
  SIRS 359
nitrogen
  balance 88
  and oxygen concentration 175
NIV *see* noninvasive ventilation
nociceptors 72
nodal/junctional rhythms 237–8
noise 24–5
noninvasive blood pressure measurement 197
noninvasive ventilation (NIV) 44
nonmaleficence 152
non-steroidal anti-inflammatory drugs *see* NSAIDs
noradrenaline (norepinephrine) 377
nosocomial infections 139–40
  causes and precaution 142–5
NSAIDs (non-steroidal anti-inflammatory drugs)
  chronic ulcers 437
  pain management 78
  in pyrexia 84
nursing perspectives 4–10
  breaking bad news 8
  nurse-patient ratios 6–7
  patient 5
  relatives 5–6
  stress 7–8
  uniforms 144
nutrition 88–97
  assessment 92
  bowel care 92–5
  clothing 144
  energy 88–90

enteral nutrition 90–1
  head injury 397
  nitrogen (protein) 88
  parenteral nutrition 91–2
  trace elements 90

obstetric emergencies 451–7
  haemorrhage 454
  pregnancy-induced hypertension 452–3
  support groups 456
  thromboembolism 453
obstructive shock 348
ocular damage 109–10
older patients 132–7
  ageism 135
  gastrointestinal 134
  hepatic dysfunction 134
  malnourishment 134
  muscle atrophy 134
  neurophysiological
    effects 133–4
  pressure sores 134
  renal problems 134
oliguria 415
oncotic and osmotic pressure, haemofiltration 425
open heart surgery 328–9
opioids 61, 75–6
oral *see* mouth care
organ donation
  donors 462–3
  live donors 464
  non-heart-beating organ donors (NHBOD) 464–5
  relatives consent 460–1, 463
organ failure *see* multiorgan dysfunction syndrome (MODS)
overdoses 489–97
  deliberate self-harm 489
  health promotion 495
  support groups 496
oxygen
  acute myocardial infarction (AMI) 317, 320
  carriage 172
  carrying fluids 369–70
  cerebral oxygenation 250
  debt 175
  dissociation curve 173–4
  haemodynamic monitoring 206
  hyperbaric 309–10
  $PaO_2$, blood analysis 190
  toxicity 175, 306
oxygenation 32
  determinants 34

PAC *see* pulmonary artery catheters
paediatrics 122–30
  airway management, initial assessment 124
  cardiovascular aspects 126
  consent 151
  ECMO 305
  endotracheal tube 49, 124
  fluid balance 126

legal aspects 128–9
neurological aspects 125
pulse rate 124
sedation 127
stabilisation 127–8
support groups 129
thermoregulation 126
pain management 71–80
  assessment 74–5
  non-opiods 78
  physiological aspects 72
  postoperative cardiac care 338–9
  psychological aspects 72–4
pancreatitis 474–9
  complications 475–6
  pathology 474–5
  symptoms 476–7
  treatment 477–8
paracetamol, overdosage 490
paralytic ileus 90
parenteral nutrition 91–2
partial pressure of gases 171–2
patient-controlled analgesia (PCA) 77–8
patient experiences
  ICU memories 25–6
  music and noise 24–5
  ventilation 35–6
PAV see proportional assist ventilation
PCA see patient-controlled
  analgesia
PCI see percutaneous cardiac interventions
PCP see pneumocystis carinii pneumonia
PDIs see phosphodiesterase inhibitors
PEA see pulseless electrical activity
PEEP see positive and expiratory pressure
pentamidine (IV nebulised) 274
peptic ulcers 436–7
percutaneous cardiac interventions (PCI) 323
percutaneous coronary angioplasty
  (PTCA) 323
percutaneous valvuloplasty 330
perfluorocarbon (PFC), liquid ventilation 308–9
perfusion and perfusion gradients 365–6
perfusion failure 346–7
perfusion pressure 197
periodontitis 101
peritoneal dialysis 423
persistent vegetative states 461
pethidine, pain management 76
PFC see perfluorocarbon
pH
  homeostasis 192
  measurement 183–4
  arterial blood gas analysis 190
philosophy, humanism 12, 14
phosphate
  hyperphophosphaemia 219
  ion $HCO_3^-$ 187
phosphodiesterase inhibitors
  (PDIs) 378
phospholipidase A 475

plaque, mouth care 100–1
plasma
  carbon dioxide 175
  ion $HCO_3^-$ 187
plasmapheresis 358–9, 429
plasma proteins 215–16
plasminogen 321
pneumocystis carinii pneumonia (PCP) 273
pneumonia
  Legionnaire's disease 301–2
  pneumocystis carinii (PCP) 273
  ventilator associated pneumonia (VAP) 140
portal vein pressure 433–4
portosystemic shunt 436
positioning
  head injury 397
  prone 290–2
positive and expiratory pressure (PEEP) 38–9
postrenal failure 416
post-traumatic stress disorder (PTSD) 25–6
potassium
  hyperkalaemia 218
  hypokalaemia 217–18
  plasma levels 217–18
pregnancy 451–2
  drugs 455
  psychological care 455
pressure limited ventilation 40–1, 290
pressure sores
  mouth care 105
  older patients 134
  skin care 115–18
    prevention 118
pressure support ventilation (PSV) 41
professionlism 502–7
  accountability 502–5
  record keeping 506
propofol 61
proportional assist ventilation (PAV) 41
prostacyclin 293, 427
prostoglandins
  $PGE_2$, analgesia 78
  prostacyclin 293, 427
  vasodilation 350
proteins, acute phase 265–6
Pseudomonas 142
PSV see pressure support ventilation
psychological care 18–28
  ARDS 293–4
  cardiac surgery 339–40
  confusion 18–19
  noise and music 24–5
  pain management 72–4
  post-traumatic stress disorder (PTSD) 25–6
  pregnancy 455
  recovery 26
  sleep 23–4
psychological distress, HIV infection 274
PTCA see percutaneous coronary angioplasty
PTSD see post-traumatic stress disorder
pulmonary artery catheters (PAC) 203–4

pulmonary hypertension 205
  reduction in ARDS 293
pulmonary oedema 290, 453
pulseless electrical activity (PEA) 245
pulse oximetry 165–7
pulse rate, children 124
pyrexia 82–6
  ecstasy overdose 493
  head injury 398
  treatment 84
pyrogens 82

radicals, free 266
Ramsay sedation scale 62–3
reactive oxygen species (ROS) 266
receptors 374–5
  types 75
record keeping see professionalism
recticulocytes 212
red blood cells (RBCs) see erythrocytes
remifentanyl, pain management 76
renal function
  acid-base balance 186
  cardiac surgery 338
  older patients 134
  see also acute renal failure
renal ischaemia, shock 347
renal replacement therapies, continuous
  (CRRT) 424
renal transplantation, numbers 464
reperfusion injury 266, 359
respiratory acidosis 184–5
respiratory alkalosis 306
respiratory compensation 192
respiratory failure
  HIV infection 273
  shock 347
  ventilation 32–4, 36
  see also acute respiratory distress syndrome
respiratory monitoring 160–9
  breath sounds 161–3
  breath waveform 163–5
  indexed measurements 165
  tactile 161
  visual 160–1
respiratory quotient 89–90
reticular activating system 21–2
rhabdomyolysis, acute renal failure 418–19
right cardiac work/index (RCW/I) 205
right ventricular stroke work/index (RVSW/I) 205
ROS see reactive oxygen species

saline
  eyecare 111
  instillation 55
saliva 99–100
salivary glands, buccal activity 100
SARS see severe acute respiratory syndrome
sclerotherapy 435
SDD see selective digestive decontamination
sedation 60–9

assessment 62–5
bolus sedation 62
children 127
hold 65
neuromuscular blockade 65–7
selective digestive decontamination (SDD) 145
Sengstaken tube, gastrointestinal bleeds 434
sensory imbalance 26
  see also patient experiences
sensory input
  reception and perception 22
  vision, hearing, touch and taste 19–21
  vision, problems 19–20
sepsis 355–61
  systemic inflammatory response syndrome (SIRS)
    355–7
  treatment 357–9
septic inflammatory response syndrome 119, 358
septic shock 351
severe acute respiratory syndrome (SARS) 298–301
  diagnosis 299
  infection 298–9
  prevention 300
  symptoms 299
  treatment 300
shivering 84
  and oximetry 166
shock 344–53
  perfusion failure 346–7
  stages 345–6
  system failure 347
  types 348–51
sickle cell (HbS) disease 178–9
sick sinus syndrome 233–4
SIMV see synchronised intermittent mechanical
    ventilation
sinus arrhythmia 231–2
sinus bradycardia 232
sinus rhythm 226
sinus tachycardia 232–3
SIRS see systemic inflammatory response syndrome
skincare 115–21
  assessment 116–18
    haemodynamic monitoring 196
  postoperative cardiac care 340
sleep
  orthodox (non-REM) sleep 23–4
  paradoxical (REM) sleep) 24
smell senses 21
sodium, hyponatraemia 217
sodium-potassium pump 263
somatostatin, gastrointestinal
    bleeds 436
spinal injury 399–400
spinal shock see neurogenic shock
sputum 161
Staphylococcus aureus
  MRSA and MSSA 141
  toxic shock syndrome 351
starches 368–9
statins, acute myocardial infarction (AMI) 322

steroids
 immunity 271
 sepsis 358
Stirling scale (pressure sore severity) 116
stress response 7–8
 acute myocardial infarction (AMI) 323–4
 intubation 51
stress ulceration 437
stretopkinase, acute myocardial infarction
 (AMI) 321
stridor, extubation 56
stroke, cartoid artery dissection 384–5
stroke volume/index (SV/I) 204
subarachnoid haemorrhage 401
sucralfate 437
suction
 closed circuit 55
 endotracheal 53–5
supraventricular tachycardia 233
Swan Ganz *see* pulmonary artery catheters
sweating 408
synchronised intermittent mechanical ventilation
 (SIMV) 40
system failure, shock 347
systemic inflammatory response syndrome
 (SIRS) 355–7

tachy-brady syndrome 233
tachydysrhythmias, cardiac postoperative care 337
tacrolimus 467
tamponade 335, 348–9
 balloon 434–5
taste and smell senses 21
TBI *see* traumatic brain injury
tears, artificial 111
TEB *see* thoracic electrical bioimpedance
technology, nursing
 perspectives 4–5
teeth care 104–5
temperature control 82–6
 cardiac postoperative care 336
 children 126
temperature measurement 83–4
thalassaemia (Cooley's anaemia) 178
thermometers 83–4
thoracic electrical bioimpedance (TEB) 204
thoracic epidural analgesia 476
thrombocytopenia and thrombosis syndrome,
 heparin-induced (HITTS) 281
thromboembolism, pregnancy-induced 453
thrombolysis, acute myocardial infarction
 (AMI) 321
thrombosis
 deep vein thromboses (DVT) 282–3
 haemodynamic monitoring 202
 heparin-induced thrombocytopenia and thrombosis
 syndrome (HITTS) 281
thrombotic thrombocytopenia purpura (TTP) 281
tidal volume 38
TIPSS *see* transjugular intrahepatic
 portosystemic shunt

tissue injury, and intracranial hypertension 250
T-lymphocytes
 helper/killer/memory cells 214
 immunity 272
tonometry, acid-base balance 188
torsades de pointes 243–4
total parenteral nutrition
 (TPN) 91
touch, sensory imbalance 20–1
toxic shock syndrome 351
TPN *see* total parenteral nutrition
trace elements 90
tracheal ulcer 51
tracheostomy 49–50
transfer of patients
 cost of intensive care 520–1
transjugular intrahepatic portosystemic shunt
 (TIPSS) 436
transplantation 459–69
 cardiac 332–3, 340–1
 donors 462–3
 ethical issues 463–4
 graft versus host disease
 (GvHD) 466
 immunosuppression 467
 live donors 464
 non-heart-beating organ donors
 (NHBOD) 464–5
 postoperative care of recipients 465–6
traumatic brain injury
 (TBI) 395
trigeminy, ventricular ectopics 241–2
trigger ventilation 39–40
troponin, acute myocardial infarction (AMI) 319
TTP *see* thrombotic thrombocytopenia purpura
tumour necrosis factor alpha (TNF$\alpha$) 265
tympanic membrane, temperature measurement 83

ultrasound 207
urea and creatinine, acute renal failure 220
urokinase
 acute myocardial infarction (AMI) 321
 haemodynamic monitoring 202

VAD *see* ventricular assist devices
vagal stimulation 231
VALI *see* ventilator associated lung injury
valve surgery 330
vancomycin, *Enterococus* (VRE) 142
VAP *see* ventilator associated pneumonia
variceal bleeding 433–6
vascular surgery 382–8
 aneurysms 383–4
 carotid artery disease 384–5
 postoperative care 385–7
vasoactive mediators 265
vasoconstrictors *see* inotropes and vasopressors
vasopressin, gastrointestinal bleeds 436
venous pressure, central (CVP) 199–200
 measurement 200–2
venous saturation (SvO$_2$), mixed 206

ventilation 32–46, 305–12
  acute respiratory distress syndrome (ARDS)
    289–92
  adaptive support ventilation (ASV) 41
  airway pressure release ventilation (APRV) 40–1
  assisted mandatory ventilation (AMV) 40
  bilevel/biphasic positive airway pressure (BIPAP) 44
  children 125–6
  continuous positive airway pressure (CPAP) 44
  dual control modes 41
  extracorporeal membrane oxygenation
    (ECMO) 305–6
  high frequency ventilation (HFV) 306–7
    jet ventilation (HFJV) 308
    oscillatory ventilation (HFOV) 307–8
    percussive ventilation 308
  hyperbaric oxygen 309–10
  independent lung ventilation 42
  inspiratory/expiratory ratio 41–2
  inverse ratio ventilation (IRV) 42, 290
  liquid ventilation 308–9
  patient care 35–6
    cardiac postoperative care 334
  physiological complications 36–7
    hepatic damage and
      dysfunction 37
    neurological 37
    respiratory 32–4, 36
  positioning, prone 290–2
  positive and expiratory pressure (PEEP) 38–9
  pressure limited ventilation 40–1, 290
  pressure regulated volume control (PRVC) 41
  pressure support ventilation 41
  proportional assist ventilation (PAV) 41
  sigh 40
  synchronised intermittent mechanical
    ventilation (SIMV) 40
  terminology 33
  tidal volume 38
  trigger ventilation 39–40
  ventilator associated lung injury (VALI) 37–8
ventilator associated lung injury (VALI) 37–8
ventilator associated pneumonia (VAP) 140
ventricular assist devices (VAD) 331–2
ventricular dysrhythmias 240–1
ventricular ectopics 241–2
  bigeminy and trigeminy 241–2
ventricular fibrillation (VF) 244
ventricular tachycardia 242–3
VF see ventricular fibrillation
vision, sensory imbalance 19–21
  problems 19–20
volutrauma 289
VRE see vancomycin, Enterococus

Waterlow scale, skincare 116
WBCs see white blood cells
weaning 42–4
white blood cells (WBCs) 212–13
  normal reference ranges 213
Wolff-Parkinson-White
  syndrome 237
wound dehiscence 340

xenografts, transplantation 465
xerostomia (dry mouth) 99

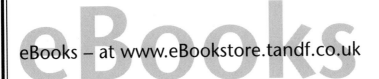